D1268226

New Drug Approval Process

DRUGS AND THE PHARMACEUTICAL SCIENCES
A Series of Textbooks and Monographs

Executive Editor

James Swarbrick
PharmaceuTech, Inc.
Pinehurst, North Carolina

Advisory Board

For Information on volumes 1–149 in the *Drugs and Pharmaceutical Science* Series, Please visit www.informahealthcare.com

FIFTH EDITION

New Drug Approval Process

edited by
Richard A. Guarino, M.D.
Oxford Pharmaceutical Resources, Inc.
Totowa, New Jersey, USA

informa
healthcare

New York   London

Informa Healthcare USA, Inc.
52 Vanderbilt Avenue
New York, NY 10017

© 2009 by Informa Healthcare USA, Inc.
Informa Healthcare is an Informa business

No claim to original U.S. Government works
Printed in the United States of America on acid-free paper
10 9 8 7 6 5 4 3 2 1

International Standard Book Number-10: 1-4200-8849-1 (Hardcover)
International Standard Book Number-13: 978-1-4200-8849-6 (Hardcover)

Library of Congress Cataloging-in-Publication Data

New drug approval process / edited by Richard A. Guarino. – 5th ed.
    p. ; cm. – (Drugs and the pharmaceutical sciences ; 190)
    Includes bibliographical references and index.
    ISBN-13: 978-1-4200-8849-6 (hardcover : alk. paper)
    ISBN-10: 1-4200-8849-1 (hardcover : alk. paper) 1. Drug approval –United States.   2. Drugs–Testing–Standards.   3. Drugs–Testing–Government policy–United States.   4. New products–Government policy–United States.
    I. Guarino, Richard A., 1935- II. Series: Drugs and the pharmaceutical sciences; v. 190.
    [DNLM: 1. Drug Evaluation–standards–United States.   2. Clinical Trials as Topic–standards–United States.   3. Drug Approval–United States.
W1 DR893B v. 190 2009 / QV 771 N5318 2009]
    RS189.N476 2009
    615'.1–dc22

                         2009007532

For Corporate Sales and Reprint Permissions call 212-520-2700 or write to: Sales Department, 52 Vanderbilt Avenue, 16th floor, New York, NY 10017.

Visit the Informa Web site at
www.informa.com

and the Informa Healthcare Web site at
www.informahealthcare.com

My sincere gratitude goes to our armed forces and my family members who sacrifice their lives to protect our nation's freedom and the principles that make America a world leader in giving mankind equal rights in their pursuit of endeavors.

Preface

Global registration of pharmaceutical drug, biologic, and device products is now the way pharmaceutical development and marketing are strategically planned. Since the publication of the fourth edition of *New Drug Approval Process*, there have been many changes in the regulations, requirements, and recommendations for international registration and approval of new products.

New Drug Approval Process, Fifth Edition offers, in detail, the necessary and vital information on how to develop and submit the research and the documentation required by worldwide agencies to obtain new pharmaceutical product approvals. The topics include a comprehensive as well as a pragmatic approach in addressing all aspects of clinical research development including statistical methodologies, global regulatory requirements for pharmaceutical product applications, and the mechanics necessary to understand and implement Good Clinical Practices (GCP), Good Laboratory Practices (GLP), and Good Manufacturing Practices (GMP).

Each contributing author is an expert in their respective field and has the knowledge and experience to educate the readers on the technical as well as the regulatory requirements for each topic presented. In addition, they also give a practical approach to resolve problems that might occur during product development. They impart their years of successes and failures in a way that the readers can take advantage of this information and apply it to their research practices and job descriptions, and can have a clear understanding of the scientific and legal responsibilities required to bring new pharmaceutical products to market.

The approach and format for assembling the specific data necessary to gain new product approvals globally have drastically changed in the past four years. The Investigational New Drug (IND) Application is still well accepted by the US FDA and will soon require to be submitted in electronic form. The same information, due to the implementation of the European Directives, is now expected in the countries belonging to the European Union and is contained in an Investigational Medicinal Product Dossier (IMPD). The New Drug Application (NDA) information is now in the format of the Common Technical Document (CTD) and is submitted to the regulatory agencies electronically termed an eCTD. These submissions as well as Biologic License Applications (BLAs), Abbreviated New Drug Applications (ANDAs), Supplemental New Drug Applications (SNDAs), and 505(b)(2) Applications are detailed. In addition, the essential components of the non and preclinical and clinical development comprising the safety and efficacy of products are presented and are integrated with the regulatory requirements necessary to expedite new product approvals. The Chemistry, Manufacturing, and Controls (CMC), pertaining to, the Quality section of the CTD, is one of the most important parts of any new product application and will be given special attention.

All aspects of Good Clinical Practices (GCP) as regulated by the US Code of Federal Regulations (CFR), the EU Directives, and the ICH Guidelines are addressed extensively in the section on Global Application of Good Clinical Practices (GCP). Investigators, Sponsors, and Monitors legal obligations for conducting clinical research are not only comprehensively covered but insights are also given on how to ensure that these disciplines can work together to expedite clinical trials. Institutional Review Boards (IRBs), Independent Ethics Committees (IECs), and Informed Consent (IC), as governed by the Declaration of Helsinki, are discussed fully. The Health Insurance Portability and Accountability Act (HIPAA) and the Privacy Laws are detailed and coordinated with how they must be considered in the Recruitment, Identification, PreScreening, Retention, Handling of Patient Data, and Use of Existing Databases of subjects participating in clinical research.

The *New Drug Approval Process, Fifth Edition,* is not only a text to educate people who plan to work in the areas of new pharmaceutical product development but also acts as a reference and guide for those personnel who have questions in specific areas of their expertise. The book addresses and details all the most recent regulations, guidelines, and procedures necessary for global registrations of new pharmaceutical products. The contributors of this book approach every topic with a practical understanding of the subject matter based on their experience gained by working in their fields of expertise. Readers will gain insights and ideas of how to apply their research and regulatory capabilities in order to bring pharmaceutical products to market more efficiently, expeditiously, and economically.

I would like to sincerely thank all the contributors who have given of their talents, time and effort in the preparation of this new edition of *New Drug Approval Process*. Again, special thanks go to my assistants, Patricia Birkner and Barbara Cannizzaro, for their perseverance in assembling this edition.

Richard A. Guarino, M.D.

Contents

xi

Contributors

Patricia Blaine   Medical Writing Corporation, Easton, Pennsylvania, U.S.A.

Mark Bradshaw   Global Consulting Partners in Medical Biometrics, Princeton, New Jersey, U.S.A.

Cai Cao   Center for Certification of Drugs, State Food and Drug Administration of China, Beijing, P.R. China

Brian J. Chadwick   LookLeft Group, New York, New York, U.S.A.

Albert A. Ghignone   AAG, Incorporated, Phillipsburg, New Jersey, U.S.A.

Rochelle L. Goodson   R. L. Goodson Consulting, Inc., Hewlett, New York, U.S.A.

Richard A. Guarino   Oxford Pharmaceutical Resources, Inc., Totowa, New Jersey, U.S.A.

Kent Hill   Biopharma Consulting Ltd., Colwyn Bay, U.K.

Earl W. Hulihan   Medidata Solutions Worldwide, New York, New York, U.S.A.

Duane B. Lakings   Drug Safety Evaluation Consulting, Inc., Elgin, Texas, U.S.A.

Peter Levitch   Peter Levitch & Associates, Bridgewater, New Jersey, U.S.A.

Daniel Liu   Medidata Solutions Worldwide, Beijing, P.R. China

Andrea Proccacino   Johnson & Johnson Pharmaceutical Research & Development, L.L.C., Titusville, New Jersey, U.S.A.

John R. Rapoza   JRRapoza Associates, Inc., Moorestown, New Jersey, U.S.A.

Max Sherman   Sherman Consulting Services, Inc., Warsaw, Indiana, U.S.A.

Evan B. Siegel   Ground Zero Pharmaceuticals, Inc., Irvine, California, U.S.A.

Helena M. Van den Dungen   Novartis Pharma AG, Basel, Switzerland

Glenn D. Watt   Medidata Solutions Worldwide, New York, New York, U.S.A.

Qingshan Zheng   Shanghai University of Traditional Chinese Medicines, Shanghai, P.R. China

synthesize compounds and pharmacologists or biologists to evaluate the leads in in vitro or in vivo models of the disease or disorder. This small group of researchers is the first project team and is commonly called a discovery project team. Their primary responsibility is to identify lead compounds or classes of compounds worthy of continued research and that are patentable, that is, having unique, previously undisclosed chemical structures. The initial effort may consist of screening existing compounds in the company's archives or libraries of compounds for activity and/or preparing new compounds with structures that are predicted to fit into the active site of the therapeutic target (or rational drug design). The primary endpoint used in this assessment is determining the biological activity or potency of the various compounds in a pharmacological model thought to be predictive of a human disease or disorder. The pharmacology results are shared with the organic or medicinal chemists, who then prepare analogues of the most active compounds to identify the pharmacophore (i.e., the chemical moiety of the compounds responsible for the biological activity) and to explore further the structural activity relationship or SAR.

Once a lead or class of leads has been identified, the discovery team commonly expands to include other scientific disciplines to more fully characterize the possibility of successfully developing the discovery leads of interest. The other disciplines include, but are not limited to:

1. Analytical chemistry to define the physical and chemical properties of the leads and to provide preliminary information on the solubility and stability of the potential drug substances.
2. Pharmacokinetics, which normally includes bioanalytical chemistry, to assess the absorption or delivery and disposition profiles of the leads in animal models using the route of administration projected for clinical studies and drug metabolism using in vitro systems to assess the extent of metabolism by the various drug metabolism enzymes.
3. Toxicology, possibly including safety pharmacology and genotoxicity, to evaluate the potential for the leads to cause adverse effects in in vitro or cell-based systems and in vivo or animal models and to determine that the dose levels that cause toxicity are substantially greater than the dose levels needed to elicit the desired pharmacologic effect.
4. Biopharmaceutics to study the formulation potential of the leads and to ensure that the compounds can be effectively delivered by the proposed clinical route of administration.

The results obtained from the preliminary or lead optimization studies conducted by these disciplines are integrated with the biological activity data obtained from the pharmacologist. If problems related to stability, delivery, metabolism, or toxicity are encountered, then the chemists use the previously generated SAR information to modify the structure of the lead without destroying the site(s) required for biological activity of the compound. The new compounds are evaluated for potency as well as to ensure that the undesirable structural attribute, which caused the observed developability problem, has been deleted or minimized. Then, the other scientific disciplines check the new lead(s) to ensure that the structural change did not adversely affect desirable characteristics (i.e., attributes) and did substantially alter the previously defined undesirable characteristics (i.e., demerits). This iterative

1   Drug Development Teams

Duane B. Lakings

Drug Safety Evaluation Consulting, Inc., Elgin, Texas, U.S.A.

INTRODUCTION

The drug discovery and development process requires the close interaction of a large number of scientific disciplines for as many as 10 to 12 years. Most pharmaceutical and biotechnology firms employ teams to guide the processes involved in taking a discovery lead through the various preclinical/nonclinical (or Safety) and clinical (or Efficacy) drug development stages for making the drug candidate into a therapeutic product. The responsibilities of these project teams include, but are not limited to:

1. Reviewing research results from experiments conducted by any of the various scientific disciplines.
2. Integrating new research results with previously generated data.
3. Planning research studies to further characterize and develop a drug candidate.
4. Preparing a detailed drug development plan, including designation of key points or development milestones, generating a timeline for completion of key research studies, and defining the critical path.
5. Monitoring the status of research studies to ensure that they are being conducted according to the timeline and critical path in the development plan and, if appropriate, modifying the plan as new information becomes available.
6. Comparing research results and development status and timelines with drug candidates under development by competitors.
7. Conducting appropriate market surveys to ensure that the development of a drug candidate is economically justified and continues to meet a medical need.
8. Reporting the status of the drug development program to management and making recommendations on the continued development of the drug candidate.

This chapter discusses the various types of project teams that are involved in the drug discovery and development process. Also included is a detailed example of a drug development logic plan for what many developmental pharmaceutical scientists consider to be the most difficult and time- and resource-consuming drug candidate to develop into a therapeutic product.

DRUG DISCOVERY PROJECT TEAM

A company makes a decision to enter into a new disease area or to expand an existing therapeutic area on the basis of new research findings, an unmet medical need, or marketing surveys. The responsible department, commonly a therapeutic disease group such as cardiovascular, CNS, cancer, infectious diseases, or metabolic diseases, assigns researchers to the new project—usually chemists to

Time involved in R&D is probably the next consideration compared to cost. Every day that a product is delayed during the R&D phases or needs additional information from regulatory agencies, before it is launched for marketing, costs the companies millions of dollars, euros, etc. Therefore, understanding exactly how to implement the correct procedures in drug, biologic, and device new product development is not only essential but can also save time and cost in bringing products to market. Basic knowledge of how and what to do, which is gained from any text, is only a foundation. It is only from experience of trial and error and constant training can one become capable of successfully achieving product submissions and approvals.

The most important recommendation that can be advanced to anyone embarking on a pharmaceutical career in R&D is that one must love and practice detail for every aspect in the process of new product development. The intricate components of developing clinical research for safety and efficacy of products, regulatory requirements for new product applications, manufacturing practice for finished pharmaceuticals, and an understanding of assurance for every aspect of the new product approval process are keys in achieving pharmaceutical product approvals by global regulatory agencies.

The fifth edition of *New Drug Approval Process* gives the reader detailed directions and is a guide on how to accomplish the intricate steps in developing pharmaceutical products for market. Specific attention, throughout the book, is based on the requirements of Good Clinical, Good Laboratory, and Good Manufacturing Practices governed by international regulations. The contributors of these chapters have many years of experience in their specialized areas and offer information based on their trials and tribulations encountered during the process of product development. The reader learns strategic advantages in the best ways to approach each phase of product development, resulting in savings of time and money. This latest edition is a must-read for all those in the pharmaceutical and related industries, as it provides the most recent rules, regulations, and guidelines essential for the approval of new pharmaceutical products worldwide.

Richard A. Guarino, M.D.

Introduction

The pharmaceutical industries developing drugs, biologics, and devices consider every new as well as an approved product a potential for international markets. Product applications and registrations, once difficult to achieve in many countries, are now evaluated by global agencies based on data meeting the requirements and guidelines governed by the International Committee of Harmonization (ICH). In the United States, pharmaceutical products have long been regulated by the US Code of Federal Regulations (CFR). For countries belonging to the European Union (EU), pharmaceutical product development now comes under the regulations of the European Union Directives (EUD). In Japan, the Pharmaceutical and Medical Safety Bureau governs pharmaceutical product development. Other countries that do not follow the CFR, the EUD, and Japanese regulations now adapt the ICH Guidelines, which are also reflected and used in the CFR, the EUD, and Japan. The international acceptance of new product development data, based on the ICH guidelines, has given pharmaceutical industries a more factual procedure and raised the incentive to register their products globally. This will result in accelerating better health care to world populations.

The ICH is largely responsible for the progress of new global pharmaceutical product development by diligently establishing ways for the international exchange and acceptance of scientific data. This committee not only presents guidelines and recommendations for the safety, efficacy, and quality components required for regulatory submissions of new products, but also outlines an easy-to-follow format for reporting these data. With the exception of some minor variations required by certain countries, the Common Technical Document (CTD) allows sponsors to submit their data to international regulatory agencies in a comprehensive way that is accepted and understood by all countries.

The cost of Research and Development (R&D) of new products, especially for prescription drugs, has become astronomical. Pharmaceutical companies are reluctant to embark on the clinical research of products if the outcome does not promise to gain a major market share. Even orphan drug development, notwithstanding the incentives offered to encourage the development of these drugs, is cautiously considered in relation to the cost of development compared to the economic projections for these drugs. Drug, biologic, and device companies are looking at every aspect of new product development with the objective of decreasing costs and time to bring their products to market. The inducement of knowing that data emanating from R&D required for new product applications can be simultaneously submitted in many countries has resulted in an enthusiasm for pharmaceutical companies to bring new products to market.

process continues until a lead compound (or a small group of leads) is identified with attributes that are considered necessary for successful nonclinical and clinical drug development and without any major demerit that would prevent successful development.

The discovery project team compiles the generated information and presents the results to the management. At this stage, the drug discovery team normally recommends that a lead candidate be entered into formal preclinical development. However, that is not always the case. In the experience of this author, the results from various scientific disciplines can be at odds with each other—with one group pushing for continued development, while another thinks that the potential for successful development is too low to justify the expenditure of additional resources. For example, the discovery and development of renin inhibitors as antihypertension agents were, and in some cases still are, being evaluated by a number of pharmaceutical companies. The discovered leads, which were structurally modified small peptides, were very potent in inhibiting renin and thus interfering with the renin-angiotensin cascade, resulting in an antihypertension effect. However, biological activity correlated and increased with the lipophilicity of the modified peptides. The most potent leads had few, if any, polar groups to provide aqueous solubility, preventing the compounds from being delivered to the intestinal wall for absorption into systemic circulation. When absorption enhancers were used to administer the leads to animal models of hypertension, the compounds had sufficient absorption to reduce blood pressure. The results from drug delivery and pharmacokinetic evaluations of these same leads showed very low absolute bioavailability, usually less than 10%, which was also quite variable, at times more than 200% of the amount absorbed. This difference in the developability potential of these discovery renin inhibitors caused a number of pharmaceutical companies to stop research in this area, whereas other companies continued their efforts to find inhibitors with acceptable delivery characteristics and without unacceptable decreases in potency. This effort has been somewhat successful with a new generation of renin inhibitors now in development.

Once the discovery project team's recommendation for preclinical development of a lead candidate is accepted by the management, this team is either disbanded or continues their efforts to discover other compounds with attributes that could identify a next-generation drug candidate. Many of the discovery project team members also become members of the more formal preclinical development project team.

PRECLINICAL DRUG DEVELOPMENT PROJECT TEAM

One of the first tasks after management's acceptance of a discovery lead as a drug candidate is the establishment of the preclinical drug development team. Commonly, the researchers from various scientific disciplines involved in the discovery project team are assigned by their departments to the new team, but not always. Some companies have defined groups that support discovery research and others that conduct nonclinical and clinical developmental studies. In this case, the newly assigned preclinical project team member needs to be "brought up to speed" by the researcher who had been providing support to the discovery team. This approach allows departments to separate the nondefinitive, or non-Good Laboratory Practice (GLP)-regulated, discovery research effort from the more definitive, or GLP-directed, drug development effort and to develop researchers with expertise in one or the other area. However, complete transfer of knowledge and experience is not always possible and "ownership" of and "champions" for a particular compound or disease area are lost. Having the same researcher or research group involved in all aspects of the drug discovery and development process provides continuity of effort but requires a possible dilution of scientific expertise. The best approach, each of which has its attributes and demerits, has been under discussion at pharmaceutical houses for years. This issue will probably continue to be a point of contention for researchers wanting to develop a specific scientific expertise or to be involved in all aspects of the drug discovery and development processes. This problem is not as prevalent at biotechnology firms or small pharmaceutical companies where researchers have to wear many hats and are commonly involved in many phases of the drug discovery and development process.

In addition to the scientific disciplines, for example, pharmacology, chemistry, toxicology, drug metabolism and pharmacokinetics, and biopharmaceutics, involved in the discovery team, the preclinical drug development team has a number of new players. These new players include, among others:

1. A management-assigned project team leader or coordinator who is responsible for the development of the drug candidate.
2. Regulatory affairs (RA) and quality assurance (QA) experts to ensure that the developmental studies meet regulatory agency requirements and are conducted according to regulatory agency regulations and guidelines, including International Conference on Harmonisation (ICH) guidelines.
3. A clinical research scientist to provide input into preclinical study designs so that the generated results support the proposed clinical program and to initiate development of clinical safety, tolerance, pharmacokinetic, and efficacy protocols and the investigator's brochure (IB).
4. An analytical chemistry researcher to develop assays, to validate the assays according to ICH guidelines, and to characterize the drug substance and proposed drug product.
5. Manufacturing scientists to scale up the synthesis of the drug candidate and provide sufficient GLP- or Good Manufacturing Practice (GMP)-quality material for regulatory-driven research studies.
6. A marketing person to determine that the drug candidate has a potential market niche in light of what other companies are developing or drugs that are already on the market for the disease indication or disorder.

One of the first charges of the preclinical development project team is to prepare a drug development plan, which lists all the studies considered necessary for the successful development of a drug candidate. Based on the disease indication (life-threatening or non–life-threatening), the drug candidate type (small organic molecule or macromolecule), the length of therapy (acute or chronic), and the route of administration (oral, intravenous, dermal, pulmonary, etc.), each of the scientific disciplines prepares a list of their proposed research studies, usually in the order to be conducted and with the predicted duration of time needed for completion. All of the studies are combined into a drug development logic plan (a sample is presented later in this chapter). The initial drug development plan is put together with key points or milestones in mind. These key points are commonly submission of a first-in-human clinical trial application or an investigational new drug (IND) submission, completion of phase 2 clinical trial studies, and submission of a marketing application or new drug application (NDA). The first plan is very detailed for the preclinical development, with less definition for the clinical and nonclinical stages of development and for the manufacturing effort.

The individual department lists are combined with the studies ordered according to time required and dependence on the results from other studies. For example, before a subchronic toxicology study can be conducted, acute toxicology study results need to be available to define dose levels and frequency of dosing; sufficient GLP- or GMP-quality drug substance and proposed drug product have to be available or will be available to dose the test species at the desired levels for the duration of the study; and acceptable analytical and bioanalytical chemistry methods should be in place to provide support for formulation assessment and toxicokinetics, which require preliminary pharmacokinetic information to determine the correct or optimal sampling times. Thus, the subchronic toxicology study does not depend only on when the toxicologist and his/her group can conduct the study but also on when other disciplines have completed supportive research studies and are available to support the toxicology effort.

Once the development studies are listed and integrated into a logic plan, the next aspect is to develop a timeline. Based on the overall plan, each department determines when they can start a proposed study and when the results of the experiment can be expected. This information is added to the development plan, and the time to completion and to reach predefined milestones, such as filing an IND or completion of phase 2 clinical studies, is determined. The timeline identifies the critical path, that is, the research studies that are rate limiting and the department or departments involved. Commonly, the departments on the critical path during preclinical development are manufacturing, then toxicology, and finally clinical. Other scientific disciplines that have a key component to the development process can also be on the critical path. Normally, management and project team leadership want the development time to be as short as possible, which is only logical and justifiable, as a single day of development time for a drug product with projected yearly sales of $365 million is worth $1 million of revenue. In addition, once a patent has been filed, each day of development time decreases the patent life by a day, reducing the overall sales revenue for a drug product. Thus, departments attempt to be off the critical path unless absolutely necessary and will often modify their projected start or completion dates for studies in order to move off the critical path. The completed drug development plan, with defined milestones and critical path, is presented to, and accepted by, management.

The drug development plan has to be a living document and subject to change or modification as results from research studies become available. Unexpected or negative data will usually require additional studies to answer or explain more fully the observations. These additional studies may, probably will, affect the development timeline and possibly the critical path. Typically, the status of a drug development project is formally presented to management on a quarterly, semiannual, or annual basis, provided no expected results or "surprises" are generated. Special meetings with management are held to present and discuss problem areas that are encountered, to make recommendations on how to overcome the problems, and to request the additional resources that may be needed to solve or correct the problem areas.

One of the final responsibilities of the preclinical drug development project team is to prepare an IND and to submit the appropriate documents to a regulatory agency, such as the FDA. As the development of the drug candidate moves into the clinic, the preclinical project team often becomes a clinical project team.

CLINICAL DRUG DEVELOPMENT PROJECT TEAM

After the IND is submitted, the project team is again expanded to include new players. Some of the old players, such as chemistry and pharmacology, have decreased roles but may continue to serve on the team to provide scientific expertise when new problems arise. The roles of many project team members substantially expand. The new players and expanded roles of members include:

1. Physicians who will conduct or be responsible for phase 1, 2, and 3 clinical trial studies or serve as medical monitors if these studies are conducted by a contract research organization (CRO).
2. Clinical research associates who will coordinate and monitor the phase 1, 2, and 3 studies and ensure that the appropriate documents, such as case report forms (CRFs), are correctly prepared.
3. Manufacturing scientists to coordinate the development of the drug substance and proposed drug product production facilities and to ensure that all the necessary manufacturing processes are in place and appropriately validated.
4. Quality control researchers to ensure that the appropriate assays are developed and validated and are in place to support the manufacturing program.
5. Statisticians to assist in designing clinical protocols and in evaluating generated results from both nonclinical and clinical studies.
6. Clinical pharmacokinetic experts to support phase 1 studies and to design and conduct pharmacokinetic studies in special populations.
7. Marketing personnel to continue evaluating the status of competitor's drug candidates and the potential of the developmental candidate to fill a medical need and to prepare for product launch.

The preclinical drug development plan is updated, with emphasis now placed on the clinical (or Efficacy) and manufacturing (or Quality) aspects, either of which could be on the critical path. The nonclinical (or Safety) program continues but, with the exception of carcinogenicity studies, is rarely rate limiting. As the results from phase 1 and phase 2 clinical trials become available, special nonclinical or even clinical studies may be needed to evaluate clinical observations. These findings may include unexpected adverse experiences (AEs) or reactions (ARs) in normal healthy volunteers or patients with the disease indication; pharmacokinetic differences between human and animal models; or correcting unforeseen problems, such as unacceptable or highly variable delivery in humans or the inability to scale up the manufacturing process using the proposed methods. For example, this author was a project team member for the development of a CNS drug candidate for anxiety. Phase 1 single-dose, dose-escalating studies in human volunteers produced no safety or tolerance issues. Thus, phase 1 multiple-dose studies were initiated and planning for phase 2 efficacy studies started. Bioanalytical chemistry analyses of clinical specimens for the parent drug and a known metabolite showed the presence of an unidentified drug metabolite. Pharmacokinetic evaluation of the new metabolite suggested that this compound had an estimated apparent terminal disposition half-life of more than seven days and thus would accumulate after multiple-dose administration of the drug candidate, possibly leading to adverse experiences. Analogues of the parent drug candidate were prepared and the metabolite was identified. Pharmacology testing showed the metabolite to be almost as biologically active as the drug candidate and, because of the accumulation aspect, was efficacious at lower doses. Toxicology evaluations demonstrated that the metabolite had a safety profile similar to that of the parent compound and thus had a better therapeutic ratio when combined with the lower dose required for pharmacological activity. Biopharmaceutical and pharmacokinetic studies showed that the metabolite had acceptable bioavailability. These results suggested that the metabolite might be a better drug candidate than the parent. A preclinical program was initiated on the metabolite and after a delay of only a few months, the metabolite entered the clinic as a drug candidate with a better chance of success than the original compound.

The final responsibility of the clinical project team is to ensure that all the research studies are appropriately documented in technical reports or scientific publications and to compile this information, along with the necessary nonclinical and clinical summaries, into a marketing application submission, such as an NDA, that is formatted in compliance with ICH guidelines on the Common Technical Document (ICH M2 and M4 guidelines). After submission, the project team, usually through the regulatory affairs department of the company, interacts with the regulatory agency and provides answers to any questions or concerns raised by the regulators. If requested, the project team designs and conducts the necessary research studies to support the submission. Once the marketing application has been approved, the final responsibility of the clinical development team is to coordinate the launch of the new therapeutic agent.

DRUG DEVELOPMENT LOGIC PLAN

One of the primary functions of the project team is to coordinate the various studies necessary for the successful development of a drug candidate and to ensure that the timeline for development is on schedule, both for time and budget. As mentioned above, this coordination is usually accomplished by preparing a detailed drug development logic plan and monitoring the research process. The required studies and the extent of the development plan depend on at least four criteria of the proposed drug candidate, which are as follows:

1. Drug candidate type (macromolecule such as a protein, polypeptide, or oligonucleotide or small organic molecule commonly referred to as a novel chemical entity or NCE).
2. Disease indication (life-threatening such as AIDS, some cancers, some cardiovascular and CNS indications, or non–life-threatening such as hypertension, diabetes, anti-inflammatory agents, antibacterial agents).
3. Therapy duration (acute, with one or a few doses being sufficient for treatment, or chronic, with prolonged administration necessary to mediate the disease process).
4. Route of administration (intravenous as a bolus injection or an infusion or nonintravenous such as oral, pulmonary, subcutaneous, intramuscular, dermal, etc.).

These four criteria form a matrix of 16 possible drug candidate types. A generic drug development plan for what most drug development scientists consider to be the most difficult drug candidate to develop successfully is shown in Appendix 1. The timelines for the various studies and their integration into a formal drug development plan are compound-specific and depend on the availability of resources within the various departments at the company or at CROs, if some of the research effort is to be outsourced. Similarly, the designation of key milestone events and the critical path are compound-specific and company-specific. However, the information provided in the sample logic plan can be used as a template to generate a logic plan for the other 15 drug candidate types. Depending on the drug candidate type, some of the listed studies, such as absolute bioavailability for a candidate to be administered intravenously or carcinogenicity studies for a candidate to be administered acutely for a life-threatening disease, may not be necessary. Other studies, such as biological potency and immunogenicity and immunotoxicity evaluations for a macromolecule, may be required.

CONCLUSION

This chapter has described the various project teams and their responsibilities, including the generation, implementation, and monitoring of a drug development plan, in the drug discovery and development processes. The large number of scientific disciplines required for the successful development of a drug candidate into a therapeutic product makes the use of project teams a common practice within the pharmaceutical and biotechnology industry. The abilities of the members to communicate the results from their research efforts and to integrate the results obtained from other disciplines into their study designs are both important and critical aspects of the project team environment.

APPENDIX 1 Drug discovery and development logic plan example

Logic Plan Drug Candidate Characteristics
A. Candidate   New chemical entity (small organic molecular)
B. Indication   Non–life-threatening disease
C. Therapy   Chronic administration
D. Dosing route   Nonintravenous

I. Drug Discovery Stage
   A. Chemistry or Synthesis
      1. Generate drug discovery lead(s) using rational approaches, such as random screening, nonrandom screening, drug metabolism, or clinical observations, or using combinatorial chemistry libraries.
      2. Modify lead(s) by identification of pharmacophore and synthesis of analogues; functional group changes; SAR of lead candidate analogues; structure modification, such as homologation, chain branching, ring-chain transformation, and bioisosterism to increase potency and therapeutic ratio; and QSAR.
      3. Determine drug–receptor interactions using techniques like molecular modeling and X-ray crystallography.
   B. Pharmacology or In Vitro and Animal Model Efficacy
      1. Using in vitro techniques, evaluate requirements for activation and dependency on dosing schedule and route of administration; calculate inhibitory concentrations, e.g., IC_{50} and IC_{90}, for each system evaluated; assess potential for resistance to lead candidate(s); determine synergistic, additive, or antagonistic drug–drug interactions during combination therapy, if appropriate; evaluate possible cytostatic or cytotoxic concentrations of lead candidate(s) on various cell types (bone marrow, stem cells, and immune system cells).
      2. Define and characterize an animal model(s) that mimics the human disease to be evaluated and determine appropriate endpoints for assessment of biological activity.
      3. Evaluate in vivo dose–response range, including dose–response comparison of lead candidates; determine pharmacologically active doses, e.g., ED_{50} or ED_{10}; and therapeutic ratio when combined with no-observable-adverse-effect level (NOAEL) or minimum-toxic-effect dose level.
      4. Conduct other in vivo evaluations including, but not limited to, dosing regimen dependency; route of administration and formulation dependency; and spectrum of activity, disease status, cross-resistance profile, combination therapy for synergy or antagonism, and special models.

II. Drug Developability Stage
   A. Preliminary Formulation Evaluation (may not be started until preclinical development is initiated)
      1. From pharmacology results and proposed clinical program, select route of administration (oral, pulmonary, intramuscular, subcutaneous, transdermal, ocular, vaginal, buccal, sublingual, etc.) and formulation type to be dosed (solution, suspension, tablet, capsule, granulation powder, microspheres, microemulsion, depot drug, etc.).
      2. Evaluate excipients, including concentration and potential for interaction.
      3. Select and evaluate formulation process(es), such as tableting, granulation, lyophilization, or microencapsulation.
      4. Prepare prototype formulation.
      5. Confirm formulation composition, including, but not limited to, drug substance content, drug substance stability, excipient levels, water, and residual solvents, using appropriately characterized methods.
      6. Measure formulation physical properties, such as hardness, size, size distribution, morphology.
      7. Measure formulation function, such as release or disintegration profile and nonrelease properties like taste masking.

(*Continued*)

APPENDIX 1   Drug discovery and development logic plan example (*Continued*)

   8. Develop and characterize stability-indicating analytical chemistry method.
   9. Define and implement preliminary solubility and stability studies on drug substance and proposed drug product.
   B. Preliminary Bioanalytical Chemistry Method Development
      1. Select bioanalytical chemistry technique (LC/MS/MS, HPLC, GC, ELISA, etc.).
      2. Select physiological matrix (plasma, serum, whole blood, urine).
      3. Characterize bioanalytical chemistry method, including sample preparation procedure, for linearity, sensitivity, specificity, precision, and accuracy.
      4. Conduct preliminary stability study of drug candidate in selected physiological matrix(ces).
   C. Preliminary Pharmacokinetic and Bioavailability Assessments
      1. Evaluate distribution and disposition in pharmacology animal model species after intravenous and proposed clinical route of administration.
      2. Evaluate pharmacokinetics and bioavailability (drug delivery) in toxicology rodent and nonrodent animal species after intravenous and proposed clinical route of administration.
   D. Toxicology
      1. Evaluate single-dose or dose-escalation acute toxicity in rodent species.
      2. Evaluate single-dose or dose-escalation acute toxicity in nonrodent species.
      3. Conduct safety pharmacology studies, if appropriate.
      4. Conduct genotoxicity evaluations, if necessary.
   E. Drug Metabolism
      1. Evaluate potential for drug metabolism by CYP450 isozymes and other enzyme systems.
      2. Study potential for conjugation, e.g., glucuronidation, sulfation, acetylation, etc.
      3. Determine extent of protein binding.

III. Preclinical Drug Development Stage
   (*Note:* If developability assessment studies listed above have not been conducted, these studies should be included in the preclinical drug development stage.)
   A. Drug Candidate Characterization
      1. Validate stability-indicating analytical chemistry method and other assays.
      2. Generate impurity profile and identify impurities in drug substance and proposed drug product.
      3. Study stress stability for drug substance and proposed drug product.
   B. Formulation Development
      1. Review preliminary pharmacokinetics and histology (local reaction) results and modify formulation, if necessary, using GLP- or GMP-quality drug substance.
      2. Characterize and optimize modified formulation for excipients, pH, processing, etc.
   C. Bioanalytical Chemistry Method Validation
      1. Validate developed method for specificity, sensitivity, range of reliable results, precision, and accuracy for each physiological matrix type and for each species.
      2. Evaluate protein binding in blood/plasma obtained from animal species and humans.
      3. Determine drug candidate stability in selected physiological matrices from time of collection to time of assay.
   D. IND-Directed Toxicology Studies
      1. Determine safety pharmacology profile in CNS, cardiovascular, respiratory, renal, and gastrointestinal systems.
      2. Evaluate genetic toxicology.
      3. Conduct local irritation studies.
      4. Determine occupational toxicology (dermal, eye irritation, skin sensitization).
      5. Perform subchronic (2- or 4-week) study in a rodent species using proposed clinical route of administration. Study should have a toxicokinetic component.
      6. Perform subchronic (2- or 4-week) study in a nonrodent species using proposed clinical route of administration. Study should have a toxicokinetic component.

(Continued)

APPENDIX 1   Drug discovery and development logic plan example (*Continued*)

7. Perform subchronic (13-week) study in a rodent species using proposed clinical route of administration. Study should have a toxicokinetic component.
8. Perform subchronic (13-week) study in a nonrodent species using proposed clinical route of administration. Study should have a toxicokinetic component.
9. Design and conduct additional confirmatory or specialized studies, as warranted.

E. Pharmacokinetics and Drug Metabolism
   1. Evaluate absolute bioavailability, distribution and disposition, and linearity of kinetics over toxicology dose range, i.e., dose proportionality, in pharmacology and toxicology animal species.
   2. Synthesize and characterize radiolabeled drug candidate.
   3. Using radiolabeled drug candidate, determine mass balance, including metabolite profiling and route(s) of elimination, in toxicology animal species.
   4. Isolate and identify major metabolites and if appropriate, evaluate pharmacological and toxicological activity of metabolites.
   5. Correlate in vitro metabolism using liver hepatocytes and other appropriate enzyme systems from animal models and humans.
   6. Provide toxicokinetic support to toxicology studies.

F. Mechanism of Action Studies
   1. Study effect on cell cycle or replication cycle.
   2. Determine intra- or extracellular site of action.
   3. Evaluate requirements for enzyme activation or inhibition for desired pharmacological response.
   4. Perform enzyme–substrate kinetic studies, if appropriate.
   5. Assess intracellular site of action using compartmentalization experiments.

G. Manufacturing Program
   1. Obtain certificates of analysis (COAs) on raw materials.
   2. Define, evaluate, and scale-up manufacturing process for drug substance.
   3. Validate formulation process procedures such as mixing, sterilization, lyophilization, closure, resolubilization.
   4. Prepare various CMC sections for first-in-human clinical trial submission or IND.
   5. Make phase 1 clinical supplies using GLP or GMP process.
   6. Test clinical supplies for composition, required characteristics, and function.
   7. Release phase 1 clinical supplies to clinic.

H. Quality Control Processes
   1. Validate analytical chemistry method(s) for drug substance, including identity tests and impurity profile.
   2. Validate analytical chemistry method(s) for proposed drug product, including impurity profile.
   3. If appropriate, validate analytical chemistry method(s) for key intermediates in drug substance manufacturing process.
   4. Develop and validated analytical chemistry methods for excipients.

I. Clinical
   1. Prepare phase 1 clinical protocol and outlines of phase 2 and 3 clinical programs.
   2. Prepare investigator's brochure (IB).
   3. Prepare and submit first-in-human clinical trial application or IND to regulatory agency.

IV. Nonclinical Drug Development Stage (conducted concurrently with Clinical Development)
   A. Chronic and Reproductive Toxicology
      1. Conduct chronic (6-month) nonrodent toxicology study.
      2. Conduct chronic (9-month) rodent toxicology study or combined rat chronic toxicity/carcinogenicity (2-year) study.
      3. Perform mouse carcinogenicity study, if necessary.
      4. Evaluate reproductive and developmental toxicity in rats or other appropriate rodent species (Segments I, II, and III).

(*Continued*)

APPENDIX 1   Drug discovery and development logic plan example (*Continued*)

5. Evaluate reproductive and developmental toxicity in rabbits or other appropriate nonrodent species (Segment II).
6. Design and conduct additional confirmatory or specialized studies, as warranted.

B. Pharmacokinetics and Drug Metabolism
   1. Using radiolabeled drug candidate, perform tissue distribution, with whole body autoradiography (WBA), in rodents after single-dose and multiple-dose (if appropriate) administration.
   2. Provide toxicokinetic support as necessary, including, but not limited to, feto-placental transfer and lacteal secretion studies to support reproductive and developmental toxicology studies.
   3. Isolate and identify metabolite(s), if appropriate, in toxicology animal species and humans.
   4. Evaluate pharmacokinetics of metabolite(s) to support pharmacological and toxicological evaluation of metabolites, if appropriate.
   5. Conduct in vitro and in vivo enzyme-induction and enzyme-inhibition studies in animal models, if appropriate.

C. Mechanism of Action
   1. Conduct additional mechanism of pharmacological action studies, if necessary.
   2. Conduct additional mechanism of toxicological action studies, if necessary.

V. Clinical Drug Development Stage (conducted concurrently with Nonclinical Development)
A. Phase 1 Safety and Tolerance Study
   1. Obtain Institutional Review Board (IRB) approval for phase 1 study.
   2. Prepare and release clinical supplies.
   3. Develop and validate bioanalytical chemistry method for drug candidate and known metabolites in human physiological fluid specimens.
   4. Conduct single-dose and multiple-dose escalation evaluation of drug candidate in normal human volunteers.
   5. Study pharmacokinetics of drug candidate and known metabolites in humans after single-dose and multiple-dose administration.
   6. Develop and validate surrogate and biochemical marker method(s), if appropriate.
   7. Design and conduct mass balance study in human volunteers using an appropriately radiolabeled drug candidate.

B. Phase 2 Efficacy Studies
   1. Prepare phase 2 efficacy study protocols and obtain IRB approval.
   2. Conduct multiple-dose evaluation of drug candidate efficacy in patients with disease indication.
   3. Determine surrogate and biochemical marker levels in human physiological fluid specimens.
   4. Design and conduct relative bioavailability studies (bridging studies) if proposed drug product used in early phase 2 is changed for later phase 2 and 3 clinical trials.

C. Phase 3 Definitive Safety and Efficacy Studies
   1. Prepare phase 3 clinical protocols and obtain IRB and regulatory agency approvals.
   2. Conduct randomized, double-blind, placebo-controlled (if appropriate) studies in patients with disease indication using at least two dose levels of proposed drug product.
   3. Perform pharmacokinetic studies in special populations (geriatric or pediatric age groups, renal or hepatic impaired patients, various ethnic groups, and drug–drug interaction studies) groups, if appropriate.
   4. Determine surrogate or biochemical marker levels in human physiological fluid specimens.
   5. Collate all information and prepare marketing application (such as NDA) for submission to regulatory agency.

(*Continued*)

APPENDIX 1   Drug discovery and development logic plan example (*Continued*)

D. Phase 4 Studies
   1. Design phase 4 protocols for product extensions for new indications or improved/modified delivery profile/route and obtain appropriate approvals.
   2. Conduct randomized, double-blind, placebo-controlled (if appropriate) studies in patients with new disease indication.
   3. Conduct relative bioavailability comparison studies for novel formulation assessment.

VI. Manufacturing (conducted concurrently with Nonclinical and Clinical Development)
   A. Raw Materials
      1. Identify critical components, intermediates, and suppliers.
      2. Negotiate supply and certify vendors.
      3. Conduct site audit for selected vendors.
      4. Determine shelf life of raw materials.
   B. Scale-Up and Engineering
      1. Identify synthesis and formulation methods, including definition of equipment, processes, scale.
      2. Define processes and validate for fill, finish, and packaging.
      3. Determine procedure for waste disposal, including appropriate environmental assessments.
      4. Determine number of batches required to support development program and product launch.
   C. Documentation
      1. Generate table of contents for manufacture and control documents.
      2. Generate appropriate standard operating procedures (SOPs).
      3. Develop validation protocols.
      4. Prepare regulatory documents, such as IND, yearly updates, and NDA.
      5. Conduct validation efforts, including preparation of progress reports.
   D. Drug Substance
      1. Define production time line for drug substance supplies for formulation development, stability, toxicology, and clinical studies.
      2. Determine characterization (content, purity, identify) and specification (acceptance and rejection) requirements.
   E. Stability
      1. Evaluate drug substance stability, including protocol preparation, approval, and study conduct.
      2. Evaluate drug product stability, including protocol preparation, approval, and study conduct.
   F. Sterilization (if appropriate)
      1. Select and evaluate sterilization methods.
      2. Select dose levels and location for sterilization.
      3. Prepare sterilization protocol and obtain necessary approvals.
      4. Develop and validate quality control methods for sterilization.
   G. Packaging and Labeling
      1. Identify each component in drug product.
      2. Define process for assemble and fill method.
      3. Generate labeling and package insert requirements.

2 FDA Approvable Indications and Other Considerations

Peter Levitch
Peter Levitch & Associates, Bridgewater, New Jersey, U.S.A.

INTRODUCTION

In selecting the appropriate and correct indication for your product candidate, whether it is a drug, biologic, or medical device it is extremely important to select one which is FDA approvable. The history of health care product development is filled with examples of potentially good products, which were studied for indications that FDA simply would not approve. This chapter will provide some guidance on selecting FDA approvable indications, along with examples of companies picking wrong indications, and the means to help you avoid making similar mistakes with candidate products. In addition, guidance in other areas related to FDA approvable indications are presented.

The health care product manufacturers, in general, have a poor track record for predicting the requirements for product approval, and an even worse record for predicting the time of FDA approval for these products. The requirements include substantial evidence of safety as well as statistically significant data to demonstrate the efficacy of a product for an approvable indication. Coupled with these data is the requirement for a complete, controlled cGMP manufactured product that is consistent, lot to lot. The safety issues for product development are clear and straightforward, including adequate numbers of subjects in studies treated with the investigational product in order to understand the frequency and severity of adverse reactions. With some biotech-derived products, the safety requirement may also include following recipients to learn the probability of sensitization to the product, or of possible subject response to treatment evidenced by the production of neutralizing antibodies to the material given. Neutralizing antibodies may, in addition to neutralizing the administered product, also neutralize any similar naturally derived substance the individual might still be producing.

But the efficacy issues remain cloudy because FDA does not offer specific recipes for approval. Although FDA often provides some guidance to industry, in many cases, specific guidance has not been issued. One reason why FDA may not have issued guidance for a specific product is that FDA may not have previously reviewed a product similar to yours and cannot offer a strategic plan or approach for the development of your product. Familiarization of FDA requirements for approval is key because industry's perception of FDA requirements is often mistaken or FDA's requirements shift higher, as FDA may follow trends rather than issue specific requirements.

BACKGROUND

The conundrum regarding FDA approvable indications had its beginnings almost 50 years ago, starting with the FDA approval of cholesterol-lowering drugs before there was any correlation with high cholesterol levels and disease. From this, industry got the wrong message, by perceiving a product claim was based on an effect and if the effect could be demonstrated, FDA would approve it. This was a fatal misconception. Shortly after the approval of one or two cholesterol-lowering drugs, nearly 50 years ago in 1962, FDA issued within the Food, Drug, and Cosmetic Act the requirement that a product be shown to be effective before it could be approved. Because effectiveness was ill defined among FDA reviewers, industry members, and academia, a more precise definition of effectiveness for products needed to be established. The immediate result required that a product had to produce patient benefit directly attributable to the administration of the product. This requirement became the standard of efficacy. In addition, it would be necessary to show a positive benefit to risk ratio in order for a product to gain FDA approval. This new standard for product approval resulted from the Drug Efficacy Study Implementation (DESI) review started about 1967. The objective of the DESI review was to remove products from the market that did not have clinical evidence of efficacy or those products that needed additional demonstration of efficacy. It is interesting to note that one of the FDA-approved cholesterol-lowering drugs, MER 29, when marketed and administered to a larger population showed a high incidence of cataract formation. This incidence of unexpected adverse events caused the FDA to ask for larger numbers of subjects to be evaluated in clinical trials before product approval and to identify any unexpected adverse events. Understanding the frequency, severity, and variety of adverse effects is often problematic in drug development. Being able to understand adverse events that may result from product administration still baffles sponsors and the Agency. For example, cholesterol-lowering drugs are still causing worrisome adverse events. Richard Peto, Oxford University, stated at a 1992 Cardio-Renal Blood Products FDA Advisory Panel meeting:

> I think that if you're trying to decide on the treatment of literally millions of subjects...then I think that it is appropriate to randomize at least tens of thousands of subjects.

Today, larger numbers of subjects are being enrolled in clinical trials. Chronically administered drugs that require 12-month continual use studies may soon be required to be evaluated for 24 months before approval is granted. Another example for FDA approval criteria is in cancer therapy. Approval in cancer studies is based on prolonged survival (extended patient life) and/or where therapy may produce an increased disease free interval, or an increased time to disease progression. Oncologists designing a study will usually be satisfied with an objective tumor response. But the tumor response may have no correlation with subject survival. In this case, FDA would perceive no subject benefit. Here is a case where academic science is different from regulatory science. If a sponsor decides to evaluate tumor response at the suggestion of an oncologist but does not also collect survival data, the product studied would probably not be FDA approved. Here the choice is to prolong survival rather than show objective tumor responses, unless of course, the tumor response did provide some measurable subject benefit, which could be measured by increased survival.

Another concept of subject benefit can be based on an early phase of the clinical development of erythropoietin. Subjects who qualified for this study met the protocol inclusion criteria of a diagnosis of end stage renal disease. They had to be on dialysis, and have hematocrit levels below 20. Subject response to treatment demonstrated an increase in hematocrit to 35 or above, patients' anemia improved or even resolved, as evidenced by real weight gain, greater exercise tolerance, and improved sleep. The medical reviewers at FDA who reviewed these data were not impressed with the results submitted. The FDA position was that hematocrit is a laboratory value, and that subjects with anemia learn to tolerate their anemia, and therefore wanted to know how the product improved this subject population. Fortunately, there were sufficient data generated to show that the subjects, who, prior to treatment, were blood transfusion dependent, but following treatment, they were transfusion independent. Center for Biologics Evaluation and Research (CBER), the FDA center which had jurisdiction over this product accepted these data as a demonstration of effective treatment in this subject population, and was additionally pleased as this product would permit saving the rare resource, blood. It was agreed that by any clinical measure, these subjects did receive a clinical benefit, but this example provides another confirmation that academic science is different from regulatory science. It was more important to reduce subject dependency on transfusions than it was to increase hematocrit to normal and alleviate the symptoms of anemia. It was fortunate the sponsor kept all the data generated during the trial. Without transfusion dependence data, this important product may not have received FDA approval.

The cited examples of an oncology trial and the erythropoietin trial emphasize the importance of assuring that a sponsor, researching an investigational product, makes certain the indication is approvable. If the product is not shown to produce subject benefit, the entire program may be lost.

CONSIDERATIONS FOR PATIENT BENEFIT OF A PRODUCT
Patient benefit is

- sometimes quite arbitrary,
- often difficult to define,
- difficult to gain FDA agreement and concurrence with, and
- often difficult to achieve once agreed upon.

While planning clinical trials it is important to know the potential benefits of your product and conceptualize what actual subject response may be demonstrated. When it is determined that subject response to treatment may actually be a clear demonstration of subject benefit, there is a good probability that product will meet FDA requirements for efficacy approval. In attempting to make certain the endpoint your product can actually produce will be FDA approvable, it becomes important to meet with FDA, to gain Agency confirmation that your concept of subject benefit coincides with FDA's requirements relative to your product. Once agreement is reached of a specific subject benefit to be achieved, there should be continuous interaction with FDA to reassure this conceptual agreement. Your protocol for your trial must reflect the benefit you wish to achieve. The design of your protocol, and the clinical endpoint(s) selected, must demonstrate your product to be effective and safe for subject benefit. The subject benefit must be derived directly from the administration of the product. Appropriate control groups should be useful to this end (see chap. 16).

Examples of subject benefit usually FDA approved:
- Increased survival
- Lower high blood pressure
- Lower high cholesterol
- Reduce inflammation, pain
- Increase diuresis
- Eliminate infection
- Diagnosis of a treatable condition

Examples of endpoints not usually FDA approved:
- Increase hematocrit
- Increase granulocytes
- Activate leukocytes
- Accelerate wound healing
- Dissolve blood clots

Another concept that is often thought of as an FDA approvable endpoint is quality of life. An improvement in quality of life is usually considered a secondary endpoint in clinical trials, and FDA is not likely to grant product approval on this finding alone. Quality of life is subjective and difficult to support with objective data, demonstrating subject benefit.

In the development program of an investigational product, it would be prudent to identify all potential indications and which indications, might be useful to subjects. From a list of potential indications, the single indication, which seems the easiest and the quickest to substantiate clinically, and an indication, which would be most readily accepted by FDA, should be the first target indication. It is important to meet with FDA and confirm that FDA agrees with the choice of the target indication (see chap. 6). Also, throughout the development of your product it is important that FDA continue to view your product as it originally was discussed. If FDA alters its position, every attempt to fine-tune your program to assure continued FDA agreement with your original plan must be discussed.

After determining and agreeing with FDA on the correct indication, make certain that the research demonstrates substantial evidence of safety and efficacy of your product for the selected endpoint. Do not dilute efforts by developing the product for other clinical indications, until the primary indication has been supported. There is a famous example of a large pharmaceutical company studying a blockbuster drug, which violated the direct research axiom. The company sponsored 115 studies on this drug, but only 20 of these studies were truly relevant for the indication the drug was intended to be used for. However, in the NDA, the company had to report the 95 non-relevant studies it had sponsored (most of which were done as favors to one clinician or another). It took the company more than a year to gather, report, and submit data from the non-relevant studies. When the NDA was submitted to CDER, it took the Agency an extra year to sort through all of the non-relevant data. This delay in product approval resulted in a loss of market share amounting to an estimated two billion dollars.

This is just one example to understand why it is important to limit the clinical research relevant to only those endpoints, which will generate relevant data that will gain Agency approval. Another important aspect in the development of a new product application is to assure that the package insert provided in the submission is not only specific about indication but is also precise in how the product can be used.

There are three major types of product indications:

1. Therapeutic
2. Prophylaxis
3. Diagnosis

Each of these major types of indications may have subdivisions which in turn may also be subdivided. The important concept to follow is that if you are claiming a therapeutic endpoint, the endpoint must show a subject benefit. With prophylaxis, you must be able to show disease prevention in an at-risk population. If diagnosis is your aim, the diagnostic information must have a real and practical value such as helping physicians determine interventional therapy for their subjects. For each of these three major types of indications, the results achieved must demonstrate a clinical or diagnostic benefit for the subject population being treated. Each clinical trial must demonstrate a clinical benefit rather than just a simple physiologic/biologic effect. A biologic effect is useless if it does not correlate with a clinical benefit. An example of a product producing information which provides no subject benefit would be the development of an in vivo imaging agent indicated to help tally the number of malignant lesions in subjects and to identify where these lesions are located. However, if the sponsor of that product never demonstrated that knowing this information would help physicians intervene in the care of these subjects, the product would not be approved. If FDA reviews a product that provides only information of academic interest, there will be no approval as there was no real benefit. Had the company studied a follow-up clinical program to guide the physician on intervention for those subjects, and had shown interventional success, the imaging agent would have provided a subject benefit and would have gained FDA approval.

SURROGATE ENDPOINTS

FDA has sometimes allowed product approvals when clinical data demonstrate safety and effectiveness for surrogate endpoints or markers. An example of surrogate markers would be objective data showing tumor response to treatment coupled with sufficient clinical data showing that the effect of the drug is a reliable marker of prolonged survival. FDA may accept both surrogate and clinical endpoints in product approval. Surrogate markers are usually considered by FDA only in serious, life-threatening conditions where the results of surrogate markers would form the basis for FDA approval. Another example is an FDA Oncology Division request that a company switch its primary endpoint, complete response, to its secondary endpoint, survival to a specific time point.

Surrogate endpoints are often acceptable to FDA if there is a strong indication that they will result in subject benefit. Surrogate markers are often based upon

- epidemiologic data,
- therapeutic results,
- pathophysiologic change, and
- other evidence (used to build a case in favor of approval).

It is to be noted that the use of a surrogate endpoint

- requires additional measures of judgment;

- surrogate markers may not be acceptable if they are only casually related to clinical outcome;
- surrogate endpoint data may show that the product has less than expected benefit; and
- product may have longer or more than expected adverse effects.

Surrogate endpoints are usually

- not for routine approval,
- acceptable for products whose clinical benefits may be well in the future, and
- useful if the product in question is for treating subjects with life-threatening conditions for which there is no alternative therapy.

Cases in which surrogate markers were not accepted by FDA include

- cardiac arrhythmia suppression trial,
- Increased cardiac output versus survival in heart failure,
- coronary artery patency versus survival in myocardial infarction, and
- bone density versus fracture rate in osteoporosis.

In summary regarding surrogate endpoints and markers, Robert Temple, M.D., when he was Director of Office of Drug Evaluation I stated:

> It seems to me the only rationale for accepting a showing that you are at least better than nothing. . .is an underlying belief that the surrogate you have is not too bad.

It seems clear from the above lists that surrogate markers can be viewed as an interim data point, one which must indicate that the clinical data generated following the time of the surrogate marker must unequivocally support subject benefit.

Today, it is usually agreed that biotechnology had its serious beginnings in the mid-1970s, resulting from technology enabling recombinant products, the use of monoclonal antibodies, and naturally derived proteins and cytokines to provide subject benefits. With only a few product types known and considered as biotechnology derived, decisions for approval of these products were relatively simple. Now however, new product types evolve frequently including DNA derivatives, or even DNA itself, antisense therapies, small interfering RNA, and many others. An IND, for peptide pulsed dendritic cells, that would have been unimaginable years ago was accepted by the FDA. There is a nonending list of possible product candidate types. But the good news is that it does not matter what the product is, or how it is manufactured, the same FDA rules apply. There will be some product types which may require additional evidence of safety in subjects, and others which may require additional characterization, or evidence of stability of the final product, but when it comes to efficacy, all products will require conclusive clinical research demonstrating subject benefit.

FDA always offers to discuss any product with a sponsor. Meetings with the FDA require very careful consideration and planning in order to assure the best possible meeting outcome, that is, of achieving your goal and have FDA concur with your development plan. (see chap. 6). The burden of almost everything at an FDA meeting rests with the sponsor. FDA is not your adversary, but it does act in its role as referee. Referees have final say, so you should position your presentation as best as you can to help FDA's final say be one that you desire. Since FDA's "big picture" agenda may be different from that of the sponsor, do not be surprised at the "requests" that will be asked of you. Some FDA requests of a sponsor may, in time, become requirements, and some early spoken "requirements" which may be dictated to you as absolute musts, may in time become requests only, or even dismissed in total. Familiarity with FDA staff members attending meetings, along with the informality in the moments following the formal meeting, may provide you with an opportunity to try to completely understand what FDA has asked for and what FDA will really require. This is the key to the success of your program. Any differences between your presentation and FDA should be resolved as early as possible. By FDA understanding any characterization issues, a mutually satisfactory resolution can be gained. Remember it is better to not ask FDA any open ended questions, because if you do, you may get a laundry list of answers or tasks that will become requirements, some impossible to complete. For example, if one is unsure on the number of subjects to include in a trial, get a biostatistical work up and present the number of subjects to FDA as being correct, and ask for FDA concurrence based upon your statistical sampling methods. Do not ask the FDA how many subjects would be required in a specific study. The sponsor should direct an FDA meeting; it should not allow FDA to direct the meeting. The meetings are held for the sponsor's needs, not for FDA needs.

PRODUCT DEVELOPMENT

No discussion of FDA-regulated products would be complete without mention of what really constitutes a well-characterized product, and how, before a product is studied in late-phase clinical trials, the sponsor has to accept that the product formulation under development must, at some point, become the final version of the product. The sooner the final product version can be identified as "final" the better. There are too many examples of "changes" that have been made to products late in their development cycle, changes which have caused delayed FDA approval. If a source material for product manufacture is too expensive to use once the product becomes commercial, do not wait until the end of phase 3 studies to introduce the replacement version. In other words, do not change a product once it is in late phase 3 clinicals (unless there is no possible alternative to change it). When someone in manufacturing decides to change the product during clinical investigations such as a different processing method or formulation and the IND or IDE for that product specifies a well-defined product, the change may invalidate the clinical results of the IND or IDE. Most often, the change is unnecessary, or if necessary, it should be made prior to phase 3 programs. If a change is made, for cost reasons or other legitimate reasons, it may be better to postpone such changes until after the initial FDA approval. Changes can be made by a supplemental application (see chap. 10).

PRECEDENTS

Precedents that exist in the annals of FDA history are very important in the overall strategic planning for product development. In reviewing precedent, it is possible to learn FDA's thinking on many issues related to product development and approval. It is possible to learn many important steps in product development by following FDA precedent. If a positive precedent was set, and it worked for a different sponsor, there is every reason to believe that the same precedent can be used in your favor.

FDA ADVISORY PANELS

When FDA believes that it may not have enough expertise among its staff to decide on the final safety and efficacy of an investigational products it calls in an Advisory Panel. These standing advisory panels, in most areas of drugs, biologics, and medical devices are comprised of expert consultants in the specific areas of the product under review. Although FDA is not bound to follow the guidance of their advisory panels, there were only a few times when a recommendation from an advisory panel was not followed by FDA. However, a negative recommendation by the panel should be assessed as a way to enhance or supplement data, and then reapply for approval. For example, an advisory panel reviewed both TPA and Urokinase at the same meeting. The panel's recommendation was for FDA to approve Urokinase, but not to approve TPA. The sponsor of TPA noted the panel's reason for its negative recommendation, and in a short time the sponsor generated the data, originally deemed deficient by the panel. The reason TPA was originally, negatively recommended by the panel is because TPA was first studied for a non-approvable indication. TPA was clinically studied for the indication of dissolving blood clots. The product did dissolve blood clots, but FDA and the panel wanted to know if dissolving blood clots provided a benefit to the infarct subjects. The sponsor generated follow-up data on its infarct study subjects and was able to show that subjects who had received TPA had beneficial, prolonged survival following the infarct, more so than subjects who did not receive TPA. The sponsor should have known by FDA discussions and meetings that dissolving blood clots alone was not an approvable indication. Because the sponsor of TPA responded and provided FDA with data to support an FDA approvable indication, TPA was approved before Urokinase.

This example of an advisory panel meeting is to emphasize that such a meeting will most likely occur in a product submission as a step toward FDA approval. When preparing for such a meeting, it behooves a sponsor to learn as much about the panel as is possible. This can be done by obtaining transcripts from prior meetings of the same panel, becoming familiar with the clinical work of the physician members of the panel. Never approach a panel member to request that he or she become an investigator of a product. If a panel member evaluates the product, then that member would be subject to recusal and could not participate in the panel because of conflict of interest.

Sponsors should prepare for an advisory panel meeting by using presenters that are well-respected and leading clinicians on the subject being discussed. Sponsor representatives should be well versed on the product and include astute regulatory persons familiar with the issues in the meeting discussions.

SPECIAL PROTOCOL ASSESSMENT (SPA)

It is possible to request and obtain a Special Protocol Assessment (SPA) from FDA or from an FDA advisory panel. The full FDA Guidance on SPAs can be obtained from the FDA website, fda.gov. Regulatory personnel representing a sponsor should be intimately familiar with this website. By correctly using this site, it is possible to learn how to save time, money, and anguish in product development. Another valuable source of clinical information is clinicaltrials.gov. This source lists almost 60,000 clinical trials, which are being conducted in about 157 countries. Valuable information to help with strategic planning, and even competitive analyses, can be obtained from this Internet connection. Also remember to use the services that provide information about companies and products that have been released through the Freedom of Information Act (see chap. 6).

CONCLUSION

In considering the large number of ongoing clinical trials, one may wonder why there are not a larger number of product approvals. Estimates exist that as few as 10% of all clinical trials generate adequate data to support clinical safety and efficacy. With all the available tools and resources, clinical trials conducted with protocols that are designed to answer objectives that can demonstrate subject benefits should be more than 90% successful. Strategic planning of product development, which truly shows clinical benefit, should result in FDA approval.

Current estimates of the time it takes from product synthesis to FDA approval range as high as 12 years. Planning the product development process, carefully, correctly, and wisely can often reduce the amount of time from bench to market.

3

Data Presentation for Global Submissions: Text and Tabular Exposition—CTD Format

Patricia Blaine

Medical Writing Corporation, Easton, Pennsylvania, U.S.A.

INTRODUCTION

Over the years, representatives of both the regulatory agencies and the pharmaceutical industry have published in pharmaceutical journals or presented at workshops many helpful suggestions to facilitate regulatory review of the Common Technical Document (CTD) or other submissions and to avoid elements that impede the review. Several authors and presenters have expressed reviewers' frustration at having to review a submission that is incoherently assembled or confusing in its presentation.

It is to the advantage of a sponsor to make the regulatory review process as effortless for the reviewer as possible. The difference in time to approval between a difficult-to-review submission and a clear, well-presented submission may be many months, as the reviewer might require the sponsor to correct the deficiencies before the review can proceed. The marketing personnel of the sponsoring company can all too readily compute the thousands and millions of sales dollars lost for every month of delay of approval or, conversely, the revenue gained from a quick review and approval. In the worst case, a submission that might be marginally acceptable on the merits of a therapeutic agent's effectiveness and safety data alone may be refused if errors in indexing, presentation, and assembly make a meaningful review tedious or even impossible. Although the Common Technical Document and other regulatory documents are now generally filed electronically, an individual reviewer will no doubt print out the assigned section(s) for ease of review.

The ideas in this chapter for improving the text and the tables in global submissions will be representative rather than comprehensive and will focus more on general methods for improving the quality of the text and tables than on specific styling conventions. Many pharmaceutical and biotech companies have their own style guides to promote uniformity and quality of documents throughout a submission. Other companies use a standard style guide, such as the *Manual of Style* published by the American Medical Association (1). Although the examples given in this chapter will be derived from the clinical area, the ideas transcend the different disciplines. Finally, it is beyond the scope of this chapter to discuss graphic presentations, which can greatly enhance the interpretation of data.

TEXT EXPOSITION

Content

The Common Technical Document contains a large amount of data comprising many electronic volumes. Although all the data collected for an individual subject or patient (or groups of subjects or patients) may be important, critical judgment must be exercised in the selection of key data for presentation and discussion within a given section of the document. Data necessary for the development of a specific thesis should be presented within the body of the document rather than placed into a remote appendix, which will impede the review. Less important data can be summarized briefly, clearly referenced in text, and placed in appendices. Additionally, data that have been collected over the years of a drug's development but add nothing to the evaluation of the effectiveness or safety of a therapeutic agent need not be presented at all. Any data submitted will have to be evaluated, so the inclusion of extraneous data will slow the review of the application. The submission should note the existence of such data and have the data available upon request of the regulatory agency.

Tone
The tone of the text should be formal without being stilted. Avoid legal language on the one hand and colloquial or informal language on the other.

Conciseness
Be mindful that regulatory reviewers must read through many volumes of global submissions to make a report on their conclusions. Having to pour through dense, inflated, entangled text to ascertain the point being made will slow the review process. Whereas scientific data are more complex and require more effort to comprehend than most general reading material, a skillful writer will ensure that the complexity derives only from the material and not from the presentation. Wordiness and needless elaborations impede the progress of the review. Also, tabular presentations rather than text are preferred to make the comparison of data easier. The following points address ways of making regulatory documents more concise:

1. Keep the language simple and straightforward. Simple language is not unscientific; rather it promotes clear, fast understanding. Edit out inflated language. For example, "prior to the initiation of the study" can be changed to the much simpler "before the study began" and "subsequent to the initial administration of study drug" can be changed to "after the first dose of study drug." Why say "The patient experienced a fall and suffered a fracture of her right hip" when "The patient fell and fractured her right hip" will convey the meaning just as well?
2. Use acronyms and initialisms to speed up the flow of text if they are easily recognized and have been spelled out at first mention. Those that may be confused with another used in the same document should be spelled out.
3. Eliminate redundancies. A careful review of the text will find many words, phrases, and even sentences that can be omitted. Sentences can often be combined by the deletion of redundant phrases, thus improving the flow of the text. Be prepared to come up against style mavens when implementing this task. For example, many "house styles" insist on units after each number in a range (e.g., 10 mg/kg–20 mg/kg). Whereas some units are brief and may not interfere with the flow of the sentence, a range such as "10 mg of iodine/mL to 20 mg of iodine/mL" would interrupt the sentence flow. This redundancy adds considerably to the length of the sentence, and the burden on the reviewer is further compounded if multiple ranges are compared within one sentence. Consider dispensing with this nicety to improve flow and comprehension.

Correctness

The textual presentation should agree with the tabular data in each section of the Common Technical Document or other global submissions; in turn, the tabular data should agree with the data source (which agrees with the case report form and other clinical documentation). This is critical to the scientific merit of the submission. When lack of agreement between in-text data and source documents is found, the entire submission may be suspect, and the reviewer will be inclined to spend much more time evaluating the raw data to be sure of the conclusions.

Consistency

Consistent punctuation, capitalization, abbreviations, and other styling conventions are much desired in any document, but use judgment before applying the consistency rule unquestioningly. Does the adherence to consistency improve the document or confound it? For example, should all section headers at the same level have the same grammatical structure or would another structure better describe the content of the section? Be critical before insisting on consistency at any cost. A pundit once said, "Foolish consistency is the hobgoblin of little minds."

Clarity

The regulatory reviewer should be able to read through an application expeditiously and not have to stop to try to discern the meaning of a textual presentation. The sponsor of the application should have someone who is familiar with the material in general, but not with the specific document, read it for clarity before submission. If a particular presentation is not clear to this reader, then most likely a reviewer will have the same problem understanding it. Clarity is facilitated by careful attention to the following:

1. *Punctuation*: In *The Art of Plain Talk*, author Rudolf Flesch said that punctuation "is the most important single device for making things easier to read" (2). Omission of punctuation marks, especially commas, can force the reviewer to reread a sentence to ascertain the meaning.
2. *Sentence structure and length*: If long sentences are needed to report equivalent statistics that will be evaluated together, it is helpful to keep the structure of the sentence straightforward and simple. In this kind of sentence, put the thrust of the sentence at the beginning, so that reviewers have a reference point for the subsequent statistics as they read them. Series items should be in order, not random, and be free of interrupting material. Vary sentence lengths to avoid boredom. If possible and feasible, use active rather than passive voice.
3. *Misplaced modifiers*: Every style book covers this topic, but the rule on avoiding misplaced modifiers is often violated. A careful reading of the text by a good editor will eliminate this error.
4. *Parallelism*: Because much of the data in a submission involves comparisons of one group with another, parallel structure is important in presenting the data. Style books for scientific writing will supply good examples of this concept.

Outline of Sections and Subsections

The clear relationship of one section to another is critical to the review of every section in the Common Technical Document or other global submission. If no definite structure is apparent, the reviewer will become lost.

The decimal system is a very popular outlining system; it is easy to use and can be set up automatically in most current word processing software applications. This author strongly advises against going beyond three or four levels in the decimal system, because it is difficult to figure out by then which level you are reading. For example, is section 3.1.2.1.2.1.1.1 on the same level as section 3.1.2.1.2.1.1 or is it a subsection of the former? If no other formatting characteristics identify the subordination of one section to another or are not recognizable as clear distinctions (e.g., all caps, bold vs. initial caps, bold), the reviewer will have difficulty in figuring out the relationship of one section to another. This is also true of another popular outlining system, the alphanumeric system, where letters and numbers alternate as section headers. After a few levels, the distinctions become obscured, and reviewers will become lost.

Indenting
Avoid indenting large sections of text. Most text should be flush to the left margin with appropriate headers to identify the section. Multiple and sequential indenting wastes space and is confusing. Short lists are appropriately indented, and conventions like indenting with bullets are useful to break up long sections of text.

Global to Specific
For any section, begin with global statements or data and then discuss the specifics. For example, in the discussion of adverse events, the overall presentation of the events should precede the presentation by severity, by relationship, by subgroup, etc. This is particularly important in the discussion of the populations evaluated in a particular document. Begin with the all-inclusive population first, then define the subpopulations. One submission this author worked on had about 10 different populations, many of which were close in numbers of patients (e.g., all patients entered, all patients treated in controlled studies, all patients treated in uncontrolled studies, patients treated with test drug in controlled studies, patients treated with active comparative agents or with placebo in controlled studies). This caused great confusion until a table was constructed to identify each population, beginning with the largest population.

TABULAR PRESENTATION
In-text tables are preferred whenever they simplify the presentation and allow for substantial reduction in text. Comprehensive multipage tables that interrupt text should be avoided, if possible, unless they are critical to the development of the thesis of the section. However, if the tables are very important, they can be placed in the same volume in an appendix. Usually, data can be collapsed to be included in the in-text table, with reference to the full table in an easy-to-locate appendix. It should be mentioned here that any tables, figures, or graphs in the appendices must have in-text references.

Information from the tables should not be repeated in the text except as part of a concluding statement about the tabular data or trends seen in the data. The commentary on data from the tables should precede the table, beginning with an introduction to the table by number and a statement identifying what type of data it contains. Additional commentary related to the table but not derived from the tabular data may follow the table.

Title

All tables require concise but descriptive titles. Sequences of tables that are similar should identify their differences very conspicuously in the title, such as at the end of the title after a colon (e.g., Treatment-Related Adverse Events: by Age; ... : by Sex; ... : by Race).

Data Source

Every table should identify the source of the data contained in it. This is usually done in a footnote to the table (e.g., Data source: Statistical Table 23, Volume XX, p. xx). The volume and page numbers will be inserted at the end of the project. Exact referencing of in-text tables will facilitate the review process.

Footnotes

Footnotes should be assigned letters (superscripted), not symbols or numbers, which can be confused with the data. Asterisks (*, **, ***) are generally reserved for levels of statistical significance. In multipage tables, footnotes should be assigned letters in the order in which they appear on the specific page of the table. Always begin such tables on a new page to avoid changing the footnotes, as the tables shift with the addition of preceding text.

Orientation

Portrait tables are always preferable to landscape tables. Remember that the reviewers will likely print out their assigned documents for review. It is cumbersome, annoying, and disruptive for a reviewer to have to move the volume around repeatedly to coordinate the text presentation with the tabular data. If data appear not to fit in the portrait orientation, try changing the axes of the table, so that the axis with more individual descriptors is vertical, whereas the axis with fewer items is horizontal (column headings). Also consider revising the table into separate sections under the same column headers, with descriptive headings for each section spanning the width of the table.

Order of Data Presentation

In multiple tables with similar data, present the data in the same order as much as possible. If the first column always has the active drug and the second column the placebo or comparative agent, then keep this order throughout the tables. In the analysis of data by demographic or disease subgroup, it is helpful to keep the subgroup of concern (e.g., women, the elderly, racial subgroups, impaired renal function) in the same column in each table.

Present Meaningful Data Together

Try to present the data that will be evaluated and compared as close together as possible rather than scattered around the table. For example, if the tabular data represent both evaluable and nonevaluable patients who have been either previously treated or previously untreated, place the evaluable patients together rather than presenting them by previous treatment.

CONCLUSION

The suggestions presented in this chapter for improving text and tables are meant to be neither complete nor sacrosanct, but simply considered. Indeed, the suggestions may be countermanded by particular constrictions and style conventions of the sponsoring company. However, the ability of the writer to look at a document through the eyes of a reviewer will reinforce the suggestions in this chapter. The goal is to speed up the review process and obtain fast approval for a new drug entity. Any suggestions that facilitate this endeavor should be welcome.

REFERENCES

1. American Medical Association. Manual of Style, 10th ed. Philadelphia, PA: Williams & Wilkins, 2007.
2. Flesch R. The art of plain talk, 1962. In: Trimble JR, ed. Writing with Style: Conversation on the Art of Writing. Englewood Cliffs, NJ: Prentice-Hall, Inc., 1975:101.

4 Technology Change—Enabling Clinical Research and Drug Development Processes

Brian J. Chadwick

LookLeft Group, New York, New York, U.S.A.

INTRODUCTION

Mapping the human genome and the collection of genotypical data (tissue specimens) supported by phenotypical data (clinical information about the patient) have *fueled the fire* of translational research and the promise of personalized medicine. While researchers warn that these marvelous scientific events have merely *peeled off yet another layer of the onion*, more than ever before, information technology is enabling innovative clinical research and drug development processes.

With these extraordinary scientific advances, the Life Sciences Industry faces many challenges on the road ahead. But significant market events continue to converge to create unprecedented opportunities for those organizations that can respond, including but certainly not limited to:

- The maturation of the disciplines of genomics and proteomics and the realization of translational research
- Continued consolidation across biopharmaceutical and related market segments in pursuit of scale economies of operation and global reach
- The ubiquity of the Internet—providing a pervasive operating environment enabling execution of eBusiness strategies that embrace all mission critical, company critical, and back officer functions
- Favorable market conditions for rapid emergence of focused biotech organizations with
  - the agility to leverage the deepening understanding of the nature of disease
  - the ability to use information technology to enhance and accelerate traditional rates of development
- The dynamic nature of this market due to economic and regulatory pressures:
  - Healthcare reform related to escalating costs and decreasing reimbursement
  - Concepts such as "pay for performance"
  - Global competition
  - Increasing medical–legal–ethical issues
  - Increasing liability across all healthcare sectors
  - Increasing demand for long-term safety data
  - Increasing demand for long-term outcomes data
  - Blurring of the lines between healthcare providers and payors
  - Explosion of available data and information
  - Changing political and regulatory environments
  - Expanding market opportunity

These events of change are pressuring life sciences companies to move toward the promise that information technology will

- enhance decision support through better access to and rapid interpretation of raw data yielding the potential for adaptive clinical trials.
- improve the velocity of new product development processes.
- improve the capacity of the new product development enterprise.
- enhance the ability to monitor long-term safety and patient outcomes.
- decrease the amount of prospective data that must be collected in support of clinical trials by leveraging the emergence of the electronic medical record (EMR) (with the potential to *reuse* some percentage of EMR data).
- improve data sharing and collaboration.
- enhance relationships—inside and outside the enterprise.

Indeed, it seems that leveraging information technology to allow individuals and groups working together to be more productive can reduce the time it takes to reach conclusions about products in the development cycle and better monitor the safety and outcomes of products on the market. Time and resources are the most significant factors when calculating the cost of drug development—and the cost of bringing a new product to market is staggering. Therefore, less time spent bringing a new product to market should translate to greater profit potential. But there is a grander goal still—and that is the promise and value of the broader concept of knowledge management.

> Knowledge Management caters to the critical issues of organizational adaptation, survival and competence in face of increasingly discontinuous environmental change.... Essentially, it embodies organizational processes that seek a synergistic combination of data and information processing capacity of information technologies, and the creative and innovative capacity of human beings.

This chapter will describe the ever-evolving variety of information technology solutions that have the potential to positively change new product development processes and meet the ongoing safety and outcomes reporting requirements for life sciences companies. The Life Sciences Industry is conservative and risk adverse by its nature and change therefore comes slowly. Yet there are sufficient events in the life sciences marketplace, which suggest that technology *change is upon us*.

PEOPLE, PROCESS—AND THEN TECHNOLOGY

Change can be challenging and costly. And human nature is often resistant to change. As employees become *knowledge workers*, those people become valuable company assets. Therefore, in order for any new information technology solution to work within an environment that has been labor and paper intensive forever, it is critical to assure that the needs of the people (users) are addressed including

- user *communication management* about technology change,
- identifying the user value proposition,
- collecting user requirements,
- user participation in the implementation of new technologies,
- investing in user training and user support, and
- driving user adoption.

Next to paying attention to the people when considering new information technologies, it is vital to understand the implications such change will have on business processes. It is important to perform a process change impact analysis. All too often technologies have been implemented without sufficient design consider- ations for integration with other technology solutions and/or business processes. While the technology clearly needs to *work* within the constraints of the highly regulated, multinational, and absolutely secure requirements of the Life Sciences Industry, the technology itself may represent only 25% of the overall impact such change brings. There is a long list of business processes—both in the internal and external enterprise—that must be proactively addressed and coincide with industry best practices, including but not limited to:

- Overall business requirements and management objectives
- Impact on staff roles and responsibilities
- Overall technology architecture and integration objectives
- Technology *future state* analysis
- Technology implementation and change management
  - Resource availability, cost, and timelines
- Quality management
  - Testing and validation
  - Standard Operating Procedures (SOPs), Business Continuity Practices (BCPs), and Work Practices (WPs)
- Regulatory compliance
  - 21 CFR Part 11, HIPAA, and Privacy rules
- Standards management
  - Local—terminology and coding
  - Global—CDISC, HL7, and other standards
- Pilot program and metrics analysis to measure success (or failure)
  - "The best test—not just a stress test"
  - Avoidance of "perpetual piloting syndrome"
- "Next steps plan" in place

Once a corporate perspective has been established, processes should be defined to evaluate vendors and their technology solutions for

- business stability;
- regulatory compliance;
- domain knowledge—experience and expertise;
- implementation processes;
- references;
- support and helpdesk capabilities;
- scalability;
- configuration, customization, integration, and optimization opportunities;
- future development plans; and
- total cost of ownership.

As vendor and information technology solution evaluation processes proceed, implementation planning should address

- user and management expectations;
- internal and external implementation resource requirements and timelines;
- validation and testing procedures;
- training, user adoption tactics, and user support requirements;
- technology administration;

- hardware qualification and procurement;
- asset management/hardware maintenance;
- roll—out plan—for the internal and external enterprise;
- change management;
- metrics to measure success (or failure); and
- return on investment (ROI) parameters.

It is *most critical* that life sciences organizations proceed down this path with appropriate executive support, financial commitment, and the necessary resources. And life sciences companies' executives must define the information they need in order to make decisions about changes to their information technology infrastructure *in a timely fashion*—with attention to *people, process—and then technology*.

TECHNOLOGY ADOPTION LIFE CYCLE

In 1999, author Geoffrey Moore wrote *Crossing the Chasm*. This book has survived the test of time in its description of the process by which a new technology is absorbed into a community.

Through his technology adoption life cycle, Moore offers a vision of how technology is absorbed into a community in phases that correspond to psychological and social profiles of population segments within the community. The most critical point in developing a high-tech market, he states, lies at the transition from an early market dominated by a few visionary customers on the technological cutting edge to a mainstream market of a larger number of customers with more pragmatic views. The latter are willing to make substantial investments in a new technology only after well-established paths to success begin to emerge.

Moore assigns the term "early market innovators" to those visionary enthusiasts who aggressively seek out the latest technological advancements and possess the skill to assess the technology's value. Innovators influence the early adopters to buy into the product concepts early in their life cycles. Early adopters, in turn, influence the next group, the early majority, to embrace the technology. This early majority combined with a late majority comprises two-thirds of the market and holds the key to the success of the technology in a community.

The Life Sciences Industry is currently in the *late majority* phase with some *early majority* stragglers. Computer modeling, combinatorial chemistry, and high throughput screening (HTS) have significantly increased the numbers of targets coming out of discovery. Preclinical (or nonclinical) development groups are using computer simulation and creating highly specific models to decrease the numbers of animals necessary to fulfill preclinical regulatory requirements. They are using animal research management systems, laboratory information management systems (LIMS), and applications that can be integrated with a variety of digital measurement tools. In clinical development, most life sciences companies are actively using a variety of solutions collectively referred to as eClinical applications in the clinical trials environment. Regulatory submissions are increasingly electronic by FDA mandate. And in the marketing environment, mobile technologies supported by websites and portals for physician encounters and direct to consumer (DTC) interactions are in play. Life sciences companies are using web-based eProcurement tools for supply chain management, learning management systems, financial and human resource management solutions, and other eBusiness applications to manage multiple back-office functions.

So *change is upon us.* Slower than other industry verticals such as financial services—reflecting the very conservative and risk adverse nature of the Life Sciences Industry—but information technology has become integral in the management of every life sciences company. Yet, the industry continues to strive to develop information technology *standards* and deal with increasingly challenging regulatory implications—further complicated by varying interpretations of these regulations. And change itself is costly. It is resource intensive and must deal with behavioral modification and human nature's resistance to change.

Technology solutions have *Crossed the Chasm*—but many have fallen into the chasm on the way across. Patience and persistence rule the day.

THE INTERNET
The Internet has changed the way we do just about everything. It provides rapid access to and exchange of information. It has become ubiquitous!

Intranets and Extranets
The Internet provides individuals and businesses a way of transferring information of every type, *quickly, easily, and inexpensively.* Corporate intranets provide an internal network for managing local applications and data. And while there are many approaches that make the Internet very secure—such as multiple firewalls, robust encryption algorithms, biometrics, . . .—there are security concerns that still make the company Intranet the preferred method of managing information technology. Having said that, a future state analysis may find client–server technologies rapidly being replaced by software as a service (SaaS) models in which less, maybe no, data is saved to the local hard drive or the local network. We may find information technology making a complete circle back to the *dumb terminal* where all data pass through an Internet cloud and are managed in professional data centers.

Two decades ago, computer users extended their environment from the desktop to the network. In the last decade, the network was extended by workgroup applications. Over the past few years, the workgroup has been extended to include all the other computers in the world through the Internet! The key to success in deploying information technology is leveraging the resources of secure global networking to help knowledge workers accomplish their jobs *quickly, easily, and inexpensively.*

The Software As a Service (SaaS) Business Model
The SaaS model is a service that provides access to applications through a secure extranet. The SaaS provider assumes all responsibility for software maintenance and upgrades, regulatory compliance, and data and document storage. Of course, life sciences companies must still maintain a proper regulatory platform and application controls. But in the SaaS model, servers, applications, and databases are co-located in two and sometimes three geographically disparate data centers through redundancy and backup procedures. Such data storage facilities have substantial physical security. This model can provide more robust security, business continuity practices, and disaster recovery processes than many corporations—especially mid-tier and smaller companies. Companies availing themselves of this service, by definition, *license rather than purchase* software applications and *rent rather than own server locations.* And this can be for a single application or for the entire IT infrastructure. Users merely need a browser. Businesses require less internal IT infrastructure.

Each company's and/or user's data are protected and accessible only by the individuals that are given permission to access that data (by the owner of that data). The SaaS model, similar in many ways to its predecessor, the Application Service Provider (ASP) model, provides *the app. on tap*—in a server-hosted environment.

Adoption of this model has been slow. Corporations and individuals alike still prefer to keep their data in their own location. But the SaaS approach, like outsourcing in general, is *coming on*. It can level the technology playing field. Smaller companies can have access to technologies without the overhead of large IT infrastructures. There is less commitment and much of the risk is shifted to the SaaS provider. This model is being explored by many large and small companies and, as mentioned previously in this chapter, the future state may find users in front of *dumb terminals* (again)—connected through secure ports to the Internet to any variety of business and personal applications.

Security

The protection of information, both corporate intellectual property and personal data, is on the top of everyone's list in a life sciences environment that increasingly depends on knowledge sharing (in real time). Although there will always be security challenges, there is more confidence than ever before in the ability to protect information. Regulations such as 21 CFR Part 11 (Title 21 Code of Federal Regulations: Electronic Records; Electronic Signatures), HIPAA, and a variety of global privacy rules, with advanced data encryption algorithms, de-identification processes, the rapidly emerging field of biometrics, and standard operating procedures for both logical and physical security hardware, software, databases, and networks are just some of the advances in security that are making the Internet a safe place to do business for life sciences companies.

Electronic signatures, especially using biometric solutions such as finger printing or retinal scanning are an important link in the security chain. Security objectives of the electronic signature are best realized through an advanced process referred to as Public Key Interface (PKI) including

- *Authentication*—the verification of the identity of an individual or organization sending information.
- *Integrity*—providing verification that a message or document is genuine and has not been manipulated or changed since its original creation (or signing).
- *Nonrepudiation*—to ensure that the originator of a message or transaction cannot subsequently disown it.

Access to data can be very granular—manageable at the *atomic level*. This means that a database administrator can allow a user access to a single data point in a huge database. This is a very powerful security feature and further enables internal and external collaboration.

HARDWARE

There are dozens of choices of popular hardware platforms, depending on the size of your business or your personal preference. Software runs your business. The hardware requirements of the software define the hardware needed. Activities of daily business or life style further define hardware requirements. Personal digital assistants or handheld computers and computer tablets have significantly improved user mobility. Wireless connectivity has made mobile computing a reality. But at the end of the day, most hardware, even stand-alone home computers (with Internet connectivity), are *networked*.

For *networked* computers, two basic types of machines exist—servers and workstations (both mobile and desktop). Servers and workstations should be as powerful and upgraded as frequently as software requirements and the budget permit. Every company should have standards in place that define minimal hardware requirements with documented installation, maintenance, backup, and disaster recovery standard operating procedures. In today's very competitive new product development marketplace, speed and processing power impact the efficiency of the knowledge worker. Management must find the balance on that delicate line between cost and productivity.

SOFTWARE

General Software Applications

Technologies (applications) that are used across industries are generally referred to as *horizontal* software. Common horizontal applications are found on the desktop computer to support general office functions and usually include word-processing and spreadsheet software as well as email. Many desktop computers also provide presentation software, project management applications, and a variety of collaboration applications for online meetings and information (data) sharing. To better enable collaboration, an emerging approach is to centralize data in a collaboration application and/or the more sophisticated data warehouse. Rather than sending data or documents via unsecured e-mail, the collaboration model locates data in a secure centralized application or database. These are secure *vaults* that can contain vast amounts of information—documents and data—from a variety of sources. And access management provides preidentified individuals with a key to those vaults that defines the data each individual can access.

The most important aspect in choosing software applications is that they provide the functionality and feature sets needed by the enterprise (or for personal use). It is also important to ensure interoperability whenever possible. And modern software applications provide better data import and export functionality than ever before.

Data Standards

Although modern software applications do provide better data import and export functionality than ever before, issues associated with interoperability and data integration still represent the most significant challenges to clinical data management. As simple as it seems, if one database uses the term *gender* and another uses the term *sex*, those data points cannot be integrated into a common dataset without first manually mapping one to the other. Multiplied by thousands of such inconsistencies makes data integration both resource intensive and time-consuming. The Clinical Data Interchange Standards Consortium (CDISC) is the primary nonprofit Life Sciences Industry group leading the charge toward data standards. The Operational Data Model (ODM) and the Study Data Tabulation Model (SDTM) are the processes driving those data standards. Further, CDISC is collaborating with the primary healthcare standards group, Health Level 7 (HL7), to make electronic medical record (EMR) data *reusable* in clinical trials. Such data standards must be achieved for true data integration to become a reality!

eDiscovery Software

Recent scientific and technological advances have introduced new paradigms for drug discovery research. The drugs developed over the last four decades have been aimed at about 500 different biological targets. With the sequencing of the human genome, numerous new biological targets are being recognized. It has been estimated that at least 10% of these could be potential targets for drugs. This creates additional decision support issues for the already *thinly spread* resources of the Life Sciences Industry.

High-throughput screening (HTS) is a system for analyzing compound libraries and natural products in order to identify leads for potential targets. "HTS arose in the 1990s as 96 microtitre plates were selected over test tubes as the receptacle of choice for biological assays". In combination with combinatorial chemistry, it resulted in a paradigm shift from knowledge-based sequential synthesis and testing to parallel processing of multiple compounds. With the objective to improve success rates and cycle times, HTS has become one of the cornerstones of drug discovery. With the advent of high-throughput approaches in genomics, combinatorial chemistry, and screening, the Life Sciences Industry should face no shortage of novel targets or promising lead compounds. Having said that, as noted earlier, many scientists see these advances as steps in an exciting direction for new discovery, but caution the industry that there are still many *layers of the onion that need to be peeled back* to unveil the secrets of gene-based therapies. And selecting the *right* new chemical entities to enter the clinical development process still requires a bit of luck and what has been referred to by some as *planned serendipity*.

ePreclinical Software

In the preclinical (nonclinical) stage of new product development, an investigational drug must be tested extensively in living organisms (in vivo) and in cells in the test tube (in vitro) to provide information about

- the pharmaceutical composition of the drug,
- its safety,
- how the drug will be formulated and manufactured, and
- how it will be administered to the first human subjects.

Regulatory agencies require testing that documents the characteristics—chemical composition, purity, quality, and potency—of the drug's active ingredient and of the formulated drug. Pharmacological testing determines effects of the candidate drug on the body. General toxicology and reproductive toxicology studies are conducted to ensure that any risks to humans are identified.

There are numerous opportunities to infuse software into the preclinical phase of new product development such as

- animal facility software management system that includes on-line IACUC, protocols, census, animal orders, and an e-mail notification system; and
- breeding colony management software that tracks projects, lines, matings and litters, injections, implantations, pedigrees, phenotypes, and genotypes.

An important requirement in selecting preclinical software solutions is the ability to interface with peripherals such as scales, automatic vital signs (i.e., arterial line), barcode readers, animal ID scanners, and others.

But the primary limitation to automating the preclinical testing environment is budget. Financial support for preclinical software solutions pales when compared to budgets to improve the clinical phases of new product development. This has resulted in a slow transition to software automation—certainly slower than in the clinical phases of new product development.

eClinical Software

So, while information technology solutions are indeed being introduced across the new product development life cycle, clinical trials are the most critical and most expensive phase of new product development. It is, therefore, the area that is receiving the most attention in attempts to increase the velocity of the new product development process and improve the capacity of the new product development enterprise. And most clinical trials are now using a host of eClinical applications and technology-based processes to improve the quality of data being collected and drive the speed of analyzing that data—to better enable decision making. This group of eClinical software solutions, unlike office applications, and like discovery and preclinical applications, is generally referred to as *vertical* software. And while large software companies have had some success in the life sciences marketplace, the idiosyncratic nature of new product development software applications has made it a challenge to *verticalize* what are otherwise *horizontal* solutions. Therefore, many of the information technology solutions at the core of drug and device development are provided by smaller vendors. And the associated increased risk of dealing with small, relatively new companies has been one of the reasons for slower uptake of such technology solutions. That increased risk results in more piloting, slower decision making, and requires greater attention to the selection and management of such *vertical* applications.

Electronic Data Capture (EDC) and Electronic Patient Reported Outcomes (ePRO)

Electronic data capture (EDC) is the generally accepted term to describe web-based collection of clinical trials data from physicians participating as investigators in a clinical trial. While these are almost exclusively web-based (online) applications, some offer hybrid functionality (combined online/offline) to reflect what is still the occasional challenge of getting an Internet connection (from hospitals that limit Internet access for nonemployees, on an airplane, . . .). Although finding an Internet connection is less a problem than ever before, it is still an issue that must be addressed when choosing such applications. But even with the occasional challenge of getting an Internet connection and a variety of user process issues, the majority of clinical trials, especially those sponsored by major biopharmaceutical companies, are using EDC as the preferred method of capturing clinical trials data. EDC provides cleaner data faster and improves the time to database lock. It is critical that EDC applications and databases are built to comply with 21 CFR Part 11 and international regulations for the protection of personal health information (PHI). EDC solutions must meet these requirements and provide robust logical and physical security to provide *regulatory grade* data to be used in support of regulatory submissions.

Another type of electronic data capture that is flourishing in the drug and device development arenas is in the area of direct-to-patient solutions such as patient diaries and quality-of-life questionnaires. This information technology group of software products is generally referred to as electronic patient reported outcomes (ePRO) solutions. While the Life Sciences Industry has been collecting this type of information for years, paper-based collection of direct patient input was never given much credibility. This was not because that data was perceived to be unimportant; rather, the paper-based approach to such data collection made that data unreliable—as such data must usually be collected at an appointed time (i.e., two hours after a dose of a medication). There was no guarantee that the information requested was indeed completed at that appointed time. There are many anecdotes of research subjects in the waiting area scrambling to complete weeks of *daily* diary data before their appointment with the physician (investigator). Nonetheless, the use of electronic tools such as the personal digital assistant (PDA) and ePRO applications have resuscitated the value that direct input from the patient can bring to assess the efficacy and safety of drugs and devices in clinical trials. ePRO technologies date and time stamp each data entry session. Alarms can be programmed to remind patients of a required time to take a medication or complete a questionnaire. That data can be sent in real time across the Internet. This approach to data collection has not only improved the value of patient reported outcomes but has also emerged as a methodology for disease management. With an eye towards improving compliance and persistence, as well as more closely managing real-time disease-related information, such as alterations in blood glucose, ePRO solutions are receiving increasing attention. There are still issues with the usability of ePRO devices. The PDA is small and requires a certain manual dexterity. And many elderly patients find these small devices a challenge to use. ePRO questionnaires must be validated tools and even with that there are still pockets of regulatory concern as to the value of patient reported information. There are viable alternatives to the PDA such as interactive voice response systems (IVRS), which use the *good old* telephone for the transmission of direct patient information. In fact, other than collecting subject-reported data, interactive voice response systems are the most popular tool used for automating subject randomization. And mobile phones are emerging as vehicles for direct-to-consumer bidirectional communication tools. All in all, advances in information technology have brought a new value to data that was always seen to be worthy of collection but until recently, there were insufficient vehicles to enable this.

Mobile devices have found other areas of value in the community of physicians involved in drug and device development as well as in general practice management. ePrescriptions, automated patient's notes, schedules, and even eDetailing (sales force effectiveness) have moved the mobile device into the daily workflow of most physicians. As this technology evolves, we can expect to see an increasing role of mobile devices in the world of drug and device development, disease management, and healthcare, in general.

Clinical Trials Management Systems (CTMS)

Clinical Trials Management Systems (CTMS) are currently receiving significant attention, as the Life Sciences Industry orients itself to the value of relationship management. Managing the business of clinical trials is as important as managing the clinical data. One could readily argue that a CTMS should be the first system to implement as the entire clinical trials process *goes electronic*. As competition for the relatively limited pool of qualified investigators continues to grow, building a database with investigator/site capabilities with objective, rather than self-reported, investigator performance metrics has strategic value. Managing the vast numbers of investigator site's business and regulatory documentation, timelines, enrollment and cost—planned versus actual—makes knowledge workers responsible for managing clinical trials more efficient and effective. These systems improve regulatory compliance, enhance resource management, and provide near real-time decision support for management. Further, the number of co-development and co-marketing partnerships is growing exponentially and the requirement to share and/or merge information about the status of ongoing clinical trials has become critically important. Most CTMS solutions offer and/or can be integrated with off-the-shelf project management tools and provide *connectors* to other eClinical and business management software solutions.

Collaboration Software

Collaboration software is any application that provides groupware functionality.

eLearning and online meeting (or virtual meeting) solutions are becoming increasingly popular as an alternative and/or adjunct to the traditional (in person) classroom or business meeting. Life sciences companies are re-evaluating the huge costs associated with training and investigators' meetings. eLearning and online meetings solutions offer a significantly less-expensive option. These software applications are evolving in two forms: self-administered web-based learning and service-based live online training and meetings. eLearning and online meetings seem to provide a rare win-win solution. Life sciences companies spend less money. Physicians and coordinators travel less. While in the past, when such meetings were held in exotic locations, today, regulatory authorities have placed more controls over the locations of investigator meetings—to eliminate inappropriate inducements for participation in a clinical trial. And that has made such travel less attractive. Equally important has become the issues of *time away from the office*, which equals lost revenue, and/or *time away from the family*, which interferes with quality of life. This is so, especially for investigators who perform multiple clinical trials each year. Further, biopharmaceutical companies have substantial staff training needs—for clinical teams in the internal and external enterprise, but especially for guiding the regulatory appropriateness of the sales professional's interactions with physicians.

eLearning applications, therefore, are often integrated with and are a key part of online meetings solutions. Again, like online meetings, eLearning has proven to be a less-expensive alternative to classroom-based learning and broadens significantly the reach of knowledge transfer. It is easier to certify that participants in clinical trials have learned. And the return on investment (ROI) is realized through reduced cost, an increased understanding of protocol requirements, better attention to regulatory compliance, and improved data quality.

Document Exchange applications are also collaboration tools. They are frequently referred to as digital workspaces. While this technology is often integrated with eLearning and online meetings applications, many CTMS solutions offer a digital workspace for the exchange and management of clinical trials documentation. Documents can be made available in centralized web-based locations to investigators and coordinators participating in clinical trials. If electronic signature technology is enabled, documents can be electronically signed and posted to the centralized site; or, they can be manually signed, scanned, and then posted into that centralized, secure website. This approach expedites the document exchange process and creates an online regulatory file cabinet.

Database Management Systems (DBMS)

In many life sciences companies the database management system (DBMS) is the center of their clinical trials data universe. Most other eClinical solutions (noted above) are expected to integrate with the corporate database management system. This can be easier said than done. Even though there are only a few significant providers of DBMS, each life sciences company historically has created its own data standards. And this can make integration with the other (disparate) eClincal systems a complex process. Having said that, importing and exporting data is improving rapidly; and CDISC is driving industry-wide adoption of data standards. DBMS are the clinical data repositories from which statistical analysis is done, reports are created, and from which ERS evolve.

Document Management Systems

Developing a new drug creates a vast amount of documentation—most of which must be included in the (electronic) new drug application submitted to Regulatory authorities. Managing such documentation is a significant task. Document management systems are very different from the documents stored in collaboration workspaces mentioned above. Document management systems must strictly control access and versioning. These systems usually work by using a library approach to documents. New documents are created and checked into a library under an appropriate heading or study name. These documents are then checked out, as approved users need to modify them, and every such transaction is logged in an audit trail. This approach ensures that only one user can modify a document at a time to maintain version control. Security controls are granular and can be set to define which users are allowed to change what documents. At any time, a document can be locked to disallow further changes. The document management system also generally provides an index of documents in the library. Through the index, a user can quickly search for documents with specific contents. Any part of any document can also be cross-referenced to other sections. These features are especially useful in preparing the ERS—the electronic version of a New Drug Application—in which volumes of paper documents can be stored electronically and readily cross-referenced. Integrated with clinical development data from a DBMS, a regulatory reviewer could have an entire NDA accessible on the desktop.

Portals and Data Warehouses

Using the metaphor of a website as a store makes a portal a shopping mall—enabling access to multiple stores (applications). Portal technology has emerged as one solution to help sort the integration problem of *connecting* otherwise not integrated, disparate eClinical applications. Future integration solutions will incorporate emerging data standards. Using tools sometimes called gadgets, portal technology allows users with proper security clearance to *reach into* multiple eClinical applications to *surface* specific data of interest to that specific user. The user can integrate that data (from multiple disparate applications) into a single report. In an age when too much data is as bad as too little data, the ability to *personalize* access to multiple applications and generate integrated reports has huge potential. The *digital dashboard* is the portal interface that facilitates the opportunity to control and report on individualized information. Portal solutions can be very expensive and therefore, to date, only major life sciences companies have been truly able to take advantage of this technology.

Most life sciences companies are in the process of developing a variety of data warehouses. The goals of a clinical data warehouse include

- establish integrated clinical operations,
- enable online review and dynamic reporting,
- enable data sharing among business divisions, and
- enable executive decision-making platform.

The complexity of integrating data from other disparate data systems and sources, such as EDC or CTMS, is related to the lack of accepted Life Science Industry data standards. But there is a bit of light at the end of this tunnel as CDISC, as noted earlier in this chapter, is leading the charge and driving the Life Sciences Industry to adopt data standards.

CONCLUSION

For information technology solutions to achieve the promise of improving the velocity of new product development processes and increasing the capacity of the new product development enterprise is clearly dependent upon *people and process—then technology.* For information technology solutions in the Life Sciences Industry to *Cross the Chasm,* software applications must enable users to do what they need to do *quickly, easily, and inexpensively.* And as standards evolve and data integration becomes easier; as personalization, workflow, and artificial intelligence improve application functionality and further enable knowledge workers—helping to drive user adoption; as younger, more computer savvy generations of knowledge workers assume leadership roles and responsibilities; and as the Internet continues to evolve—the Life Sciences Industry will reap the benefits of innovative information technology solutions. *Change is upon us.*

As technology is playing a major role in most life sciences companies, attempts are being made to make the new product development process faster and less expensive. But the investment has been, and will continue to be, significant. The return on that investment is that *technology change is, indeed, enabling clinical research and drug development processes.*

5 Working with a Contract Research Organization (CRO)

Duane B. Lakings

Drug Safety Evaluation Consulting, Inc., Elgin, Texas, U.S.A.

PART I: CONTRACT RESEARCH ORGANIZATIONS

INTRODUCTION

The use of contract research organization (CROs) or contract service organizations (CSOs) in discovery, nonclinical, clinical, and manufacturing drug development programs—or "outsourcing," as the process is commonly referred to by the industry—is a common practice of most, if not all, pharmaceutical and biotechnology companies. At present, more than 450 CROs exist in the United States and Europe with others being started or already available in Asia, and the use of their services for all aspects of the drug discovery and development process is rising. The growth of outsourcing is expected to continue, with some CROs offering an almost, but not quite, complete drug development support system, from synthesis and characterization of the drug substance to conducting phase 3 safety and efficacy human clinical trials, and preparing marketing applications, such as an New Drug Application (NDA), documents for submission to regulatory agencies. Other CROs specialize in selected aspects of the drug characterization process, offering services in such areas as pharmacology animal model development and implementation, formulation development and drug substance and proposed drug product stability testing, bioanalytical chemistry method development and validation, or clinical trial protocol preparation and study support, such as site and investigator selection or data management.

This chapter discusses the processes commonly used to select a CRO for the nonclinical and clinical stages of drug development and the requirements for obtaining an appropriately completed study at a CRO. The processes and requirements for outsourcing the manufacturing program for a drug substance and the preparation and testing of a proposed drug product are also areas of high growth and a number of contract manufacturing organizations (CMOs) offer these services. However, the outsourcing of manufacturing processes, including the preparation of the chemistry, manufacturing, and control (CMC or Quality) sections for regulatory submissions, is not covered in this chapter even through the processes described in this chapter can be applied to these types of CROs or CMOs.

NONCLINICAL CONTRACT RESEARCH ORGANIZATIONS

A pharmaceutical or biotechnology company identifies a lead compound that has potential for mediating a human disease or disorder and then conducts the required Good Laboratory Practice (GLP)-regulated preclinical safety (safety pharmacology, pharmacokinetic, and toxicology) studies to submit a first-in-human clinical trial application (such as an Investigational New Drug or IND submission), followed by the nonclinical (or Safety) and clinical (or Efficacy) studies necessary for a marketing application submission. For several reasons, corporate management may decide to have some or all of these studies performed at a CRO. The drug development project team is informed of this management decision and is usually given the responsibility of coordinating the outsourcing program, as well as any internal research studies, and ensuring that the drug development program stays on time and on track. For a small biotechnology company, this responsibility may fall on the shoulders of a single individual or a small group of two or three researchers, each of whom need to have a good understanding of each of the scientific disciplines for which outsourced studies are being considered. A common practice for many biotechnology firms is to contract with a consultant or a consulting firm to assist in the outsourcing effort, including the design of the research studies to be outsourced, the selection and management of the service providers, and the review of generated results and study reports.

The first requirement for a successful program at CROs is to identify which research studies or aspects of the nonclinical drug development program are to be conducted at a CRO. Then, the projected timeline for initiation and completion of the studies are needed, so that results and technical or study reports are available at the appropriate time for decision making and for regulatory agency submissions. As discussed in the chapter on project teams, a well-constructed drug development plan provides much of this information. The project team members whose scientific disciplines are part of the outsourcing program are typically assigned as scientific experts and the project team coordinator is given the responsibility for contractual arrangements. These subproject teams need to first identify and then select the appropriate CRO or CROs to conduct the desired research studies. These teams also need to appropriately monitor the CRO(s) to ensure that the studies are being conducted as designed and described in the study protocol and that the generated results are appropriately recorded in both the study records and the study report. The following sections provide more details on the CRO selection and monitoring processes for nonclinical drug development research studies.

CRO Identification and Selection

After a pharmaceutical or biotechnology company, commonly referred to as the sponsor, has decided to use CROs to support some or all of the nonclinical research effort in a drug development program, management or the project team responsible for the development of the drug candidate assigns individuals to identify and select the appropriate CROs. The steps in a selection process should include, but are not limited to

1. Preparing the study designs for each of the research studies to be outsourced. The more details provided in the study designs, the better. The CROs will use the provided information to prepare a draft study protocol and a proposal with time and cost estimates. Examples of two study designs are shown in Table 1.
2. Determining which CROs should be considered as potential contractors. This aspect of the selection process is discussed in more detail below.
3. Soliciting cost and time proposals for each study design from each CRO. Generally, three to five CROs that have the necessary expertise to complete the study successfully are requested to submit proposals for each study design.

TABLE 1   Study Design Examples for Contract Research Organization Time and Cost Proposal
Preparation

| 28-Day toxicology in a nonrodent species |

Purpose: To evaluate the toxicology of a protein test article in a nonrodent species after
every-other-day subcutaneous dosing for 28 days.

Test species	Beagle dog
Test article	Protein therapeutic
Dose levels	300, 100, 30, and 10 μg/kg plus vehicle control
Frequency	Every other day (EOD), 14 doses total
Administration	Subcutaneous, bolus injection; dosing solutions to be prepared daily; duplicate aliquots of each formulation level collected predose and postdose for the 1st, 7th, and 13th dose to be analyzed (using a validated analytical chemistry method to be transferred to the service provider) for test article concentration
Number	Three animals per sex per dose group with four dose groups and a vehicle control group (30 animals total)
Evaluation	Clinical signs of toxicity during in-life phase including general health, body weight, food consumption; clinical pathology (standard hematology, clinical chemistry, urinalysis parameters, and immunotoxicity) predose and after 4th, 7th, and 14th doses; gross pathology including selected organ weights; histopathology at all dose levels
Toxicokinetics	Blood specimens collected after the 1st, 7th, and 13th dose to be analyzed (using a validated bioanalytical chemistry method to be transferred to the service provider) for test article concentration to assess extent of exposure and potential gender differences
Antibodies	Blood specimens collected prior to the 1st, 7th, and 14th dose to be analyzed (using a developed assay to be transferred to the service provider) for antibodies to the test article
Timeline	Projected start date and estimated completion date

| Absolute bioavailability, pharmacokinetics, and dose proportionality in a nonrodent species |

Purpose: To evaluate the absolute bioavailability and pharmacokinetics, including dose
proportionality, of a small organic molecule drug candidate in a nonhuman primate.

Test species	Rhesus monkey
Test article	Small organic molecule, molecular weight <350
Route	Intravenous, 100, 30, 10, and 3 μg/kg (or other dose range) Oral, 1000, 300, 100, and 10 μg/kg (or other dose range)
Frequency	Multiple using balanced, cross-over design with 7-day washout period between doses
Administration	Intravenous, slow bolus injection at about 1 mL/min Oral, gavage Duplicate aliquots of each formulation collected predose and postdose to be analyzed (using a validated analytical chemistry to be transferred to the service provider) for test article concentration
Number	Equal to number of doses in cross-over design
Specimens	Blood for plasma; sufficient number to characterize the absorption, distribution, and disposition phases of the test article Possible series: 0, 5, 10, 20, 30, 45, 60, 90, 120, 180, 240, 360, 480, 720, and 1440 min for intravenous doses and 0, 15, 30, 45, 60, 90, 120, 150, 180, 240, 300, 360, 480, 720, and 1440 min for oral doses Urine; sufficient number of intervals to characterize the rate and extent of urinary elimination of the test article Possible series: 0–2, 2–4, 4–8, 8–12, and 12–24 hr for both routes of administration

(Continued)

TABLE 1 Study Design Examples for Contract Research Organization Time and Cost Proposal Preparation (*Continued*)

Bioanalytical	Validated assay for plasma and urine specimens from rats to be cross species validated by the service provider
Stability	Test article stability in collected specimens to be determined from time of collection to projected time of analysis
Analyses	Individual analytical runs to include all specimens of a given matrix for an individual animal or 30 plasma unknowns per run
Timeline	Projected start date and estimated completion date

4. Evaluating the proposals, which includes determining if the CRO understands the study design, and selecting those CROs to be considered further. At times, CROs will recommend additions to a study design, which may or may not improve the overall study and could provide additional information for the complete characterization of the drug candidate. When this occurs, the sponsor needs to critically evaluate the expanded study and determine if the increased costs and, possibly, extended study duration justify the additions to the study design.
5. Scheduling and conducting pre-award site visits to ensure that the CROs are qualified and have the facilities and personnel necessary to conduct the research studies. These site visits should include assessments of GLP compliance, standard operating procedures (SOPs), and computer validation.
6. Negotiating time and cost for completion of the research studies. The original estimate in the proposal is usually not the final cost of conducting a research study at a CRO. Those CROs still on the short list should be asked to provide their "best and final" cost, the dates they can actually initiate the study, and the date they project the draft final report will be available for review. Some consulting firms specialize in this phase of interacting with CROs and will negotiate with the CROs for the sponsor, thus relieving the sponsor of the problems that can occur by pushing for the best price.
7. Selecting the CROs and awarding the contracts for each study to be outsourced.

The number of sponsor person–hours required for the identification and selection process depends on the size of the research program to be contracted. Normally, a minimum of one to two person–weeks is necessary to evaluate three to four CROs for each research study to be outsourced. This effort can be substantially reduced by the placement of more than one study at a CRO. Many biotechnology companies and some pharmaceutical firms use consultants or consulting firms to assist them in the CRO selection process. However, these sponsors need to ensure that the consultants have expertise both in scientific disciplines for the studies being outsourced and knowledge of how CROs operate. A common mistake is to hire a consultant with expertise in the disease area of the drug candidate but not in the nonclinical drug development process, or conversely, in regulatory compliance but not in the science necessary to successfully characterize a drug candidate. The sponsor should evaluate and select consultants who have the necessary knowledge of drug development and contract research to enhance the chance of a successful outsourcing program.

Pharmaceutical and biotechnology companies commonly use one of three strategies to identify CROs. These strategies can be designated virtual company, preselected, and special study.

Virtual Company Strategy

The virtual company strategy is used by companies, mostly biotechnology firms and many United States and European subsidiaries of Asian pharmaceutical firms that do not have the infrastructure or resources to conduct GLP-compliant nonclinical research studies necessary to support regulatory agency submissions. The primary benefit of this outsourcing approach is that the various expertises, such as toxicologist, pathologist, and drug metabolism expert, and the infrastructure, such as facilities, quality assurance unit, and GLP compliance, needed to support regulated studies can be devoted to completing nonclinical development studies. This means the sponsoring company does not have to build the in-house groups and facilities necessary for ensuring GLP compliance and thus can avoid costly time delays. A primary limitation to this strategy is that the sponsoring company can be vulnerable to poor CRO selection or to mismanagement by the CRO. However, by using experts or consultants appropriately to assist in the identification and selection process and the monitoring aspects, discussed in the following section, a sponsor can usually avoid this limitation.

Preselected Strategy

In the preselected strategy, the first choice of many large and mid-sized pharmaceutical houses, a limited number—usually three to six—of CROs are prequalified to support a sponsor's possible nonclinical drug development needs. The qualification process usually includes a detailed site visit to review the CRO's facilities, staff, and GLP compliance and to determine which types of nonclinical research studies, such as toxicology, drug metabolism, and formulation development, can be placed at the CRO. At times, long-term contracts are defined in which the CRO guarantees the sponsoring company a certain level of resources to be available to support projects and the sponsor guarantees to provide a sufficient number of research studies to effectively use the committed resources. This strategy can provide a synergistic working relationship between the sponsoring company and the CRO, which in essence becomes an integral part of the development processes of the sponsor. The major drawback to the preselected CRO strategy is the unnecessary limitation of outsourcing. If a fairly large number of CROs, say 30, have the necessary expertise to conduct a nonclinical study or group of studies but the sponsoring company prequalified list contains only three CROs with the required expertise, the other 27 are not considered, even though some of these CROs may be able to complete the studies faster and cheaper or may have superior expertise and experience in the drug candidate's therapeutic area.

Special Study Strategy

The final strategy, the special study strategy, is used by some sponsoring companies to place single or a few nonclinical research studies with a CRO. If a company's internal resources are usually, but not always, sufficient to meet their nonclinical drug development needs, this strategy provides a means to have a critical study completed to meet the timeline on a drug development plan. However, some companies use the special study strategy for all their nonclinical drug development needs and then attempt to integrate the results for the independent studies into a drug development story. For a company with substantial drug development expertise, this strategy may work but requires considerable effort in identifying and selecting CROs, in monitoring the various CROs, and in synthesizing the results from the various research studies. Contract research organizations are generally not in favor of this strategy because they become only "a pair of hands," having little understanding of the overall development program, and thus cannot provide the sponsoring company with their considerable expertises.

Whichever strategy is used, the sponsor should carefully select the CRO to conduct a nonclinical drug development study. One poorly conducted study can delay the drug development process until the study has been repeated and the results integrated into the overall story. If this delay is for a research study on the critical path, the projected time for regulatory agency submission has to be changed, thus delaying the date of approval for marketing and resulting in lost revenue for the sponsoring company.

CRO Monitoring

The identification and selection process is only the first step. The second aspect involves monitoring and managing the CROs to ensure that the outsourced research studies are conducted according to the study protocol, that the results are obtained with appropriate techniques and procedures, and that the generated data are correctly recorded and documented in the study report. Monitoring studies at CROs should include, but are not limited to:

1. Reviewing and approving the study protocols prepared by the CROs and detailing the procedures to be followed to complete the study designs. The study protocol should provide information on all aspects of the study. Commonly included items in a nonclinical study protocol are listed in Table 2.
2. Monitoring various aspects during the research phase of each study. Each item listed in Table 2 is a possible point for potential study monitoring. Monitoring will ensure that the data collected are appropriately documented and do not contain "surprises" that can prevent the results from being used to support submissions to regulatory agencies.
3. When "surprises" do happen, and most outsourced studies will have at least one "surprise," interacting with the CRO to characterize the problem or protocol deviation and to effectively correct the "surprise" or to amend the study protocol to document the problem and the solution.
4. Assisting in the evaluation and interpretation of results to ensure that the data are analytically acceptable and correctly correlated to tell the story of the experimental results.
5. Reviewing technical reports to ensure that the information provided accurately reflects the generated results, documents any deviation from the study protocols, and gives appropriate conclusions.

The number of person–hours required to appropriately monitor a research study conducted by a CRO again depends on the size of the outsourced research program. Normally, a minimum of one person–week for each in-life phase month of a research study is required and includes the time necessary to review and approve the study report. As noted above, some firms use consultants or consulting firms to assist with CRO monitoring and management and to ensure that the studies are

TABLE 2 Nonclinical Study Protocol Items Commonly Included in a CRO Conducted Research Study

Protocol title	Descriptive title of the nonclinical research study
Objective	Purpose of conducting the study
Study location	Where and by whom the study is to be conducted
Sponsor	Company that is sponsoring the study
Study monitor	Sponsor's agent who is responsible for monitoring the study
Personnel	CRO senior staff, including the individual assigned as Study Director, who will responsible for the various aspects of the study
Study dates	Dates when the study is scheduled to be initiated, when the in-life phase is to be completed, and when the draft final report is to be available for review
Compliance	Statements on which regulations, such as 21 CFR 58 for FDA GLP compliance, will be followed and on Animal Care Committee protocol that will be reviewed.
Test article	Information on the drug substance, which commonly includes the test article name or number, identification criteria, physical description, who is responsible for test article characterization, the concentration(s) to be used, recommended storage conditions, inventory maintenance, formulation procedures, reserve samples, retention samples, analyses for content and homogeneity (if necessary), disposition, and safety precautions.
Test species	Information on the animal species to be studied, animal husbandry procedures such as housing, food, water, contaminants, environment conditions, acclimation, and justification of selection.
Study design	Description of the number of test species groups, the dosage level to be administered to each group, the test article concentration or amount to be administered, the number of animals of each sex in each dose group.
Assignment	Statement on how animals will be assigned or randomized to each of the dose groups
Dose preparation	Description of how the test article will be prepared for administration to the test species
Route of dosing	Statements on how the test article will be administered, the frequency of dosing, and a justification for the selected route and dose levels
Clinical observations	Descriptions on how frequently the test species will be observed and what specific clinical signs are to be recorded in addition to unspecified signs
Body weights	Information on how often the test species will be weighed during the in-life phase of the study
Food consumption	Information on how food consumption will be determined
Physical examination	Description of how often physical examinations will be conducted and by whom
Blood collection	Information on when blood specimens will be collected for hematology, clinical chemistry, and toxicokinetics
Hematology	Description of hematology tests to be conducted
Clinical chemistry	Description of clinical chemistry parameters to be determined
Toxicokinetics	Description of how blood specimens are to be processed and analyzed for test article concentration, including information on the testing laboratory, assay procedure, and storage and shipping procedures

(Continued)

TABLE 2 Nonclinical Study Protocol Items Commonly Included in a CRO Conducted Research Study (*Continued*)

Euthanasia	Information on how the test species will be sacrifice at the end of the in-life phase of the study
Moribund or found dead animals	Statements on how animals found moribund or dead during the in-life phase will be handled
Necropsy	Information on the procedures to be used during necropsy
Organ weights	Description on which organs are to be weighed and the procedures used to prepare organs for weighing and fixing for histopathological examination
Histopathology	Statements on which dose levels, if not all dose levels, and which tissues will be examined and how the information will be recorded by the pathologist doing the reading
Statistical analysis	Information on the statistical tests that will be performed on the results
Reports	Description of what information will be included in the study report to be submitted to the sponsor
Raw data	Information on how, where, and for how long raw data will be stored
Approvals	Signatures of a sponsor representative, commonly the study monitor, the Study Director, and a corporate officer of the CRO

conducted according to GLP Regulations. These consultants should be specialists in the scientific disciplines for the conducted studies. Having a toxicologist or pharmacologist consultant monitor the bioanalytical chemistry program to support a pharmacokinetic research study could result in an assay that is inappropriately validated or implemented and thus not capable of analyzing collected physiological fluid specimens (e.g., plasma, serum, urine) for drug and drug metabolite concentrations.

CONCLUSION

This part of the chapter has provided information on the selection and monitoring aspects of conducting nonclinical research studies at CROs. By carefully evaluating and selecting CROs and then managing these service providers during and after the study, the sponsoring firm can obtain the information needed to successfully characterize a drug candidate and to prepare the necessary submissions to regulatory agencies. A close partnering between the sponsor, or its designated agents, and the CRO is very important to ensure that the research studies are conducted as designed and within the planned time frame and budget.

PART II: CLINICAL CONTRACT RESEARCH ORGANIZATIONS

INTRODUCTION

The clinical portion of a drug development program constitutes the most time-consuming and costly phase of drug development. Even large pharmaceutical companies sometimes find themselves understaffed and thus unable to effectively complete some aspects of a particular clinical drug development program. This situation is even more acute in most small pharmaceutical and biotechnology companies. If senior management in the sponsor company is not willing to support permanent increases in staff to accommodate the program's needs or if sufficient numbers of qualified staff cannot be recruited and hired soon enough, the sponsor will frequently turn to a CRO specializing coordinating clinical trials for the solution. The trend in using clinical CROs is increasing and thus managers and directors of clinical programs need to adopt to this new way of conducting clinical research programs.

When properly selected and managed, clinical CRO services can provide a cost-effective solution and thereby enhance the ability of the sponsor team to achieve the corporate goals that are typically defined by time and budget constraints. However, if the sponsor–CRO relationship is mismanaged, valuable time and money will be wasted. A common reason for failure, probably the most common, is ineffective communication among the various parties. Effective communication between the sponsor and CRO has to occur at all stages of the relationship, including:

1. At the onset, when the scope of the clinical project is being defined and a CRO is being chosen to support some or all aspects of a clinical trial.
2. During the conduct of the project, which includes monitoring the clinical trial sites and the collection and evaluation of the generated data for inclusion into the clinical study report (CSR).
3. After completion of the study, when the CSR is being drafted either by the sponsor, the CRO, or a scientific/medical writer.

Each of these phases of the relationship will be discussed in turn, with an emphasis on ways to achieve effective communication and a successful relationship.

DEFINING THE SCOPE AND CHOOSING A CLINICAL CRO

An entire clinical development program usually spans several years and includes many individual clinical studies. Most sponsors will use CROs for some portion of the clinical development program but rarely for creating the overall clinical drug development plan. Nevertheless, if a particular CRO has established experience in a particular therapeutic area or human disease or disorder, this service provider may be helpful in providing an independent assessment of draft plans prepared by the sponsor.

CROs can provide services for clinical trials whether they are the relatively simple phase 1 safety, tolerance, and pharmacokinetic studies or the more complex multicenter phase 3 efficacy and safety studies. Table 3 identifies specific activities that may be considered for outsourcing of clinical research. These activities are grouped according to four major categories: management of the study conduct at clinical sites, data management, data evaluation, and summarization.

The scope of the work to be outsourced is driven by the specific needs of the sponsor. In some instances, most or all aspects of a particular clinical study will need to be outsourced. In other instances, CROs are needed to provide only specific services to complement an almost complete team within the sponsor company. The bulk of the contracts awarded to CROs deal with one or more of the more labor-intensive portions of clinical research, such as clinical monitoring of study investigation sites, data entry, programming for data listings and summary tables, and writing CSRs.

TABLE 3 Scoping Out the Project

Prepare or review overall clinical development plan
Management of clinical trial study conduct
Protocol writing
Site selection
Investigator meetings
Monitoring
Site initiations and close-outs
Primary and secondary monitoring
GCP audits
Data management
Case report form (CRF) design
Database design
Data entry
Data evaluation
Programming for data listing and summary tables
Statistical analyses and interpretation
Data summarization
Medical interpretation
Scientific writing of clinical study report (CSR)

Whatever be the scope of the project, clear communication of the exact work plan is enhanced by the sponsor providing a detailed description of the activities and the expectations of the CRO. Merely listing activities, as presented in Table 3, is grossly inadequate and will result in numerous iterations in contract proposals as the CROs request more specific instructions and rework their proposals according to the newly provided information that should have been shared with the original project scope. Some questions to be considered when providing details of the work plan and deciding which CRO to select are as follows:

1. Does the CRO have experience in the particular therapeutic area and/or disease indication or disorder under development? This is not always an absolute requirement but may be strength when comparing CROs, particularly for clinical trials that are designed to evaluate efficacy in patients.
2. Does the CRO have access to the subject or patient population needed for the clinical trial? For example, some CROs maintain specific patient pools, such as patients with hepatic impairment or renal impairment, often needed for clinical pharmacology studies.
3. If the study being outsourced is a pharmacokinetic or clinical pharmacology study, does the CRO have bioanalytical chemistry laboratory facilities and expertise appropriate for the analysis of plasma, serum, or other physiological fluid specimens for the desired analyte(s)? Can bioanalytical chemistry methods developed and validated by the sponsor be transferred to their laboratories and validated or will samples be shipped to the sponsor or to another CRO that has the necessary method(s) up and running for analysis?
4. If the CRO is to prepare the detailed clinical protocol, are there other protocols from the same program that can be used as a template?
5. Does the sponsor want the CRO to assist or participate in the investigator meeting?

6. If the CRO will be monitoring the clinical study at the clinical site(s), will they be doing all of the monitoring for all sites and the other groups (e.g., bioanalytical chemistry laboratory, clinical chemistry, and hematology laboratory) that will be providing support to the clinical trial or will some sponsor personnel also be monitoring?

7. If the trial is international, can the CRO provide monitoring services (or other services) in all jurisdictions? If a decision is made to work with separate CROs in each country, the sponsor needs to recognize the effort needed for coordination of all CROs.

8. Will the CRO be providing primary or secondary monitoring, or both?

9. When will the CRO get involved with clinical trial sites—before site initiation or after selection and initiation are completed by the sponsor?

10. Who will be negotiating the investigator grants for each clinical site, the CRO or the sponsor?

11. Will the CRO be asked to conduct GLP and Good Clinical Practice (GCP) audits for selected clinical sites and other groups supporting the clinical trial?

12. If the CRO is to design the case report forms (CFRs), does the sponsor have a set from a similar study that can be used as a template?

13. If the CRO will be asked to design the database, will the CRO need to standardize certain aspects with existing databases to allow them to be combined later? If so, the sponsor should provide some details on the required structure.

14. Has the sponsor established data conventions for other studies in the clinical program for a particular drug candidate that will need to be followed for this new study?

15. What are the standard procedures of the CRO for handling queries and corrections to the database?

16. What audit trail will be created to document data conventions and database corrections?

17. Has the CRO ever been audited by the FDA or other regulatory agency?

18. Will an independent GCP audit of the CRO's activities be undertaken?

19. If the CRO is being asked to program data listings and summary tables, how many such listings and tables are expected? Does the sponsor have templates or examples from other clinical studies in the same program?

20. Are the final deliverables clear to all parties? For example, does the sponsor expect to receive the programs (for example, the SAS code) used to run the statistical analyses?

21. Does the CRO have experienced staff to provide statistical or medical interpretation of the data?

22. If the CRO is to write the CSR, does the sponsor have a standard template to be followed?

23. What word processing program is required? What are the expectations regarding in-text tables? Can they be imported directly from SAS, for example, or will significant word processing be required for new formats?

24. How many drafts are expected for a CSR?

25. What are the time constraints for the activities being outsourced? Which dates are not negotiable? Which are subject to some flexibility?

26. Can the CRO offer assurance that the necessary personnel will be dedicated to the project?

27. What is the experience level of the specific individuals at the CRO who will be assigned to the project?
28. Can the CRO provide names of previous clients with whom the sponsor can speak directly and privately?
29. What are the provisions in the proposed contract that deal with cost overruns and substantial increases in workload above what was originally anticipated?
30. What are the procedures for changing the scope of the project?
31. Does the CRO have the capacity to add more resources to the project, if necessary?
32. How important is this project to the CRO? Is there a risk that the project will suffer because of competition for CRO resources for higher status projects from other clients?
33. What are the provisions in the contract for dealing with poor performance by the CRO?
34. Are the financial terms of the contract acceptable to the sponsor? How much is paid up front versus upon completion of the major milestones defined in the contract?
35. Should the financial terms include penalties for significantly missed milestones or incentives for milestones completed ahead of schedule?
36. If the CRO is providing only selected activities to support a clinical study, how will the overall project be managed? Will a formal joint project team be established with regular meetings?
37. How frequently will status reports be required from the CRO? Do these reports need to be written or verbal?
38. Will all contact be directed through one person in the sponsor company? How accessible to the CRO will other key personnel in the sponsor company be?

WORKING WITH THE CRO

The start-up of the relationship with a CRO requires a considerable amount of time from sponsor personnel to ensure that the scope of the work is fully understood and that standards are clear and appropriately documented. This highly interactive phase of the relationship may be ill-timed, unfortunately, because most companies decide to use CROs only after all possibilities of using internal resources have been exhausted, which often means that the sponsor personnel themselves have been stretched to their limits. The sponsor staff may have a tremendous desire to "hand off" the project completely, and as quickly as possible, to the CRO but this will not be in the best interest of the sponsor or the project.

Although working with a CRO can be an efficient way to expand the clinical project's human resources rapidly, the sponsor needs to recognize that substantial internal resources will still be needed. With such significant investments (both time and money) in clinical programs, the sponsor's management team needs to ensure that sufficient personnel exist in-house to oversee the performance of the CRO and to interact with the CRO when "surprises" happen to effectively evaluate and correct the unexpected happenings.

Usually, one individual in the CRO and one in the sponsor company are given project management responsibilities for the contract activities. However, this should not be interpreted narrowly to mean that all communication has to go through these two individuals. Other individuals in each organization should have direct access to their counterparts in the other company for clarification of specific details. Joint working teams that discuss the details of the project at the level of implementation will enhance the quality of the communication between the sponsor and CRO and increase the likelihood of the project's success.

The most effective working relationships are forged when the sponsor views the CRO staff as an extension of the sponsor's own in-house team. If the CRO is providing supplemental services to complement an in-house study team (for example, providing additional clinical monitors or handling the data management and statistics for a clinical trial that is monitored by the sponsor), then regularly scheduled joint team meetings will foster effective communication and standardization of efforts. Face-to-face meetings are ideal but not always possible, given the geographic distances existing between some parties. Teleconferences and videoconferences can be very effective. If the CRO is responsible for the entire conduct of a study, then regular (and frequent) update meetings are necessary to review progress and modify the activities as necessary to achieve the time and cost goals.

Even with the best intentions and careful review of the contract, either party may find that part of the way through the conduct of the activities the scope (and perhaps the timeline and cost estimates) needs to be revised. Provisions for how to approach such discussions should be provided in the contract, and these discussions may be best handled by senior management of the sponsor and the CRO to preserve the working relationships of the members of any joint working teams.

Returning to the clinical activities listed in Table 3, some thoughts on the level of support that is realistic to obtain from CROs are as follows. A number of the labor-intensive activities, such as monitoring, auditing, database management, programming for listings and tables, and statistical interpretation, are relatively easy to outsource. Many CROs will have the necessary experience and capacity for these activities.

Protocol writing and CRF design go hand in hand and most CROs have the capability to handle these activities. But the sponsor should lead the strategic discussions on the study design and the statistical plan, taking into consideration the overall clinical development plan, which may include other indications, and the commercial objectives of the company. A high level of sponsor involvement in designing the study will increase the "ownership" of the project by the internal clinical project team, even if 95% of the activities for running the clinical trial are handled by one or more CROs. This ownership is important to maintain throughout the clinical trial because in the end, the sponsor personnel will be defending the data to regulatory authorities, such as the FDA.

Some CROs can be very helpful in identifying qualified clinical investigational sites if the CRO has previous experience in a particular therapeutic area and/or human disease or disorder. This can be of great use to small companies that are just starting their first or second clinical development programs.

The process of data summarization, encompassing both medical and scientific interpretation and scientific writing, can be one of the more challenging aspects of a clinical developmental program. The greater the level of sponsor involvement in these activities, the more internal ownership is reinforced and the sponsor is better able to defend the data. CROs can still play an important role in these steps. CROs that have medically trained personnel with expertise in particular therapeutic areas can be an excellent resource for small companies that may have no internal medical staff. Similarly, CROs that have personnel trained in statistics or pharmacokinetics can be an excellent resource for sponsors without these expertises.

Highly skilled medical writers are currently a limited commodity and difficult to recruit for most companies (both sponsors and CROs). Furthermore, the writing process itself is very time-consuming. For both these reasons, companies are seeking these experts more and more through contract services, where the scientific writer is either an independent contractor or an employee of another CRO. If the sponsor has no medical writers, then having the CRO or an independent scientific writer to complete the CSR might be best. However, the sponsor should seek medical interpretation from the sponsor clinical team, as necessary. If the sponsor does have experienced medical writers, but the volume of work is too much for this group, then a CRO or an independent contractor could provide valuable assistance for the most labor-intensive parts of the writing, for example, by providing first and second drafts of the CSR. The sponsor team could then take over the CSR and provide the finishing "polish" on the interpretation of the data and standardization with reports for other clinical trials in the same program.

CONCLUSION

An effective relationship with a CRO is, in some ways, like a marriage. The key to success is open and honest communication, clear division of responsibilities, and patience while the relationship evolves into maturity. Once a match has been made, knowledge acquired in the first successful project can carry forward to subsequent contracts and efficiencies are then realized for both organizations. Many companies are finding advantages in considering long-term relationships with desirable CROs, in which both parties provide some level of commitment to future projects, even before the exact details of those projects are known. Both parties benefit from such arrangements. The CRO can better manage personnel requirements when future contracts are guaranteed and the sponsor has the security of knowing that qualified resources will be available to support clinical drug development needs on various programs.

6 Industry and FDA Liaison

Richard A. Guarino

Oxford Pharmaceutical Resources, Inc., Totowa, New Jersey, U.S.A.

INTRODUCTION

Experienced Drug Regulatory Affairs (DRA) personnel are essential in the process of new product development. They are largely responsible for establishing a liaison with their counterparts at the U.S. Food and Drug Administration (FDA) and other regulatory agencies globally. This chapter will center on the regulatory affairs activities in the United States and describe the function and liaison services of the FDA. Emphasis will be on their responsibility for the review and approval of Investigational New Drug Applications (INDs), New Drug Applications (NDAs), and Biologic License Applications (BLAs).

The European Drug Regulatory Process can be found in chapter 24, "European CT Directive: Implementation and Update."

The FDA is an agency within the Public Health Service (PHS), which in turn is a part of the Department of Health and Human Services (DHHS). The FDA regulates over $1 trillion worth of products, which account for 25 cents of every consumer dollar spent annually by American consumers. The FDA touches the lives of virtually every American, every day, for it is FDA's job to see that the food we eat is safe and wholesome, the cosmetics we use will not harm us, the medicines and medical devices we use are safe and effective, and radiation-emitting products such as microwave ovens will not cause harm. Feed and drugs for pets and farm animals also come under FDA scrutiny. The FDA also ensures that all of these products are labeled truthfully with the information people need to understand what they are consuming and how to use them properly.

The FDA is one of our nation's oldest consumer protection agencies dating back to 1862. It employs over 12,000 employees who monitor the safety, manufacturing, import, transport, storage, and sale of products each year. It does so at a cost to the taxpayer of about $.03 per person per day with an overall budget exceeding $2.1 billion. First and foremost, FDA is a public health agency, charged with protecting American consumers by enforcing the Federal Food, Drug, and Cosmetic Act and several related public health laws. To carry out this mandate of consumer protection, FDA has 120 residential inspection posts throughout the country, 13 laboratories, 9 regional offices, 19 district offices, and over 1100 investigators and inspectors who visit more than 16,000 facilities a year covering the country's 135,885 plus FDA-regulated businesses.

Inspections and Legal Sanctions

The FDA investigators and inspectors ensure that products are made correctly and labeled truthfully. As part of their inspections, they collect about 80,000 domestic and imported product samples for examination by FDA scientists or for label checks. If a company is found violating any of the laws that FDA enforces, FDA can encourage the firm to correct the problem voluntarily or to recall a faulty product from the market. A recall is generally the fastest and the most effective way to protect the public from an unsafe product.

When a company cannot or will not voluntarily correct a public health problem with one of its products, FDA has legal sanctions it can bring to bear. The agency can go to court to force a company to stop selling a product and to have items already produced seized and destroyed. When warranted, criminal penalties, including prison sentences, are sought against manufacturers and distributors.

About 3000 products a year are found to be unfit for consumers and are withdrawn from the marketplace, either by voluntary recall or by court-ordered seizure. In addition, about 30,000 import shipments a year are detained at the port of entry because the goods appear to be unacceptable.

Scientific Expertise

The scientific evidence needed to backup FDA's legal cases is prepared by the agency's 2100 scientists, including 900 chemists and 300 microbiologists, who work in 40 laboratories in the Washington, D.C., area and around the country. Some of these scientists analyze samples to see, for example, if products are contaminated with illegal substances. Other scientists review test results submitted by companies seeking agency approval for drugs, vaccines, food additives, coloring agents, and medical devices. The FDA operates the National Center for Toxicological Research at Jefferson, Arkansas, which investigates the biological effects of widely used chemicals. The agency also runs the Engineering and Analytical Center at Winchester, Massachusetts, which tests medical devices, radiation-emitting products, and radioactive drugs.

Assessing risks for drugs and medical devices, weighing risks against benefits is the primary objective of FDA's public health protection duties. By ensuring that products and producers meet certain standards, FDA protects consumers and enables them to know what they are buying. For example, the agency requires that drugs and biologics both prescription and over-the-counter be proven safe and effective. The agency must determine that a drug or biologic produces the benefits it is supposed to without causing side effects that would outweigh the benefits.

Product Safety

Another major FDA mission is to protect the safety and wholesomeness of foods. The agency's scientists test samples to see if any substances, such as pesticide residues, are present in unacceptable amounts. If contaminants are identified, FDA takes corrective action. They also set labeling standards to help consumers know what is in the foods they buy. The nation's food supply is protected in yet another way, as FDA sees that medicated feeds and other drugs given to animals raised for food are not threatening to the consumer's health.

The safety of the nation's blood supply is another FDA responsibility. The agency's investigators routinely examine blood bank operations, from record-keeping to testing for contaminants. The FDA also ensures the purity and effectiveness of agents such as insulin and vaccines.

Medical devices are classified and regulated according to their degree of risk to the public. Devices that are life-supporting, life-sustaining, or implanted, such as pacemakers, must receive agency approval before they can be marketed.

The FDA's scrutiny does not end when a drug or device is approved for marketing; the agency collects and analyzes tens of thousands of reports each year on drugs and devices after they have been put on the market to monitor for continued reproducibility of the product and any unexpected adverse effects that might be reported when a product is consumed by larger populations.

Cosmetic safety also comes under FDA's jurisdiction. The agency can have unsafe cosmetics removed from the market. The dyes and other additives used in drugs, foods, and cosmetics are subject to FDA scrutiny. The agency must review and approve these chemicals before they can be marketed.

Presently (as an January 20, 2009) the FDA is headed by Acting Commissioner Frank Torti, MD of Food and Drug. However, as of March 14, 2009 Margaret Hamburg, MD was named the new Commissioner and Joshua Sharfstein, MD was named Deputy Commissioner. The commissioner is appointed by the President of the United States, confirmed by the U.S. Senate, and serves at the President's discretion. The office of the Commissioner oversees all of the Agency's activities.

FDA'S MAJOR PROGRAM CENTERS
The FDA is divided into many centers; each center comprising a division with specific regulatory responsibilities. The main centers are as follows:

CDER—Center for Drug Evaluation and Research
CBER—Center for Biologics Evaluation Research
CDRH—Center for Devices and Radiologic Health
CFSAN—Center of Food Safety and Applied Nutrition
CVM—Center for Veterinary Medicine
NCTR—National Center for Toxicological Research

The Center for Drug Evaluation and Research (CDER)
The responsibility for reviewing new pharmaceutical products is the major responsibility of CDER. Until recently some of these duties were shared with CBER. However, because of the increasing number of products that are being developed in the crucial areas of vaccines and blood safety and other biologic scientific areas such as gene therapy and tissue transplantation, this responsibility will now be directed solely to CBER. Therefore, CDER will now be responsible for all pharmaceutical products including Dental and most Biologics. CDER is now organized into various divisions and offices—each one responsible for new drug approval process according to the expertise of the personnel assigned to that division. As of January 2001, there are 16 review divisions within CDER (including the Division of Over-the-Counter drug products) that are responsible for reviewing all Investigational New Drugs (INDs), New Drug Applications (NDAs), and chemistry and efficacy Supplemental New Drug Applications (SNDAs). Deciding which division will be assigned to a particular IND or NDA depends solely on the indication for the new drug. Divisions are organized on the basis of therapeutic uses for new products, and the divisions are staffed with experts in a particular pharmacotherapeutic area. The current divisions include Cardiorenal; Neuropharmacological; Oncology;

Pulmonary; Metabolic and Endocrine; Reproductive and Urologic; Gastrointestinal and Coagulation; Anesthetic, Critical Care, and Addiction; Medical Imaging and Radio-pharmaceutical; Antiviral; Anti-infective; Special Pathogen and Immunologic; Anti-inflammatory, Analgesic, and Ophthalmologic; and Dermatologic and Dental Drug Products and now Biologics.

The 16 divisions are grouped among one of five Offices of Drug Evaluation (ODE). The ODE I, for example, has administrative control for the divisions of Cardiorenal, Neuropharmacological, and Oncologic Drug Products. The Division of Drug Marketing, Advertising, and Communications (DDMAC) is also a part of this Office. The organizational chart for CDER and its component parts is usually updated quarterly, and these updates may be found on the Internet at: http://www. fda.gov/cder/cderorg.htm. The Center for Drug Evaluation and Research is organized into three main offices: the Office of the Center Director (OCD), the Office of Review Management (ORM), and the Office of Pharmaceutical Science (OPS).

The OCD encompasses the executive operations staff, regulatory policy staff, the ombudsman, and the equal employment opportunity and diversity management staff. The executive operations staff provides support to the OCD, including coordinating executive and legislative activities, managing the preparation and coordination of center-level meetings, and responding to written correspondence from constituents. The regulatory policy staff initiates, develops, and reviews regulations, policies, procedures, and guidances that affect the drug review process. This includes creating and publishing CDER's Manual of Policies and Procedures, preparing *Federal Register* notices for publications, and responding to citizen petitions. The primary mission of the ombudsman is to receive complaints, investigate and act on them, mediate disputes, and, in general, attend to problems involving interpersonal working relationships.

The ORM develops and implements drug review management and scientific policies, including prescription drug user–fee policies. With support from the OPS on chemistry and manufacturing controls and biopharmaceutical issues, this office reviews all INDs and NDAs for human drugs, except generic drug applications. In addition, ORM evaluates for safety and effectiveness NDAs for OTC drug products and handles prescription drug switches to OTC drug status. It develops and implements safety and effectiveness standards for prescription and OTC drug products and provides direction and policy formulation for pharmacology and toxicology issues.

The OPS provides scientific and regulatory support in several areas. It develops and implements review management and scientific policies pertaining to the generic drug review process. It also is the office providing the management and scientific policies pertaining to the new drug review process for chemistry, manufacturing, and controls; clinical pharmacology; and biopharmaceutics for both INDs and NDAs. Other OPS activities include developing and implementing policies and directing programs through applied regulatory research; developing and implementing standards for generic drugs and new drugs that enhance the drug development and regulatory review processes; and providing scientific oversight of CMC and sterility sections of INDs, NDAs, and supplements. The office also oversees microbiology, biopharmaceutics, and clinical pharmacology aspects of regulatory submissions.

All drugs, upon FDA receipt of an IND filing, are classified on the basis of their anticipated indication(s) for use and assigned to one of the 16 divisions. In addition to the director in charge, each division has personnel with responsibilities in scientific review areas. For each IND or NDA, a "drug review team" is established to provide the appropriate expertise to allow for a judgment regarding the drug's overall acceptance based on its safety, clinical efficacy, and manufacturing information, provided to the FDA by the sponsor of the drug application.

The CDER drug review team members apply their individual, special technical expertise to review INDs or NDAs.

Each review division employs a team of *chemists* responsible for reviewing the chemistry, manufacturing, and controls sections of drug applications. In general terms, chemistry reviewers address issues related to drug identity, manufacturing control, and analysis. The reviewing chemist evaluates the manufacturing and processing procedures for a drug to ensure that the compound is adequately reproducible and stable. If the drug is either unstable or not reproducible, then the validity of any clinical testing would be undermined, because one would not know what was really being used in patients, and, more importantly, IND trials could pose significant risks to participants.

At the beginning of the chemistry and manufacturing section, the drug sponsor should state whether it believes the chemistry of either the drug substance or the drug product—or the manufacturing of either the drug substance or the drug product—present any potential human risk. If so, these risks should be discussed, with steps proposed to monitor them.

In addition, sponsors should describe any chemistry and manufacturing differences between the drug product proposed for clinical use and that used in the animal toxicology trials that formed the basis for the sponsor's conclusion that it was safe to proceed with the proposed clinical trial. How these differences might affect the safety profile of the drug product should be discussed? If there are no differences in the products, that should be stated.

The *pharmacology/toxicology* review team is staffed by pharmacologists and toxicologists evaluating the results of animal testing and attempt to relate animal drug effects to potential effects in humans. In the area of pharmacology and drug disposition, an application should generally contain (a) a description of the pharmacologic effects and mechanism(s) of action of the drug in animals and (b) information on the absorption, distribution, metabolism, and excretion of the drug. For toxicology studies, the types of studies needed depend on the nature of the drug but will typically include short- and long-term studies, including the potential for drugs to induce birth defects or cancer in humans.

Medical/clinical reviewers, often called medical officers, are almost exclusively physicians. In rare instances, nonphysicians are used as medical officers to evaluate drug data. Medical reviewers are responsible for evaluating the clinical sections of submissions, such as the safety of the clinical protocols in an IND or the results of this testing as submitted in the NDA. Within most divisions, clinical reviewers take the lead role in the IND or NDA review and are responsible for synthesizing the results of the animal toxicology, human pharmacology, and clinical reviews to formulate the overall basis for a recommended agency action on the application.

During the IND review process, the medical reviewer evaluates the clinical trial protocol to determine (a) if the participants will be protected from unnecessary risks and (b) if the trial design will provide data relevant to the safety and effectiveness of the drug. Under federal regulations, proposed phase 1 studies are evaluated almost exclusively for safety reasons. Since the late 1980s, FDA reviewers have been instructed to provide drug sponsors with greater freedom during phase 1, as long as the investigations do not expose participants to undue risks. In evaluating phase

2 and 3 investigations, however, FDA reviewers also must ensure that these studies are of sufficient scientific quality to be capable of yielding data that can support marketing approval.

Other reviewers include *statisticians, microbiologist,* and *biopharmaceutical experts.* Statisticians evaluate the statistical relevance of the data in the NDA, with the main tasks being to evaluate the methods used to conduct studies and those used to analyze the data. The purpose of these evaluations is to give the medical officers a better idea of the power of the findings to be extrapolated to the larger patient population in the country.

Clinical microbiology information is required only in NDAs for anti-infective drugs. Because these drugs affect microbial, rather than human physiology, reports on the drugs' in vivo and in vitro effects on the target microorganisms are critical for establishing product effectiveness.

An NDA's microbiology section usually includes data describing:

- the biochemical basis of the drug's action on microbial physiology.
- the drug's antimicrobial spectra, including results of in vitro preclinical studies demonstrating concentrations of the drug required for effective use.
- any known mechanisms of resistance to the drug, including results of any known epidemiologic studies demonstrating prevalence of resistance factors.
- clinical microbiology laboratory methods needed to evaluate the effective use of the drug.

Pharmacokineticists/biopharmaceuticists evaluate the rate and extent to which the drug's active ingredient is made available to the body and the way it is distributed in, metabolized by, and eliminated from the human body.

All team members work together to assure that the label and the labeling are accurate and provide clear instructions to health care practitioners and consumers.

A key member of the review team is the project manager (PM), formerly called the consumer safety officer or CSO. The PM evaluates regulatory information to determine compliance with current policies and regulations. In addition, project managers orchestrate and coordinate the drug review team(s) interactions, efforts, and reviews, and they serve as the CDER review team's primary contact with the drug industry (FDA meetings etc.). They may be considered as the liaison between the FDA and industry.

The total full-time equivalent staff working in CDER is around 2000. The number of FDA staff has increased in recent years as a result of the Prescription Drug User Fee Act (PDUFA) of 1992. The renewal of PDUFA in the FDA Modernization Act (FDAMA) of 1997 and the PDUFA Renewal Act—FDA Revitalization Act (FDARA), a five-year renewal of the PDUFA in September 2007 (see http://www.fda.gov/ohrms/dockets/98fr/07-5052.htm for details).On average, each of the five ODEs have about 135–145 employees. Because there are essentially three divisions per office, the average staff in a particular division is about 45–50, including clerical, secretarial, and project management support. Updates of these organizational charts may be found on the Internet at http://www.fda.gov/cder/cderorg.htm.

CONTACTS AND COMMUNICATIONS WITH FDA

All the FDA divisions' primary goal is to work collaboratively and cooperatively with industry, academia, and others to improve new product development and to expedite the review process. It also strives to provide consumers and health care providers with drug information that is vital to improve the public health. The topics listed below provide an overview of the various means of communicating with the FDA divisions.

Consumer/Industry Inquiries

The FDA is dedicated to ensure that all persons involved in new product development, or who depend upon drug regulation excellence, have the information needed to research, develop, review, market, dispense, prescribe, or use products safely and effectively.

To enhance the communications aspect of this process, the Center created the Division of Communications Management (DCM). This division enhances information exchange, strategic communications planning, and the development of communications products and initiatives. The DCM works to ensure that pharmaceutical industry representatives, health care professionals, government officials, and consumers have easy and open access to information and are educated about the drug regulation process and the benefits and risks of drugs.

Any of these individuals or groups may request information on specific drugs, guidance documents, publications, or general information such as a description of the drug approval process.

There are a number of ways in which consumers and industry representatives can communicate with or obtain reliable, current, and up-to-date information from the Center.

1. The newest, easiest method for getting information is the Center's world wide web homepage http://www.fda.gov/cder or cber.
2. For more specific or complex drug or biologic inquiries, individuals may telephone the Drug Information Branch for CDER at 301-796-3400 or CBER at 800-835-4709 or send an electronic mail message at druginfo@fda.hhs.gov or dib@cder.fda.gov, or dib@cber.fda.gov.

   Other sources of information include:

1. The FDA's Office of Public Affairs (OPA) at 301-796-3123

   In addition, consumers and industry representatives can contact

FDA Freedom of Information Staff at http://www.fda.gov/foi
FOI for CDER at http://www.fda.gov/cder/foi
FOI for CBER at http://www.fda.gov/foi
FDA MedWatch Office at 1-800-FDA-1088

Industry/FDA Meetings

FDA meetings are extremely important and should be requested judiciously by sponsors. Project managers (PMs) or, Consumer Safety Officers (CSOs), a large percentage of who were former FDA field investigators, are responsible for coordinating FDA/sponsor/industry meetings. Their other duties include acting as the contact point between the division and the regulated industries, preparing minutes of FDA/industry meetings, and assisting the division with the FDA advisory committee meetings.

Meeting Requests

The first step to request a FDA meeting is to telephone the project manager assigned to the IND or NDA. The need for a meeting should be explained, a statement about the general topic of the meeting should be described, and an idea of when the meeting can be scheduled should be offered. The project manager will likely return the call and indicate if a meeting will be granted or not. In addition, if it is feasible, the objective of the meeting might be able to be resolved over a conference call. However, if a face-to-face meeting at the FDA is necessary, a letter from the sponsor or e-mail should be sent to the appropriate division confirming that the meeting has been granted with the date and time. In turn the project manager will also send a letter to the sponsor confirming the type of meeting, the date, time, and where the meeting will take place. The names and titles of those representatives of the sponsor who will be attending the meeting and the proposed agenda with the topics to be discussed should be included in the letter. Typically, depending on the meeting type it will be four to eight weeks after the initial telephone contact with FDA before the meeting date will take place. If the meeting requires FDA review of material, most meetings do, the premeeting documents (information package) should be submitted to that division based upon their request of when they would like to have the information package before the meeting date. If the information to be discussed is already on file with FDA, this should be spelled out in a letter to the division explicitly pointing out, in detail, by submission number, what documents in an IND or NDA should be referred to. It is always appropriate to contact the project manager within the division by telephone to reconfirm the meeting about two weeks before the established meeting date. In February 1999, CDER issued a draft guidance document entitled: Formal Meetings With Sponsors and Applicants for PDUFA Products. It may be found on the Internet at http://www.fda.gov/cder/guidance/2125fnl.pdf.

FDA/Industry Meetings

There are three categories of meetings that industry can request of the agency. They are typically known as Type A, B, or C meetings.

Type A meetings are considered the most important. These are meetings immediately necessary for a delayed development program sometimes called a (critical path meeting). Type A meetings usually occur to dispute issues that arise during new drug development, meeting to resolve clinical holds that FDA has deemed necessary, or at times they may pertain to protocol assessments after the FDA has critiqued the submitted protocols. These meetings are usually scheduled 30 days from FDAs receipt of a written request for a meeting. If the sponsors' request a date beyond the 30 days, the meeting should occur no later than 14 days after the date requested.

Type B meetings are those that usually occur for a pre-IND, an End-of-Phase 1 (EOP1), an End-of-Phase 2 (EOP2), a Pre-NDA, or BLA Conference. All of these meetings will be honored by the FDA. These meetings are usually scheduled 60 days from the time the agency received the written request. If the sponsor requests a date beyond 60 days, the meeting should occur no later than 14 days after the date requested.

Type C meetings are any other meetings not falling into Type A or B meetings. These are meetings that pertain to review of human drug applications. These meetings are usually scheduled within 75 days of the agencies receipt of the written request. If a sponsor requests a date beyond 75 days, the meeting should be scheduled to occur no later than 14 days after the date requested.

Pre-IND/Preclinical Meetings

Prior to initiating clinical studies, the sponsor needs to demonstrate evidence that the compound is biologically active, and both the sponsor and the FDA need data demonstrating that the drug is reasonably safe for initial administration in humans; hence the filing of an IND. Preclinical meetings are occasionally conducted with the appropriate division that would review the IND or the drug marketing application, and these meetings are typically requested by the sponsor of a drug. Meetings at such an early stage in the process are sometimes useful opportunities for open discussion about testing phases, data requirements, and any scientific issues that may need to be resolved prior to IND submission. At these meetings, the sponsor and the FDA will discuss and agree that the design and results of the animal data that will be submitted in the pharmacology and toxicology sections of the IND will satisfy the FDA reviewers for the sponsor to initiate human testing. Other discussions may also revolve about the types of clinical testing that would best demonstrate the safety and efficacy of the drug in humans.

It is sometimes difficult to know when it is necessary or prudent to request a pre-IND conference with the FDA prior to the filing of an IND. This decision frequently depends on the history and completed research of the new compound. If one is dealing with a new chemical entity that has been synthesized in the United States and on which minimal preclinical and clinical investigations have been conducted, there is seldom a need to review data with the FDA prior to submitting the IND. There are, however, exceptions to this statement. They reflect the nature of the proposed indication, the use of new technology (e.g., recombinant DNA techniques), the expected human toxicity based on animal data, the design of the initial clinical trials, or appropriate efficacy criteria to be monitored.

On the other hand, an IND may be submitted for a compound that has been developed overseas and may even be marketed in one or more offshore countries. In this case, the data comprising the IND will be more voluminous. Many preclinical reports will need to be evaluated and summarized, and a large number of clinical reports and perhaps a significant amount of published literature may need to be reviewed, summarized, and presented to regulatory personnel. It is also possible that the sponsor has accumulated sufficient data on the compound from these sources to support calculations regarding both its safety and initiation of an IND with a phase 2 clinical investigation. Any or all of the above circumstances point to a discussion with appropriate division staff prior to IND filing—a staff that may help the FDA as well as the drug's sponsor. In the course of such a meeting, some agreement should be reached on a phase of clinical investigation that will be acceptable to the FDA for the initial study protocols to be included in the original IND submission. The FDA will then be alerted to the filing and can plan to review the IND armed with the prior information received during the meeting.

In preparing for a pre-IND meeting, the sponsors regulatory representative should provide the FDA with summary documents of the subjects to be discussed. The question of confidentiality must be carefully considered. With no IND filing reference number, the information submitted should be general in nature. Complete details of the synthesis and chemical structure should not be provided. It is usually sufficient to vaguely describe the compound and identify it by a code number.

The only division in CDER with an established policy regarding pre-IND consultation meetings is the Division of Anti-viral Drug Products (DAVDP). Established in 1988, the DAVDP pre-IND Consultation Program is a proactive strategy designed to facilitate informal early communications between DAVDP and potential sponsors of new therapeutics for the treatment of AIDS and life-threatening opportunistic infections, other viral infections, including soft tissue transplantation. Pre-IND advice may be requested for issues related to drug development plans; data needed to support the rationale for testing a drug in humans; the design of nonclinical pharmacology, toxicology, and drug-activity studies; data requirements for an IND application; and regulatory requirements for demonstrating safety and efficacy. All potential drug sponsors/developers working in the antiviral area are encouraged to initiate contact with the division as early in the drug development process as possible, so that they will have the opportunity to consider the recommendations of DAVDP in planning their preclinical and clinical development programs. The individual to contact is the project manager assigned to your project within the DDAVP.

End-of-Phase 2 Meeting (EOP2)
The primary focus of "end-of-phase 2" meetings is to determine whether it is safe to begin phase 3 testing. This is also the time to plan protocols for phase 3 human studies and to discuss and identify any additional information that may be required to support the submission of an NDA. It is also intended to establish an agreement between the agency and the sponsor of the overall plan for phase 3 and the objectives and design of particular studies. These meetings avoid unnecessary expenditures of time and money because data requirements have been clarified. Minutes of these meeting with special attention to attendees, agreements, recommendations, and conclusions are of vital importance when the NDA is submitted. Often, by the time the NDA data is completed and ready to be submitted to the FDA, many of the attendees that were at the end-of-phase 2 meeting will not be same people who will be reviewing and accepting the NDA data.

One month before the end-of-phase 2 meeting or when the project manager designates when the review materials should be sent to the division, the sponsor should submit the background information and summary protocols for phase 3 program. This information should include data supporting the claim of the new drug product, chemistry data, animal data and any proposed additional animal data, results of phase 1 and 2 studies, statistical methods to be used, specific protocols for phase 3 trials, as well as a copy of the proposed labeling for the drug, if available. This summary provides the review team with information needed to prepare for a productive meeting.

In the past, only selected NDA candidate drug sponsors were encouraged to request an end-of-phase 2 conference. However, FDA now encourages all holders of an IND for new chemical entities to request this important conference. Depending on the workload of the division and the members of the FDA that are responsible for review of the IND information, the meetings may take up to four to eight weeks before they can be scheduled. However, requests for a meeting for an end-of-phase 2 conference may be easier to arrange if the conference requested is for one of the following:

1. new molecular entities for a high-priority review drug,
2. drugs with important toxicity problems,

3. a compound representing a moderate therapeutic gain but not assigned as a high-priority drug, or
4. a marketed drug with an important new indication under study

Preparing for an End-of-Phase 2 Meeting

There are a number of checkpoints worth observing in preparation for the end-of-phase 2 conference. These key elements may include:

1. Ascertain that there have not been pauses in clinical studies between phase 1 and phase 2. The FDA's policies regarding no pauses apply to the usual situation in which research on a drug progresses without serious adverse effects. This statement does not, however, take precedence over the FDA's responsibility, when necessary, to stop or limit clinical trials for reasons of safety. (Summary phase 1 data along with the necessary chronic toxicity reports should be submitted to support the safety of phase 2 studies when they are initiated.)
2. There should be no pause between phases 2 and 3 clinical studies. For maximum benefit, the end-of-phase 2 conference should be timed as close as possible to the start of the phase 3 program.
3. There is no clearcut dividing line between phase 2 and 3. (The latter usually includes well-controlled clinical trials governed by the phase 2, but in larger populations, under controlled conditions.) The sponsor of an IND should carefully determine the time when late phase 2 results have been clearly defined (efficacy has been essentially demonstrated statistically to a sufficient degree of confidence based on the final dose and the projected safety profile of the product) and the drug is ready for phase 3 development. At this point, with phase 3 plans defined, a meeting with FDA is appropriate.
4. To aid in the review of phase 2 data, the sponsor must prepare a summary separately presenting the results and conclusions for each investigation or multicenter trials; conclusions should be supported by appropriate statistical analyses. When results from more than one institution or investigator are presented under a single protocol, the information should be summarized so that data from each investigator or institution can be readily identified outside the pooled analysis.
5. Be prepared to provide the following items for the end-of-phase 2 conference for each protocol used in the Phase 2 program:
   (a) Tables showing the number of patients (*i*) randomly assigned for each treatment category according to the protocol, (*ii*) actually entered into each treatment category, (*iii*) lost to follow-up or prematurely withdrawn from the trial, and (*iv*) summarized by pertinent selection criteria.
   (b) A list explaining why patients were lost to follow-up or prematurely withdrawn from the trial for each investigator. The number of days that each of the patients spent in the trial also should be submitted.
   (c) A summary of the pertinent procedures used to obtain baseline information, measurements of effectiveness, and safety tests performed according to each applicable test or measure. Also prepare a table showing the frequency of testing, the unit of measurement, and the number of patients actually checked as of the reported date. Be sure to include normal values for each laboratory that measured the laboratory tests.

(d) For each investigator, summarize baseline and final results of the trial in terms of the appropriate variables used to measure safety and effectiveness of the drug under investigation.

(e) A statement describing whether statistical analysis has been applied in evaluating the data and justification of the adequacy of such analysis based on the statistical handling section of each protocol.

(f) If requested, submit the "hard copy" or "electronic copy" of raw data used in the summary report. Clinical records or case report forms should be organized and identified for convenient reference and review. If data is presented as, electronic submissions, pre-established formats with the FDA division should be agreed upon before the data are submitted.

The end-of-phase 2 conference should examine and appraise the adequacy of the phase 2 trials with respect to answering essential questions about the safety and effectiveness in humans for the claimed indications. The safety of the final dose selected, balanced with the efficacy results reported with that dose should be agreed upon before proceeding to phase 3 trials. The suitability of the phase 3 protocols, the completeness of the animal toxicity and pharmacology studies, and the manufacturing and controls data should all be finalized at the end of the phase 2 conference.

To address these and related matters, appropriate personnel from the company and the FDA should be present. The FDA will have medical reviewers and a statistician to attend all meetings. Whether a pharmacologist, chemist, or microbiologist needs to attend these sessions will depend on the items on the agenda. An FDA consultant may be invited, or a review of the consultant's data may be presented in his or her absence. The sponsor may also bring to the meeting one or more consultants. Minutes of the conference will be prepared by the FDA. In conjunction with these minutes, the sponsor should prepare their minutes of the meeting and send them to the project manager (PM) of FDA as soon as they get back from the meeting. The PM then will have time to review the sponsors' minutes and compare them with the tape recording of the meeting, which will not be available to the sponsor. Important conclusions or agreements can then be brought to the attention of the PM before the PM completes their minutes that might have a different interpretation for the PM. These minutes are circulated to all the attendees of the meeting before they are sent to the sponsor.

Finally, the draft meeting guidance discussed in this chapter should be reviewed.

End-of-Phase 2 Conference—Summary

When a firm has reached the end-of-phase 2, it should contact the appropriate division at the FDA to arrange for a conference. All clinical data should be summarized, tabulated, and statistically analyzed, as described. These data, together with any additional preclinical and manufacturing and controls data, and plans and protocols for phase 3 should be submitted at least one month in advance of the scheduled meeting or as agreed upon with the PM of that division. A copy containing only clinical data, as a rule, and the proposed protocols for phase 3, should be provided for the FDA statistician. The submission should also include any specific questions the firm wishes to discuss.

Discussions should be limited to those indications of the drug that the sponsor intends to claim. Agreements should be reached at the conference on the adequacy of, or deficiencies in, the submitted data, or the proposed protocols for phase 3 program. Specific proposals for correcting deficiencies, for performing additional trials, or for not performing what might be considered an excess of studies should be reviewed and agreed to. The minutes of the conference and the follow-up letter from the sponsor will serve as a permanent record of these agreements. Barring new and significant scientific developments, a major improvement in the state of the art, unforeseen circumstances occurring during further investigation of the drug, or major inaccuracies in the summarized data noted after full review of the NDA, these agreements shall have the same status as advisory opinions in which they are binding on the FDA. The execution of the agreed upon trials, nevertheless, does not guarantee approval of the subsequent NDA. Any NDAs submitted after end-of-phase 2 conferences that are deficient in satisfying the recorded or subsequently modified agreements still may require additional trials to be considered for NDA approval. FDA commitments will not necessarily be considered binding if the sponsor fails to comply with agreed-upon commitments.

Pre-NDA/BLA/CTD Meetings
The purpose of a pre-New Drug Application (NDA)/pre-Biologic License Application (BLA)/ and Common Technical Document (CTD) format meeting is to discuss the presentation of data (both paper and electronic) in support of an application, to identify and resolve any potential refuse-to-file issues, and to review the proposed marketing application. The meeting should be requested at least six months prior to the planned submission date of the application. The deadline date of the information package to be submitted to the FDA for the meeting should be established with the PM. The data from the sponsor should include:

• A summary of clinical studies to be submitted in the NDA.
• The proposed format for organizing the submission, including acceptable methods for presenting the data (electronic submissions).
• Any outstanding CMC issues discussed at the EOP2 meeting including finalization of any contractors, suppliers, etc., relationship of manufacturing, formulation, and packaging used in the phase 3 trials, product intended for marketing, any comparability trials completed, adequate stability data protocols, whether or not all manufacturing facilities will be ready for inspection, and any regulatory or other issues that are now resolved.

The meeting is conducted to identify studies the sponsor is relying on as adequate and well controlled in establishing the safety and effectiveness of the product and to help the FDA reviewers to become acquainted with the general information to be submitted. Each division has different formats in which the data is reviewed and these should be discussed to facilitate the review time. Once the application is filed, an additional meeting may also occur 90 days after the initial submission of the application to discuss issues that are uncovered by the FDA during their initial review.

Advisory Committee Meetings
All of the FDA's current advisory committees are scientific and technical committees. Advisory committees have been established to advise and make recommendations on issues related to the agency's regulatory responsibilities. The primary role of FDA advisory committees is to provide independent expert scientific advice

to the agency in its evaluation of regulated products, and to help make sound decisions based on the reasonable application of good science. The committees are advisory in nature, and final decisions on all NDA issues presented to an advisory committee are made by the FDA. Members of an advisory committee consist of individuals with recognized expertise and judgment in a specific field who have the training and experience necessary to evaluate information objectively and to interpret its significance under various, often controversial, circumstances. Advisory committees weigh available evidence and provide scientific and medical advice on the safety, effectiveness, and appropriate use of products under FDA jurisdiction. Another role is to advise the agency on general criteria for evaluation and on broad regulatory and scientific issues that are not related to a specific product. Although advisory committees have a prominent role in the product approval stage, they are sometimes used earlier in the product development cycle and may be invited to consider postmarketing issues.

The charter of each of the advisory committees provides for at least one member to represent the consumer perspective. Consumer representatives make a valuable contribution by raising concerns that might not be otherwise addressed before products come to the marketplace. As they participate in the advisory committee process, consumer members become more knowledgeable about FDA issues and products that are often on the cutting edge of new research and technology. They gain the experience of working with nationally recognized scientific experts.

The current CDER drug advisory committees include the following:

Anesthetic and Life Support Drugs
Anti-Infective
Antiviral Arthritis
Cardiovascular and Renal
Dermatologic
Drug Abuse
Endocrinology and Metabolic
Fertility and Maternal Health
Gastrointestinal
Generic
Medical Imaging
Over-The-Counter (OTC)
Oncology
Peripheral and Central Nervous System
Psychopharmacologic
Pulmonary-Allergy
Reproductive Health

At times, CDER and CBER may especially want a committee's opinion about a new drug or biologic, a major indication for an already approved drug, or a special regulatory requirement being considered, such as a boxed warning in a drug's labeling. Committees may also advise these FDA divisions on necessary labeling information or help with guidelines for developing particular kinds of drugs. They may also consider questions such as whether a proposed trial for an experimental drug should be conducted or whether the safety and effectiveness information submitted for a new drug is adequate for marketing approval.

In October 1998, FDA published a guidance for industry entitled *Advisory Committees: Implementing Section 120 of the Food and Drug Administration Modernization Act of 1997*. This document provided guidance for industry on changes to the policies and procedures being used by CDER regarding advisory committees in response to section 120 of the FDA Modernization Act of 1997 (FDAMA). This section of the FDAMA directed FDA to establish panels of experts, or to use already-established panels of experts, to provide scientific advice and recommendations to the agency regarding the clinical investigation of drugs or the approval for marketing of drugs. The FDA has defined the term "panel of experts" to mean "advisory committees."

Section 120 of FDAMA amended section 505 of the FD&C Act by adding section 505(n). This new section includes provision for the following: (a) additional members to be included in new advisory committees, (b) new conflict of interest considerations, (c) education and training for new committee members, (d) timely committee consideration of matters, and (e) timely agency notification to affected persons of decisions on matters considered by advisory committees.

Advisory Committee Meetings can be very advantageous to sponsors who are filing an NDA for similar drug categories. It would behoove these sponsors to attend Advisory Committee meetings. The sponsor should get to know the Advisory Committee members and what the Advisory Committee is looking for in evaluating a product. Sponsors should carefully assess the issues that are important to the Advisory Committee and make careful notes as to their concerns. Heed to their recommendations and consider them seriously when they are developing their products.

FDA INITIATIVES TO SPEED DRUG APPROVAL
The FDA has instituted several programs designed to hasten the drug approval process for effective drugs. Pharmaceutical regulatory professionals should be aware of any and all ways that can be recommended to their research and management staff for more rapid drug approval. These FDA alternatives to expedite new drug approval are described below.

Subpart E in Section 312 of the Code of Federal Regulations establishes procedures to expedite the development, evaluation, and marketing of new therapies intended to treat people with life-threatening and severely debilitating illnesses, especially where no satisfactory alternatives exist.

Accelerated Development/Review Program
The first is the accelerated development/review program. Accelerated development/review (see Federal Register, April 15, 1992) is a highly specialized mechanism for speeding the development of drugs and biological products that promise significant benefit over existing therapy for serious or life-threatening illnesses. This process incorporates several novel elements aimed at making sure that rapid development and review are balanced by safeguards to protect both the patient and the integrity of the regulatory process.

Accelerated development/review can be used under two special circumstances: (a) when approval is based on evidence of the product's effect on a "surrogate end point" and (b) when the FDA determines that safe use of a product depends on restricting its distribution or use. A surrogate end point is a laboratory finding or physical sign that may not be a direct measurement of how a patient feels, functions, or survives but is still considered likely to predict therapeutic benefit for the patient.

The fundamental element of this process is that the manufacturers must continue testing after approval to demonstrate that the drug indeed provides therapeutic benefit to the patient. If not, the FDA can withdraw the product from the market more easily than usual.

Treatment IND

Treatment INDs (see Federal Register, May 22, 1987) are used to make promising new drugs available to desperately ill patients as early in the drug development process as possible. The FDA will permit an investigational drug to be used under a treatment IND if there is preliminary evidence of drug efficacy and the drug is intended to treat a serious or life-threatening disease, or if there is no comparable alternative drug or therapy available to treat that stage of the disease in the intended patient population. In addition, these patients are not eligible to be in the definitive clinical trials, which must be well under way, if not almost finished.

An immediately life-threatening disease means a stage of a disease in which there is a reasonable likelihood that death will occur within a matter of months, or in which premature death is likely without early treatment. For example, advanced cases of AIDS, herpes simplex encephalitis, and subarachnoid hemorrhage are all considered immediately life-threatening diseases. Treatment INDs are made available to patients before general marketing begins, typically during phase 3 studies. Treatment INDs also allow FDA to obtain additional data on the drug's safety and effectiveness.

FDA Guidance Documents/Guidelines

A regulatory professional must be aware of the guidance documents that FDA has made available to assist industry to understand expectations regarding drug development and the approval process. The website providing the complete list of FDA guidances is updated almost daily. It may be accessed at http://www.fda.gov/cder/guidance/index.htm.

The FDA comprehensive list of all guidances available is found on the Internet at http://www.fda.gov/cder/guidance/.

The FDA guidance page is subdivided into the following sections for ease of use: advertising; biopharmaceutics (final and draft); chemistry (final and draft); clinical/antimicrobial (draft); clinical/medical (final and draft); compliance (final and draft); generics (final and draft); industry letters; information technology; international congress on harmonization (final and draft); IND; labeling; microbiology; modernization act; OTC; pharm/tox; and procedural.

FREEDOM OF INFORMATION ACT (FOIA)

Freedom of information is another important way in which the public may readily obtain information from the FDA. The FDA has a guidance handbook published intended to facilitate requests for both public information and records not originally prepared for distribution by the FDA. This handbook has been updated in response to the Electronic Freedom of Information Act (FOIA) amendments of 1996.

Obtaining Public Information

Certain documents that are prepared for public distribution—press releases, consumer publications, speeches, and congressional testimony—are available from the FDA without having to file an FOI request. Many of these documents are available on FDA's Internet site (http://www.fda.gov/). Consumers with questions about FDA-related matters also may write to the Office of Public Affairs/FDA, 5100 Paint Branch Parkway, College Park, MD 20740-3835, or call (301) 436-2335.

Obtaining Information Through FOI

The Freedom of Information Act allows anyone to request copies of records not normally prepared for public distribution. It pertains to existing records only and does not require agencies to create new records to comply with a request. It also does not require agencies to collect information they do not have or to do research or analyze data for a requestor. In addition, FOI requests must be specific enough to permit an FDA employee who is familiar with the subject matter to locate records in a reasonable period.

Under FOIA, certain records may be withheld in whole or in part from the requestor if they fall within one of nine FOIA exemptions. Of these nine, six of these exemptions most often form the basis for the withholding of information by the FDA:

Exemption 2 protects certain records related solely to the FDA's internal rules and practices.

Exemption 3 protects information that is prohibited from disclosure by other laws.

Exemption 4 protects trade secrets and confidential commercial or financial information.

Exemption 5 protects certain interagency and intra-agency communications.

Exemption 6 protects information about individuals in personnel, medical, and similar files when disclosure would constitute a clearly unwarranted invasion of privacy.

Exemption 7 protects records or information compiled for law enforcement purposes when disclosure (a) could reasonably be expected to interfere with enforcement proceedings, (b) would deprive a person of a right to a fair trial or an impartial adjudication, (c) could reasonably be expected to constitute an unwarranted invasion of personal privacy, (d) could reasonably be expected to disclose the identity of a confidential source, (e) would disclose techniques and procedures for law enforcement investigations or prosecutions, or would disclose guidelines for law enforcement investigations or prosecutions, if such disclosure could reasonably be expected to risk circumvention of the law, or (f) could reasonably be expected to endanger the life or physical safety of an individual.

In the event, the FDA relies on one or more FOIA exemptions to deny a requestor access to records; a letter stating the reasons for denying the records will be sent to the requestor. The letter will also notify the requestor of the right to appeal the agency's denial determination. More specific information on these exemptions and on other aspects of the FOIA programs are contained in the FDA's FOIA implementation regulations codified in 21 CFR Part 20.

How to Make a FOI Request

All FOI requests must be in writing and should include the following information:

1. Requestor's name, address, and telephone number.
2. A description of the records being sought. The records should be identified as specifically as possible. A request for specific records that are releasable to the public can be processed much more quickly than a request for "all information" on a particular subject. Also fees for a more specific and limited request will generally be less. Information on major information systems maintained by the FDA can be obtained by using the Department of Health and Human Services Government Information Locator Service (GILS) site. This information may be useful in narrowing a request.
3. Separate requests should be submitted for each item of information.
4. A statement concerning willingness to pay fees, including any limitations.

All FOI requests must be in writing. The FDA does not accept FOI requests sent by e-mail. Requests should be mailed to Food and Drug Administration, Office of Management Programs, Division of Freedom of Information (HFI-35), 5600 Fishers Lane, Rockville, MD 20857. Or requests may be sent by fax to (301) 443-1726. If there are problems sending a fax, call (301) 443-2414.

Fees

Requestors under FOIA may have to pay fees covering some or all of the costs of processing their request. Requestors may want to include the maximum dollar amount they are willing to pay. If the fees exceed the maximum amount stated, FDA will contact the requestor before filling the request. Requestors are generally billed for fees after their requests have been processed; however, if total fees are expected to exceed $250.00, the FDA may require payment in advance for processing.

Requests received on or after January 1, 2009, fees are as follows:

1. Commercial use requestors
   Review time: $22.00, $45.00, and $81.00 per hour, depending upon the grade level of the FDA employee filling the request. No charges for search time will be assessed.
   Duplication: $.10 per page for standard-size paper or actual cost per page for odd-size paper.
   Compact Disc: $1.00 each.
   Certifications: $10 each.
   Computer charges: actual cost for time involved.
   Electronic forms/formats: actual cost for form/format requested.
2. Noncommercial use requestors, such as representatives of the news media, and educational and noncommercial scientific institutions. No search, review, or duplication charges will be assessed.
   Duplication charges are issued at the same rates listed above, with no charge for first 100 pages of duplication.
3. Other requestors, including consumers
   Duplication charges are issued at the same rates listed above, with no charge for the first 100 pages of duplication. No charge for search or review time will be assessed.

Requestors should not send payment with their requests. They will be billed if the total processing charges are $25 or more. If you send a personal check, it will be converted into an electronic funds transfer. You may also pay your invoice by ACH (electronic check) or Credit Card online at the following Website: https://fdasfinapp8.fda.gov/OA_HTML/irecLogin.jsp.

SUMMARY

FDA and Sponsor Liaison is an art that is developed over years of experience gained from understanding Regulations, Guidelines, and recommendations from regulatory experts. It is vital that regulatory personnel attend meetings, conferences, and courses on all aspects of regulatory issues on the process of new product development. Regulatory requirements differ for each country where a sponsor intends to market regulated products. The variations in the acceptance of global new product submissions are tremendous since the implementation of ICH guidelines and the European Directives. The regulatory agencies around the world are constantly faced with the challenge of reviewing international data that must meet the legal regulatory requirements used in the process of new product development. However, the CTD format has lessened the burden of required data for new products. The highest recommendation that one can bestow on all personnel in the regulatory profession is to heed to the regulations, follow guidelines as close as possible, and submit valid data following required and legal regulatory principles. Listed below are statements that can help guide regulatory personnel to measure their success in new product submissions and even direct their thinking in adapting new procedures that might expedite agencies' approval for new products:

1. How expeditiously are the sponsors' submissions reviewed by FDA and other agencies around the world compared with other pharmaceutical manufacturers?
2. How many filings require follow-up submissions with additional data? Would adequate review prior to the initial filing have disclosed the deficiencies cited by agency reviewers?
3. What additional steps can be implemented to speed the product review or support process?
4. Is there an accord between the Drug Regulatory Department (DRA) representatives and regulatory agencies personnel?
5. How difficult is it to arrange meetings with agency staff members? Can the relationship be improved?

A knowledge of how global regulatory agencies operate is essential to the success of a DRA department. All dealings with regulatory agencies must be well conceived and adequately planned. Without knowledge, conception, planning, and an understanding of how the other half works, significant delays in drug approval frequently and painfully occur. Whether the regulatory goal is to speed the approval process for a new product or to keep a product on the market, the firm must know how best to work with all regulatory agencies involved. Will patience work? Should there be a legal confrontation? Should the commissioner be involved? These and other questions must be addressed and constructively resolved by the regulatory professional.

7 Nonclinical Drug Development: Pharmacology, Drug Metabolism, and Toxicology

Duane B. Lakings

Drug Safety Evaluation Consulting, Inc., Elgin, Texas, U.S.A.

INTRODUCTION

The discovery and development of a novel therapeutic agent, whether a small organic molecule (novel chemical entity or NCE) or a macromolecule such as a protein and oligonucleotide, require scientific expertise from a number of different disciplines and an enormous amount of time and money. While humans may be the ultimate test species to ascertain the safety and efficacy of a potential new therapeutic agent, research studies in animal models are necessary to determine whether a drug candidate has a pharmacological property that might mediate a human disease process or disorder and that the test article does not have a toxicity profile that could cause adverse experiences in humans at pharmacological doses. Present estimates suggest that about 10 to 12 years and more than $1000 million or $1 billion (with this cost including the amount expended on drug candidates that "died" during development) are needed to successfully discover and develop a novel therapeutic agent. Figure 1 presents the relationship between the dollars spent and time of development. As shown, the drug discovery and preclinical phases are relatively inexpensive compared to that for the clinical and nonclinical phases of development.

Historically, for every 100 compounds with acceptable biological activity in in vitro pharmacology systems or in animal models of a human disease or disorder and tested for toxicity in animals, only one has the necessary pharmacology and preclinical safety (safety pharmacology, pharmacokinetics, and toxicology) profiles for evaluation in humans. Of those compounds tested in humans, only about 1 in 10 is successfully brought to the marketplace. This poor rate of success has been attributed to a number of factors, including that animals are not truly predictive of biological activity and/or safety in humans. The problem, however, may be (most likely is) that insufficient time and resources are devoted to characterize a discovery lead or drug candidate in pharmacology, drug metabolism, and toxicology animal models to first select the compound with the desired drug-like attributes needed for successful development and then to critically evaluate the results from preclinical animal studies to ensure that a compound with developability problems does not enter into clinical studies until those demerits are resolved. Instead of a rush from the first sign of biological activity in an in vitro pharmacology test to clinical trail evaluation, careful design, conduct, and interpretation of preclinical pharmacology, pharmacokinetic, and toxicology animal studies will detect "loser" candidates much earlier. These assessments will allow precious time and resources to be devoted in finding development candidates with a better chance than 1 in 10 of successfully completing clinical studies and becoming a marketed therapeutic agent. Being able to identify the 999 losers of the 1000 discovery leads that have

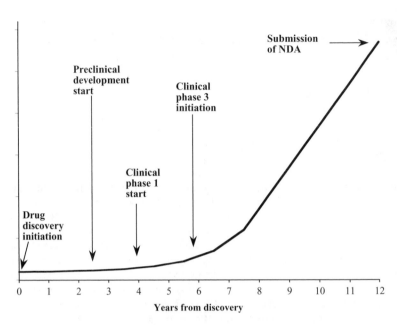

FIGURE 1   Time and cost profile for the discovery and development of a drug candidate.

a potentially desirable biological activity but that have safety "issues" as early as possible in the development process will save substantial time and resources.

This chapter describes the biological aspects of the nonclinical research programs of the drug development process. The chapter has been organized along the timeline for the nonclinical drug discovery and development process, with the major subsections being pharmacology or drug discovery, developability assessment, preclinical or pre-IND development, and nonclinical or post-IND development. The information presented should help drug development researchers in designing experiments to evaluate discovery leads and drug candidates as they progress from drug discovery through the nonclinical research studies required for successful drug development and to determine which nonclinical research studies need to be conducted in order to support regulatory agency submissions.

OVERVIEW OF DRUG DISCOVERY AND DEVELOPMENT

Normally, the biological aspects of the drug discovery and development processes can be subdivided into four distinct stages. The first is drug discovery, in which the pharmacology or biological activity of a discovery lead is explored in in vitro models or more appropriately in defined and characterized animal models, showing that the compound, or class of compounds, mediates a disease process and thus has potential human therapeutic benefit. This stage should also include preliminary studies to characterize the developability, which may include studies on delivery, metabolism, acute toxicity, preliminary pharmacokinetics, and initial formulation development, of a lead candidate or to select the optimal lead from a group of compounds with similar pharmacological properties (1,2). The second stage consists of preclinical development in which the safety, including safety pharmacology, acute and subchronic toxicology, pharmacokinetics, drug metabolism, and deliverability, of a drug candidate are studied in animal models. Additional pharmacology studies may also be conducted during this stage to optimize the route and frequency of administration, to determine the pharmacological mechanism of action, and to further explore the candidate's pharmacology profile for other possible disease indications. During the early (phase 1 and 2) clinical studies, the third stage of the process includes the initial human experiments to define the drug candidate's safety and tolerance and pharmacokinetics in normal volunteers and the candidate's efficacy in patients. In addition, the nonclinical research program is continued to extend the scientific database on the toxicity, metabolism, and delivery of the drug candidate. The final, fourth stage involves definitive safety and efficacy (phase 3) clinical studies in humans; carcinogenicity and reproductive and developmental toxicology studies in animals with supportive toxicokinetic experiments; metabolite isolation and identification to compare the metabolism profile of a drug candidate in humans and toxicological animal species; and, where appropriate, human pharmacokinetic studies to evaluate potential changes in the extent and duration of delivery and disposition profiles caused by age, gender, race, interaction with other drugs, disease state, and hepatic and renal dysfunction. Figure 2 shows the interactions among these various biological stages. Each of these areas may also include a number of special experiments designed to confirm and extend results on a drug candidate's pharmacology, pharmacokinetic and drug metabolism, and toxicology profiles.

PHARMACOLOGY

The drug discovery process has undergone enormous changes during the past few years. After years of first synthesizing individual compounds, then purifying and obtaining physical and chemical characterization of the new chemicals, and finally testing the NCEs in in vitro and in vivo pharmacology models of a particular human disease, the pharmaceutical and biotechnology industry attempted to use combinatorial chemistry to generate large libraries of compounds, which were then screened for activity using high-throughput screening (HTS) techniques. However, the combinatorial chemistry compounds that showed some biological activity for a given target were generally unacceptable as drug candidates because the active sites of the targets were lipophilic and thus the more active discovery leads were also highly lipophilic and thus were delivered across membranes in insufficient concentrations to effectively mediate a disease process where the target was expressed in the body. The industry has now turned to rational drug design as a way to generate organic compounds that have chemical structures that fit into the active site of a target protein or receptor. This rational drug design approach requires that the target be isolated and the three-dimensional structure, including the active site, determined so that organic compounds with chemical structures that fit into and bind with the active site can be modeled and then synthesized.

The rationally designed organic compounds are then screened for biological activity, usually first in an in vitro system, in which a known biochemical process, which is thought to mimic a human disease or disorder, is agonized or antagonized. Those chemical structures with the optimal (usually the highest) biological activity are designated as discovery leads. These leads may have acceptable biological activity but frequently do not have the necessary attributes to become successful drug candidates. One of more common problems with the leads is that they do not

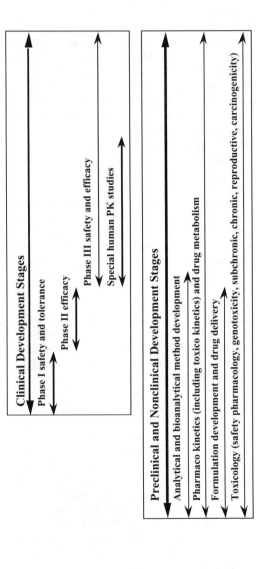
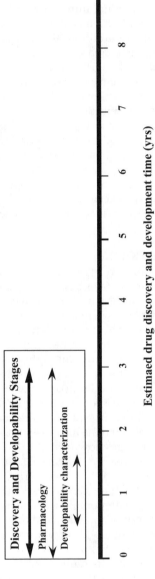

FIGURE 2 Interaction and timing of the various stages in the biological aspects of the drug discovery and development process.

have sufficient aqueous solubility to be delivered to the membranes that have to be crossed in order to reach the organ system that contains the target for the disease to be mediated. Thus, the organic chemist and the pharmacologist work together to identify the structure moieties that are necessary for biological activity. The moieties are termed the pharmacaphore and cannot be substantially changed without causing significant decreases in biological activity. However, while the pharmacaphore cannot be changed, other structural groups can be added or removed from the chemical structure to modify the physicochemical properties of the leads and thus make the leads more "drugable."

After a sufficient quantity of the biologically active compounds discovered during the screening process have been synthesized, purified, identified, and characterized, additional studies are conducted to more fully evaluate the pharmacology of the lead. This more classic approach to evaluate the biological potency of a lead is referred to as structural activity relationship (SAR) assessment. An important requirement in SAR determination is having or developing an animal model that correlates to, or mimics, a disease or disorder in humans. Developing these animal models can be time-consuming and expensive and is often complicated by the fact that the model may not simulate the disease as manifested in humans. Many important human diseases, including psychoses, depression, Alzheimer's disease, AIDS, and many cancers, do not yet have predictive animal models. After the animal model has been characterized, various dose levels of the lead(s), identified from the in vitro pharmacology screens and possibly modified during SAR evaluations, are administered to the test species and a dose–response curve is generated. The most commonly used endpoint is the dose that provides a 50% response (the ED_{50}). Structural analogues of the lead(s) are frequently synthesized and tested in the same model to generate a family of curves with varying biological potencies or ED_{50}s. The lead with the greatest biological activity is frequently selected for further development. However, at this point, many unanswered questions exist. Some of these concerns are

1. Does the animal model reflect, in most or all aspects, the disease in humans?
2. Is the delivery or extent of exposure of all the leads similar so that the generated dose–response curves accurately predict the compound with the greatest in vivo potency?
3. Are the route and frequency of administration and the formulation used to dose the test species similar to those proposed for human evaluation?
4. Do the leads have similar pharmacokinetic and drug metabolism profiles so that the durations of exposure to the pharmacologically active compounds are similar?
5. Do any of the leads produce unacceptable toxicity in organs or physiological systems not involved in the desired pharmacology of the compounds?

Before the more formal and definitive preclinical development begins, attempts should be made to answer as many of these questions as possible. The following section discusses the developability experiments that can be conducted relatively quickly and cheaply to ascertain whether the lead(s) has the necessary biopharmaceutical, or drug-like, characteristics needed for further development and does have any major demerits that would prevent successful development.

DEVELOPABILITY ASSESSMENT

Completed drug discovery research studies indicate that a compound, or class of compounds, mediates a disease process and has potential as a human therapeutic agent. Is this lead compound now ready to be transferred from the discovery area to a preclinical development group? Should additional, nondefinitive experiments be conducted to more fully characterize the properties of the lead candidate? If more studies are considered necessary, what experiments should be done?

This section describes some of the biological research experiments that could, and in most cases should, be conducted to evaluate the potential of a lead compound to become a developmental candidate or to select the optimal compound from a group of discovery leads. Figure 3 shows where these developability experiments fit into the drug discovery and development process. These nondefinitive developability studies may also uncover problems that have to be resolved before the more definitive preclinical development studies required to support an IND submission are started and before the clinical protocols to evaluate the safety, pharmacokinetics, and efficacy of the drug candidate in humans are designed.

Before the preclinical drug development program is begun and because each discovery program is company and compound specific, a number of questions should be asked and answered so that the research studies, both types and designs, may be planned effectively and the timelines for their completion can be determined. These questions include:

1. What is the human disease indication for the proposed drug candidate?
2. What is the proposed route and frequency of dosing for the candidate in human clinical studies?
3. What is the estimated pharmacological active substance concentration in physiological fluids and how long should that concentration be maintained so that the desired biological response can be obtained?
4. What, if any, are the biological markers that may be useful for monitoring toxicity or therapeutic effectiveness in nonclinical and clinical studies?
5. What definitive preclinical studies need to be completed before a human clinical program can be initiated?

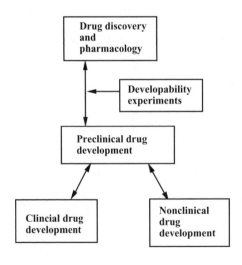

FIGURE 3 How drug developability experiments fit into the drug discovery and development process?

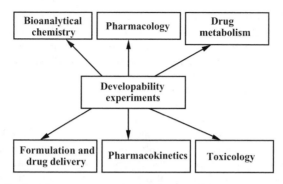

FIGURE 4 Scientific disciplines necessary for drug developability assessment.

6. What is the projected timeline for the completion of the preclinical studies and for submission of the first-in-human clinical trial application or an Investigational New Drug (IND) submission?

Additional questions need to be considered, including whether the drug candidate can be synthesized and purified in sufficient quantity to support a development program, how to document and validate these manufacturing processes, how to characterize and document the identity of impurities present in the drug substance and the proposed drug product, and how to determine the stability of the drug substance and the proposed drug product. However, these questions are outside the scope of this discussion.

At least six scientific disciplines are involved in the developability characterization of a discovery lead or group of leads. As shown in Figure 4, these disciplines are in vivo pharmacology, bioanalytical chemistry (BAC) method development, nonclinical formulation assessment and delivery, animal pharmacokinetics, drug metabolism, and toxicology. The following sections discuss each of these scientific disciplines in more detail. The discussion is for a single discovery lead. If more than one lead is being evaluated to select the lead with the most drug-like properties, which depends on a variety of factors such as disease indication, route and frequency of dosing, etc., for further development, similar experiments should be conducted on each lead and the results are compared to determine which lead has the desired attributes without any major demerits and thus has the "best" chance of being a successful drug candidate.

Pharmacology

Preliminary pharmacology evaluations in in vitro systems or animal models will have shown that a lead interacts with a biological process suggestive of human therapeutic benefit. Depending on the design and extent of these early studies, additional pharmacology studies may be needed to further characterize the dose, or physiological fluid concentration, response curve using the proposed clinical route and frequency of administration. If possible, these pharmacology studies should be conducted in at least two species to show that the biological response is not species dependent. The ED_{50} dose should be determined and that value should be divided into the no-observable-adverse-effect-level (NOAEL) dose in the same animal species, described in the section on toxicology, to estimate a therapeutic ratio

(TR), or index. If TR is one or less, a lead will most likely elicit adverse effects in addition to the beneficial response. Unless the lead is for the treatment of a life-threatening disease, such as AIDS, some cancers, or certain CNS indications, a low TR is a warning sign that the lead may not have the necessary properties for further development. A TR of five, preferably 10 or more, indicates that a lead will most likely produce the desired pharmacological response before causing any dose-limiting toxicities.

If possible, these developability pharmacology studies should be conducted with dosing to steady state unless the frequency of dosing to be used in clinical trials is as a single-dose therapeutic. The number of doses required to reach steady state depends on the lead's pharmacokinetic profile in the same animal model. These multiple-dose studies provide information on the frequency of dosing necessary to maximize the biological response. This is particularly important for compounds that inhibit an enzymatic system or are effective only during certain phases of the cell cycle.

These pharmacology evaluations assist in the selection of dose levels and route and frequency of administration for preliminary and definitive toxicology studies and for initial phase 1 safety, pharmacokinetic, and tolerance human clinical trials. If the effective pharmacological dose is unknown, under dosing and achieving no therapeutic response or over dosing and being unable to define a dose that produces minimal or acceptable toxic effects are undesirable possibilities. In such cases, the development of a potential beneficial therapeutic agent could be inappropriately discontinued.

Bioanalytical Chemistry Method Development

If not already available, a BAC method needs to be defined and characterized for the quantification of the lead in physiological fluids. This assay can then support experiments in some of the other scientific disciplines involved in assessing the developability of the lead and, after appropriate validation, the preclinical, non-clinical, and clinical development of a selected drug candidate. For preliminary studies, a BAC method should be characterized to demonstrate the range of reliable results, the lower and upper limits of quantification, specificity, accuracy, and precision. In addition, evaluations on the matrix to be used (blood, plasma, serum) should be conducted and the stability of the lead in the selected matrix should be determined.

The first step in characterizing a BAC method is to select the analytical technique. For a compound with a molecular weight of less than 2000, instrumental methods such as LC/MS/MS (a very sensitive and specific technique and the most common method employed by the pharmaceutical industry), or HPLC and GC with a variety of detectors, including ultraviolet, fluorescence, flame ionization, and electron capture, may be used. A macromolecule (large peptide, protein, or oligonucleotide) may require an ELISA or RIA method. Samples in assay diluent and in a physiological fluid and over a large concentration range should be analyzed to show that the technique produces an appropriate signal to detect the analyte and to determine the potential interference caused by the matrix, that is, assay specificity. The ability to quantify a lead in a physiological fluid may depend on the matrix. For example, serum is a poor choice when the analyte interacts with clotting factors. The matrix that gives the best recovery and has the least interference when the compound is added to whole blood should be selected.

The specificity of an assay evaluates the potential interferences from matrix components and from the different animal species to be used in pharmacology and toxicology experiments. Samples from each species to be studied are analyzed neat (with no added compound) and fortified with known amounts of the lead and the results are calculated using a standard curve prepared in assay diluent. The response obtained from the neat samples indicate the level of interference from each matrix, and the calculated amounts in the fortified samples show the difference in absolute recovery from the matrix compared to that with the candidate in buffer. If the absolute recovery is low, that is, less than 50%, and/or highly variable, that is, greater than 25%, the assay may not have the desired characteristics to quantify the lead in collected specimens. Additional development should be expended on such a method so that the assay will provide reliable results that can be used to evaluate the pharmacokinetic profile of the lead in animals.

Acceptable results from the above experiments suggest whether a BAC method should be able to quantify a lead in a physiological matrix. The range and reliability of quantification are assessed through the preparation and analysis of standard curves, prepared in either diluted or undiluted matrix, and multiple samples fortified at two or more concentrations. The standard curve responses that can be described by a mathematical equation (linear, quadratic, sigmoidal) define the range of reliable results. The lower limit of quantification (LLOQ) is the lowest signal that can be accurately measured above background and should not be confused with the limit of detection (LOD), which is the lowest level that can be detected. The upper limit of quantification (ULOQ) is the highest signal that can be defined by the response curve. The fortified or quality control samples provide information on precision, defined as the ability to obtain similar calculated concentrations from samples containing the same amounts of analyte, and accuracy, which is the ability to predict the actual concentration of the analyte in a sample.

The ability to measure a lead in a physiological fluid is not useful if the compound is unstable during collection, processing, storage, or sample preparation. Thus, a nondefinitive stability study should be conducted to ensure that the compound does not degrade in blood during processing to obtain plasma or serum, during the time (hours, days, and weeks) and under the conditions (room temperature, refrigerated, frozen at $-20°C$ or $-80°C$) that specimens may be stored until analyzed, and during sample preparation. The design of stability experiments is usually compound specific. The results ensure that measured concentrations in unknown specimens reflect the amount of the lead present at the time of collection.

Successful completion of the above experiments will characterize BAC methods for use in evaluating a lead in animal models. If a lead is selected for further development, the method will need to be validated (3,4) for each matrix and for each species before being used to support definitive toxicology, drug metabolism, and pharmacokinetic studies.

Early Nonclinical Formulation Development and Delivery

Nonclinical formulation definition and the drug delivery characteristics of a lead are not usually studied in detail during the transition from discovery to development. The experiments necessary to define an acceptable formulation depend on the proposed clinical route of administration and usually require substantial quantities, that is, milligram or gram amounts, of the lead. For a compound to be administered by intravenous injection or infusion, the formulation needs to be compatible with blood so that the lead does not precipitate when administered and has minimal local toxicity. Leads that are highly lipophilic or have limited aqueous solubility are the most likely compounds to have these types of problems. A low extent of, or a high variability in, absorption can cause problems for leads administered by other routes, such as oral, subcutaneous, and dermal. For compounds that are poorly absorbed, the amount reaching the site of action may be insufficient to elicit or to maintain a desired pharmacological response. If the absorption is variable and the TR is low, a toxic response may be observed in some animals. Experiments conducted by the author have shown that when the extent of absorption is 50% or more and the variability of absorption is less than 50% of the amount absorbed, which gives a 25% to 75% range of absorption, the lead should have acceptable bioavailability for further development. For leads with an extent of absorption less than 25% of the administered dose or a variability of absorption of more than 100% of the amount absorbed, other formulations with absorption enhancers or solubilizers might be evaluated to improve the drug delivery profile. If improvement in the drug delivery profile is not possible, the chances that a lead with low, variable absorption will become a therapeutic product are greatly reduced. The candidacy of such a compound should be carefully considered.

An analytical chemistry method should be developed and validated for the quantification of a lead in nonclinical formulations and should predict whether the compound degrades from the time of preparation to the time of dosing. A method with this ability is a stability-indicating assay. The physical and chemical properties of the lead usually suggest a technique (heat, light, pH) that can degrade the compound. Samples stored under nondegrading and degrading conditions are assayed by the stability-indicating assay and, if possible, by another technique that can also determine if the original compound is present in the sample. If the lead is not stable, formulation excipients possibly can be added to prevent the degradation, or the formulations can be maintained under conditions that provide sufficient stability for testing in animal models. However, when a lead has limited stability in nonclinical formulations, the development of a clinical formulation with a sufficient shelf life for marketing is problematic. Again the candidacy of such a compound should be carefully considered.

For proteins and other large molecules, degradation may include changes in the secondary or tertiary structure, provided that rearrangement back to the original, biologically active structure does not occur. Stability-indicating assays for macromolecules should assess structural changes that cause reductions in biological activity. However, a protein may have a number of amino acids removed from one or both ends of the molecule and still retain some, and possibly all, biological activity relative to that for the intact protein. This chemically modified peptide may have a different delivery profile or be more toxic than the parent protein. Structural modifications may not be apparent if biological activity alone is used to determine the amount of the macromolecule in a formulation. Thus, experiments to demonstrate that an assay method is stability-indicating need to be carefully designed and conducted. For macromolecules, a specific chemical assay, such as HPLC or ELISA, and a biological potency assay may be necessary to determine the concentration and stability of a compound in a formulation.

The stability-indicating assay should be used to determine the amount of the lead in nonclinical formulations used for dosing animals in preliminary pharmacokinetic, drug metabolism, and toxicology studies. For single-dose studies, samples from each formulation at each dose level can be collected before dosing and after the completion of dosing. For multiple-dose studies, samples from each formulation used can be collected before the first dose and after the last dose or at selected other times. Results from these analyses ensure that the formulations contain the desired amount of the lead, that the concentrations do not change during the dosing period, and that the animals are receiving the appropriate dose levels.

Without an acceptable nonclinical formulation, the extent and variability of delivery may make interpretation of results from developability studies meaningless and could prevent the continued development of a potentially useful therapeutic agent.

The best formulation is of little use if the lead is not effectively delivered to the site of biological action. One of the primary reasons for discovery leads being not successful drug candidates is the limited or insufficient transport across various membranes from the site of dosing to the site of activity. Only compounds administered intravenously to mediate a disease indication expressed in the cardiovascular system do not have to cross at least one membrane in order to reach the site of action. Thus, assessments of a lead's ability to cross membranes should be conducted as early as possible. Many pharmaceutical companies use delivery potential as a key indicator for whether or not a discovery lead should move into preclinical development.

A number of in vitro models are available to evaluate the delivery potential of a lead. For a lead to be administered orally, the Caco-2 model is still the most commonly employed system, but other models are also available. The Caco-2 cells mimic the cell wall of the GI tract and can be used to estimate the rate and extent of diffusion across membranes. Recently, a lipophilic membrane technique has been defined and shown to be equally predictive of passive diffusion transport across membranes. Other in vitro systems are available to evaluate transport across other membrane types, including the blood–brain barrier, the lung, and the skin.

As most membranes are lipophilic in nature, a lead has to have some lipophilic characteristics in order to effectively diffuse into and across the membrane. However, in order to reach the membrane, the lead has to be dissolved in the surrounding media, which is aqueous. Thus, the lead also needs some hydrophilic properties in order to have sufficient aqueous solubility to be transported to the membrane. An estimate of a lead's ability to have both the lipophilic and hydrophilic characteristics necessary for effective delivery, primarily from the GI tract, can be determined from the chemical structure of the compound and by using what is commonly called Lipinski's Rules of Five, which are four rules with cut off numbers that are 5 or multiples of 5. These rules are:

1. A molecular weight of less than 500 Da.
2. A log P (octanol–water coefficient) of less than 5.
3. Hydrogen-bond donors (sum of hydroxyl and amine groups) less than 5.
4. Hydrogen-bond receptors (sum of nitrogen and oxygen atoms) less than 10.

Although these rules may be somewhat predictive of a lead's ability to cross membranes, not all compounds having the desired characteristics are orally absorbed or effectively transported across membranes, and laboratory experiments are required to determine if a lead will effectively be delivered to the site of biological action.

Preliminary Animal Pharmacokinetics

The first animal pharmacokinetic study confirms that the BAC method is useful in characterizing the absorption and disposition profiles of the lead. The animal species for this study is usually the same as used in in vivo pharmacology evaluations, most likely a rodent. A study design for a lead that has pharmacological activity when administered orally to rats may consist of dosing at least two rats with intravenous bolus injections at a dose level between 25% and 50% of the pharmacologically active dose and dosing at least two rats orally at the pharmacologically active dose and another two rats at 10 times that dose. Serial blood samples, collected from each rat and processed to obtain the desired physiological fluid, are analyzed by the BAC method. The plasma concentration versus time profiles after intravenous dosing provides preliminary information on the distribution and disposition kinetics of the lead. These intravenous results certify that the assay method is useful for quantifying the lead in specimens obtained from animals, predict the concentration range that can be expected in animal specimens, and assist in determining the sampling times to be used in more definitive animal pharmacokinetic experiments. The plasma concentration versus time profiles after oral dosing provides preliminary information on the absorption kinetics and the absolute bioavailability of the lead. The design of additional animal pharmacokinetic studies depends on the results of the preliminary animal pharmacokinetic study, the theoretic kinetic profile needed to produce the desired pharmacology response, and the results from preliminary toxicology experiments.

For most drug development programs, toxicology studies in two or more species are necessary. In this case, preliminary animal pharmacokinetic studies should be conducted in each species projected for use in animal safety studies. If differences in delivery or disposition exist between species and result in an enhanced or decreased toxicology profile, the pharmacokinetics may explain, in part, the different toxicology profiles. If possible, physiological fluid specimens should be obtained from animals in the preliminary toxicology studies to determine the extent and uniformity of exposure, which is termed toxicokinetics. Normally, three or four specimens from each animal are sufficient for toxicokinetic evaluations but this level of sampling may not be possible for all studies. A single specimen at one collection time can be obtained from one or two animals in a dose group and the other animals in that dose group can be sampled at other times. Analyses of these specimens provide data on the extent of exposure but not on the uniformity of exposure within a dose group. For multiple-dose studies, specimens are usually obtained after the first dose and after the last, or next to last, dose. The results provide information on possible changes in exposure and on the accumulation potential of the lead or drug candidate and can be used to design multiple-dose animal pharmacokinetic and tissue distribution studies. If the change in disposition or accumulation is substantial, modification of the dosing regimen may be necessary to obtain the desired concentration time profile after dosing to steady state.

Preliminary Drug Metabolism

The number and design of drug metabolism studies needed to characterize the fate of a drug candidate in the body depend on the results from preliminary animal pharmacokinetic and toxicology studies. Commonly, the results from these in vivo experiments are not available during earlier developability assessments and in vitro drug metabolism evaluations are utilized to determine the metabolic stability and the extent of metabolism of a lead and to compare the extent of metabolism among various species, including humans. These in vitro experiments can be conducted in a variety of systems, including CYP450 isozymes (the enzymes responsible for most oxidative metabolism of drugs), microsomes, hepatocytes, or liver slices. As hepatocytes contain both phase 1 (oxidative, hydrolysis, and reduction) and phase 2 (conjugation) metabolism systems and can be relatively easily obtained from pharmacology and toxicology animal species and from humans, many researchers select this model for the first assessment of metabolism. If the results from hepatocytes show extensive metabolism, additional in vitro experiments are usually conducted first in microsomes to ascertain if oxidative metabolism is present and then in isolated CYP450 isozymes to determine which enzyme, or enzymes, is responsible. Extensive metabolism is not necessarily a "death knell" for a lead. If rapid clearance from the body is a desired attribute for effectively treating a disease indication, metabolism to inactive metabolites may be advantageous. However, for most disease indications, extensive metabolism may prevent delivery of a pharmacologically active substance to the site of biological activity in sufficient concentration to produce the desired response. Thus, a lead that is extensively metabolized may not be a successful drug candidate.

Another reason for conducting in vitro metabolism studies early is to determine if species differences are present. Evaluating metabolism in the pharmacology and proposed toxicology animal species and in humans assists in selecting the species that are similar, at least in metabolism, to humans for definitive toxicology studies. If an animal species has limited metabolism while humans may have extensive metabolism, pharmacological and/or toxicological metabolites may be responsible for some, or all, of the biological activity or adverse effects in humans and these responses would not be observed in the animal model. Conversely, if an animal species has extensive or different metabolism compared to humans, the safety profile in that species would probably not be predictive of safety in humans.

If desired, which is sometimes the case when metabolism is extensive, the metabolites generated from in vitro systems can be isolated and identified. After preparation of sufficient quantities for additional testing, these metabolites can be evaluated for pharmacological and/or toxicological potential. This author, like many drug development researchers, has found metabolites with equal or greater biological activity when compared to that for the parent compound. At times, these pharmacologically activity metabolites have more drug-like attributes than those of the parent and can be developed either as a replacement of the parent compound or as a second-generation drug candidate.

Acute Toxicology Studies

Toxicology studies are conducted to define the safety profile of a drug candidate and include definition of the NOAEL dose, maximum tolerated dose (MTD), potential organs of toxicity, and potential biochemical markers to detect and track toxic events. Most developmental compounds that do not become therapeutic products have unacceptable toxicity in animals and/or humans. Before the definitive toxicology studies needed to support an IND submission are initiated, a number of in vitro and animal experiments can be conducted to characterize the potential toxicity of the lead. These early toxicology evaluations are usually conducted in the same species as used in pharmacology evaluations. As mentioned earlier, the lowest dose that has no apparent toxicity, or an acceptable level of toxicity, is compared with the dose that gives the desired pharmacological response in the same animal species to obtain a therapeutic ratio or index for that species.

A toxicology program to obtain toxicological characterization of a discovery lead should be accomplished through close interaction with the efforts of other scientists conducting developability experiments. Before drug safety studies are conducted, a sufficient quantity of the lead should be available and characterized so that testing is conducted with a known compound. If the lead requires formulation before dosing, the formulation should be the same for each study. If a change in the synthesis, purification, or formulation is necessary to improve the biopharmaceutical properties of the lead or the drug delivery profile, then some of the early toxicology studies should be repeated with the new formulation to determine whether the safety profile has been altered. These early safety studies do not need to be, but in many cases are, conducted according to Good Laboratory Practice (GLP) Regulations requirements. However, these experiments should be designed and conducted as close as possible to the processes used for definitive, GLP-compliant toxicology studies. Then, the results will be scientifically defensible and useful in predicting the toxicity expected from the GLP-compliant studies. Examples of the early toxicology studies needed to characterize a lead, or a drug candidate selected based on pharmacological activity and not evaluated using developability assessment studies, include the following.

In Vitro Toxicology Assessments

When a number of discovery leads have been identified and need to be further evaluated to select the optimal lead for further evaluations, the potential for toxic effects may be determined using in vitro techniques, such as cell-based systems or microarrays. By incubating various concentrations of the leads with cells, such as the pharmacological target cell, hepatocytes, neurons, kidney cells and measuring an adverse effect, such as cell death (cytotoxicity) or change in cellular function or release of a biological marker [such as glutathione S-transferase (GST) or lactate dehydrogenase (LDH)] considered predictive of toxic effect, the leads can be stratified as to toxicological potential. Similarly, microarrays that have systems considered predictive of toxic events can be used to determine which leads "turn on" these systems. While most, if not all, toxicologists think these in vitro systems cannot be used to predict toxicology in animal models or humans, the results may be useful in evaluating a group of discovery leads to determine which lead may have a more acceptable profile compared to that of the others.

Acute or Single-Dose Tolerability Studies

To evaluate the qualitative and quantitative single-dose toxicity of a lead, a single dose at a number of dose levels is administered by the proposed clinical route and the animals are observed for 14 days after dosing. This acute study is not an LD_{50} study, which is not needed for overall risk assessment according to an International Conference on Harmonisation (ICH) guideline (5). This ICH guideline suggests that the drug candidate dose levels include at least one that produces pharmacological activity and one that causes overt evidence of major or life-threatening toxicity and that a vehicle control group is included. The acute toxicity study should evaluate both the intravenous route (if feasible) and the intended clinical route of administration, unless the clinical route is intravenous. The studies should be conducted in two relevant mammalian species, one of which is not a rodent, and unless scientifically unjustifiable, should use equal numbers of male and female animals for each species evaluated. The test species is observed for 14 days after dosing and, as with all toxicology studies, all signs of toxicity with time of onset, duration of symptoms, and reversibility are recorded. Also, the time to first observations of lethality is recorded. Gross necropsies are performed on all animals sacrificed moribund, found dead, or terminated after 14 days of observation and the results are presented by dose group. An evaluation of results should include all observations made and a discussion of the toxicological findings and their implications to humans, taking into account the pharmacology of the lead, the proposed human therapeutic use and dose, and experience with related drugs. The highest no-toxic-effect dose and the highest nonlethal dose are noted.

Dose-Range–Finding Studies
The doses for definitive toxicology studies are defined in dose-range–finding studies. These experiments usually include four dose levels, with the highest level being the dose that did not cause substantial acute toxicity effects, and a vehicle control group, and they are conducted in each species proposed for use in definitive toxicology studies. For rodents, dose groups usually have 6 to 10 animals, 3 to 5 animals per sex. For nonrodent species, normally beagle dogs or nonhuman primates, the number of animals in each dose group is commonly 4 or 6, 2 or 3 animal per sex per group. Endpoints for dose-range–finding studies may include, but are not limited to, weight loss, activity changes, clinical chemistry changes, and histology and pathology evaluations at necropsy. The primary goal of these studies is to determine an MTD. The route of administration and the frequency and duration of dosing are determined from the expected clinical use of the compound.

Pilot, 14-Day Studies
A dose level that causes toxic changes, such as morbidity or salivation, and one that produces the NOAEL dose are determined during 14-day studies. For a lead or drug candidate to be used for a non–life-threatening clinical indication, at least two animal species are tested, one rodent (usually the rat) and one nonrodent. The information gained by these studies is used to model the definitive GLP-compliant toxicology studies so that these experiments are conducted with a cost-efficient design and are data productive. These early toxicology studies can also evaluate the potential for antibody production, if the lead might be antigenic, and clinical chemistry changes in physiological parameters (electrolyte or biochemical imbalances, changes in liver enzymes). These data may identify potential biological markers that can be used in definitive toxicology and clinical studies to evaluate and possibly predict adverse effects.

Organs that are the targets of toxicity may be identified during the above toxicology studies by a full histology workup of animals in each dose group and from the results obtained from the analyses of clinical chemistry samples (discussed in more detail in the preclinical toxicology section). The level of the lead in the identified target organs of toxicity can be determined by the drug metabolism group in an attempt to correlate the observed toxicity with high or accumulated concentrations of the compound, providing a potential toxicodynamic correlation. If possible, investigations into the biochemical mechanism of identified toxicity should be initiated. Results from these experiments can provide insight into potential toxicities in definitive toxicology studies, identify biological markers that predict a toxic event, and suggest conditions in human patients where administration of the lead or drug candidate is contraindicated. If results from the early toxicology studies show that a lead has an unacceptable level of toxicity, the development candidacy of such a compound should be carefully considered.

Safety Pharmacology and Genotoxicity

If desired, the safety of a lead can be further assessed by conducting safety pharmacology and/or genotoxicity studies, which are described in more detail in the section on preclinical development. These studies, which are to be completed prior to the initiation of human clinical testing, are more commonly conducted after selection of a drug candidate. However, if some discovery leads are considered "equal" after other developability assessment experiments have been completed, the results from safety pharmacology or genotoxicity studies may be able to identify the "optimal" lead or determine that some leads do not have the desired profile and should not be selected as the drug candidate.

Drug Development Candidate Selection

Many discovery leads are transferred to the preclinical development process with insufficient characterization to assess their development potential. This lack of knowledge usually results in poorly designed experiments that are not data productive and that, in many cases, have to be repeated when the drug candidate shows unexpected toxicity, low and variable delivery, instability or solubility problems, or unacceptable pharmacokinetic and drug metabolism profiles. In all too many cases, the recognition of these problem areas results in termination of development for a potentially useful therapeutic agent. At best, the problems encountered cause a delay, at times substantial, in the development of a candidate, while additional studies are conducted to elucidate the causes of the problems and minimize their effect. Then, the definitive preclinical development experiments have to be repeated.

The developability assessment experiments in six scientific disciplines shown in Figure 4 can more fully characterize a discovery lead before the compound enters the definitive preclinical, then the nonclinical and clinical, drug development processes. The experimental designs could also be used, with minor modifications, to evaluate a group of compounds and thus to select the lead with the best characteristics, that is, the most drug-like attributes and the least demerits, for further development. With appropriate planning and commitment of resources, these studies can usually be completed in three to six months if major problems are not encountered in one or more of the scientific areas.

If these developability assessment experiments are completed as part of the transition from discovery to development, compounds that do not have the characteristics necessary to become therapeutic agents can be identified early and prevented from entering the most costly and time-consuming development process. Analogues of a compound with unacceptable characteristics or demerits can be evaluated to find a development candidate that has more optimal properties. In addition, the results from the developability studies will allow the preclinical development studies to be designed and conducted in a timely, cost-efficient manner and thus most likely allow the candidate to have an earlier entry into the clinic.

PRECLINICAL DRUG DEVELOPMENT

Before entering into a clinical evaluation program, a drug candidate is subjected to a number of preclinical studies to further define and characterize its safety profile in animals. The results from the pharmacology, developability, and preclinical studies are documented in technical reports or scientific publications and used to prepare a regulatory agency submission for the initiation of human clinical trials. Most of the preclinical studies, described in the sections below, and nonclinical studies, discussed in the following section, need to be conducted in compliance with GLP Regulations.

If the experiments described in the developability assessment section have not been completed (as is the case for many drug development programs), many of these studies should be conducted after the drug candidate has been selected. The results from these early or preliminary studies are needed to effectively design the more definitive preclinical studies, particularly the toxicology and drug metabolism evaluations needed to support an IND submission.

Good Laboratory Practice

Research studies, particularly safety pharmacology, genotoxicity, and toxicology studies, intended for submission to a regulatory agency are to be conducted according to GLP Regulations, as published by regulatory authorities in all the leading pharmaceutical markets, such as the United States (the FDA Regulations applicable to GLP are provided in Title 21 Code of Federal Regulations, Part 58), European Community, and Japan. GLP Regulations are very similar worldwide; however, researchers are cautioned to review the regulations for the planned marketing area(s) to ensure that the completed studies are in compliance.

GLP Regulations concern standard methods, facilities, and controls used in conducting preclinical and nonclinical laboratory studies and are used to assure the quality and integrity of generated data. The standards relate to both the design and the conduct of the research studies and the qualifications of the personnel and facilities involved with all aspects of the experiments. The GLP Regulations necessitate that

1. SOPs are written for all routine or standard practices in the laboratory.
2. All personnel, including management, involved with the studies are sufficiently trained and experienced to perform their assigned functions.
3. An adequate number of personnel are available to conduct the various aspects of the studies.
4. The facilities and equipment are appropriately designed and maintained.
5. A group, commonly called the quality assurance unit or QAU, monitors and checks the results from the studies to ensure that the experiments are conducted in compliance with the regulations.

Bioanalytical Chemistry

The BAC method, defined and characterized during developability assessment, can be used to support definitive pharmacokinetic and toxicology studies after the assay has been appropriately validated for each physiological matrix and each species to be evaluated. The validation experiments need to address and define acceptance and rejection criteria for the range of reliable results, the lower limit (and if appropriate as for an ELISA or RIA method, the upper limit) of quantification, accuracy, precision, specificity, and recovery and should include appropriate stability studies. These stability studies will ensure that the analyte is stable in the physiological matrix from the time of collection to the time of analysis. Guidelines for validation of a BAC method have been published (3,4). The validated BAC method should be documented in a test assay procedure and supported by appropriate SOPs. Also, the results from the validation experiments should be documented in a technical report and included in the IND submission.

Pharmacokinetic and Bioavailability Experiments

Pharmacokinetic and bioavailability (absolute and relative) experiments are usually designed and conducted to evaluate dose proportionality over the dose range used, or expected to be used, in toxicology studies in rodents and nonrodents and possible species-to-species differences in pharmacokinetic profiles. With the incorporation of one or two intravenous dose levels into the study protocol, the drug candidate's absolute bioavailability or F can also be determined and information on the linearity of absorption, distribution, and disposition kinetics can be obtained. If more than one drug formulation is to be used in toxicology studies (e.g., an oral solution for rodent studies and tablets or drug in capsules for dosing the larger, nonrodent species), relative bioavailability experiments comparing the formulations can determine if the extent of delivery is similar or different and thus can make extrapolation of pharmacology and toxicology results between animal species meaningful and useful in designing the later nonclinical studies and phase 1 safety, pharmacokinetic, and tolerance studies in humans.

Drug Metabolism

Drug metabolism or ADME evaluations determine absorption (how a compound gets into the body), distribution (where the compound goes in the body), disposition (how long the compound stays in the body), metabolism (whether the compound is changed and to what), and elimination (how the compound is removed or cleared from the body) or the fate of a compound in the body.

Drug metabolism experiments in animal species used or to be used in toxicology studies are conducted using an appropriately labeled compound, usually a radioactive isotope such as carbon-14. At times, drug metabolism studies are conducted with a less than desirable radiolabel, such as ^{125}I on a protein or ^{3}H at a potentially exchangeable site on an NCE. However, the results obtained from these studies can be misleading, reflecting the distribution and disposition of the label and not the drug candidate or its metabolites. For more reliable results, the radiolabeled compound should be radiochemically pure and stable and should have a specific activity high enough to be measurable after dosing. Also, the label needs to be in a chemical structural position where it does not affect the physical, chemical, or pharmacological properties of the candidate and is not lost during phase 1 (oxidation, reduction, cleavage) or phase 2 (conjugation) metabolism. Before animals are dosed, the radiochemical purity needs to be evaluated and the stability in physiological matrices should be studied. If the radiolabel is nonmetabolically removed from the compound, the results from the drug metabolism experiments, or other studies using the labeled compound, will have little, if any, meaning or usefulness in the determination of the metabolic fate of the drug candidate.

If the candidate has a slow disposition phase, suggesting distribution into some extravascular tissues or organs, or if the early toxicology experiments identify potential organs of toxicity, a preliminary mass balance combined with tissue distribution study can be designed to evaluate the radioactivity level versus time profiles in selected tissues, such as liver, kidney, fat (for a lipophilic candidate), muscle, skin, heart, and brain and to determine the primary route(s) and rate(s) of elimination. The results from this preliminary metabolism study can also be used to more effectively design (i.e., selection of time points and matrices for evaluation) the definitive mass balance and tissue distribution studies needed for supporting regulatory agency submissions.

The total radioactivity minus the parent compound concentration (determined by the BAC method for the drug candidate) in a specimen (plasma, serum, urine, bile) estimates the amount of metabolites present. If the difference is minimal and does not change over time, the extent of metabolism is low. For plasma or serum specimens, a small difference indicates that metabolites are not present in systemic circulation. For bile or urine specimens, high levels of radioactivity suggest a primary route of elimination for the parent and its metabolites. For a drug candidate cleared primarily by metabolism, a preliminary metabolite profile in urine and bile can determine the amount of each potential metabolite. When the level of a metabolite in a matrix is high, that is, greater than 5% of the parent in the same matrix at the same collection time, attempts to isolate and identify the metabolite should be undertaken and the results should be compared with those from in vitro drug metabolism studies, if conducted. After sufficient quantities of the metabolites are available, the metabolite's pharmacological and toxicological activity potential can be evaluated, providing possible additional information on the pharmacological and toxicological mechanism of action for the drug candidate.

One of the first metabolism studies conducted should be protein binding in animal and human physiological fluids. The pharmacological and toxicological activity of a drug candidate is usually attributed to the free or unbound fraction in systemic circulation and not to the total drug content, which includes both free and bound drug. The unbound drug is the species that passes through the cell walls of blood vessels and is distributed to various organs, including the pharmacological and toxicological sites of actions. The free and bound fractions of a drug candidate are in equilibrium so that when the free drug is removed from systemic circulation (either distributed to tissues or eliminated in excreta), the bound drug disassociates to maintain the free-to-bound ratio. A drug candidate that is highly and tightly bound, for example, more than 95%, to blood proteins may not have sufficient distribution to attain the necessary concentration at the site of action to elicit the desired pharmacological effect. If this is the case, a BAC method that quantifies unbound drug may be needed so that the pharmacokinetic profile of the free fraction can be evaluated. For a drug with a protein binding of less than 95%, the amount of free drug and the equilibrium process generally provide a good correlation between total drug concentration in systemic circulation and pharmacological or toxicological responses.

The two most common drug metabolism studies are mass balance and tissue distribution. Mass balance studies are usually conducted in both the rodent and the nonrodent species used for toxicology evaluations, whereas tissue distribution is performed only in the rodent. For mass balance, a radiolabeled compound is administered to the test species and urine, feces, and, if necessary, expired air are

TABLE 1 Tissues Collected at Necropsy and Prepared for Hisopathological Evaluation

Tissue	Tissue
Adrenal glands	Pancreas
Aorta	Pituitary gland
Bone marrow (sternum)	Prostate gland (males)
Brain (usually at least three levels)	Rectum
Cervix/vagina (females)	Salivary gland (Manidibular)
Epididymides (males)	Sciatic nerve
Esophagus	Skeletal muscle
Eyes with optic nerve	Skin from the abdomen
Femur with articular surface	Spinal cord (usually at least three levels)
Gallbladder	Spleen
Heart	Thymus
Large intestine (including cecum and colon)	Thyroid and parathyroid (when in same section)
Testes (males)	Tongue
Small intestine (including duodenum, jejunum, and ileum)	Stomach (including cardia, fundus, and pylorus)
Kidneys	Trachea
Liver	Uterus (females)
Lungs with bronchi	Urinary bladder
Lymph nodes	Gross lesions
Lacrimal gland	Seminal vessels (males)
Mammary gland (females)	Vertebra
Ovaries (females)	Injection site (if appropriate)

collected at intervals and counted for total radioactivity. Commonly used intervals are 0–4, 4–8, 8–12, 12–24, and then daily, up to 168 hours or until more than 95% of the administered dose has been excreted by the kidney, liver, or lung. Depending on the pharmacokinetic profile of the candidate, other collection intervals can be selected to give a better picture of the excretion profile. For tissue distribution, a radiolabeled compound is administered to the test species, and after predefined times, usually 2, 4, 8, 24, and 48 hours, the test species is sacrificed, and tissues are collected, processed, and counted for total radioactivity. The tissues commonly evaluated are similar to those collected during necropsy in toxicology studies (listed in Table 1) plus the carcass. A routine aspect of most tissue distribution studies, in fact a technique that is being used by many pharmaceutical companies to replace tissue distribution studies, is quantitative whole body autoradiography (QWBA). Recent advances in QWBA allow this technique to quantify low levels of radioactivity in tissues and to even determine the radioactivity levels in substructures of tissues. Some researchers think that QWBA should (will) completely replace the classic tissue distribution study to profile the organs and systems that are exposed to and may accumulate the drug candidate and its metabolites.

These preclinical drug metabolism studies may also include metabolite profiling in plasma, selected tissues, urine, and bile to assess the distribution and disposition of potentially important metabolites, such as those having a level 5% or greater relative to the parent compound. Metabolite profiling requires a technique to separate the parent compound from its metabolites and other endogenous compounds. For small organic molecules, HPLC is usually the method of choice. For macromolecules, gel or capillary electrophoresis techniques can be defined with sufficient resolution capability to separate the compounds. Those metabolites representing more than 5% of the parent compound are usually identified with such techniques as mass spectrometry and nuclear magnetic spectroscopy. After identification, those metabolites that might elicit a pharmacological or toxicological response can be synthesized and tested in appropriate animal models. Many novel drugs have been discovered during metabolite characterization of drug candidates. These new compounds may have attributes, such as better extent of delivery, longer or shorter disposition kinetics, less potential for accumulation, better clearance properties, or less toxicity, that make them better drug candidates than the parent compound.

Toxicology

Before human clinical trials can be initiated, a number of toxicology studies need to be completed and documented in the IND submission. In addition to the studies listed above for toxicology developability assessment, preclinical toxicology studies include local tolerance, genotoxicity, safety pharmacology, and subchronic toxicology tests.

One of the most troublesome aspects in interpretation of toxicology results is determining whether these data are predictive of safety in humans. Often, animal toxicology may not correlate with human safety because the observed adverse effects are species specific. For example, HMG-CoA reductase inhibitors induce cataracts, potentially a drug-candidate–killing effect, in beagle dogs but not in rats or monkeys. Human clinical use of these therapeutic agents also has not shown this adverse experience, suggesting that the beagle dog is susceptible to this problem but other species are probably not. Species specificity is sometimes discovered early in the development of a drug candidate, such as the drug developability phase discussed earlier, and can be used to design the early human trials to ascertain if humans also manifest the observed toxicity.

Local Tolerance

An ICH guideline (5) indicates that local tolerance evaluations are to be conducted in animals using the route of administration proposed for human clinical testing and that these evaluations are to be performed before human exposure. The assessment of local tolerance may be part of other toxicity studies, such as acute and subchronic toxicology studies in rodents and nonrodents.

Genotoxicity

Registration for marketing of pharmaceuticals requires an assessment of the drug candidate's genotoxic potential. An revised ICH guideline (6) has been issued for genotoxic testing, which includes in vitro and in vivo studies that are designed to determine if a compound induces genetic damage either directly or indirectly and by any of a number of mechanisms. Positive genotoxic compounds have the potential of being human carcinogens or mutagens, that is, these drug candidates may induce cancer or heritable defects.

Three tests are recommended to evaluate the genotoxicity potential of a drug candidate: (a) a test for gene mutation in bacteria (the Ames test); (b) an in vitro cytogenetic evaluation of chromosomal damage by use of mammalian cells, such as human lymphoblastoid TK6, CHO, V79, and AS52 cells, or an in vitro mouse lymphoma L5178Y cell line tk assay; and (c) an in vivo study for chromosomal damage in rodent hematopoietic cells. Drug candidates that give negative results in these three tests are usually considered to have demonstrated an absence of genotoxic activity. Depending on the proposed therapeutic use, positive compounds may need to be, probably should be, tested more extensively.

Safety Pharmacology

Safety pharmacology involves assessing the effects of a drug candidate for pharmacological activity on the functions of various organ systems other than the target organ or tissue system. Normally the organ systems that are evaluated are the cardiovascular, central nervous, and respiratory systems. Depending on the physical and chemical characteristics of the candidate and the route of administration, other systems to be evaluated include the renal/urinary, autonomic nervous, and gastrointestinal systems. Safety pharmacology studies on a drug candidate need to be conducted (7) before human exposure and may be additions to other toxicology studies or separate studies. Many companies include some safety pharmacology assessments as part of subchronic toxicology studies. These assessments may include, but are not limited to, ECG or other cardiovascular parameters, neurological behavior, and ophthalmology. If the results suggest potential changes in these organ systems, more detailed safety pharmacology studies are necessary to further define and characterize the potential adverse effects. Of particular concern are changes in cardiovascular parameters, such as QT interval prolongation. When QT interval prolongation is present in animals, companies will need to conduct special clinical trials to further explore this adverse effect in humans.

Subchronic Toxicology

The FDA and most other regulatory agencies require subchronic toxicity studies in two species, one of which is a nonrodent, before human clinical trials are initiated. The recommended duration of the subchronic toxicity studies is related to duration of exposure during the proposed clinical trials. An ICH guideline (5) suggests the minimum duration of toxicity studies, shown in Table 2, needed to support phase 1, 2, and 3 clinical trials in which humans are to be exposed to the drug candidate for varying durations.

The two most common species used in subchronic toxicology studies are the rat and the dog. The most common strain of rat used within the pharmaceutical and biotechnology industries is the Charles River CD rat, which is Sprague-Dawley

TABLE 2 Duration of Multiple Dose Toxicology Studies Needed to Support Phase 1, 2, and 3 Clinical Trials

	Minimum duration of toxicity study	
Duration of clinical trial	Rodents	Nonrodents
Single dose	2–4 wk[a]	2 wk
Up to 2 wk	2–4 wk[a]	2 wk
Up to 1 mo	1 mo	1 mo
Up to 3 mo	3 mo	3 mo
Up to 6 mo	6 mo	6 mo
Greater than 6 mo	6 mo	Chronic

Note: Support for phase 3 clinical trails in Europe and for marketing in all regions required longer minimum duration toxicology studies than those listed in the table.
[a] In Europe and the United States, 2-week studies are the minimum duration. In Japan, 2-week nonrodent and 4-week rodent studies are needed.

derived and an outbred strain. Some companies use the Fisher 244 albino rat, which is an inbred strain, because this strain does not grow as large as the Charles River CD rat. Other rodent species sometimes used for subchronic toxicity include the mouse and the hamster. The beagle dog, purebred and specifically bred for research, is the most common nonrodent species used in toxicology assessments. Cynomolgus and rhesus monkeys are also used as the nonrodent toxicology species, primarily by the biotechnology industry developing macromolecule therapeutics but also more and more frequently by pharmaceutical firms evaluating NCEs. The rabbit, which is commonly one of the species used in reproduction toxicology evaluations, has also been used as the nonrodent species for subchronic testing. For drug candidates to be administered dermally, the mini-pig is commonly employed as the skin of this animal species is similar to that of humans and thus provides a similar rate and extent of transport of a drug candidate across the skin.

During the past few years, significant advances have been made for effective dosing regimens of animals in toxicology studies. The most common route of administration for human therapy is oral, usually as tablets or capsules. Other routes include intravenous, pulmonary, dermal, subcutaneous, intramuscular, rectal, nasal, and buccal. Whatever the proposed route of administration for humans, the preclinical animal toxicology studies should use the same route of delivery and frequency of dosing (once a day or qd, twice a day or bid, three times a day or tid, or once a week as may be necessary for some macromolecules). For rodents, oral dosing of tablets or capsules is not usually possible but daily, or more frequent, oral gavage dosing as a solution or a suspension is a now standard technique. For larger species, the tablets or capsules can be placed in soft gelatin capsules and dosed. Present-day technology allows continuous infusion of both rodent and nonrodent species for evaluation of drug candidates to be administered as intravenous infusions. For other routes of administration (especially pulmonary, nasal, and dermal) special techniques and drug candidate formulations may be necessary to ensure that the test species is appropriately exposed to the test article.

Whenever possible, the proposed clinical formulation should be used in preclinical toxicology evaluations, because formulation excipients can be important in the extent and duration of delivery (which is frequently correlated with the dissolution profile of the solid dosage form) and in local tolerance. For oral dosing to rodents, the solid clinical formulation can be ground and the appropriate amount dissolved or suspended in water or other vehicle prior to gavaging. The most common dosing volume for rodents is 10 mL/kg but other volumes can be used. The volume administered should be uniform for all dose groups, including the vehicle control group.

For rodent subchronic studies, 10 to 25 animals/sex/group are used, with the smaller groups used for shorter (2–4 weeks) studies and the larger groups for longer-term (more than 13 weeks) studies. If an interim sacrifice or a reversibility phase, which is a drug-free recovery phase of two or four weeks or possibly longer, is incorporated into the study design, an extra 10 animals/sex are commonly added to each dose group, including the vehicle control group. For nonrodent subchronic studies, the number of animals/sex/group is usually three to six, depending on the length of the study, the expected toxicology profile, and the recovery phase.

Dose selection for subchronic and chronic toxicology studies should be based on the results from acute toxicity studies, dose-range finding studies, and pharmacokinetic evaluations. The three typical dose levels are (a) a no-toxic-effect level or

NOAEL, which should be at least equivalent to, and hopefully a multiple of, the proposed human dose (after conversion to the human equivalent dose or HED for that species); (b) a dose level that produces a significant toxic effect in clinical observations, clinical chemistry and hematology parameters, clinical pathology (including organ weight and gross pathology), or histopathological changes; and (c) a dose level between these two. The high dose level should be sufficient to identify the major organs of toxicity and to identify the toxicological effects in those organs. Whenever possible, the toxic effects in organs should be compared and correlated with changes in clinical chemistry and hematology parameters in order to identify potential markers for toxicity for monitoring during clinical trials on a drug candidate.

Formulation Analyses

Analyses of formulations for a drug candidate content are conducted to ensure that doses administered to animals in toxicology, pharmacokinetic, and drug metabolism studies have the proper amount of the drug candidate. Before these analyses are performed, a stability-indicating analytical method that can quantify the drug candidate in the formulation needs to be defined and validated (8) for sensitivity, linearity, precision, accuracy, and robustness. If the dosing formulation is changed between studies, revalidation of the analytical method for application to the new formulation is necessary.

For acute toxicity, single-dose pharmacokinetic and single-dose drug metabolism studies, formulations for each dose level, including the vehicle control, are commonly analyzed before and after administration. If no apparent change in the drug candidate content is detected, the animals are assured to have been dosed with the appropriate amount of the compound. For subchronic and chronic studies, including carcinogenicity studies, and multiple-dose pharmacokinetic and drug metabolism experiments, formulations for each dose level are analyzed for drug candidate content before the first dose, at predefined times during the course of the study, and after the last dose. If the length of the study requires that the formulations be prepared periodically, such as once a week or every other week, content analyses need to be performed on some of the new formulations to ensure that the method of preparation provides a uniform drug candidate content. If the drug content in a formulation drops below or is above a predefined acceptance criteria (usually a range of 95–105% is considered acceptable), that formulation should not be used for dosing animals.

Toxicokinetics

For many years, the dose levels of a drug candidate administered to the test species in the various dose groups of a toxicology study were used to correlate the observed toxic effects with the drug candidate and to show that the effects increased with increasing dose. The administered dose levels were assumed to predict, and be proportional to, the amount of drug candidate that was in the body. However, for drug candidates that are poorly absorbed, have variable rate and extent of absorption, or show saturable absorption as the dose level increases, the administered dose has been shown not to be a uniform predictor of toxicity. Ensuring that test species have an increased exposure to the drug candidate, as the dose levels increase, has become a critical, and now standard, aspect of toxicology studies. Equally important is determining that the extent and duration of exposure are or are not changed after multiple-dose administration and that male and female animals are or are not exposed to similar levels of the drug candidate. An ICH guideline (9) describes the generation of toxicokinetic data to support the development of a drug candidate. The objectives of toxicokinetics include:

1. Describing the systemic exposure in each of the test species used in toxicology studies and showing how exposure relates to dose level and the time course of the study.
2. Correlating the extent of exposure with toxicological findings and contributing to the assessment of these findings to clinical safety.
3. Supporting the choice of test species and treatment regimen for nonclinical toxicology studies.
4. Along with toxicity results, providing information on the appropriate design for subsequent nonclinical toxicity studies and human clinical trials.

Toxicokinetic data, considered an integral part of a nonclinical program, can be obtained from the test species in a toxicology study or in specially designed supportive studies. The primary focus of toxicokinetic data is to assist in the interpretation of toxicity results and not for characterizing the basic pharmacokinetic parameters of the drug candidate being studied. Not all toxicology studies need to include a toxicokinetic component but most do have. If the extent and duration of exposure of a drug candidate in a particular formulation for a given test species have been generated for the dose level range to be used in a toxicity study, additional toxicokinetic evaluations may not be necessary. Toxicology studies, which are usefully supported by toxicokinetics, include single-dose studies for which results from preliminary pharmacokinetic studies may be applicable; multiple-dose studies, in which toxicokinetic data may predict whether multiple-dose pharmacokinetic studies are necessary; reproductive studies, which may use different test species that have an altered absorption and disposition profile due to pregnancy; and carcinogenicity studies, in which the test species may be dosed differently compared to other toxicology studies and changes in exposure can occur because of age.

Hematology, Clinical Chemistry, and Histopathology

Three important aspects for detecting and understanding the adverse effects observed during a toxicology study are hematology and clinical chemistry assays and histopathology evaluation of tissues collected at necropsy. Hematology parameters commonly evaluated include those listed in Table 3. These parameters should be determined periodically during the toxicity study, with the number of

TABLE 3 Hematology Parameters Evaluated During Toxicology Studies

Parameter	Abbreviation
White blood cell count	WBC
Red blood cell count	RBC
Hemoglobin concentration	HGB
Hematocrit	HCT
Mean corpuscular volume	MCV
Mean corpuscular hemoglobin	MCH
Mean corpuscular hemoglobin concentration	MCHC
Platelet count	PLT
Prothrombin time	PT
Activated partial thromboplastin time	aPTT

TABLE 4 Clinical Chemistry Parameters Evaluated During
Toxicology Studies

Parameter	Abbreviation
Total protein	TP
Triglycerides	TRI
Albumin	Alb
Globulin	Glob
Albumin/globulin ratio	A/G
Glucose	GLU
Cholesterol	CHOL
Total bilirubin	TBILI
Urea nitrogen	BUN
Creatinine	CREAT
Creatine phosphokinase	CPK
Alanine aminotransferase	ALT
Aspartate aminotransferase	AST
Alanine phosphatase	ALK
Gamma-glutamyltransferase	GGT
Lactate dehydrogenase	LDH
Calcium	Ca
Phosphorus	Phos
Sodium	Na
Potassium	K
Chloride	Cl

evaluations depending on the length of the study. Clinical chemistries routinely determined include those listed in Table 4. Urinalysis may also be performed but is usually limited to nonrodents and should include microscopic examination of sediment. Pretreatment clinical chemistry analyses and the number of determinations per group should be the same as for hematology. Depending on the pharmacology and toxicology profile of a drug candidate, other biological marker analyses can be included in addition to hematology and clinical chemistry evaluations. Results from these additional tests can provide information on physiological parameter changes caused by the drug candidate in animal models and may be used to evaluate pharmacological and toxicological effects during human clinical studies.

Tissues collected at necropsy and prepared for histopathological evaluation include those previously listed in Table 1. Routine sectioning and examination are recommended for all tissues from rodent and nonrodent animals used in subchronic and chronic studies. Requirements for special histopathology examination depend on adverse effects that are indicated by in-life clinical observations changes and are usually on a case-by-case basis. Electron microscopy (EM) is a useful extension of light microscopic evaluation in determining morphological alteration of cellular structures not otherwise clearly visualized. Selected specimens can be processed for EM examination when use of this technique is justified. The application of EM to all tissues is considered impractical and unnecessary.

Immunogenicity
Many proteins, polypeptides, oligonucleotides, and other large molecules are immunogenic and/or immunotoxic in the animal models used in pharmacology and toxicology evaluations. According to an ICH guideline (10), the potential for

antibody formation should be determined during the conduct of subchronic toxicology studies to aid in the interpretation of results from these and later studies. Antibodies that are formed are characterized as to titer, number of responding animals, neutralizing or nonneutralizing, change in pharmacological or toxicological response, complement activation, and immune complex formation and deposition. If the observed immune response neutralizes the pharmacological or toxicological effects of the drug candidate, modification of the study design may be warranted. Because the induction of antibody formation in animal models is not predictive of a similar response in humans, no special significance to animal antibody formation should be ascribed unless the interpretation of results from pharmacology or safety studies is compromised. However, if antibodies are formed during animal studies, the potential for antibody formation in humans should be assessed during early clinical development to ensure that antibodies will not adversely affect the pharmacological profile and do not increase the potential toxicity of the drug candidate in humans. Similarly, the potential of a macromolecule drug candidate to be immunotoxic needs to be assessed during toxicology studies. A drug candidate that produces immunotoxicity in animals will usually also show some immunotoxicity in humans.

NONCLINICAL DRUG DEVELOPMENT
After a drug candidate enters into human clinical testing, information on the pharmacokinetics and toxicology of the compound in the relevant species (humans) finally becomes available. The results from pharmacology, developability, and preclinical drug development experiments should be re-evaluated in light of this new information to ascertain if the animal models were predictive of the efficacy, safety, and pharmacokinetics in humans. If the animal results are extrapolative to humans, the remaining nonclinical animal studies are fairly straightforward and are conducted to provide supportive information on the safety of the drug candidate. However, if the early animal data do not extrapolate to the human situation, additional animal experiments should be designed and conducted to better and more fully understand the observed pharmacology and toxicology in humans. Considering the expense in both time and money to conduct nonclinical drug development studies, most pharmaceutical and biotechnology companies meet with the appropriate regulatory agencies to discuss the study designs and protocols and how dose levels were selected to avoid nonacceptance of regulatory agency submissions later on.

Pharmacokinetics
Unless justified from pharmacokinetic results from humans, only a few types of additional animal pharmacokinetic studies are conducted during nonclinical development. Types of animal pharmacokinetics that might be performed include:

1. Multiple-dose pharmacokinetics to assess accumulation or changes in clearance caused by enzyme induction or inhibition.
2. Bioavailability comparison when the formulation used in early toxicology or human studies is changed to alter the delivery profile of the drug candidate.
3. Drug candidate metabolite distribution and disposition evaluations.
4. Effect of food and time of feeding on the extent and duration of absorption.
5. Drug–drug interaction if the animal model is considered predictive of humans.

Drug Metabolism

After initiation of human clinical studies, drug metabolism studies are continued to build the database to show that the results from the animal models used to demonstrate the pharmacology and toxicology of the drug candidate can be extrapolated to the human situation. The most common drug metabolism studies conducted during nonclinical drug development are single-dose and/or multiple-dose tissue distribution, additional characterization and evaluation of metabolites, and studies such as fetal-placental transfer and lacteal secretion, which are designed to support reproductive and developmental toxicology evaluations.

Although most regulatory agencies agree that a single-dose tissue distribution study in rodents is needed to support the development of a drug candidate, and that this study often provides sufficient data on the distribution of the compound, a multiple-dose tissue distribution study may yield additional information (11). This study, for which no consistent requirement currently exists, may be appropriate when:

1. The apparent half-life of the drug candidate or a metabolite in organs or tissues significantly exceeds the apparent terminal disposition half-life in plasma and is more than twice the dosing interval in toxicity studies.
2. When the steady-state concentrations of the drug candidate or a metabolite in systemic circulation, usually first detected from toxicokinetic results from multiple-dose toxicology studies, are substantially higher than predicted from single-dose pharmacokinetic studies.
3. When the drug candidate is being developed for site-specific targeted delivery.
4. When histopathology changes that were not predicted from shorter-term toxicology studies, single-dose tissue distribution studies, or pharmacology studies are observed.

The study design for multiple-dose tissue distribution studies is usually compound and result specific and thus is determined on a case-by-case basis.

Reproductive and developmental toxicology studies are conducted to reveal the effect of the drug candidate on mammalian reproduction and whether potential reproductive risks may exist for humans. These reproductive studies commonly use pregnant rats and rabbits as the test species. To ensure that the dams and the fetuses are appropriately exposed to the drug candidate and metabolites (12), the dams can be dosed with radiolabeled compound and the amount of radioactivity that crosses the placenta and into the fetuses at various times after dosing determined. If little or no radioactivity is detected in the fetuses, then the ability of animal reproductive studies to predict risks in humans has to be questioned in humans, because humans may have a different delivery profile compared to that observed in animal models. Similarly, the exposure of the drug candidate to nursing pups can be ascertained after the dam is dosed with radiolabeled compound and the amount of radioactivity excreted in the milk is determined. If little or no radioactivity is detected in the dam's milk, then potential risk to nursing humans cannot be ascertained. When reproductive toxicology studies show no apparent effect, fetal-placenta transfer and lacteal secretion studies can be used to certify these findings and demonstrate that the animals were appropriately exposed to the drug candidate.

Toxicology
Chronic Studies
Regulatory agencies require chronic toxicity studies in two species, one of which is a nonrodent, for drug candidates that are to be administered to humans for more than three months (13). The two basic reasons for conducting chronic studies are to produce a toxic effect and to define a safety factor. The study should provide a dose–response relationship to effects resulting from prolonged exposure to the drug candidate and should reveal adverse effects that require a long exposure to be expressed or that are cumulative.

Chronic studies often can be conducted in species whose metabolism is most similar to that of humans, because early human evaluations most likely have been completed before these chronic studies are initiated. The rat is the most common rodent species used in chronic studies, whereas the beagle dog and nonhuman primates are the usual nonrodent species. The dog, a carnivore, often metabolizes compounds differently from humans and should be used with caution. However, nonhuman primates have not been shown to have metabolic systems any closer to humans than most other laboratory animals. Monkeys are the preferred species for macromolecules because they are similar to humans in anatomy and physiology.

The duration for chronic toxicology studies depends on the projected duration of administration to humans (Table 2). The present consensus according to an ICH guideline (5) and usually acceptable to the FDA is that six-month rodent and nine-month nonrodent studies are sufficient for drug candidates intended for long-term human use, provided the candidate is studied in rats, or other appropriate species, to evaluate the potential for tumor production, that is, a carcinogenicity study.

Dose selection for chronic studies is very important, because regulatory agencies want one dose to be the NOAEL and another to show frank toxicity. Several approaches are available to select doses, as described in the section on carcinogenicity studies. However, the most common approach historically has been to use the MTD as the high-dose level for chronic toxicology studies. The MTD has been defined as the dose that, at a minimum, suppresses body weight gain by approximately 10%. The mid- and low-dose levels are based on the MTD and have usually been one quarter of the MTD for the mid-dose and one-eighth of the MTD for the low dose. Using this approach, the low dose (based on HED equivalents) may be substantially above, but could even be below, the expected human therapeutic dose.

Reproductive and Developmental Toxicology
Reproductive and developmental toxicology studies are designed and conducted to reveal any effect of a drug candidate or a metabolite on mammalian reproduction and to ascertain the potential risks to humans. These studies evaluate male and female fertility, embryo and fetal death, parturition and the newborn, the lactation process, care of the young, and the potential teratogenicity of the drug candidate. Historically, these reproductive parameters have been evaluated in three types of studies, generally referred to as segment I, segment II, and segment III. Segment I evaluates fertility and general reproductive performance in rats. Segment II, commonly conducted in rats and rabbits, determines the embryo toxicity or teratogenic effects of the drug candidate. Segment III, designated the perinatal and postnatal study and normally conducted only in rats, assesses the effects of the drug candidate on late fetal development, labor and delivery, lactation, neonatal viability, and

growth of the newborn to sexual maturity. Other rodents and nonrodent species, such as mice, guinea pigs, mini-pigs, ferrets, hamsters, dogs, and nonhuman primates, have been used to evaluate the reproductive toxicity of drug candidates.

According to an ICH guideline (12), the combination of studies selected needs to allow exposure of mature adults and all stages of development from conception to sexual maturity to conception in the following generation. This integrated sequence has been subdivided into various stages, which are designated (A) premating to conception, (B) conception to implantation, (C) implantation to closure of the hard palate, (D) closure of the hard palate to the end of pregnancy, (E) birth to weaning, and (F) weaning to sexual maturity. Using these designations, segment I evaluates stages A and B of the reproductive process, segment II studies stages C and D, and segment III detects adverse effects during stages C to F. A common practice is to combine segments I and III into a single study and conduct separate segment II studies in rats and rabbits.

Segment I studies, designed to evaluate fertility and general reproductive performance (stages A and B), use sexually mature male and female rats. Male fertility is determined by premating dosing of at least four weeks and with dosing continuing throughout the mating period. Histopathology of the testes and sperm analysis is used to detect effects on spermatogenesis (12). Female fertility is determined by premating dosing of at least 14 days with dosing continuing during the mating period. A mating ratio of 1 to 1 is recommended, and documentation should allow identification of both parents of a litter. Copulation is evaluated daily by vaginal smears or by observation of the copulatory plug. Day 0 of gestation is when proof of copulation is discovered. Half of the females are sacrificed at a point after mid-pregnancy, usually day 13 of gestation, and are examined for the number and distribution of embryos in each uterine horn, embryos undergoing resorption, and the presence of empty implantation sites. Males are sacrificed at any time after mating and assurance of successful induction of pregnancy. The other half of the females are allowed to deliver normally and the litter size, number per litter alive or dead, and any abnormal observations during gross examination are noted.

Segment II, or teratology, studies are designed to ascertain if a drug candidate has potential for embryotoxicity or teratogenic effects (stages C and D) and are conducted in a rodent and nonrodent species. The drug candidate is administered during the period of organogenesis, which is usually considered gestation day 6 to 15 for mice and rats and gestation day 6 to 18 for rabbits. Fetuses are delivered by Cesarean section a day or two before anticipated parturition. For rats, half of the fetuses are examined for visceral alterations and the other half are evaluated for skeletal abnormalities. For rabbits, microdissection techniques for soft tissue alterations allow all of the fetuses to be examined for both soft tissue and skeletal abnormalities.

Segment III studies are usually conducted only in rats and are designed to evaluate effects on perinatal and postnatal development of pups and on maternal function (stages C to F). The drug candidate is administered to the dams from implantation to the end of lactation (stages C to E). At the time of weaning, normally one male and one female offspring per litter are selected for rearing to adulthood and mating to assess reproductive competence. These offspring can also be evaluated by use of behavioral and other functional tests for the study of physical development, sensory functions and reflexes, and behavior. The dams and other pups are sacrificed at the time of weaning and evaluated histopathologically.

As with most toxicology studies, three dose levels and a vehicle control group are recommended for reproductive studies. Commonly, a dose-range–finding study, which can incorporate toxicokinetic evaluation, is conducted in pregnant animals, which may be more susceptible to toxic effects, to define the dose levels, one of which should produce frank signs of toxicity and another that should be a no-toxic-effect dose. As noted earlier, drug metabolism studies are sometimes conducted to demonstrate that the dams and the fetuses have been appropriately exposed to the drug candidate and metabolites.

Carcinogenicity
Carcinogenicity studies encompass most of the test species' life span and are designed to measure tumor induction in animals and to assess the relevant risk in humans (14). These studies are normally conducted concurrently with phase 3 human clinical trials and are required by regulatory agencies when human exposure to a drug candidate is anticipated to be more than six months. For drug candidates being developed to treat certain life-threatening diseases, carcinogenicity studies may be concluded after marketing approval but should be started during human clinical testing. Carcinogenicity studies should be initiated earlier in the drug development process when

1. the drug candidate or a known metabolite is structurally related to a known carcinogen.
2. a special aspect of the drug candidate's biological action (e.g., members of the therapeutic class have shown a positive carcinogenic response) causes concern.
3. the drug candidate produces toxicities in early studies that are indicative of pre-neoplastic changes.
4. the drug candidate or a metabolite shows evidence of accumulation in organ systems.
5. mutagenicity tests suggest that the drug candidate may be a potential carcinogen.

Some companies combine chronic toxicity and carcinogenicity studies in the rat by appropriately increasing the sizes of each dose group but this approach is not recommended.

Mice and rats, with life spans of approximately 18 and 24 months, respectively, are normally used in carcinogenicity studies because of economy of these species, their susceptibility to tumor induction, and the large database available on their physiology and pathology. If other nonclinical or clinical results suggest that the rodent is an inappropriate model, carcinogenicity studies in other species, such as the dog for the development of birth control drugs, can be conducted. An ICH guideline (15) suggests that one rodent (usually the rat) carcinogenicity study plus one other study, commonly a study in a transgenic mouse model such as the p53+/− deficient model, may be sufficient to ascertain the carcinogenicity potential of a drug candidate.

When feasible, the route of exposure in the test species should be the same as the clinical route of administration. An alternative route may be used if this route gives similar metabolism and systemic exposure, particularly to relevant organs, such as the lung for inhalation agents, as the clinical route. Supportive drug metabolism and toxicokinetic data are generally required for selection of an alternative route of administration.

Standard carcinogenicity studies are generally inappropriate for biotechnology-derived pharmaceuticals (10). Macromolecules, unless they are endogenous substances used as replacement therapy, may need to be evaluated for carcinogenic potential if indicated by treatment duration, clinical indication, and patient population. A variety of approaches, such as the ability to support or induce proliferation of transformed cells or to simulate growth of normal or malignant cells expressing a receptor for the drug candidate, can be used to assess risk and are usually compound specific. The study designs and protocols to evaluate carcinogenicity potential of macromolecules should be discussed with the appropriate regulatory agencies before the evaluations are initiated.

Dose selection for carcinogenicity studies has been a topic of discussion for many years. According to an ICH guideline (16), the selected doses (a) should provide a test species exposure to the drug candidate that allows an adequate margin of safety over the human therapeutic exposure, (b) are tolerated without significant chronic physiological function impairment and are compatible with good survival, (c) are guided by a comprehensive set of animal and human data that focus on the properties of the drug candidate and the suitability of the test species, and (d) permit data interpretation in the context of proposed clinical use. In all cases, appropriate dose-ranging studies, usually of 90-day duration, need to be conducted.

The approaches that may be appropriate and are acceptable for dose selection include toxicity-based endpoints such as the MTD, pharmacokinetic endpoints, saturation of absorption, pharmacodynamic endpoints, maximum feasible dose, and additional scientifically defensible endpoints. For toxicity-based endpoints, general study design characteristics to establish the MTD include that:

1. The rodent species/strains with metabolic profiles as similar as possible to that of humans should be used.
2. Dose-ranging studies should be conducted for both males and females for all strains and species to be tested in the carcinogenicity bioassay.
3. Dose selection is generally determined from 90-day studies with the route and method of administration that will be used in the bioassay.
4. Selection of an appropriate dosing schedule and regimen should be based on clinical use and exposure patterns, pharmacokinetics, and practical considerations.
5. Both the toxicity profile and any dose-limiting toxicity should be characterized, with consideration given to the occurrence of preneoplastic lesions or tissue-specific proliferative effects and disturbances in endocrine homeostasis.
6. Changes in metabolite profile or alterations in metabolizing enzyme activities (induction or inhibition) over time should be understood to allow for appropriate interpretation of results from the studies.

Systemic exposure of the drug candidate in the test species that represents a large multiple of human exposure, based on the area under the plasma concentration versus time curve (AUC), at the maximum proposed human daily dose may be used for carcinogenicity study dose selection. The AUC is the most comprehensive pharmacokinetic endpoint, because this value includes both the plasma concentrations of the drug candidate and the residence time in vivo. For pharmacokinetic endpoints to be used for dose selection, the information needed to establish the recommended 25-fold ratio of rodent to human normalized (using mg/m^2 dose levels or HED equivalents) AUC include that:

1. Rodent pharmacokinetic data are derived with the use of the test species strains, the route of administration, and dose ranges planned for the carcinogenicity study.
2. BAC methods, which have been appropriately validated, are used to determine plasma concentrations of the drug candidate in both rodents and humans.
3. Pharmacokinetic data are derived from studies of sufficient duration to take into account potential time-dependent changes in pharmacokinetic parameters, which may be detected from toxicokinetic results obtained during the 90-day dose-ranging studies.
4. Documentation is available on the similarity of metabolism between the test species and humans.
5. In the assessment of exposure, scientific judgment is used to determine whether the AUC comparison is based on data for the parent, parent and metabolite(s), or metabolite(s), and justification for the decision is provided.
6. Interspecies differences in protein binding are taken into consideration when relative exposure is estimated.
7. Human pharmacokinetic data are obtained from studies encompassing the maximum recommended human daily dose.

For saturation of absorption to be used for dose selection, information that the absorption process has been saturated using the intended route of administration is necessary. These data can usually be obtained during well-designed pharmacokinetic studies that evaluate linearity of absorption and dose proportionality using the route and frequency of dosing projected for human clinical studies.

The use of pharmacodynamic end points for high-dose selection is considered to be highly compound specific and is considered for individual study designs on the basis of scientific merit. The high dose should produce a pharmacodynamic response in the test species that precludes further dose escalation but does not produce disturbances of physiology or homeostasis that would compromise the validity of the carcinogenicity study. Examples of such pharmacodynamic endpoints include hypotension and inhibition of blood clotting.

The use of maximum feasible dose for dose selection is usually applicable only to studies using dietary administration of the drug candidate. When routes other than dietary administration are used, the high dose may be limited because of practicality and local tolerance. The use of pharmacokinetic endpoints for dose selection should significantly decrease the need to select the high dose for carcinogenicity studies based on feasibility criteria.

The mid and low doses for a carcinogenicity study are to provide information for assessing the relevance of the study findings to humans. The low dose (in HED equivalents) should be equal to, or a multiple of, the maximum dose proposed for human testing. The rationale for the selection of the low and mid dose needs to be provided on the basis of pharmacokinetic linearity and saturation of metabolic pathways, human exposure and therapeutic dose, pharmacodynamic response in the test species, alteration in the normal physiology of the test species, mechanistic information and the potential for threshold effects, and the unpredictability of toxicity progression observed in other toxicology studies.

CONCLUSION

This chapter has provided information on the nonclinical aspects of the drug development process. As described, the biological stages of nonclinical development normally proceed linearly (a) from drug discovery, when the pharmacology of a discovery lead is evaluated in in vitro systems and/or animal models to show that the compound has the potential to mediate a human disease, (b) to developability assessment, which provides preliminary data on the pharmacokinetics, drug delivery, and toxicology of the discovery lead to ascertain if the compound has the necessary attributes and without substantial demerits to enter the drug development process, (c) to preclinical evaluations, when the necessary drug safety studies are conducted to support the submission of an IND for a first-in-human clinical trial, and (d) finally to nonclinical studies, which extend information on the metabolism and toxicity of the drug candidate and show that the earlier animal studies are predictive of human pharmacological and toxicological responses. Careful design, conduct, and interpretation of the results from these nonclinical research experiments normally determine which discovery leads have the necessary attributes to become marketed human therapeutic products. These experiments can be used to "weed out" those candidates that have unacceptable pharmacology or toxicology profiles before, or shortly after, the initiation of human clinical testing, but definitely before the start of phase 3 clinical studies, which are the most expensive aspect of drug development in terms of both time and dollars (Fig. 1). If most, or at least many, of the estimated 999 out of 1000 "loser" candidates can be detected earlier in the drug development process and dropped from further evaluation, the precious time and resources needed to support clinical and nonclinical drug development studies can be devoted to drug candidates that have a greater potential of successfully completing the studies necessary for the submission of a marketing application or an NDA.

REFERENCES

1. Lakings DB. Making a successful transition from drug discovery to drug development, part 1. Biopharmaceutics 1995; 8(7):20–24.
2. Lakings DB. Making a successful transition from drug discovery to drug development, part 2. Biopharmaceutics 1995; 8(8):48–51.
3. FDA Guidance for Industry. Bioanalytical Method Validation, 2001.
4. Viswanathan CT, Bansal S, et al. Workshop/Conference Report—Quantitative Bioanalytical Methods Validation and Implementation: Best Practices for Chromatographic and Ligand Binding Assays. AAPS J 2007;9(1)Article 4:E30–E42.
5. ICH Harmonised Tripartite Guideline (M3[R2]). Nonclinical Safety Studies for the Conduct of Human Clinical Trials for Pharmaceuticals. www.ich.org.
6. ICH Harmonised Tripartite Guideline (S2 [R1]). Genotoxicity Testing and Data Interpretation for Pharmaceucticals Intended for Human Use. www.ich.org.
7. ICH Harmonised Tripartite Guideline (S7a). Safety Pharmacology Studies for Human Pharmaceuticals. www.ich.org.
8. ICH Harmonised Tripartite Guideline (Q2[R1]). Validation of Analytical Procedures: Text and Methodology. www.ich.org.
9. ICH Harmonised Tripartite Guideline (S3a). Note for Guidance on Toxicokinetics: The Assessment of Systemic Exposure in Toxicity Studies. www.ich.org.
10. ICH Harmonised Tripartite Guideline (S6). Preclinical Safety Evaluation of Biotechnology-Derived Pharmaceuticals. www.ich.org.

11. ICH Harmonised Tripartite Guideline (S3b). Pharmacokinetics: Guidance for Repeated Dose Tissue Distribution Studies. www.ich.org.
12. ICH Harmonised Tripartite Guideline (S5 [R2]). Detection of Toxicity to Reproduction for Medicinal Products. www.ich.org.
13. U.S. FDA's proposed implementation of ICH safety working group consensus regarding new drug applications. Federal Register 1992; 57 (73):13105–13106.
14. ICH Harmonised Tripartite Guideline (S1a). Guidelines on the Need for Carcinogenicity Studies of Pharmaceuticals. www.ich.org.
15. ICH Harmonised Tripartite Guideline (S1b). Testing for Carcinogenicity of Pharmaceuticals. www.ich.org.
16. ICH Harmonised Tripartite Guideline (S1c[R2]). Dose Selection for Carcinogenicity Studies of Pharmaceuticals. www.ich.org.

8

The Investigational New Drug Application (IND), the Investigational Medicinal Product Dossier (IMPD) and the Investigator's Brochure (IB)

Richard A. Guarino

Oxford Pharmaceutical Resources Inc., Totowa, New Jersey, U.S.A.

OVERVIEW

The Federal Food, Drug, and Cosmetic Act prohibits the shipment of a new drug into interstate commerce unless there exists an approved NDA or an effective IND application for that drug. In the European Union countries and countries that follow the EU Directives, the equivalent information that is required for a new product application is an effective Investigational Medicinal Product Dossier (IMPD). For those countries, which wish to conduct clinical research in the United States, an IND is required regardless of the proposed phase of clinical trial. Thus, even phase 1 trials to be conducted in the United States on volunteer subjects require the prior submission of an IND before that trial may be undertaken.

The requirements for the format and content of the IND application, as well as the requirements governing the use of the IND, are provided in Title 21 of the Code of Federal Regulations (21 CFR), Section 312. Unlike an NDA, the FDA does not formally "approve" an IND submission. If the FDA reviewers believe that the proposed clinical trial(s) submitted in the IND are acceptable from a safety and risk versus benefit viewpoint, the IND is in "effect," and the product that is the subject of that IND may be shipped in interstate commerce for the purpose of conducting specific clinical trials. Drugs shipped under an IND have specific labeling requirements, and false or misleading statements, as well as any claims regarding safety and efficacy, are prohibited. In countries requiring an IMPD, consisting of information on the quality and manufacturing of the investigational product, available toxicological and pharmacological studies and results from previous clinical trials or its use are considered as an authorized product. Some Member States (see chap. 24) may require different information on the history and development on the quality requirements.

This chapter will provide information that is necessary to achieve a successful IND submission to the FDA in the United States. It will focus on the differences between the requirements for an IND submitted to permit a phase 1 trial as contrasted to IND submissions intended to support phase 2 or 3 clinical research. It will also review the information available that should be included in an IMPD. Finally, detailed requirements for the investigator's brochure, the document that summarizes the known safety and efficacy information about the investigational product that will be submitted to potential investigators, IRBs/IECs, and as part of the IND/IMPD will be addressed.

THE INVESTIGATIONAL NEW DRUG APPLICATION

Introduction
An IND may be submitted to the FDA by a commercial organization (the "sponsor") or by a clinical investigator (often referred to as an Investigator IND). The sponsor or investigator may not commercially distribute or test market an investigational new drug, nor may an investigation be unduly prolonged after the finding that the results of the investigation appear to establish sufficient data to support a marketing application. Under certain defined circumstances described in 21 CFR Part 312.7, a sponsor may charge the patient for an investigational drug, but this is atypical and can be done only after written approval from the FDA.

General Information Regarding INDs
Exemptions
The clinical investigation of a drug product that is lawfully marketed in the United States is exempted from the requirements of an IND, providing all of the following apply: (a) the investigation is intended neither to be reported to the FDA as a well-controlled trial in support of a new indication for use nor to be used to support any other significant change in the labeling for the drug, (b) if the drug that is undergoing investigation is lawfully marketed as a prescription drug product, the investigation is not intended to support a significant change in the advertising for the product, (c) the investigation does not involve a route of administration nor dosage level or use in a patient population or other factor that significantly increases the risks (or decreases the acceptability of the risks) associated with the use of the drug product, and (d) the investigation is conducted in compliance with the requirements for IRB/IEC approval and the requirements for informed consent as discussed elsewhere in this book.

Labeling Requirements for an Investigational New Drug
Labeling for a drug covered by an IND will be discussed under the Chemistry, Manufacturing, and Control requirements for part 7 of the IND; however, independent of the use or indication for the drug and independent of the dosage form, all immediate packages of drug product supplied to a patient involved in an investigational trial require the following statement: "Caution: New Drug—Limited by Federal (or United States) law to investigational use." Additionally, the label or labeling (including the investigator's brochure) shall not bear any statement that is false or misleading to possibly represent the investigational new drug as being safe or effective for the purposes for which it is being investigated.

Waivers
In rare instances, the FDA may grant a waiver to the requirements for an IND on the basis of a justified request from the sponsor. Acceptable justification may include an explanation of why the sponsor's compliance is unnecessary or cannot be achieved or a description of an alternative means of satisfying the requirement. The FDA may grant such a request for a waiver if it determines that the sponsor's noncompliance would not pose a significant or unreasonable risk to the human test subjects.

Preconsultation Program

At this time, only one division within the Center for Drug Evaluation and Research, the Division of Antiviral Drug Products (DAVDP), has established a pre-IND consultation program. This program, established in 1988, is a proactive strategy designed to facilitate informal early communications between DAVDP and the potential sponsor of new therapeutics for the treatment of AIDS and life-threatening opportunistic infections, other viral infections, and soft tissue transplantations. Pre-IND advice may be requested for issues related to drug development plans, data needed to support the rationale for testing a drug in humans, the design of non-clinical pharmacology, toxicology, and drug-activity trials, data requirements for IND applications, and regulatory requirements for demonstrating safety and efficacy. Details on requesting information about this program or on how to participate in this preconsultation program may be found on the Internet.

For INDs to be submitted to other divisions, on the sponsor's request, the FDA will provide advice on specific matters relating to an IND. Examples may include advice on the adequacy of technical data to support an investigational plan, on the design of a clinical trial, and on whether proposed investigations are likely to produce the data and information needed to meet requirements for a marketing application. It should be noted, however, that unless the communication is accompanied by a clinical hold, FDA communications with a sponsor regarding pre-IND information is solely advisory and does not require any modification in the planned or ongoing clinical investigations or response to the agency.

Binders for IND Submissions

Presently the FDA has specific requirements for the type and color of binders in which an IND may be submitted. However, future IND submission format and binder requirements may change when and if the INDs will be required to be submitted in a CTD format. All INDs and IND amendments are submitted to FDA in triplicate. The original IND submission (copy 1) is to be submitted in a red binder, and copies 2 and 3 are submitted in green and orange binders, respectively. Effective April 1, 1998, sponsors may call the U.S. Government Printing Office (GPO) to order FDA IND, ANDA, and Drug Master File binders. The red binder is Form No. 2675, and the green and orange binders are Form No. 2675a and 2675b, respectively. The GPO may be contacted by telephone at (202) 512-1800 or by mail at U.S. Government Printing Office, Washington, D.C. 20404–0001. In either instance, reference should be made to Program #B511-S. Details on the required specifications for the FDA's binders may also be obtained from the Internet at http://www.fda.gov/cder/ddms/binders.htm.

Address for IND Submissions

An initial IND submission is to be sent in triplicate to the Central Document Room, Center for Drug Evaluation and Research, Food and Drug Administration, 5901-B Ammendale Road, Beltsville, MD 20705–1266. Upon receipt of the IND, the FDA will inform the sponsor which one of the divisions in the Center for Drug Evaluation and Research or the Center for Biologics Evaluation and Research is responsible for the IND.

Once the IND is in effect, amendments, reports, and other correspondence relating to matters covered by the IND should be directed to the appropriate division. The outside cover or cover letter of each submission should state what is contained in the submission, for example "IND Application," "Protocol Amendment," etc.

Specific address information relating to submission of applications for products subject to the licensing provisions of the Public Health Service Act of July 1, 1944, urokinase products, plasma volume expanders, coupled antibodies, and biological products that are also radioactive drugs are described in 21 CFR Part 312.140.

Availability for Public Disclosure of IND Data

The manner in which FDA handles requests for disclosure of information to the public under the Freedom of Information Act is described in 21 CFR Part 312.130. The existence of an IND will not be disclosed by the FDA unless it has previously been publicly disclosed or acknowledged by the sponsor. However, upon request, the FDA will disclose to an individual to whom an investigational new drug has been given a copy of any IND safety report relating to the use in the individual.

Phases of Clinical Investigations

As noted previously, the FDA has recently clarified the requirements for an IND intended for phase 1 clinical trials compared with trials that are designed for phase 2 or 3 clinical programs. Table 1 provides information regarding the differences between the phases of investigation with respect to the size and scope of the particular phase. A more detailed description of the phases of investigation may be found in 21 CFR Part 312.21.

Phase 1 includes the initial introduction of an investigational new drug into humans. These trials are typically closely monitored and may be conducted in patients or in normal volunteer subjects. They are designed to determine the metabolism and pharmacologic actions of the drug in humans and the side effects associated with increasing doses and sometimes to gain early evidence on effectiveness. The results of the phase 1 program concerning the drug's pharmacokinetic and pharmacologic effects will be obtained to permit the design of well-controlled and scientifically valid phase 2 trials.

Phase 2 includes the controlled clinical trials conducted to evaluate the appropriate dose-range and effectiveness and safety of the drug for a particular indication in patients with the disease or condition under trial and to determine the common short-term side effects and risks associated with the drug. Phase 2 trials are typically

TABLE 1 Phases of Clinical Investigation

Phase	No. of patients	Length	Purpose	% Of drugs successfully tested[a]
1	20–100	Several months	Mainly safety	70
2	100 Up to several hundred	Several months to 2 yr	Some short-term safety, dosage, and effectiveness	33
3	Several hundred to several thousand	1–4 yr	Safety, dosage, and effectiveness	25–30

[a]For example, of 100 drugs for which IND applications are submitted to the FDA, about 70% will successfully complete phase 1 trials and go on to phase 2; about 33% of the original 100 will complete phase 2 and go to phase 3; and 25% to 30% of the original 100 will clear phase 3 (and, on average, about 20% of the original 100 will ultimately be approved for marketing).

well controlled, closely monitored, and conducted in a relatively small number of patients, usually involving no more than 100 to 200 subjects.

Phase 3 programs comprise expanded controlled and uncontrolled trials. They are performed after preliminary evidence, suggesting that a knowledge of the proper dosage and effectiveness of the drug has been obtained, usually based on the results of the phase 2 trials and are intended to gather the additional information in large patient populations about effectiveness and safety needed to evaluate the overall benefit–risk relationship of the drug and to provide an adequate basis for physician labeling.

Phase 1
INDs for Phase 1 Trials

The FDA has recently assessed means to increase the efficiency of the drug development process without sacrificing the long-standing safety and efficacy standards expected by the public for their drug products to meet.

In November 1995, CDER and CBER issued a Guidance for Industry entitled, Content and Format of Investigational New Drug Applications for Phase 1 Trials of Drugs, Including Well-Characterized, Therapeutic, Biotechnology-Derived Products. This guidance clarified the requirements for data and data presentation related to the initial entry into human trials in the United States of an investigational drug, including well-characterized, therapeutic, biotechnology–derived products. The FDA emphasized that the IND regulations allowed a great deal of flexibility in the amount and depth of various data to be submitted in an IND, depending in large part on the phase of investigation and the specific human testing being proposed. In some cases, the extent of that flexibility had not been appreciated by industry. Thus, the guidance was developed to clarify many of the phase 1 IND requirements to help expedite entry of new drugs into clinical testing by increasing transparency and by reducing ambiguity, inconsistencies, and the amount of information submitted, while providing the FDA with the data it needs to assess the safety of the proposed phase 1 trial. According to the guidance, if the suggestions specified in the document are followed, typical IND submissions for phase 1 trials usually should not be larger than two to three 3-inch binders.

The most significant clarifications in the guidance document are (a) the explicit willingness of the FDA to accept an integrated summary report of toxicology findings based on the unaudited draft toxicologic reports of completed studies as initial support for human trials and (b) specific manufacturing data appropriate for a phase 1 investigation. Because of the manufacturing and toxicologic differences between well-characterized, therapeutic, biotechnology-derived products and other biologic products, the FDA emphasized that the guidance applies only to drugs and well-characterized, therapeutic, biotechnology-derived products. For products not covered by this phase 1 guidance, it is recommended that the center responsible for the product be contacted for specific information.

Requirements for Protocols

The regulation requires submission of a copy of the protocol for the conduct of each proposed clinical trial. However, the regulations were changed in 1987 specifically to allow phase 1 trial protocols to be less detailed and more flexible than protocols for phase 2 or 3 trials. This change recognized that these protocols are part of an early learning process and should be adaptable as information is obtained, and that the principal concern at this stage of development is that the trial be conducted for safety. The regulations state that phase 1 protocols should be directed primarily at providing an outline of the investigation: an estimate of the number of subjects to be included; a description of safety exclusions; and a description of the dosing plan, including duration, dose, or method to be used in determining dose. In addition, such protocols should specify in detail only those elements of the trial that are critical to subject safety, such as (a) necessary monitoring of vital signs and blood chemistries and (b) toxicity-based stopping or dose adjustment rules. The regulations also state that modifications of the experimental design of phase 1 trials that do not affect critical safety assessments are required to be reported to FDA only in the IND Annual Report.

Requirements for CMC Information

The IND regulations emphasize the graded nature of manufacturing and control information that is required to be submitted. Although in each phase of the investigation, sufficient information should be submitted to assure the proper identification, quality, purity, and strength of the investigational drug, the amount of information needed to make that assurance will vary with the phase of the investigation, the proposed duration of the investigation, the dosage form, and the amount of information otherwise available. For example, although stability data are required in all phases of the IND to demonstrate that the new drug substance and drug product are within acceptable chemical and physical limits for the planned duration of the proposed clinical investigation, if very short-term tests are proposed, the supporting stability data also can be very limited.

It is recognized that modifications to the method of preparation of the new drug substance and dosage form, and even changes in the dosage form, are likely as the investigation progresses. Emphasis in an initial phase 1 CMC submission should generally be placed on providing information that will allow evaluation of the safety of subjects in the proposed trial. The identification of a safety concern or insufficient data to make an evaluation of safety is the only basis for a clinical hold based on the CMC section.

Reasons for concern may include (a) a product made with unknown or impure components, (b) a product possessing chemical structures of known or highly likely toxicity, (c) a product that cannot remain chemically stable throughout the testing program proposed, (d) a product with an impurity profile indicative of a potential health hazard or an impurity profile insufficiently defined to assess a potential health hazard, or (e) a poorly characterized master or working cell bank.

In addition, for preclinical trials to be useful in assuring the safety of human trials, sponsors should be able to relate the drug product being proposed for use in a clinical trial to the drug product used in the animal toxicology trials that support the safety of the proposed human trial.

The following information will usually suffice for a meaningful review of the manufacturing procedures for drug products used in phase 1 clinical trials. As will be discussed later in this chapter, additional information should ordinarily be submitted for review of the larger-scale manufacturing procedures used to produce drug products for phase 2 or 3 clinical trials or as part of the manufacturing section of an NDA.

The CMC Section Introduction. At the beginning of this section, the sponsor should state whether it believes (a) the chemistry of either the drug substance or the drug product, or (b) the manufacturing of either the drug substance or the drug product presents any signals of potential human risk. If so, these signals of potential risks should be discussed. The steps proposed to monitor for such risk(s) should be described or the reason(s) why the signal(s) should be dismissed should be discussed. In addition, sponsors should describe any chemistry and manufacturing differences between the drug product proposed for clinical use and the drug product used in the animal toxicology studies that formed the basis for the sponsor's conclusion that it was safe to proceed with the proposed clinical trial. How these differences might affect the safety profile of the drug product should be discussed? If there are no differences in the products, that should be stated.

The Drug Substance. It should be noted that references to the current edition of the USP-NF may be used to satisfy some of the requirements of this section, when applicable. Information on the drug substance should be submitted in a summary report containing the following items:

1. *Description*: A brief description of the drug substance and some evidence to support its proposed chemical structure should be submitted. It is understood that the amount of structure information will be limited in the early stage of drug development.
2. *The name and address of its manufacturer*: The full street address of the manufacturer of the clinical trial drug substance should be submitted.
3. *Method of preparation*: A brief description of the manufacturing process, including a list of the reagents, solvents, and catalysts used, should be submitted. A detailed flow diagram is suggested as the usual, most effective presentation of this information. However, more information may be needed to assess the safety of biotechnology-derived drugs or drugs extracted from human or animal sources.
4. *Tests and analytical methods*: A brief description of the test methods used should be submitted. Proposed acceptable limits supported by simple analytical data (e.g., IR spectrum to prove the identity and HPLC chromatograms to support the purity level and impurities profile) of the clinical trials material should be provided. Submission of a copy of the certificate of analysis is also suggested. The specific methods will depend on the source and type of drug substance (e.g., animal source, plant extract, radiopharmaceutical, other biotechnology-derived products). Validation data and established specifications ordinarily need not be submitted at the initial stage of drug development. However, for some well-characterized, therapeutic, biotechnology-derived products, preliminary specifications and additional validation data may be needed in certain circumstances to ensure safety in phase 1.
5. *Stability data*: A brief description of the stability trial and the test methods used to monitor the stability of the drug substance should be submitted. Preliminary tabular data based on representative material may be submitted. Neither detailed stability data nor the stability protocol should be submitted.

The Drug Product. It should be noted that references to the current edition of the USP-NF may be used to satisfy some of the requirements of this section, when applicable. Information on the drug product should be submitted in a summary report containing the following items:

1. *A list of all components*: A list of usually no more than one or two pages of written information should be submitted. The quality (e.g., NF, ACS) of the inactive ingredients should be cited. For novel excipients, additional manufacturing information may be necessary.
2. *Quantitative composition*: A brief summary of the composition of the investigational new drug product should be submitted. In most cases, information on component ranges is not necessary.
3. *The name and address of the manufacturer*: The full street address(es) of the manufacturer(s) and packager of the clinical trial drug product should be submitted.
4. *Method of manufacturing and packaging*: A diagrammatic presentation and a brief written description of the manufacturing process should be submitted, including the sterilization process for sterile products. Flow diagrams are suggested as the usual, most effective presentations of this information.
5. *Acceptable limits and analytical methods*: A brief description of the proposed acceptable limits and the test methods used should be submitted. Tests that should be submitted will vary according to the dosage form. For example, for sterile products, sterility and nonpyrogenicity tests should be submitted. Submission of a copy of the certificate of analysis of the clinical batch is also suggested. Validation data and established specifications need not be submitted at the initial stage of drug development. For well-characterized, therapeutic, biotechnology-derived products, adequate assessment of bioactivity and preliminary specifications should be available.
6. *Stability testing*: A brief description of the stability trial and the test methods used to monitor the stability of the drug product packaged in the proposed container/closure system and storage conditions should be submitted. Preliminary tabular data based on representative material may be submitted. Neither detailed stability data nor the stability protocol needs to be submitted.
7. *Placebo*: If any placebo dosage form is to be used in the phase 1 trial, diagrammatic, tabular, and brief written information should be submitted.
8. *Labeling*: A mock-up or printed representation of the proposed labeling that will be provided to investigators in the proposed clinical trial should be submitted. Investigational labels must carry a "caution" statement as stated earlier. The required statement reads: "Caution: New Drug—Limited by Federal (or United States) law to investigational use."
9. *Environmental assessment*: The FDA believes that the great majority of products will qualify for a categorical exclusion. Sponsors who believe that their investigational product meets the exclusion categories under 21 CFR 25.24 should submit a statement certifying that their product meets the exclusion requirements and request a categorical exclusion on that basis. (For INDs submitted to CDER, it is recommended to review the FDA guidance entitled: *Guidance for Industry for the Submission of Environmental Assessments for Human Drug Applications and Supplements*, November, 1995.)

Pharmacology and Toxicology Information

Pharmacology and drug distribution: This section of the phase 1 IND should contain, if known, (a) a description of the pharmacologic effects and mechanism of action of the drug in animals and (b) information on the absorption, distribution, metabolism, and excretion of the drug. The regulations do not describe the presentation of these data. A summary report, without individual animal records or individual trial results, usually suffices. In most circumstances, five pages or less should be adequate for this summary. To the extent that such studies may be important to address safety issues or to assist in evaluation of toxicology data, they may be necessary; however, lack of this potential effectiveness information generally should not be a reason for a phase 1 IND to be placed on clinical hold.

Toxicology—integrated summary: The IND regulations require an integrated summary of the toxicologic effects of the drug in animals and in vitro. The particular trials needed depend on the nature of the drug and the phase of human investigation. The regulations are not specific due to the nature of the report of toxicology data needed in an IND submission and the nature of the trial reports upon which the report submitted to the IND is based. Also, the IND regulations are silent on whether the submitted material should be based on (a) "final, fully quality-assured" individual trial reports or (b) earlier, unaudited draft toxicologic reports of the completed trials. In the past, most sponsors have concluded that a submission based on final, fully quality-assured individual trial reports is required, and a substantial delay in submission of an IND for several months is often encountered to complete such final, fully quality-assured individual reports from the time the unaudited draft toxicologic reports of the completed trials are prepared.

Moreover, although the regulation does not specifically require individual toxicology study reports to be submitted, referring only to an integrated summary of the toxicologic findings, the requirement for a full tabulation of data from each trial suitable for detailed review has led most sponsors to provide detailed reports of each trial.

Although the GLP and quality assurance processes and principles are critical for the maintenance of a toxicology trial system that is valid and credible, it is unusual for findings in the unaudited draft toxicologic report of the completed trials to change during the production of the "final," quality-assured individual trial reports in ways important to determine whether use in humans is safe.

Therefore, for a phase 1 IND, if final, fully quality-assured individual trial reports are not available at the time of IND submission, an integrated summary report of toxicologic findings based on the unaudited draft toxicologic reports of the completed animal studies may be submitted. This integrated summary report should represent the sponsor's evaluation of the animal studies that formed the basis for the sponsor's decision that the proposed human trials are safe. It is expected that the unaudited draft reports that formed the basis of this decision might undergo minor modifications during final review and quality assurance auditing. Full toxicology department individual trial reports should be available to the FDA, upon request, as final, fully quality-assured documents within 120 days of the start of the human trial for which the animal study formed part of the safety conclusion basis. These final reports should contain in the introduction any changes from those reported in the integrated summary. If there are no changes, that should be clearly stated at the beginning of the final, fully quality-assured report.

If the integrated summary is based upon unaudited draft reports, sponsors should submit an update to their integrated summary by 120 days after the start of the human trials identifying any differences found in the preparation of the final, fully quality-assured trial reports and the information submitted in the initial integrated summary. If no differences were found, that should be stated in the integrated summary update. In addition, any new findings discovered during the preparation of the final, fully quality-assured individual trial reports that could affect subject safety must be reported to the FDA as an IND safety report.

Usually, 10 to 15 pages of text with additional tables as needed should suffice for the integrated summary. It should represent a perspective on the completed animal studies at the time the sponsor decided that human trials were appropriate. Use of visual data displays (e.g., box plots, histograms, or distributions of laboratory results over time) will facilitate description of the findings of these trials. The summary document should be accurate contemporaneously with the IND submission (i.e., it should be updated so that if new information or findings from the completed animal studies have become known since the sponsor's decision that the proposed human trial is safe, such new information should also be included in the submitted summary).

The integrated summary of the toxicologic findings of the completed animal studies to support the safety of the proposed phase 1 human investigation should ordinarily contain the following information:

1. A brief description of the design of the trials, dates of performance, and any deviations from the design in the conduct of the trials. Reference to the trial protocol and protocol amendments may be adequate for some of this information.
2. A systematic presentation of the findings from the animal toxicology and toxicokinetic trials. Those findings that an experienced expert would reasonably consider as possible signals of human risk should be highlighted. The format of this part of the summary may be approached from a "systems review" perspective (e.g., CNS, cardiovascular, pulmonary, gastrointestinal, renal, hepatic, genitourinary, hematopoietic, immunologic, and dermal). If a product's effects on a particular body system have not been assessed, that should be noted. If any well-documented toxicologic "signal" is not considered evidence of human risk, the reason should be given. In addition, the sponsor should note whether these findings are discussed in the Investigator's Brochure.
3. Identification and qualifications of the individual(s) who evaluated the animal safety data and concluded that it is reasonably safe to begin the proposed human trial. This person(s) should sign the summary attesting that it accurately reflects the animal toxicology data from the completed trials.
4. A statement of where the animal trials were conducted and where the records of the trials are available for inspection, should an inspection occur.
5. A declaration that each trial subject to GLP regulations was performed in full compliance with GLPs or, if the trial was not conducted in compliance with those regulations, a brief statement of the reason for the noncompliance and the sponsor's view on how such noncompliance might affect the interpretation of the findings.

It should be noted that the information described in the last three points may be supplied as part of the integrated summary or as part of the full data tabulations described in the next section.

Toxicology—full data tabulation: The sponsor should submit, for each animal toxicology study that is intended to support the safety of the proposed clinical investigation, a full tabulation of data suitable for detailed review. This should consist of line listings of the individual data points, including laboratory data points, for each animal in these studies along with summary tabulations of these data points. To allow interpretation of the line listings, accompanying the line listings should be either (a) a brief (usually a few pages) description (i.e., a technical report or abstract including a methods description section) of the trial or (b) a copy of the trial protocol and amendments.

In conclusion, this section has been included to assist sponsors who are preparing an IND submission for a phase 1 trial in the United States. Emphasis was provided on the requirements for submission of chemistry and manufacturing data for the drug substance and the drug product, and for information to be submitted regarding the pharmacologic and toxicologic assessments of the new drug candidate.

If a sponsor has conducted phase 1 trials outside of the United States and believes that there are adequate human safety trials already available, it may not be necessary to conduct any phase 1 trials in the United States. In such a case, the sponsor would prepare an IND and include in the initial IND submission a clinical protocol for phase 2 or 3. This IND, because it will involve exposure of more patients to the drug for the purposes of safety testing as well as efficacy evaluations, will require a greater level and depth of manufacturing and nonclinical data.

IND Submissions Assessments

As noted in the previous section, the FDA's review of phase 1 submissions focuses on assessing the safety of those investigations. The review by the FDA for submissions of phase 2 and 3 trials will also include an assessment of the scientific quality of the clinical investigations and the likelihood that the investigations will yield data capable of meeting statutory standards for marketing approval.

The central focus of the initial IND submission will be on the general investigational plan and the protocols for specific human trials. Subsequent amendments to the IND that contain new or revised protocols should build logically on previous submissions and should be supported by additional information, including the results of animal toxicology trials or other human trials as appropriate. Annual reports to the IND will serve as the focus for reporting the status of trials being conducted under the IND and should update the general investigational plan for the coming year.

An IND goes into effect 30 days after the FDA receives the IND, unless the FDA notifies the sponsor that the investigations described in the IND are subject to a clinical hold. It is possible, but not usual, that there may be earlier notification by the FDA that the clinical investigations in the IND may begin. When the initial IND is filed, the FDA will notify the sponsor in writing of the date it receives the IND.

A sponsor may ship an investigational new drug to investigators named in the IND (a) 30 days after the FDA receives the IND, or (b) on earlier FDA authorization to ship the drug. Of course, an investigator may not administer an investigational new drug to human subjects until the IND goes into effect and there is compliance with the applicable requirements for protection of human subjects, as described by the IRB and IC regulations.

Form FDA 1571

INDs and each amendment to an IND are to be submitted in triplicate and must include a completed copy of the two-page Form FDA 1571. A copy of this form is shown in Figure 1. This form and many other FDA forms may be downloaded from

DEPARTMENT OF HEALTH AND HUMAN SERVICES FOOD AND DRUG ADMINISTRATION **INVESTIGATIONAL NEW DRUG APPLICATION (IND)** *(TITLE 21, CODE OF FEDERAL REGULATIONS (CFR) PART 312)*	*Form Approved:* OMB No. 0910-0014. *Expiration Date: May 31, 2009* *See OMB Statement on Reverse.* **NOTE:** No drug may be shipped or clinical investigation begun until an IND for that investigation is in effect (21 CFR 312.40).

1. NAME OF SPONSOR	2. DATE OF SUBMISSION

3. ADDRESS *(Number, Street, City, State and Zip Code)*	4. TELEPHONE NUMBER *(Include Area Code)*

5. NAME(S) OF DRUG *(Include all available names: Trade, Generic, Chemical, Code)*	6. IND NUMBER *(If previously assigned)*

7. INDICATION(S) *(Covered by this submission)*

8. PHASE(S) OF CLINICAL INVESTIGATION TO BE CONDUCTED: ☐ PHASE 1 ☐ PHASE 2 ☐ PHASE 3 ☐ OTHER _____ *(Specify)*

9. LIST NUMBERS OF ALL INVESTIGATIONAL NEW DRUG APPLICATIONS (21 CFR Part 312), NEW DRUG OR ANTIBIOTIC APPLICATIONS *(21 CFR Part 314)*, DRUG MASTER FILES *(21 CFR Part 314.420)*, AND PRODUCT LICENSE APPLICATIONS (21 CFR Part 601) REFERRED TO IN THIS APPLICATION.

10. ***IND submission should be consecutively numbered. The initial IND should be numbered "Serial number: 0000." The next submission (e.g., amendment, report, or correspondence) should be numbered "Serial Number: 0001." Subsequent submissions should be numbered consecutively in the order in which they are submitted.***	SERIAL NUMBER

11. THIS SUBMISSION CONTAINS THE FOLLOWING: *(Check all that apply)*

☐ INITIAL INVESTIGATIONAL NEW DRUG APPLICATION (IND) ☐ RESPONSE TO CLINICAL HOLD

PROTOCOL AMENDMENT(S):
☐ NEW PROTOCOL
☐ CHANGE IN PROTOCOL
☐ NEW INVESTIGATOR

INFORMATION AMENDMENT(S):
☐ CHEMISTRY/MICROBIOLOGY
☐ PHARMACOLOGY/TOXICOLOGY
☐ CLINICAL

IND SAFETY REPORT(S):
☐ INITIAL WRITTEN REPORT
☐ FOLLOW-UP TO A WRITTEN REPORT

☐ RESPONSE TO FDA REQUEST FOR INFORMATION ☐ ANNUAL REPORT ☐ GENERAL CORRESPONDENCE

☐ REQUEST FOR REINSTATEMENT OF IND THAT IS WITHDRAWN, INACTIVATED, TERMINATED OR DISCONTINUED ☐ OTHER _____ *(Specify)*

CHECK ONLY IF APPLICABLE

JUSTIFICATION STATEMENT MUST BE SUBMITTED WITH APPLICATION FOR ANY CHECKED BELOW. REFER TO THE CITED CFR SECTION FOR FURTHER INFORMATION.

☐ TREATMENT IND 21 CFR 312.35(b) ☐ TREATMENT PROTOCOL 21 CFR 312.35(a) ☐ CHARGE REQUEST/NOTIFICATION 21 CFR312.7(d)

FOR FDA USE ONLY

CDR/DBIND/DGD RECEIPT STAMP	DDR RECEIPT STAMP	DIVISION ASSIGNMENT:
		IND NUMBER ASSIGNED:

FORM FDA 1571 (4/06)   PREVIOUS EDITION IS OBSOLETE.   **PAGE 1 OF 2**

PSC Media Arts (301) 443-1090   EF

FIGURE 1

12.   **CONTENTS OF APPLICATION**
                       This application contains the following items: *(Check all that apply)*

☐ 1. Form FDA 1571 *[21 CFR 312.23(a)(1)]*
☐ 2. Table of Contents *[21 CFR 312.23(a)(2)]*
☐ 3. Introductory statement *[21 CFR 312.23(a)(3)]*
☐ 4. General Investigational plan *[21 CFR 312.23(a)(3)]*
☐ 5. Investigator's brochure *[21 CFR 312.23(a)(5)]*
☐ 6. Protocol(s) *[21 CFR 312.23(a)(6)]*
   ☐ a. Study protocol(s) *[21 CFR 312.23(a)(6)]*
   ☐ b. Investigator data *[21 CFR 312.23(a)(6)(iii)(b)]* or completed Form(s) FDA 1572
   ☐ c. Facilities data *[21 CFR 312.23(a)(6)(iii)(b)]* or completed Form(s) FDA 1572
   ☐ d. Institutional Review Board data *[21 CFR 312.23(a)(6)(iii)(b)]* or completed Form(s) FDA 1572
☐ 7. Chemistry, manufacturing, and control data *[21 CFR 312.23(a)(7)]*
   ☐ Environmental assessment or claim for exclusion *[21 CFR 312.23(a)(7)(iv)(e)]*
☐ 8. Pharmacology and toxicology data *[21 CFR 312.23(a)(8)]*
☐ 9. Previous human experience *[21 CFR 312.23(a)(9)]*
☐ 10. Additional information *[21 CFR 312.23(a)(10)]*

13. IS ANY PART OF THE CLINICAL STUDY TO BE CONDUCTED BY A CONTRACT RESEARCH ORGANIZATION? ☐ YES ☐ NO

IF YES, WILL ANY SPONSOR OBLIGATIONS BE TRANSFERRED TO THE CONTRACT RESEARCH ORGANIZATION? ☐ YES ☐ NO

IF YES, ATTACH A STATEMENT CONTAINING THE NAME AND ADDRESS OF THE CONTRACT RESEARCH ORGANIZATION, IDENTIFICATION OF THE CLINICAL STUDY, AND A LISTING OF THE OBLIGATIONS TRANSFERRED.

14. NAME AND TITLE OF THE PERSON RESPONSIBLE FOR MONITORING THE CONDUCT AND PROGRESS OF THE CLINICAL INVESTIGATIONS

15. NAME(S) AND TITLE(S) OF THE PERSON(S) RESPONSIBLE FOR REVIEW AND EVALUATION OF INFORMATION RELEVANT TO THE SAFETY OF THE DRUG

I agree not to begin clinical investigations until 30 days after FDA's receipt of the IND unless I receive earlier notification by FDA that the studies may begin. I also agree not to begin or continue clinical investigations covered by the IND if those studies are placed on clinical hold. I agree that an Institutional Review Board (IRB) that complies with the requirements set fourth in 21 CFR Part 56 will be responsible for initial and continuing review and approval of each of the studies in the proposed clinical investigation. I agree to conduct the investigation in accordance with all other applicable regulatory requirements.

16. NAME OF SPONSOR OR SPONSOR'S AUTHORIZED REPRESENTATIVE

17. SIGNATURE OF SPONSOR OR SPONSOR'S AUTHORIZED REPRESENTATIVE

18. ADDRESS *(Number, Street, City, State and Zip Code)*

19. TELEPHONE NUMBER *(Include Area Code)*

20. DATE

(**WARNING:** A willfully false statement is a criminal offense. U.S.C. Title 18, Sec. 1001.)

Public reporting burden for this collection of information is estimated to average 100 hours per response, including the time for reviewing instructions, searching existing data sources, gathering and maintaining the data needed, and completing reviewing the collection of information. Send comments regarding this burden estimate or any other aspect of this collection of information, including suggestions for reducing this burden to:

Department of Health and Human Services
Food and Drug Administration
Center for Drug Evaluation and Research
Central Document Room
5901-B Ammendale Road
Beltsville, MD 20705-1266

Department of Health and Human Services
Food and Drug Administration
Center for Biologics Evaluation and Research (HFM-99)
1401 Rockville Pike
Rockville, MD 20852-1448
Please DO NOT RETURN this application to this address.

"An agency may not conduct or sponsor, and a person is not required to respond to, a collection of information unless it displays a currently valid OMB control number."

FORM FDA 1571 (4/06)   **PAGE 2 OF 2**

FIGURE 1

the Internet at the following location: http://www.fda.gov/opacom/morechoices/fdaforms/default.html.

The form contains 20 subitems, each of which must be completed. Items 1, 2, 3, 4, 7, 8, 14, 15, 18, 19, and 20 are self-evident and need no further elaboration. Comments on the remaining items will help formulate the IND.

Item 5 requires the name of the drug. It is cautioned that all names and codes that appear in the IND documentation be added in this space. It is not uncommon that, in the very early stages of preclinical development, a code name is used. As the drug advances in the preclinical stage, a generic name or modified code name may be used. If the early pharmacology or toxicology reports refer to the drug by the earlier code name, this too should be included in item 5.

Item 6, the IND number, will not be inserted at the time of the submission of the initial IND filing. Once the IND is filed, the FDA will assign an IND number, and the sponsor will be notified in writing of this number. From that point forward, every communication between the sponsor and the FDA should include this IND number.

A list of numbers of all referenced applications is needed in item 9. This list will include any referenced drug master files or references to other existing INDs or NDAs on file with the FDA. If the CMC section of the IND refers to the DMF of a container manufacturer for a particular container-closure system, the DMF number and, if possible, the specific pages within that DMF containing information on the container-closure system being used, should be referenced. Similarly, if a previously filed IND or NDA contains pharmacologic or toxicologic data that support the safety of the present IND submission, reference by IND or NDA number, date, volume, and page numbers should be provided in this item.

Each IND submission is serially numbered. It should be noted that the initial filing of the IND is considered the "000" filing. Once the IND is filed, each amendment to the IND is given a progressively increasing serial submission number from 001 upward. When writing to the FDA about previous filings, the serial submission number may be used to reference the communication.

The appropriate box(es) briefly describing the submission should be checked in item 11. It is possible that one IND amendment may contain protocol amendments and information amendments. In such a case, the applicable boxes are marked. If the filing is for the initial IND, a response to a clinical hold, an initial or follow-up IND safety report, a response to an FDA request for information, an annual report, or general correspondence, the appropriate box should be checked. Finally, there is a box if the sponsor is requesting reinstatement of an IND that has been withdrawn, inactivated, terminated, or discontinued.

The second page of the form FDA 1571 contains items 12–20. Item 12 is a checklist table of contents. Any of the 10 items constituting this table of contents and contained in the specific IND submission for which the form is being prepared should be checked. An initial IND will most likely have all or a majority of the boxes checked. A protocol amendment will have items 1 and all or some of the items 6a–6d checked.

The transfer of obligations of GCP from a sponsor to a Contract Research Organization (CRO) is described in detail in 21CFR Part 312.52. A sponsor may transfer responsibility for any or all parts of the GCP obligations to a CRO. Any such transfer is to be described in writing. Conversely, any CRO that assumes any obligation of a sponsor for the requirements of GCP shall comply with the regulations and are subject to the same regulatory actions as a sponsor for failure to comply with their assumed obligations. Thus, the purpose of item 13 of the form FDA 1571 is to inform the FDA of whether any part or all of a clinical trial is to be performed by a CRO, and to identify whether the sponsor has transferred the obligations of compliance with GCP to that CRO. Finally, if the response is affirmative, the name and address of the CRO must be provided as part of the IND submission.

Items 16, 18, and 19 are to be completed only if the sponsor of the IND does not have a physical presence in the United States. It is not uncommon for a foreign-based company to sponsor an IND. However, when this occurs, the FDA must have the name, address, and telephone number of a contact person within the United States, as the FDA usually will not contact an overseas company directly. The contact person named by the sponsor may be either a representative within a United States affiliate office or a consultant working on behalf of the foreign sponsor.

IND Content and Format

As shown in Figure 1, item 12 of the form FDA 1571 outlines the 10 parts of the IND. This section will detail the requirements for each of those parts and provide illustrations and examples of the items to be presented in the IND. It must be emphasized again that the information to be provided in the following sections represents more complete IND data to support a clinical program in phase 2 or 3. The lesser requirements for phase 1 trials have been discussed previously.

Table of Contents. Once the IND has been formatted and assembled, a detailed table of contents should be prepared. Depending on the size of the initial IND filing, this table of contents may be contained only in volume 1 or preferably included as the first pages of each of the IND volumes. The table of contents should be sufficiently detailed so that an FDA reviewer can easily access any specific topic or report contained in the IND. It is also preferable to sequentially number the IND for each volume, rather than to sequentially number the entire IND. Thus, in reference to a specific report or in cross-referencing, it is necessary to provide the volume number and the page number.

The table of contents may have the following headings:

IND Part   Title of Information Provided   Volume   Page

Part 3: Introductory Statement and General Investigational Plan. On the Form FDA 1571, the introductory statement appears as part 3 and the general investigational plan appears as part 4 in item 12 of the contents of application (Fig. 1). This is inconsistent with the requirements as detailed in 21 CFR Part 312.23, inasmuch, as the introductory statement and general investigation plan are listed only as part 3. Part 4 in the CFR is listed as "Reserved." Thus, the option exists to combine these parts or to present them as separate entities. It is not important which way it is handled. The important thing is to have a clear and concise section, because, as the introduction to the IND, this section is likely to be read not only by the IND reviewers but also by the division director and others within the division. It is recommended that combining parts 3 and 4 is the preferred format.

The introductory statement and general investigational plan will contain the following:

1. A brief introductory statement giving the name of the drug and all active ingredients, the drug's pharmacologic class, the structural formula of the drug (if known), the formulation of the dosage form(s) to be used, the route of

administration, and the broad objectives and planned duration of the proposed clinical investigation(s).

2. A brief summary of previous human experience with the drug, with reference to other INDs if pertinent, and to investigational or marketing experience in other countries that may be relevant to the safety of the proposed clinical investigation(s).

3. If the drug has been withdrawn from investigation or marketing in any country for any reason related to safety or effectiveness, identification of the country(ies) where the drug was withdrawn and the reasons for the withdrawal.

4. A brief description of the overall plan for investigating the drug product for the following year. The plan should include the following: (a) the rationale for the drug or the research trial, (b) the indication(s) to be studied, (c) the general approach to be followed in evaluating the drug, (d) the kinds of clinical trials to be conducted in the first year after the submission (if plans are not developed for the entire year, the sponsor should so indicate), (e) the estimated number of patients to be given the drug in those trials, and (f) any risks of particular severity or seriousness anticipated on the basis of the toxicologic data in animals or prior trials in humans with the drug or related drugs.

Part 5: The Investigator's Brochure. This will be covered as a separate topic in this chapter.

Part 6: Protocols and Other Clinical Trial Information. It is necessary to provide at least one protocol in the initial IND submission. If more than one trial is planned, a protocol for each planned trial should be submitted. Protocols for trials not submitted initially in the IND should be submitted as a protocol amendment in a future IND serial submission. As noted in the discussion of phase 1 INDs, these protocols may be less detailed and more flexible than protocols for phase 2 and 3 trials. In phases 2 and 3, detailed protocols describing all aspects of the trial should be submitted. A protocol for a phase 2 or 3 investigation should be designed in such a way that if the sponsor anticipates that some deviation from the trial design may become necessary as the investigation progresses, alternatives or contingencies to provide for such a deviation are built into the protocols at the outset. For example, a protocol for a controlled, short-term trial might include a plan for an early crossover of nonresponders to an alternative therapy.

The requirements for clinical protocols are described in detail in chap. 16 of this book; however, there are seven components that must be included in a clinical protocol to ensure that adequate and well-controlled trials meet regulatory requirements:

1. A statement of the objective must include evaluations of safety, and for phases of clinical research requiring evaluations of efficacy, these should be based on the use of an investigational product for a specific diagnosis.

2. The method or methods of statistical analysis must be precisely designed.

3. When possible, a valid comparison with a control group so that the results are unbiased.

4. Method of subject selection must be based on a diagnosis as determined by a medical history and confirmed by precise inclusion and exclusion criteria.

5. When double-blind randomization is used, subject randomization to product assignment must be carefully selected to guard against bias during subject assessments.

6. Methods of subject assessments and the instruments used for the same must reflect:
   - the degree of subject safety and efficacy without bias;
   - laboratory, clinical, and mechanical assessments;
   - selection of valid objective and subjective evaluation forms.
7. Assure that an adequate number of subjects are entered into a clinical trial in order to derive statistical results that are significant to prove safety and efficacy.

This section can be best assembled by preparing various subparts. Part 6 (a) will be the complete and signed clinical protocol written in compliance with the above suggestions. Part 6 (b) can be the completed and signed Form FDA 1572— Statement of Investigator. A copy of this form is provided in Figure 2. This subpart can also contain the curriculum vitae of the principal investigator. It is up to the discretion of the sponsor as to whether it wishes to file the curricula vitae of all subinvestigators. However, for the sake of minimizing the size of the IND, the FDA is generally in agreement with a statement that all of the curricula vitae of subinvestigators are on file and any or all of the vitae are available upon request. Part 6 (c) is a good place to provide the curricula vitae of the individuals named in items 14 and 15 of the Form FDA 1571, that is, the individual(s) responsible for monitoring the conduct and progress of the clinical investigations and the individual(s) responsible for review and evaluation of information relevant to the safety of the drug.

It should be emphasized that there is no requirement to provide the FDA at the time of the IND submission with copies of a specimen case report form or a specimen informed consent document (ICD). However, an ICD review is at the discretion of the review division but, in most cases, ICDs should be reviewed as part of the review of an IND submission when the review of the proposed investigational use raises a particular concern about the adequacy of informed consent. For example, review of an ICD is warranted when:

- Unusual toxicity is associated with the trial drug.
- The trial population is particularly vulnerable.
- The trial design is unusual for the therapeutic class.
- CDER is in a better position than the IRB/IEC to assess whether the ICD adequately addressed a particular concern based on proprietary data.

In the above situations the review division will assess the adequacy of the ICD in addressing any safety issue or matter of trial design and the elements identified in the 21 CFR 50.25.

Finally, on the introduction page to this section or in the cover letter, it is always a good idea to emphasize that the clinical trial supplies will not be shipped by the sponsor until there is written documentation in hand to demonstrate IRB approval, and that the drug will not be shipped to the clinical trial site until after the 30-day review period of the initial IND filing.

Part 7: Chemistry, Manufacturing, and Control Data. This section is also easier to review and better formatted with the use of subparts. Any number of approaches are acceptable; however, one logical formatting technique is to provide the CMC data for the drug substance as subpart (a), data for the drug product as subpart (b), information relating to any placebo formulations as subpart (c), labeling as subpart (d), and finally all environmental assessment information as subpart (e).

DEPARTMENT OF HEALTH AND HUMAN SERVICES FOOD AND DRUG ADMINISTRATION **STATEMENT OF INVESTIGATOR** *(TITLE 21, CODE OF FEDERAL REGULATIONS (CFR) PART 312)* (See instructions on reverse side.)	Form Approved: OMB No. 0910-0014. Expiration Date: May 31, 2009. *See OMB Statement on Reverse.* **NOTE:** No investigator may participate in an investigation until he/she provides the sponsor with a completed, signed Statement of Investigator, Form FDA 1572 (21 CFR 312.53(c)).

1. NAME AND ADDRESS OF INVESTIGATOR

2. EDUCATION, TRAINING, AND EXPERIENCE THAT QUALIFIES THE INVESTIGATOR AS AN EXPERT IN THE CLINICAL INVESTIGATION OF THE DRUG FOR THE USE UNDER INVESTIGATION. ONE OF THE FOLLOWING IS ATTACHED.

    ☐ CURRICULUM VITAE   ☐ OTHER STATEMENT OF QUALIFICATIONS

3. NAME AND ADDRESS OF ANY MEDICAL SCHOOL, HOSPITAL OR OTHER RESEARCH FACILITY WHERE THE CLINICAL INVESTIGATION(S) WILL BE CONDUCTED.

4. NAME AND ADDRESS OF ANY CLINICAL LABORATORY FACILITIES TO BE USED IN THE STUDY.

5. NAME AND ADDRESS OF THE INSTITUTIONAL REVIEW BOARD (IRB) THAT IS RESPONSIBLE FOR REVIEW AND APPROVAL OF THE STUDY(IES).

6. NAMES OF THE SUBINVESTIGATORS *(e.g., research fellows, residents, associates)* WHO WILL BE ASSISTING THE INVESTIGATOR IN THE CONDUCT OF THE INVESTIGATION(S).

7. NAME AND CODE NUMBER, IF ANY, OF THE PROTOCOL(S) IN THE IND FOR THE STUDY(IES) TO BE CONDUCTED BY THE INVESTIGATOR.

FORM FDA 1572 (5/06)   PREVIOUS EDITION IS OBSOLETE.   **PAGE 1 OF 2**

PSC Graphics (301) 443-1090 EF

FIGURE 2

8. ATTACH THE FOLLOWING CLINICAL PROTOCOL INFORMATION:

☐ FOR PHASE 1 INVESTIGATIONS, A GENERAL OUTLINE OF THE PLANNED INVESTIGATION INCLUDING THE ESTIMATED DURATION OF THE STUDY AND THE MAXIMUM NUMBER OF SUBJECTS THAT WILL BE INVOLVED.

☐ FOR PHASE 2 OR 3 INVESTIGATIONS, AN OUTLINE OF THE STUDY PROTOCOL INCLUDING AN APPROXIMATION OF THE NUMBER OF SUBJECTS TO BE TREATED WITH THE DRUG AND THE NUMBER TO BE EMPLOYED AS CONTROLS, IF ANY; THE CLINICAL USES TO BE INVESTIGATED; CHARACTERISTICS OF SUBJECTS BY AGE, SEX, AND CONDITION; THE KIND OF CLINICAL OBSERVATIONS AND LABORATORY TESTS TO BE CONDUCTED; THE ESTIMATED DURATION OF THE STUDY; AND COPIES OR A DESCRIPTION OF CASE REPORT FORMS TO BE USED.

9. COMMITMENTS:

I agree to conduct the study(ies) in accordance with the relevant, current protocol(s) and will only make changes in a protocol after notifying the sponsor, except when necessary to protect the safety, rights, or welfare of subjects.

I agree to personally conduct or supervise the described investigation(s).

I agree to inform any patients, or any persons used as controls, that the drugs are being used for investigational purposes and I will ensure that the requirements relating to obtaining informed consent in 21 CFR Part 50 and institutional review board (IRB) review and approval in 21 CFR Part 56 are met.

I agree to report to the sponsor adverse experiences that occur in the course of the investigation(s) in accordance with 21 CFR 312.64.

I have read and understand the information in the investigator's brochure, including the potential risks and side effects of the drug.

I agree to ensure that all associates, colleagues, and employees assisting in the conduct of the study(ies) are informed about their obligations in meeting the above commitments.

I agree to maintain adequate and accurate records in accordance with 21 CFR 312.62 and to make those records available for inspection in accordance with 21 CFR 312.68.

I will ensure that an IRB that complies with the requirements of 21 CFR Part 56 will be responsible for the initial and continuing review and approval of the clinical investigation. I also agree to promptly report to the IRB all changes in the research activity and all unanticipated problems involving risks to human subjects or others. Additionally, I will not make any changes in the research without IRB approval, except where necessary to eliminate apparent immediate hazards to human subjects.

I agree to comply with all other requirements regarding the obligations of clinical investigators and all other pertinent requirements in 21 CFR Part 312.

INSTRUCTIONS FOR COMPLETING FORM FDA 1572
STATEMENT OF INVESTIGATOR:

1. Complete all sections. Attach a separate page if additional space is needed.

2. Attach curriculum vitae or other statement of qualifications as described in Section 2.

3. Attach protocol outline as described in Section 8.

4. Sign and date below.

5. FORWARD THE COMPLETED FORM AND ATTACHMENTS TO THE SPONSOR. The sponsor will incorporate this information along with other technical data into an Investigational New Drug Application (IND).
   INVESTIGATORS SHOULD NOT SEND THIS FORM DIRECTLY TO THE FOOD AND DRUG ADMINISTRATION.

10. SIGNATURE OF INVESTIGATOR	11. DATE

(**WARNING:** A willfully false statement is a criminal offense. U.S.C. Title 18, Sec. 1001.)

Public reporting burden for this collection of information is estimated to average 100 hours per response, including the time for reviewing instructions, searching existing data sources, gathering and maintaining the data needed, and completing reviewing the collection of information. Send comments regarding this burden estimate or any other aspect of this collection of information, including suggestions for reducing this burden to:

Department of Health and Human Services	Department of Health and Human Services	"An agency may not conduct or sponsor, and a
Food and Drug Administration	Food and Drug Administration	person is not required to respond to, a collection
Center for Drug Evaluation and Research (HFD-143)	Center for Biologics Evaluation and Research (HFM-99)	of information unless it displays a currently valid
Central Document Room	1401 Rockville Pike	OMB control number."
5901-B Ammendale Road	Rockville, MD 20852-1448	
Beltsville, MD 207052-1266		

Please DO NOT RETURN this application to this address.

FORM FDA 1572 (5/06)   PAGE 2 OF 2

FIGURE 2

The emphasis of this part of the IND is to assure the proper identification, quality, purity, and strength of the investigational drug. As noted earlier in the section on the phase 1 IND, the amount of information needed to make that assurance will vary with the phase of the investigation, the proposed duration of the investigation, the dosage form, and the amount of information otherwise available. The FDA recognizes that modifications to the method of preparation of the new drug substance and dosage form and changes in the dosage form itself are likely as the investigation progresses. Therefore, as noted, the emphasis in an initial phase 1 submission should generally be placed on the identification and control of the raw materials and the new drug substance. Final specifications for the drug substance and drug product are not expected until near the end of the investigational process.

Having said this, as drug development proceeds and as the scale or production is changed from the pilot-scale production appropriate for the limited initial clinical investigations to the larger-scale production needed for expanded clinical trials, the sponsor should submit information amendments to update the initial information submitted on the chemistry, manufacturing, and control processes with information appropriate to the expanded scope of the investigation.

At the time of this writing, details on the different levels of data suggested for an IND for the drug substance and drug product may be found in a preliminary draft guidance published by the FDA. The draft guidance is entitled "INDs for Phase 2 and 3 trials of Drugs, Including Specified Therapeutic Biotechnology-Derived Products—CMC Content and Format" dated February 1999.

Subpart (a)—Drug Substance: This section will contain a description of the drug substance, including its physical, chemical, or biological characteristics; the name and address of its manufacturer; the general method of preparation of the drug substance; the acceptable limits and analytical methods used to assure the identity, strength, quality, and purity of the drug substance; and information sufficient to support stability of the drug substance during the toxicologic trials and the planned clinical trials. Reference to the current edition of the USP-NF may satisfy relevant requirements in this section.

By the time the clinical program has entered phase 3, the sponsor should provide a full description of the physical, chemical, and biological characteristics of the drug substance. For example, most of the following should be evaluated and submitted: solubility and partition coefficient, pK_a, hygroscopicity, crystal properties/morphology, thermal evaluation, X-ray diffraction, particle size, melting point, and specific rotation stereochemical consideration. Proof of structure should include information on elemental analysis, conformational analysis, molecular-weight determination and spectra for IR, NMR (1H and 13C), UV, MS, optical activity, and single crystal data (if available). For peptides and proteins, amino acid sequence, peptide map, and secondary and tertiary structure information should be available.

For the description of the synthesis or preparation of the drug substance, a detailed flow diagram containing chemical structures (including relevant stereochemical configurations), intermediates (either in situ or isolated), and significant side products, solvents, catalysts, and reagents should be submitted. For biotech or natural products, fermenters, columns, and other equipment/reagents should be identified. By late phase 2 or early phase 3, the synthetic process should be almost completely characterized, and the IND should therefore be able to contain a step-by-step description of the synthesis or manufacturing process, including the final recrystalization of the drug substance. The description should indicate the batch size (range) and descriptions of the types of equipment in which reactions will be carried out. Relative ratios of the reactants, catalysts, and reagents, as well as general operating conditions (time, temperature, pressures), are to be provided. Identification of steps at which all in-process controls are performed (with a complete description of the analytical methods and tentative acceptance criteria to be provided in the Process Control section) is also necessary.

Subparts (b) and (c)—Drug Product and Placebo: These sections require the submission of a list of all components. This may include reasonable alternatives for inactive compounds used in the manufacture of the investigational drug product and placebo, including those components intended to appear in the drug product and those that may not appear but are used in the manufacturing process and, where applicable, the quantitative composition of the investigational drug product, including any reasonable variations that may be expected during the investigational stage; the name and address of the drug product manufacturer and packager; a brief general description of the manufacturing and packaging procedure for the product; the acceptable limits and analytical methods used to ensure the identity, strength, quality, and purity of the drug product; and information sufficient to ensure the product's stability during the planned clinical trials. Reference to the current edition of the USP-NF may satisfy certain requirements in this subpart. There also should be a brief general description of the composition, manufacture, and control of any placebo used in a controlled clinical trial.

By the time the drug product is in phase III, trials should be included to demonstrate the inherent stability of the drug product, and the ability to detect potential degradation products should be available. The analytical method should use a validated stability-indicating assay.

Subpart (d)—Labeling: A copy of all labels and labeling to be provided to each investigator should be submitted in the IND. This would include a mockup or printed representation of the proposed labeling and labels that will be provided to investigators to be used on the drug container. The investigational labels must also carry the standard "caution statement" as previously discussed.

Subpart (e)—Environmental Analysis Requirements: A claim for categorical exclusion under 21 CFR Section 25.30 or 25.31 or an environmental assessment under 21 CFR Section 25.40 should be provided.

Part 8: Pharmacology and Toxicology Information. This section of the IND must contain adequate information about pharmacologic and toxicologic trials of the drug involving laboratory animals or any trials conducted in vitro, on the basis of which the sponsor has concluded that it is reasonably safe to conduct the proposed clinical investigations. The kind, duration, and scope of animal and other tests required vary with the duration and nature of the proposed clinical investigations. Guidelines are available from the FDA that describe ways in which these requirements may be met. Such information is required to include the identification and qualifications of the individuals who evaluated the results of such trials and concluded that it is reasonably safe to begin the proposed investigations and a statement of where the investigations were conducted and where the records are available for inspection. As drug development proceeds, the sponsor is required to submit informational amendments, as appropriate, with additional information pertinent to safety.

With regard to formatting, this part of the IND may be divided into the following sections: Subpart (a): Pharmacology and Drug Disposition; Subpart (b)(i): Toxicology—Integrated Summary; Subpart (b)(ii): Full Toxicological Reports; and Subpart (c): Good Laboratory Practices Statement.

Subpart (a)—Pharmacology and Drug Disposition: This section should describe the pharmacologic effects and mechanism(s) of action of the drug in animals and information on the absorption, distribution, metabolism, and excretion of the drug, if known.

Subpart (b)(i)—Toxicology: Integrated Summary: An integrated summary of the toxicologic effects of the drug in animals and in vitro should be written. Depending on the nature of the drug and the phase of the investigation, the description is to include the results of acute, subacute, and chronic toxicity tests; tests of the drug's effects on reproduction and the developing fetus; any special toxicity test related to the drug's particular mode of administration or conditions of use (e.g., inhalation, dermal, or ocular toxicology); and any in vitro trials intended to evaluate drug toxicity.

If the drug is to be studied in females of child-bearing potential in phase 2, complete investigations of the effect of the drug on fertility and reproductive performance should be a part of the IND submission.

Subpart (b)(ii)—Full Toxicologic Reports: For each toxicology trial that is intended primarily to support the safety of the proposed clinical investigation, a full tabulation of data suitable for detailed review should be submitted. The full reports must be quality assured by the QA Unit of the laboratory that conducted the testing.

Subpart (c)—GLP Statement: For each nonclinical laboratory trial subject to the GLP regulations under 21 CFR Part 58, a statement that the trial was conducted in compliance with the good laboratory practice regulations, or, if the trial was not conducted in compliance with those regulations, a brief statement of the reason for the noncompliance.

Part 9: Previous Human Experience. All previous human experience with the drug must be summarized. The information is required to include the following:

Subpart (a): If the investigational drug has been investigated or marketed previously, either in the United States or in other countries, detailed information about such experience relevant to the safety of the proposed investigation or to the investigation's rationale should be provided. If the drug has been the subject of controlled trials, detailed information on such trials that is relevant to an assessment of the drug's safety and effectiveness for the proposed investigational use should also be provided. Any published material that is relevant to the safety of the proposed investigation or to an assessment of the drug's effectiveness for its proposed investigational use should be provided in full. Published material that is less directly relevant may be supplied by a bibliography.

Subpart (b): If the drug is a combination of drugs previously investigated or marketed, the information required in the above section should be provided for each active drug component. However, if any component in such a combination is subject to an approved marketing application or is otherwise lawfully marketed in the United States, the sponsor is not required to submit published material concerning that active drug component unless such material relates directly to the proposed investigational use (including publications relevant to component–component interaction).

Subpart (c): If the drug has been marketed outside the United States, a list of the countries in which the drug has been marketed and a list of the countries in which the drug has been withdrawn from marketing for reasons potentially related to safety or effectiveness must be included.

Part 10: Additional Information. This section is necessary in only a small percentage of INDs to provide information on special topics, as listed below.

Drug Dependence and Abuse Potential: If the drug is a psychotropic substance or otherwise has abuse potential, a section describing relevant clinical trials and experience and trials in test animals is to be submitted.

Radioactive Drugs: If the drug is a radioactive drug, sufficient data from animal or human trials to allow a reasonable calculation of radiation-absorbed dose to the whole body and critical organs upon administration to a human subject are to be submitted. Phase 1 trials of radioactive drugs must include trials that will obtain sufficient data for dosimetry calculations.

Other Information: A brief statement of any other information that would aid evaluation of the proposed clinical investigations with respect to their safety or their design and potential as controlled clinical trials to support marketing of the drug.

Protocol and Information Amendments

As noted previously, the sponsor is required to wait 30 days after the submission of the IND before clinical investigations with the new drug may be instituted. Once the IND is in effect, all additional data and information submitted to that IND will be provided in the form of Protocol and Information Amendments, provided as sequentially numbered serial submissions.

Protocol Amendments: It is the obligation of the sponsor to amend the IND to ensure that the clinical investigations are conducted according to protocols included in the IND application. This section will describe the provisions under which new protocols may be submitted and the changes in previously submitted protocols that may be made.

New Protocol: Whenever a sponsor intends to conduct a trial that is not covered by a protocol already contained in the IND, the sponsor shall submit to the FDA a protocol amendment containing the protocol for the trial. Such a trial may begin without delay provided two conditions are met: (a) the sponsor has submitted the protocol to FDA for its review and (b) the protocol has been approved by the IRB with responsibility for review and approval of the trial.

Changes in a Protocol: A sponsor shall submit a protocol amendment describing any change in a phase 1 protocol that significantly affects the safety of subjects or any change in a phase 2 or 3 protocol that significantly affects the safety of subjects, the scope of the investigation, or the scientific quality of the trial. Examples of changes requiring an amendment under this paragraph include:

1. Any increase in drug dosage or duration of exposure of individual subjects to the drug beyond that in the current protocol or any significant increase in the number of subjects under trial.
2. Any significant change in the design of a protocol (such as the addition or deletion of a control group).

3. The addition of a new test or procedure that is intended to improve monitoring for, or reduce the risk of, a side effect or adverse event or the deletion of a test intended to monitor safety.

New Investigator: A sponsor shall submit a protocol amendment when a new investigator is added to carry out a previously submitted protocol. Once the investigator is added to the trial, the investigational drug may be shipped to the investigator, and the investigator may begin participating in the trial. The sponsor shall notify the FDA of the new investigator within 30 days of the investigator's being added.

It is important to note the distinction in timing of submissions to the IND for a protocol amendment and the addition of a new investigator. A sponsor must submit a protocol amendment for a new protocol or a change in protocol *before* its implementation. Protocol amendments to add a new investigator or to provide additional information about investigators may be grouped and submitted at 30-day intervals. When several submissions of new protocols or protocol changes are anticipated during a short period, the sponsor is encouraged, to the extent feasible, to include these all in a single submission.

Information Amendments: A sponsor shall report in an information amendment essential information on the IND that is not within the scope of a protocol amendment, IND safety reports, or annual report. Examples of information or data requiring an information amendment include new toxicology, chemistry, or other technical information or a report regarding the discontinuance of a clinical investigation. Information amendments to the IND should be submitted as necessary but, to the extent feasible, not more than every 30 days.

IND Safety Reports

Effective April 6, 1998, the FDA changed definitions associated with adverse experience reporting and the time frame for when IND safety reports must be provided to the FDA in relation to their occurrence.

At present, the following definitions of terms apply to this section:

Associated with the use of the drug means that there is a reasonable possibility that the experience may have been caused by the drug.

Disability: A substantial disruption of a person's ability to conduct normal life functions.

Life-threatening adverse drug experience means any adverse drug experience that places the patient or subject, in the view of the investigator, at immediate risk of death from the reaction as it occurred, that is, it does not include a reaction that, had it occurred in a more severe form, might have caused death.

Serious adverse drug experience means any adverse drug experience occurring at any dose that results in any of the following outcomes: death, a life-threatening adverse drug experience, in-patient hospitalization or prolongation of existing hospitalization, a persistent or significant disability/incapacity, or a congenital anomaly/birth defect. Important medical events that may not result in death, be life-threatening, or require hospitalization may be considered a serious adverse drug experience when, based upon appropriate medical judgment, they may jeopardize the patient or subject and may require medical or surgical intervention to prevent one of the outcomes listed in this definition.

An example would be blood dyscrasias or convulsions that do not result in in-patient hospitalization.

Unexpected adverse drug experience means any adverse drug experience, the specificity or severity of which is not consistent with the current investigator brochure; or, if an investigator brochure is not required or available, the specificity or severity of which is not consistent with the risk information described in the general investigational plan or elsewhere. For example, under this definition, hepatic necrosis would be unexpected (by virtue of greater severity) if the investigator brochure only referred to elevated hepatic enzymes or hepatitis. "Unexpected," as used in this definition, refers to an adverse drug experience that has not been previously observed (e.g., included in the investigator brochure) rather than from the perspective of such experience not being anticipated from the pharmacological properties of the product.

Review of safety information: An IND sponsor must review all information relevant to the safety of the drug obtained from any source, foreign or domestic, including information derived from any clinical or epidemiological investigations, animal investigations, commercial marketing experience, reports in the scientific literature, and unpublished scientific papers, as well as reports from foreign regulatory authorities that have not already been previously reported to the FDA by the sponsor.

There are two types of IND safety reports, written and telephone/facsimile reports. A written IND safety report is required for any adverse experience associated with the use of the drug that is both serious and unexpected; or for any finding from tests in laboratory animals that suggests a significant risk for human subjects including reports of mutagenicity, teratogenicity, or carcinogenicity. A telephone/facsimile report is required for any unexpected fatal or life-threatening experience associated with the use of the drug. The written report should be made as soon as possible but in no event later than 15 calendar days after the sponsor's initial receipt of the information. The report must clearly indicate the contents as an "IND Safety Report." A telephone/facsimile report must occur not more than seven calendar days after receipt of the initial information. Any follow-up information obtained after initial notification must be submitted as soon as the relevant information is available.

In the written IND safety report, the sponsor shall identify all safety reports previously filed with the IND concerning a similar adverse experience, and provide an analysis of the significance of the adverse experience in light of the previous, similar reports.

FDA offers the opportunity for the sponsor to make a disclaimer to each IND safety report. The letter of transmittal of the initial and any follow-up reports should state that the information submitted does not necessarily reflect a conclusion by the sponsor or FDA that the report or information constitutes an admission that the drug caused or contributed to an adverse experience. A sponsor need not admit, and may deny, that the report or information submitted by the sponsor constitutes an admission that the drug caused or contributed to an adverse experience.

Annual Reports

In order to keep the FDA up-to-date with the progress of the IND, all sponsors are required to provide an annual report to the IND review division. This must be done within two months of the anniversary date that the IND went into effect. The annual report should be brief but summarize the progress of the investigations with the new drug.

This section will describe the information required for an annual report.

For each individual trial, it is necessary to provide a brief summary of the status of each investigation in progress and each trial completed during the previous year. The summary is required to include the following information for each trial:

1. The title and protocol number of the trial, its purpose, a brief statement identifying the patient population, and a statement as to whether the trial is completed.
2. The total number of subjects initially planned for inclusion in the trial; the number entered into the trial to date, *tabulated by age group, sex, and race*; the number whose participation in the trial was completed as planned; and the number who dropped out of the trial for any reason; the requirement for tabulation by age, group, sex, and race is a new annual report requirement effective February 1998.
3. If the trial has been completed or if interim results are known, a brief description of any available trial results.

The annual report will also contain summary information obtained during the previous year's clinical and nonclinical investigations including:

1. A narrative or tabular summary showing the most frequent and most serious adverse experiences by body system.
2. A summary of all IND safety reports submitted during the past year.
3. A list of subjects who died during participation in the investigation, with the cause of death for each subject.
4. A list of subjects who dropped out during the course of the investigation in association with any adverse experience, whether or not thought to be drug related.
5. A brief description of what, if anything, was obtained that is pertinent to an understanding of the drug's actions, including, for example, information about dose response, controlled trials, and bioavailability.
6. A list of the preclinical trials (including animal trials) completed or in progress during the past year and a summary of the major preclinical findings.
7. A summary of any significant manufacturing or microbiological changes made during the past year.

A description of the general investigational plan for the coming year to replace that submitted one year earlier should be submitted, as well as any revised Investigator's Brochure. If the drug is in phase 1, a description of any significant phase 1 protocol modifications made during the previous year and not previously reported to the IND in a protocol amendment should be identified. If applicable, a brief summary of significant foreign marketing developments with the drug during the past year, such as approval of marketing in any country or withdrawal or suspension from marketing in any country, is to be submitted. Finally, if desired by the sponsor, a log of any outstanding business with respect to the IND for which the sponsor requests or expects a reply, comment, or meeting may be included.

Clinical Holds and Withdrawal of an IND

The last thing a regulatory professional wants to receive from the FDA is the notification that, for one or more reasons, the IND has been placed on "clinical hold."

When this occurs, a sponsor is not allowed to initiate or continue the clinical trial until the FDA has responded in writing that the clinical hold has been removed and the research program may begin. Thus, a clinical hold is an order issued by the FDA to the sponsor to delay a proposed clinical investigation or to suspend an ongoing investigation. The clinical hold order may apply to one or more of the investigations covered by an IND. When a proposed trial is placed on clinical hold, subjects may not be given the investigational drug. When an ongoing trial is placed on clinical hold, no new subjects may be recruited to the trial and placed on the investigational drug; patients already in the trial should be taken off therapy involving the investigational drug unless specifically permitted by the FDA in the interest of patient safety.

Typically, a clinical hold is imposed prior to a phase 1 investigation if the FDA believes that human subjects are or would be exposed to an unreasonable and significant risk of illness or injury; if the clinical investigators named in the IND are not qualified by reason of their scientific training and experience to conduct the investigation described in the IND; if the Investigator's Brochure is misleading, erroneous, or materially incomplete; or if the IND does not contain sufficient information to assess the risks to subjects of the proposed trials. A clinical hold may occur during phase 2 or 3 for any of these reasons or if the FDA believes the plan or protocol for the investigation is clearly deficient in design to meet its stated objectives.

Details on the FDA's policy for the IND process and review procedures, including the handling of clinical holds, are presented in the FDA Manual of Policies and Procedures MAPP No. 6030.1, dated May 1, 1998. This document provides the general review principles for investigational new drugs, policies, and procedures for issuing and overseeing clinical holds of INDs and policies and procedures for processing and responding to sponsors' complete responses to clinical holds.

With regard to withdrawal of an IND, this may be done at any time by a sponsor without prejudice. If a decision is taken to withdraw an IND, the FDA shall be notified in writing of this decision, all clinical investigations conducted under the IND shall be ended, all current investigators shall be notified, and all stocks of the drug shall be returned to the sponsor or otherwise disposed of at the request of the sponsor. If an IND is withdrawn for safety reasons, the sponsor shall promptly inform the FDA, all participating investigators, and all reviewing IRBs of the reasons for such withdrawal.

THE INVESTIGATOR'S BROCHURE

Introduction
The Investigator's Brochure (IB) is an important document, which is not only required as a part of the IND but also prepared for presentation to potential clinical investigators and ultimately for presentation to the investigator's IRB/IEC. The IB is a compilation of the clinical and nonclinical data on the investigational product that are relevant to the trial of the product in human subjects. Its purpose is to provide the investigators and others involved in the trial with the information to facilitate their understanding of the rationale for, and their compliance with, many key features of the protocol, such as the dose, dose frequency/interval, methods of administration, and safety monitoring procedures. The IB also provides insight to support the clinical management of the trial subjects during the course of the

clinical trial. The information should be presented in a concise, simple, objective, balanced, and nonpromotional form that enables a clinician or potential investigator to understand it and make his or her own unbiased risk-benefit assessment of the appropriateness of the proposed trial. For this reason, a medically qualified person should generally participate in the editing of an IB, but the contents of the IB should be approved by the disciplines that generated the described data.

The Efficacy Committee of the International Conference on Harmonization has prepared a final guidance (E6) entitled: *Good Clinical Practice: Consolidated Guideline*. This document was issued by the FDA in April 1996, by both the Center for Drug Evaluation and Research and the Center for Biologics Evaluation and Research. This document should be consulted prior to completion of the final IB.

It is expected that the type and extent of information available will vary with the stage of development of the investigational product. If the investigational product is marketed and its pharmacology is widely understood by medical practitioners, an extensive IB may not be necessary. In this situation, a basic product information brochure, package insert, or labeling may be an appropriate alternative, provided that it includes current, comprehensive, and detailed information on all aspects of the investigational product that might be of importance to the investigator. If a marketed product is being studied for a new indication, an IB specific to that new use should be prepared.

The IB should be reviewed at least annually and revised as necessary in compliance with a sponsor's written procedures. The revised version should be included in the IND annual report. More frequent revision may be appropriate depending on the stage of development and the generation of relevant new information. However, in accordance with GCP, relevant new information may be so important that it should be communicated to the investigators, and possibly to the IRB/IEC and the FDA, before it is included in a revised IB.

Generally, the sponsor is responsible for ensuring that an up-to-date IB is made available to the investigator(s), and the investigators are responsible for providing the up-to-date IB to the responsible IRB/IEC.

The following provides the information that should be included in the IB:

1. *Title Page*
   This should provide the sponsor's name, the identity of each investigational product (i.e., research number, chemical or approved generic name, and trade name(s) where legally permissible and desired by the sponsor), and the release date. It is also suggested that an edition number and a reference to the number and date of the edition it supersedes be provided.
   TITLE PAGE OF INVESTIGATOR'S BROCHURE (Example)
   Sponsor's Name:
   Product:
   Research Number:
   Name(s): Chemical, Generic (if approved)
   Trade Name(s) (if legally permissible and desired by the sponsor)
   Edition Number:
   Release Date:
   Replaces Previous Edition Number:
   Date:

2. *Confidentiality Statement*
    The sponsor may wish to include a statement instructing the investigator/recipients to treat the IB as a confidential document for the sole information and use of the investigator's team and the IRB/IEC.
3. *Contents of the Investigator's Brochure*
    The IB should contain the following sections, each with literature references where appropriate:
    a. *Table of Contents*
        TABLE OF CONTENTS OF INVESTIGATOR'S BROCHURE (An Example)
            Confidentiality Statement (optional)
            Signature Page (optional)
        1. Table of Contents
        2. Summary
        3. Introduction
        4. Physical, Chemical, and Pharmaceutical Properties and Formulation
        5. Nonclinical Trials
            5.1. Nonclinical Pharmacology
            5.2. Pharmacokinetics and Product Metabolism in Animals
            5.3. Toxicology
        6. Effects in Humans
            6.1. Pharmacokinetics and Product Metabolism in Humans
            6.2. Safety and Efficacy
            6.3. Marketing Experience
        7. Summary of Data and Guidance for the Investigator
            NB: References on
            1. Publications
            2. Reports [These references should be found at the end of each chapter Appendices (if any)]
    b. *Summary*
        A brief summary (preferably not more than two pages) should be given, highlighting the significant physical, chemical, pharmaceutical, pharmacologic, toxicologic, pharmacokinetic, metabolic, and clinical information available that is relevant to the stage of clinical development of the investigational product.
    c. *Introduction*
        A brief introductory statement should be provided that contains the chemical name (and generic and trade name(s) when approved) of the investigational product(s), all active ingredients, the investigational product(s) pharmacologic class and its expected position within this class (e.g., advantages), the rationale for performing research with the investigational product(s), and the anticipated prophylactic, therapeutic, or diagnostic indication(s). Finally, the introductory statement should provide the general approach to be followed in evaluating the investigational product.
    d. *Physical, Chemical, and Pharmaceutical Properties and Formulation*
        A description should be provided of the investigational product substance(s) including the chemical and structural formula(s), and a brief summary should be given of the relevant physical, chemical, and pharmaceutical properties.

To permit appropriate safety measures to be taken in the course of the trial, a description of the formulation(s) to be used, including excipients, should be provided and justified if clinically relevant. Instructions for the storage and handling of the dosage form(s) also should be given. Any structural similarities to other known compounds should be mentioned.

e. *Nonclinical Trials*

The results of all relevant nonclinical pharmacology, toxicology, pharmacokinetic, and investigational product metabolism trials should be provided in summary form. This summary should address the methodology used, the results, and a discussion of the relevance of the findings to the investigated therapeutic and the possible unfavorable and unintended effects in humans.

The information provided may include the following, as appropriate, if known or available:

Species tested

Number and sex of animals in each group

Unit dose [e.g., milligram/kilogram (mg/kg)]

Dose interval

Route of administration

Duration of dosing

Information on systemic distribution

Duration of postexposure follow-up

Results, including the following aspects:

– Nature and frequency of pharmacological or toxic effects

– Severity or intensity of pharmacological or toxic effects

– Time to onset of effects

– Reversibility of effects

– Duration of effects

– Dose response

Tabular format/listings should be used whenever possible to enhance the clarity of the presentation.

The following sections should discuss the most important findings from the trials, including the dose response of observed effects, the relevance to humans, and any aspects to be studied in humans. If applicable, the effective and nontoxic dose findings in the same animal species should be compared (i.e., the therapeutic index should be discussed). The relevance of this information to the proposed human dosing should be addressed. Whenever possible, comparisons should be made in terms of blood/tissue levels rather than on an mg/kg basis.

Nonclinical Pharmacology: A summary of the pharmacologic aspects of the investigational product and, where appropriate, its significant metabolites studied in animals should be included. Such a summary should incorporate trials that assess potential therapeutic activity (e.g., efficacy models, receptor binding, and specificity), as well as those that assess safety (such as special trials to assess pharmacologic actions other than the intended therapeutic effect(s)).

Pharmacokinetics and Product Metabolism in Animals: A summary of the pharmacokinetics and biological transformation and disposition of the investigational product in all species studied should be given.

The discussion of the findings should address the absorption and the local and systemic bioavailability of the investigational product and its metabolites, and their relationship to the pharmacologic and toxicologic findings in animal species.

Toxicology: A summary of the toxicologic effects found in relevant trials conducted in different animal species should be described under the following headings where appropriate:

- Single dose
- Repeated dose
- Carcinogenicity
- Special trials (such as, irritancy and sensitization)
- Reproductive toxicity
- Genotoxicity (mutagenicity)

f. *Effects in Humans*

A thorough discussion of the known effects of the investigational product(s) in humans should be provided, including information on pharmacokinetics, metabolism, pharmacodynamics, dose response, safety, efficacy, and other pharmacologic activities. Where possible, a summary of each completed clinical trial should be provided. Information should also be provided regarding results from any use of the investigational product(s) other than in clinical trials, such as from experience during marketing.

Pharmacokinetics and Product Metabolism in Humans: A summary of information on the pharmacokinetics of the investigational product(s) should be presented, including the following, if available:

1. Pharmacokinetics (including metabolism, as appropriate, and absorption, plasma protein binding, distribution, and elimination)
2. Bioavailability of the investigational product (absolute, where possible, or relative) using a reference dosage form
3. Population subgroups (e.g., sex, age, and impaired organ function)
4. Interactions (such as, product–product interactions and effects of food)
5. Other pharmacokinetic data (e.g., results of population trials performed within clinical trial(s)).

Safety and Efficacy: A summary of information should be provided about the investigational product's safety (including metabolites, where appropriate), pharmacodynamics, efficacy, and dose response that were obtained from preceding trials in humans (healthy volunteers or patients). The implications of this information should be discussed. In cases where a number of clinical trials have been completed, the use of summaries of safety and efficacy across multiple trials by indications in subgroups may provide a clear presentation of the data. Tabular summaries of adverse drug reactions for all the clinical trials (including those for all the studied indications) would be useful. Important differences in adverse drug reaction patterns/incidences across indications or subgroups should be discussed.

The IB should provide a description of the possible risks and adverse drug reactions to be anticipated on the basis of prior experiences with the product under investigation and with related products.

A description should also be provided of the precautions or special monitoring to be done as part of the investigational use of the product.

Marketing Experience: The IB should identify countries where the investigational product has been marketed or approved. Any significant information arising from the marketed use should be summarized (such as, formulations, dosages, routes of administration, and adverse product reactions). The IB should also identify all the countries where the investigational product did not receive approval/registration for marketing or was withdrawn from marketing/registration.

g. *Summary of Data and Guidance for the Investigator*
This section should provide an overall discussion of the nonclinical and clinical data and should summarize the information from various sources on different aspects of the investigational product, wherever possible. In this way, the investigator can be given the most informative interpretation of the available data, with an assessment of the implications of the information for future clinical trials.

Where appropriate, the published reports on related products should be discussed. This could help the investigator to anticipate adverse drug reactions or other problems in clinical trials.

The overall aim of this section is to provide the investigator with a clear understanding of the possible risks and adverse reactions, and of the specific tests, observations, and precautions that may be needed for a clinical trial. This understanding should be based on the available physical, chemical, pharmaceutical, pharmacologic, toxicologic, and clinical information on the investigational product. Guidance should also be given to the clinical investigator on the recognition and treatment of possible overdose and adverse drug reactions, based on previous human experience and on the pharmacology of the investigational product.

THE INVESTIGATIONAL MEDICINAL PRODUCT DOSSIER (IMPD) AND REQUIRED DOCUMENTATION TO CONDUCT CLINICAL RESEARCH IN THE EU

Introduction

The European Union (EU) Clinical Trials Directive issued on May 1, 2001, became national law on May 1, 2004 (see chapt. 24). The Directive describes the regulatory and ethical review processes and the information which now have to precede the initiation of clinical trials in the EU. This information has to be submitted to and approved by the Competent Authorities (CA) and the IECs of each Member State (MS) where the trials will be implemented. The information will be submitted in a document termed Investigational Medicinal Product Dossier (IMPD). This Dossier will basically be composed of the information as was previously presented for the IND. The difference being that the format for the information presented in an IMPD, where possible should be provided under the heading and arranged in the order given in The Rules Governing Medicinal Product in the European Union Volume 2,

Notice to Applicant Volume 2B Presentation and Content of the Dossier, Common Technical Document. The IMPD should contain information to justify the quality of any Investigational Medicinal Product (IMP) to be used in a clinical trial and include information on reference products and placebo. The document should also provide data from nonclinical trials and any information on the previous clinical use of the IMP or justify in the application why information is not provided. Although separate IMPDs need to be submitted to each MS in which a trial is to be performed, the content and format for these submissions are common with some additional regional requirements.

Although the IMPD comprises the main component of the documentation provided to each MS in order to obtain permission to initiate clinical trials, there are other documents that need to accompany the IMPD before approval is granted by the competent authorities of each MS. Before submitting an application to the MS, with the following list of documents, it is advisable to check the requirements for each MS, as they may vary from country to country. The Investigators Brochure is a very comprehensive document that contains much of the information in the IMPD. Therefore an applicant may either provide a stand alone IMPD or cross-refer to the IB for the preclinical and clinical parts of the IMPD providing the IB has sufficient detail to allow assessors to reach a decision about the potential toxicity of the IMP and safety of its use in the proposed trial. The following should accompany the IMPD:

- Receipt of confirmation of EudraCT number (see chap. 24)
- Covering letter
- Application form
- List of all CAs where application has been submitted
- Copy of IEC approval or comments
- Any letters of concern received from any MS
- Copy of any scientific advice
- A letter of authorization for use when applicant is not the sponsor
- Confirmation that CA will accept application in English
- Informed consent form
- Subject information (if any)
- Arrangement for recruitment of subjects
- Protocol with any amendments
- Summary of protocol in the national language
- Peer review of trial if available
- Ethical assessment by principal investigator
- Investigators Brochure (IB) (see IND for detail)
- Report of any trial with same IMP
- Example of label in the national language

Overall Content of the IMPD

An IMPD should include summaries of information related to the quality, manufacture, and control of the IMP. Data from nonclinical trials and from its clinical use, if any, should also be included. As with the recommended format of the IND presentation of the data in tabular form with brief narratives of the main points is acceptable. Although the format, as stated in the above reference, is recommended, it is not mandatory and the list is exhaustive. Sponsors are advised to use this detailed guidance as a starting point in their IMPD submissions. The following is a listing of the data that should be included in the IMPD:

a. Quality data including summaries of chemical pharmaceutical and biological data on the IMP. Data should be based on the IMPs to be used for a clinical trial whose manufacture complies with the principle of Good Manufacturing Practice (GMP) Applicants should also supply the following:
    *   A copy of the manufacturing authorization stating the scope of the authorization if the IMP is manufactured in the EU and does not have a marketing authorization in the EU.
    *   If the IMP is not manufactured in the EU and does not have a marketing authorization in the EU
        *   Certification of the Qualified Person that the manufacturing site works in compliance with GMP at least equivalent to EU GMP
        *   Certification of the GMP status of any active biological substance
        *   Copy of the importer's authorization
b. Nonclinical pharmacology and toxicology data including summaries of nonclinical pharmacology and toxicology data for any IMP to be used in the clinical trial or justify why they have not.
c. Previous clinical trial and human experience data section providing summaries of all available data from previous clinical trials and human experience with the proposed IMPs.
d. Overall risk and benefit assessment section should provide a brief integrated summary that critically analyses the nonclinical and clinical data in relation to the potential risks and benefits of the proposed trial. The test should identify any trials that wee terminated prematurely and discuss the reasons. Any evaluation of foreseeable risks and anticipated benefits for trials on minors or incapacitated adults should be taken into account.

Simplified IMPD

A simplified IMPD may be submitted if information related to the IMP has been assessed previously as part of a marketing authorization in any MS of the Community or as part of a clinical application to the CA concerned. The test should include a discussion of the potential risks and benefits of the proposed trial. Where appropriate, sponsors are allowed to cross-reference to the IMPD submitted by another applicant and held by the CA. This may require a letter from the other applicant to authorize the CA to cross-reference their data. The sponsor should have relevant information about this IMP that can be included in the investigator's brochure. In addition, an appropriate and adapted content of the IMP dossier may be allowed occasionally by the CA, provide that it is justified and agreed before the application is submitted.

CONCLUSIONS

This chapter has been prepared to describe in some detail the requirements of an IND application and the content of an IMPD. Emphasis has been placed on the different requirements for the clinical trial of a product in a phase 1 situation compared with a more advanced stage of drug research, that is, phases 2 and 3. Information relating to the submission of IND protocol and information amendments and IND annual reports has also been included. Finally, the newest guidance relating to the writing and content for an IB based on the International Conference on Harmonization has also been provided in detail. The content of detailed information to be submitted in an IND and an IMPD is interchangeable. Presently, these submissions are referenced in the CTD format.

9   New Product Applications for Global Pharmaceutical Product Approvals: U.S. NDA Vs. Global CTD Formats

Richard A. Guarino

Oxford Pharmaceutical Resources, Inc., Totowa, New Jersey, U.S.A.

INTRODUCTION

Submitting a New Drug Application (NDA) to the FDA and to other international agencies requires a meticulous, well-indexed, comprehensive, and readable prepared document. In the United States, the applicant's responsibility is to submit data that will satisfy the U.S. requirements of the Food, Drug, and Cosmetic Act, the Code of Federal Regulations (CFR), and the International Committee on Harmonisation (ICH) guidelines. In the European Union where a Sponsor intends to register their pharmaceutical products, the European Directives must be adhered to along with the ICH guidelines. In addition to these requirements, as of January 2008, the FDA in cooperation with ICH indicated that all NDAs are to be submitted in an electronic Common Technical Document (eCTD) format following the ICH M2 and M4 guidelines for Modules 1, 2, 3, 4, and 5 (1). These ICH guidelines specify the format for the presentation of generated data on Safety, Efficacy, and Quality for all international new product submissions (2). The United States, European Union, and Japan regulations are very similar on what should be submitted in a new product application. The only difference is for specific requests that must be addressed according to each countries requirement for the submission of new product applications (see chap. 24).

As a Sponsor plans and follows the formatting of the CTD, there must be a clear understanding of how to separate the most essential data from supporting material. The FDA Regulations, ICH guidelines, and meetings with the FDA and other agencies during the development stages, that is, particularly the pre-NDA submission conference, are all invaluable for the applicant to resolve any unforeseen problems that might arise from the FDA and other agency reviews, owing to the nature of the product or data submitted in an application.

GENERAL OVERVIEW OF NEW DRUG APPLICATIONS

There are no shortcuts in the preparation of an NDA even in the new CTD/eCTD format. The items highlighted in this chapter encompass information that can take literally thousands of pages of detailed explanation. To help prevent delays until approval is granted, the Sponsor of a new product application must meticulously organize the submission, check and recheck every fact, explain all omissions, and summarize all relevant information in an accurate, clear, concise, and complete manner. One author, experienced in submitting NDAs, has stated that: "Every NDA is a learning experience. A trial that was sophisticated when planned 3 years ago may seem less than adequate when subjected to the harsh glare of tomorrow's advisory committee review." It is of extreme importance for a Sponsor to anticipate and minimize time-consuming problems that can delay the approval process.

In the United States all NDAs, including abbreviated NDAs (ANDAs) and supplemental NDAs (SNDAs), must contain the information required in 21 CFR 314.50. This information is synonymous with that outlined in the format recommendations of the CTD; the only difference is that the CTD format is more precise and detailed. This gives the applicant more direction on how and what information is to be submitted. In the past, the NDA format required that two copies of the application were required: an archival and a review copy. In addition, an optional field copy could be submitted to expedite a Chemistry, Manufacturing, and Control (CMC) review. With the eCTD format only one electronic copy is necessary. This single copy of the electronic portions of a submission should be sent to the appropriate document room facility. FDA District offices have access to documents submitted in electronic format. Therefore, when sending a submission in electronic format, a Sponsor need not provide any documentation to the FDA Office of Regulatory Affairs District Office (Field copy). It is important to note that no copies should be sent directly to the reviewer or review division. Electronic documents that bypass the controls for electronic files described in 21 CFR 11 are not considered official documents for review. In the past when paper NDAs were submitted, it was recommended that the Sponsor deliver a desk copy of the summary volumes directly to the division reviewer.

An NDA format of an application for a new drug product would generally contain a signed FDA 356 h (5) form (www.fdaforms), an index, a summary, five or six technical sections, case report tabulations of subject data, case report forms, drug samples, and labeling. The organization of the content was generally left up to the applicant. The CTD format spells out exactly in what order these items should be submitted and where in the application the items are to be located. ANDAs and Biological License Applications (BLAs) are also addressed in the ICH guidelines; however, they usually contain only some of the above items and the information will be limited to what is needed to support that particular application (see chap. 10).

RETROSPECTIVE OVERVIEW OF THE NDA IN THE UNITED STATES (REVIEW AND ARCHIVAL COPIES)

The Paper NDA—Required Information
Prior to the CTD format, NDA submissions in the U.S. were comprised, for new drug and biologic submissions, a review and archival copy each containing a copy of Volume 1 with the contents of:

1. Cover letter that confirms agreements or understandings between the FDA and the applicant. This letter cited any relevant correspondence or meetings by date and topic, and identifies one or more persons of the Sponsor that the FDA could contact regarding the application and any other important information the applicant wished to convey to the FDA about the application.
2. Application Form (FDA 356 h). This application form, which serves as a cover sheet for the application, contains basic identifying information about the applicant and the drug product. Importantly, it obligates the applicant to comply with applicable laws and regulations including: GMP Regulations (21 CFR 210 and 211), GLP Regulations (21 CFR 58), GCP Regulations (21 CFR 312), labeling regulations (21 CFR 201), prescription drug advertising regulations (21 CFR 202),

regulations on making changes in an application (21 CFR 314.70314.71, and 314.72), regulations on reports (21 CFR 314.80 and 314.81), local, state, and federal environmental impact laws.

3. An overall summary of the components to be included in the NDA.
4. FDA Form 3397—User fee cover sheet, should be included in the first volume (User fee ID number can be obtained from FDA Central Document Room).
5. Financial Disclosure Forms: 3454 (no financial interest) and 3455 (financial interest) must be completed and included.
6. The Debarment Certification Statement

If the person signing the application does not reside or have a place of business within the United States, the application must contain the name and address of a representative agent or other authorized official who resides or maintains a place of business within the United States (many CROs or consulting firms act as the legal agent for foreign pharmaceutical companies not having an established office in the United States).

FDA 356 h form, Items 1, 2, and 3 listed on this application were to be bound together in a single volume. Items 4 to 12 were submitted in separately bound volumes in the order in which they are listed. Patent information on the applicant's drug (item 13) and a patent certification with respect to the drug (item 14) were submitted separately and were attached to the application form.

All Investigational New Drug Applications (INDs) (3), Drug Master Files (DMFs), and any other applications that are referenced in an NDA were to be identified in the space provided on the 356 h application form.

The information cited above is still required in the U.S. NDA. However, this information is now submitted in Module 1 in the CTD format. [FDA Guidance for Industry: Providing Regulatory Submissions in Electronic Format—Human Pharmaceutical Product Applications and Related Submissions Using the eCTD Specification (2006) and FDA eCTD Module 1 Specification Version 1.2 (2006) (4).]

General Format
An understanding of what comprised the detail components of a paper NDA format can enhance and ensure that the information submitted in a CTD format will meet CFR requirements. In addition, by comparing the paper NDA format to the CTD electronic format will demonstrate the advantages of using the eCTD format for global submissions.

Index: The comprehensive index would be composed of the volume and page number for the summary, the technical sections, and any supporting information. The index serves as a detailed table of contents for the entire application. It was prudent for the Sponsor to keep additional copies of the index and have them available if regulatory, clinical, or other company personnel were contacted by an agency reviewer with questions.

Each technical review section would have a copy of the overall index and an individualized table of contents based on the relevant portions of the application.

As stated above, NDA regulations (21 CFR 314.50) required the submission of an archival copy and a review copy with an optional field copy.

Contents of the Archival Copy

This was a complete copy of an application submission and was intended to serve as a reference source for FDA reviewers to locate information not contained in the section of the review copy assigned to them. This archival copy also served as a reference source for other FDA officials and as the repository of the copies of tabulations and clinical study case report forms.

After approval, the archival copy was retained by FDA and served as the sole file copy of the approved application. Certain parts of the archival copy would be accepted on microfiche, another suitable microform system, or by electronic (computer) means. Imagine the volume of paper that was and is stored in the FDA archives. The eCTD will now eliminate the need for this voluminous storage.

Contents Review Copy

The review copy of an application was divided into five (or six) sections containing the technical and scientific information required by FDA reviewers. Each of the technical sections of the review copy was separately bound and would go the reviewer in charge of that specific section, for example, clinical, pharmacology, statistics, etc. Each section of the review copy also contained a copy of Volume 1.

Other NDA Submission Requirements

The procedures used by the FDA to file and retrieve material from the document rooms where applications are kept required that applicants used colored folders (or "jackets") to bind the specific sections of the review copy. The archival volume all bore the same color.

For example, Archival copy—Light Blue, Review copy: Chemistry, Manufacturing, and Controls (CMC) section—Red, Nonclinical pharmacology and toxicology section—Yellow, Human pharmacokinetics and bioavailability section—Orange, Microbiology section—White, Clinical data section—Light Brown, Statistical section—Green, Field Copy—Maroon.

All applications were bound on the left side of the page using the United States standard size loose-leaf page ($8^{1}/_{2} \times 11$). Both sides of the page could be used for the presentation of information and data, provided Information and data on both sides were not obscured in the binding; Legibility was not impaired because of bleeding of the copy through the page; and Pages were in correct order and accurately numbered.

Pagination/Volume Size/Identification

Any method of pagination could be used, as long as the paging and indexing permitted rapid access to the entire submission. It is important that all pages in the application were numbered and that the numbering of the review copy pages were the same as the numbering of the corresponding pages in the archival copy. Numbering of the volumes for the technical sections of the review copy had to be the same as that used for the volumes of the archival copy. *Volumes submitted in hard copy form had to be no more than 2-in. thick.* The front cover of each volume bore name of applicant, drug, and NDA number that was obtained from FDAs central document room (if not previously assigned) and clearly written in waterproof marking pen or on typed, stick-on labels.

Packing Cartons

The box size of $14 \times 12 \times 9^1/_2$ was recommended for shipment of applications to FDA. Because ANDAs are handled and stored separately, smaller boxes may be appropriate for them. An exterior label indicated the contents by applicant's name, drug name, and volume numbers; it was also important to identify which cartons contain the archival copy and which one the review copy.

Overall Comments

Understanding the logistics of the administrative part of an NDA submission will give you an idea of how much effort had to go into the organization of a submission, no less the format in the reporting of the data. This tedious and time-consuming process required a large number of personnel who were trained to do detail and precision review of every page of every volume in the submission of a new product application. It required tons of paper processing and facilities to house these volumes at the company as well as at the Agency. The eCTD format eliminates all of these processes and gives Sponsors as well as Agency reviewers information of the new product submissions that can be electronically transmitted and retrieved in a format that is globally accepted. The ease in which reviewers can electronically confirm questions from one discipline to another is invaluable. The ICH guidelines pertaining to CTD and eCTD format for new product submissions have revolutionized the way data is presented and reviewed by agencies worldwide.

U.S. NDA VS. CTD FORMAT

As stated the old format used for an NDA in the United States followed FDA Form 356 h. The items listed on this form were used as a guide by almost all pharmaceutical industries when submitting NDAs and BLAs to the FDA. The 356 h form will still be submitted in an NDA application. However, the format of data submitted in a new product application will now follow the CTD/eCTD format. The information will be organized in five (6) Modules (see chap. 11 CTD/eCTD). The overall content in an eCTD format reflects all the information as outlined in the Form 356 h. Whereas, the system and the organization of the data in the old NDA format was left up to the Sponsor; the CTD format specifies how the submission is to be paginated and organized. The ICH guidelines outlining the format of the CTD is much more specific and details what information is to be included in each Module of new product applications.

All countries that follow the CTD format will have an interchange of information that will be consistent and therefore easily reviewed in the process of new product approvals.

The specific contents of Module 2, 3, 4, and 5 are clearly stated in chapter 11, "The CTD and eCTD for the Registration of Pharmaceuticals for Human Use," however, the region specific items that a Sponsor must include in a new product submission should be included in Module 1.

Region Specific Documentation

Even though the CTD format will facilitate the ease in reviewing a new product submission from country to country, each country has specific requirements that must be addressed. Module 1 is where these requirements should be addressed. Every effort should be placed on scheduling a meeting to discuss these specific requirements of the particular region where an application is to be submitted. The conclusions and the outcomes of these meetings should be incorporated in Module 1.

Listed below are items to be considered for the content of Module 1. Note that each of these items can follow the specific requirements of the country where the new product application is to be submitted.

A. Administration Information and Prescribing Information
    The eCTD backbone document information files (see www.fda.gov/CDER/ regulatory/ersr/eCTD.htm). The specifications for creating the electronic technical document (eCTD) backbone file for Module 1 can be found at this web site. This backbone file for Module 1 includes information for each file submitted in Module 1. The file information is provided within an XML element called the leaf element. The leaf elements are organized using the Module 1 headings. These headings are named and organized according to the subject matter of the information contained in the file. The heading information is provided as an XML element called header in this specification. The Module 1 eCTD Backbone File also includes administrative information about each submission, which is provided in the administration element. Because Module 1 eCTD Backbone File may be used in a wide range of applications and related submission types, a specific submission may not use all of the possible heading elements. Headers should be organized to suit the specific files for each submission.
B. Cover Letter (optional)
    If the sponsor decides to include a cover letter, it is recommended to include the following information:
    1. A description of the submission including appropriate regulatory information.
    2. A description of the submission including the approximate size of the submission (e.g., 2 GB), the format that was used for the DLT tapes, and the type and number of the electronic media used, if applicable.
    3. A statement that the submission is computer virus free with a description of the software; version and company used to check the files for viruses.
    4. Contact names of the Sponsor's regulatory and technical personnel.
    5. Any agreements made between the Sponsor and Agency.
C. Labeling
    Labeling documents are to be included in Module 1 and should contain the following:
    a. Labeling history summarizing any labeling changes as a single PDF file including the following information:
        • Complete list of the labeling changes being proposed in the current submission and an explanation for the changes.
        • Date of the last approved labeling.
        • A history of all the changes since the last approved labeling with a description of why changes were made.
        • List of any supplements pending approval that may affect the current label submission.
    b. Content of Labeling

Guidance for Industry on Providing Regulatory Submissions in Electronic Format is also cited in the eCTD Backbone Files specifications for Module 1 and includes the following:

c. Draft Labeling

d. Draft Carton and Container Labels

e. Annotated Draft Labeling Text: This is an extremely important part of the labeling requirements. A presentation of the proposed text of the labeling for the product, with each statement made referenced back to the data in the technical sections that support the statement. For each statement, claim, caution, or related group of statements, the proposed text of the package labeling must be annotated and referenced to the Module and document page number of the information in the summaries as well as the technical sections of the application that support each of the package labeling claims. In the United States, the format of labeling must follow that described in 21 CFR 201.57 and will form the basis for the advertising and promotion of the drug product. Any adverse experiences that appear in the nonclinical and clinical data but are not reflected in the labeling must be explained and must take into account the pharmacology of related drugs.

f. Draft Labeling Text

g. Label Comprehension Studies

h. Labeling History

i. Final Labeling

j. Final Package Insert (package inserts, patient information, medication guides)

k. Final Labeling Text

l. Listed Drug Labeling

m. Annotated Comparison with Listed Drug

n. Approved Labeling Text for Listed Drug

o. Labeling Text for Reference Listed Drug

p. Investigational Drug Labeling

q. Investigation Brochure

r. Foreign Labeling: If the product of the NDA is marketed outside the United States, regardless of the dosage form, strength, salt, ester or complex of the drug, the marketing history and labeling of the product should be addressed. This should include a list of the countries in which the product is marketed, with the dates of marketing, and a list of any countries in which the drug has been withdrawn for any reason related to safety or effectiveness.

s. End Labeling

D. Labeling Samples

Each labeling sample (e.g., carton labels, container labels, package inserts) should be provided as individual PDF files. The samples should include: all panels, be provided in their actual size, and reflect the actual color proposed for use.

E. Advertisements and Promotional Material

Advertisements and promotional material should be submitted to the appropriate regulatory authority. Do not mix submissions of advertisements and promotional labeling with submissions containing other types of information.

Each promotional piece should be provided as an individual PDF file. The reviewer should be able to view the entire layout at one time. For three dimensional objects a digital image of the object in sufficient detail should be provided. Information adequate to determine the size of the object should also be included. A dimensional piece shown flat can also be submitted. If cover letters are included with a submission of advertising and promotional material, they should be provided as individual PDF files and indicate for the reviewer any additional important information that needs priority review.

All references should be submitted as an individual PDF file. Hypertext links for references may be used.

F. Marketing Annual Reports

If there are any requests for postmarketing study commitments, each study should be described with projections of when the commitments will be fulfilled.

G. Information Amendments

Documents that are provided in information amendments should be included in the appropriate module using the appropriate heading to describe the subject matter. In the case when information amendments do not fit appropriately under any heading in the CTD, the documents should be placed in Module 1 under the heading "information amendment". For information not covered under Modules 2 to 5, a separate PDF file for each item covered should be provided. Documents that apply to more than one module should be placed under the heading "Multiple module information amendments."

FORMATS FOR NEW PRODUCT APPLICATIONS

The specifics of a U.S. NDA format of the information requested was never clearly defined as is in the CTD format. The Sponsors in the United States referred to the Code of Federal Regulations (CFRs) as their guide for including specific information under the headings listed in Form 356 h, with the aspiration that the FDA Division reviewing the submission would be satisfied with the information. It was also difficult for a U.S. Sponsor to submit the same information compiled in a U.S. NDA when trying to register the product in another country. This was mainly due to the unfamiliarity of the countries reviewing process to a U.S. NDA format. With the ICH guidelines on how new product submissions should be formatted, this is a concern of the past. Hopefully, this will be key for global registrations and approval of health care products more rapidly and economically.

Below is a listing of items that were included in a U.S. NDA submission. It is assuring to know that the information for new product submissions listed in the U.S. CFR reflect all the items addressed in the ICH CTD guidelines for new product submissions. However, the CFR's require many items that are still not clarified in the ICH CTD guidelines. For some U.S. NDA submissions, the content of these items should be discussed with the appropriate division of the FDA in order to clarify their inclusion and importance in a new product submission in the CTD/eCTD format.

The following is a list of items requested for U.S. NDA submissions but not yet addressed in the CTD/eCTD format. These items are listed on page 2 of form 356 h (5) (www.fdaforms).

Although some of these items are addressed in the information to be included in Module 1, listed below are some specific items that pertain only to U.S. NDA submissions:

- Patent information on any patent, which claims the drug.
- A patent certification with respect to any patent, which claims the drug.
- Establishment description.
- Debarment certification.
- User Fee Cover Sheet.
- Financial Information, Financial Disclosure forms.
- Certification of the information submitted in the U.S. NDA (see details on Form 356 h: fdaforms).
- Signature of Responsible Official or Agent. (If it is a submission by a foreign company that does not have an office in the U.S.A., a U.S. Agent and address of the same must be appointed.)

Overall Comments Between an NDA and CTD Format

As discussed, the CTD format is a precise document as compared to the NDA format. The CTD gives specific information as to what is to be incorporated in each section. However, there are certain parts of the CTD that do not give information that will give the agency reviewers a more in-depth feeling of the data in the submission. The following information is to help the composers of a CTD add some in-depth clinical information that will aid the agencies in the review of new product applications. These suggestions can be incorporated in Module 1 or in other Modules according to the information categories.

Listing of IND and NDA Investigators

Assure that a complete alphabetical list of all the names and addresses of all known investigators that the applicant supplied with the drug substance or product. In addition, all dosage forms used by these investigators should be stated.

Background/Overview of Clinical Investigations

This is a very important part of the clinical data section of a CTD. It provides the medical reviewer with a summary of how the product was researched and developed. Because of the time required for the clinical development of a product, many times agency reviewers assigned to a project have changed. As a result, the CTD may be reviewed by a new set of individuals who are unfamiliar with the history of the development of the project. It is also possible that the standards for research in the particular field may have changed and what was standard clinical practice when the clinical studies were initiated is no longer the method of choice for studying the particular class of drugs. In this section, a Sponsor is given the opportunity to describe the general approach and rationale used in developing the clinical data. This discussion should include how information derived from clinical pharmacology studies led to critical features in the design of clinical studies. The basis for the critical design features of the clinical trials as well as their suitability and selection of major clinical endpoints should also be discussed. Any Agency drug-class or other guidelines used in designing the studies and the rationale for any deviations from the guidelines should be discussed.

Agency/Sponsor discussions concerning issues related to the development of the clinical program, major agreements reached, and any important differences between these agreements and the ultimate conduct of the clinical studies must be referenced. The selection of areas of special interest for study and analysis, and effectiveness or safety issues raised by drugs/products of the same pharmacologic or therapeutic class warrant discussion. Any specific questions raised by the results of the clinical trials or by experience with related drugs and not answered by the clinical studies should be cited together with an explanation as to how the Sponsor plans to handle these issues. Any planned studies in support of an additional indication also should be noted.

Clinical Pharmacology
In the overall summary of the clinical pharmacology, information should include data relevant to clinical use of the drug, such as dose–response or blood concentration response data, duration of action data, and potential problems that can be associated with the observed patterns of metabolism or excretion (see chap. 11 on CTD).

Controlled Clinical Studies
Before a detailed discussion of the information to be included in this section presented, it is useful to review the definition of adequate and well-controlled studies. Approval of a new drug requires substantial evidence of effectiveness. Substantial evidence is defined in the United States under the Federal Food, Drug, and Cosmetic Act as well as in the ICH guidelines and EU Directives as follows:

> "evidence consisting of adequate and well-controlled investigations by experts qualified by scientific training and experience to evaluate the effectiveness of the drug/biologic involved, on the basis of which it could fairly and responsibly be concluded by such experts that the drug will have the effect it purports or is represented to have under the conditions of use prescribed, recommended, or suggested in the proposed labeling. The requirement for well-controlled investigations has been interpreted to mean that the effectiveness of a drug should be supported by more than one well-controlled trial and carried out by independent investigators."

In the United States, approval of new submissions for certain products (particularly products for life-threatening disorders or for which no acceptable therapy is presently available) may be based on a single pivotal clinical trial. This thrust is based on the FDA Modernization Act (FDAMA) of 1997. Section 115 of FDAMA (6) states that the "substantial evidence" of efficacy requirement may be satisfied by *one* adequate and well-controlled clinical investigation supported by confirmatory evidence. The FDA issued a guidance on when one phase 3 trial would suffice for product approval in May 1997.

Study Reports
The CTD does not comment on the content of reports for clinical studies and how they should be submitted. Therefore, for studies intended to support effectiveness, full reports (as described in the ICH E3 guideline) are required; for others, an abbreviated report may be acceptable.

As a guide in preparation of a report Synopsis, a brief (one-page) summary of the study is required.

For a comprehensive summary for studies, a detailed description of the study design and results should include the following:

a. Investigator
b. Study objectives
c. Detailed of design
d. Subject selection and rejection criteria
e. Clinical observations and laboratory measurements
f. Evaluation criteria
g. Planned statistical analyses
h. Method of eliciting adverse experiences
i. Comparability of treatment groups for demographic and other variables
j. Analysis of results of safety and effectiveness
k. Detailed accounting of subjects entered/excluded from the study
l. The dosage and duration of treatment

When special clinical and laboratory measures are used for the study, a rationale for the use of these tests as well as an explanation for the significance of the results must be fully addressed.

Safety Information
Remember to include in the safety information a summary of adverse experiences by frequency and body system and by dose level and dosing duration. Subjects who died or who left the study prematurely because of an adverse experience should be described in detail, and the role of the drug should be evaluated for each reaction. The safety analysis should consider abnormal laboratory values as well as adverse experiences, and the following points should be kept in mind:

a. Is the subject receiving several different medications simultaneously?
b. Are the subject's complaints totally subjective, for example, headache, nausea, dizziness? Many of these often appear in healthy volunteers taking placebo.
c. The evaluation of adverse experiences is dependent in great part on the extent of the control of the study.
d. The effect of the environment in which the study was conducted—acute medical ward versus outpatient clinic.
e. Examination of subject's history and careful follow-up of subject; authentication of facts.

Uncontrolled Clinical Studies
Uncontrolled studies will not, in general, be useful in contributing to substantial evidence of effectiveness of a drug, but they can provide support for controlled clinical studies and provide safety information. However, any subject who receives any dose of the proposed drug product must be included in the overall evaluation of safety data.

Other Studies and Information
It is important to remember when planning your CTD that any additional information obtained by the applicant from any source, foreign or domestic, that is relevant to the evaluation of the efficacy and safety of the product should be included. It may include results of controlled or uncontrolled clinical trials of uses of the drug other than those claimed in the application, commercial marketing experience, and

reports in the literature or otherwise obtained, other than those cited in the controlled trials and uncontrolled trials in Module 5.

ORGANIZING COMMON TECHNICAL DOCUMENTS SUMMARIES

Chapter 11 details the information that should be contained in Module 2, the most important part of a CTD submission. However, there are points that should be emphasized within the integrated summaries of Quality, Safety, and Efficacy. Listed below are some helpful suggestions of issues that must be covered in the summary submissions and may ensure a more comprehensive understanding of the data for Agency reviewers.

Quality

1. Drug Substance: Description Including Physical and Chemical Characteristics and Stability:
   a. Names: established generic name, synonyms, code designations, proprietary (brand name or trademark) name, identification number (chemical abstract service registry number) and chemical name. The applicant should not designate or reference a drug or ingredient by a proprietary name because at times a similarity in spelling or pronunciation may be confused with the proprietary name or the established name of a different drug already available in the global marketplace. It is to be noted that in the United States the FDA discourages the use of fanciful proprietary name for a drug or any ingredient that might imply that the drug or ingredient has some unique effectiveness or composition when, in fact, the drug or ingredient is a common substance, readily recognized when the drug or ingredient is listed by its established name.
   b. Physical and Chemical Characteristics: Besides describing these characteristics, where applicable, provide information on isomers, polymorphs, pKa values, and pH. Refer to standards used to elucidate the structure of the drug substance.
   c. Stability: Stability data should be submitted for the drug substance in the container in which it is packaged. (This is only done on request from the Agency.) In the method of manufacture flowcharts many are used to present this information.
2. Drug Product:
   a. Composition and Dosage Form should state each active and inactive ingredient in the drug product in the form in which the drug product is to be distributed. Any novel excipient needs to be described in detail.
   b. Manufacture, if more than one entity (i.e., manufacturing group) is involved in any part of the process, describes the responsibilities of each.
   c. Specifications and Analytical Methods: Describe as with the drug substance the acceptable specifications for the drug product and the test method used to assure the specifications. Cite any official compendia methods used.
   d. Beside the container/closure used, safety closure systems should be detailed.
   e. Stability, remember beside stability for the expiration date submit stability for the drug product in the container in which it will be marketed. Stability data must include stability data from three separate batches of the proposed drug product at each dosage strength and for each formulation type

[(i.e., tablet and capsule, etc.) for expiration date to be used on marketing containers].

f. Investigational Formulations for each clinical trial, bioavailability and pharmacokinetic trials, clinical pharmacology trials, and dose tolerance trials conducted during the investigational phases of the product must have the quantitative compositions and lot number of each finished dosage form used in these trials submitted in the Quality summary. Each formulation must be cross-referenced to the trial report and any differences in formulations must be explained.

Safety (Nonclinical Pharmacology, Pharmacokinetics, and Toxicology) Summary

In the nonclinical pharmacology, pharmacokinetics, and toxicology or Safety summary, all studies conducted on the drug candidate must be listed. Provide an overview of the data from these studies with emphasis on notable adverse effects and dose relationships, species similarities and differences, possible gender differences, and identified mechanisms for pharmacological and toxicological effects. The discussion should center on the appropriateness and adequacy of the data in support of the drug's proposed therapeutic uses.

Tabular summaries (as described in the ICH M4S guideline) should be used that permit identification and comparison of the pertinent observations.

It is recommended that the studies for this section be presented as follows:

1. Pharmacology studies. Further subgroup by type of test with studies that support the pharmacologic activity of the drug first, followed by secondary pharmacodynamic studies, safety pharmacology studies, and pharmacodynamic drug interaction studies (if conducted).
2. Pharmacokinetic or ADME (absorption, distribution, metabolism, excretion) studies. Animal species should be presented under each group by the smallest (mouse) up to the largest (monkey, dog, or minipig). The route of administration should be presented under each species tested and the treatment group under each route of administration. For special toxicity studies, such as irritation and hemolysis studies tabulate data as appropriate. An example of the format would be: The first route presented would be the projected clinical route followed by the routes that are not the clinical route, for example:

Mouse
   (1) Oral
      (a) Untreated control, (b) Vehicle control, (c) Etc.
   (2) I.V.
      (a) Untreated control, (b) Vehicle control, (c) Etc.

Rat
   (1) Oral
      (a) Untreated control, (b) Vehicle control, (c) Etc.
   (2) I.V.
      (a) Untreated control, (b) Vehicle control, (c) Etc.

In summarizing the pharmacokinetic and ADME studies, tabulate species, strain, and dose comparison data by the following:

- Peak concentration, half-life, and so forth
- Plasma protein binding
- Tissue distribution/accumulation
- Enzyme induction or inhibition
- Metabolites
- Excretion pattern and characteristics

The absorption, distribution, metabolism, and excretion in the species used in the toxicology studies should be discussed and justified. Quantitative or notable qualitative differences in ADME between the various animal species and humans should be discussed, as well as any references to observed species differences in toxicity and extrapolation of the findings to humans. The significance of these findings to the interpretation of the results of the carcinogenicity, bioassay, and other nonclinical toxicity studies should be considered.

3. Toxicology—acute toxicity studies. Tabulate species, sex, age, dose range, pharmacologic actions and interactions with other drugs, routes of administration, vehicle, toxic signs, lethal dose, time of death, etc.
4. Toxicology—repeat-dose toxicity studies (subchronic and chronic). Provide a table of studies including species and strain, number of animals, sex, age, dose, dose schedule, and route of administration. Notable treatment and dose-related changes in survival, percent weight gain, toxic signs, hematology, clinical chemistries, urinalysis, organ weight, gross pathology, and histopathology should be provided. Toxicokinetic information should also be summarized.
5. Carcinogenicity studies. The following information should be included:
   (a) For each treatment group, the number of animals entered and surviving 12, 15, 18, 21, and 24 months.
   (b) A summary table of tumor occurrences with deaths and sacrifices combined, organized by body system, tumor type, and dose level.
   (c) In the above table, each tumor shown to have a statistically significant dose response (positive or negative) at the $P = 0.05$ level (one-sided) using a mortality-adjusted statistical test of dose response over the entire study time unadjusted for multiple comparisons or multiple testing should be indicated. Calculated P values for the significant dose–response test for each of these tumors should be included.
6. Special toxicity studies should briefly describe why they were done and how the results answer any questions that might arise from the agency's review.
7. Reproduction studies. For *reproduction* studies, tabulate fertility and reproductive performance studies (segment I), and perinatal and postnatal studies (segment III) if differences are observed from controls. Teratology study data (segment II) should be tabulated showing differences and similarities in gross viscera and skeletal anomalies.
8. Mutagenicity studies.
   For *mutagenicity* studies, data should be presented in the following order:
   A. In vitro nonmammalian cell system
   B. In vitro mammalian cell system
   C. In vivo mammalian system

Human Pharmacokinetics and Bioavailability Summary

The human pharmacokinetic and bioavailability summary should include the following:

1. A brief description of each bioavailability study of the drug in humans, by type, objective, design, analytical and statistical method used, and results.
2. A brief description of the pharmacokinetic characteristics of the active ingredient(s) and the performance of the dosage form, integrating conclusions from the bioavailability and pharmacokinetic studies and from clinical studies performed. Information on volume of distribution, half-life, routes and rates of excretion, and metabolism of each dosage form studied, and the proportionality of absorption and disposition profiles over the therapeutic dose range should be included. If pertinent, a comparison with the bioavailability of other dosage forms should be provided. Any identified differences in pharmacokinetics among subject subgroups should be cited (age, gender, renal status, etc.).
3. A description of the dissolution profile of the drug should be included and compared with the bioavailability of that dosage form in humans.

Microbiology Summary

For anti-infective drugs, provide a summary of the results of the microbiologic studies conducted with the drug. This should include the following:

1. A brief description of the known mechanisms of action together with structural or other similarities to known families of antimicrobial drugs.
2. A brief description of the antimicrobial spectrum of action and a summary of the results of in vitro susceptibility testing demonstrating the concentrations of the drug required for effective use.
3. A brief description of known mechanisms of resistance to the drug and results of any in vitro studies regarding resistance or any known epidemiologic studies that demonstrate prevalence of resistance factors.
4. A brief description of the clinical microbiology laboratory test method needed for effective use of the drug.

Clinical Data Summary and Results of Statistical Analysis (Module 2)

The clinical data summary (as discussed in the ICH M4E guideline for Section 2.7) and results of statistical analyses are divided into several parts as presented below. This section is probably the most scrutinized by the FDA's and other global agencies clinical reviewers. It is the basis of efficacy and safety that will determine a new pharmaceutical product approval. Note that the clinical summary section [2.7] is to provide only factual information on the clinical trials conducted on the proposed drug product. The clinical overview section [2.5] is to summarize why the proposed drug product should be approved based on the generated results (see chap. 11).

Clinical Pharmacology

Describe the phase 1 studies that establish human tolerance to the drug, absorption, distribution, and elimination kinetics, blood concentrations as a function of time after dosing, the metabolic profile, drug interactions, dependence, and pharmacologic effects at various doses. Although it is usual to test the drug during phase 1 studies in normal (healthy) subjects, if a drug has dramatic biochemical or pharmacologic effects tailored to address a specific disease state, phase 1 studies are conducted only in individuals with such a disease state. A careful explanation in this section should be prepared.

Conclusions drawn from this group of studies must be carefully summarized. This summary should provide the critical findings, especially those relevant to clinical use of the drug (e.g., dose–response or blood concentration-response data, duration of action, and any specific potential problems associated with metabolism or excretion). There should be a complete discussion of data pertinent to other common important pharmacologic properties, including cardiac electrophysiologic effects, hemodynamic effects, anticholinergic effects, and effects on the central nervous system. Any effects related to age or sex or other demographic characteristic should be highlighted.

Overview of Clinical Studies

The objective of all clinical studies is to produce clear and well-documented evidence that a new drug candidate is effective and safe when used in the manner intended. The clinical experience that the Sponsor is submitting (see GCP chap. 21 must provide assurance of the care taken in the evaluation of the drug product. This assurance must be passed on to Agency reviewers in the summary of the clinical evaluation.

In the United States, the overview should reference any specific FDA guidelines used and any FDA/Sponsor discussions held on major issues, such as an end-of-phase 2 conference etc. If conferences were held with other international agencies, these should also be referenced. The critical features of the trials should be explained, including duration, study design, and particular advantages or potential problems examined. If there is pertinent clinical literature (controlled or uncontrolled clinical studies or reports on subjects), a review may be helpful. (The sponsor may want to comment on literature pertaining to closely related drugs that provide insight into potential problems or areas of special interest for the proposed drug product.)

It is important to comment on all studies conducted on the product, even those that were not completed or are ongoing, or studies of claims other than those for which approval is being sought.

A tabular presentation of studies by protocol, investigator, study design (e.g., randomized, double-blind, open, parallel, crossover), drug or other treatment used for comparison (if any), number of subjects, age, sex, dose, and duration of dosing. Location of study report and CRFs should also be included.

Controlled Clinical Studies

All controlled studies, whether they provide positive, equivocal, or negative evidence, must be included:

a. A table of all completed studies sponsored by the applicant, including domestic studies and foreign studies, as well as those from published or unpublished papers or other sources. Provide the protocol number (where available), reference to any published report, investigator(s), study design (e.g., double-blind, open, parallel, crossover), the formulation and dosage used, number of subjects, demographics of subjects, dose and duration of therapy, and location of the clinical report and CRFs.
b. A short narrative of each study is to include information on the study design, conduct, and analysis. This section should be of sufficient detail to allow the reader to understand what the dose was and what data were collected and

analyzed for efficacy and safety determinations. Quantitative results should be provided, and the statistical methodologies, specific endpoints used, and any subject inclusion and exclusions should be described.

c. An analysis of each study and all the studies as a whole is considered necessary to demonstrate how the conducted studies relate to each claim of effectiveness. If some studies are considered more important than others, this should be noted and an explanation given. Any pooled analyses should be explained and presented. Any major inconsistencies or areas needing further exploration should be identified. Dose–response and dose-duration/dose-frequency information as well as any differences in response among subgroups should be included.

Uncontrolled Clinical Studies
This section covers the following:

a. A table of studies similar to that included in the controlled clinical studies section of the summary. The information should include the protocol number or other identifier, conditions studied, formulation and dosage, number of subjects, age and sex, duration of therapy, and location of the full report in the clinical data section.
b. A brief narrative description of the design and results of each study, including effectiveness results and adverse experiences.
c. An overall analysis of these studies with the conclusions of the results.

N.B.: Note for 95% of submissions of new product applications Uncontrolled or Open Studies will not support effectiveness of the product but will add to safety evaluations.

Other Studies and Information
A brief description of any studies not included in the clinical pharmacology, controlled clinical studies, or uncontrolled clinical studies sections should be included here. These may include studies and publications not directly related to the claims sought in the application but that provide pertinent safety information. Analyses of marketing experience or epidemiologic data may also be included in this section.

Safety Summary—General Safety Conclusions
This section should cover the following information:

1. Extent of Exposure
    The extent of drug exposure and the number of subjects exposed to the drug for various periods and at various doses.
2. Adverse Experiences & Adverse Reactions
    Data from controlled and uncontrolled studies should be integrated to provide estimated rates of adverse experiences. The tables of adverse experience rates, including the more serious or frequent experiences, should be compiled (see chap. 19 on ADR reporting). It is useful to analyze results from controlled and open studies separately and distinguish short-term use from longer-term studies. Any differences in rates of reported adverse experiences (AEs) related to dose, duration of therapy, and subject characteristics should be identified. Data related to drug–drug interactions should also be included. An analysis of subjects who left the study prematurely because of an AE or who died while on

this study drug should be included. For potentially serious adverse experiences (SAEs), not drug related and justified through disclaimers, should be discussed in this section. In addition, steps in premarketing or postmarking follow-up should take into account this SAE to ensure it is not study drug related.

3. Clinical Laboratory Data

    Provide a short summary of these data, noting clinically significant trends and statistically significant changes. The summary should compare the proposed drug product with active control drug or placebo and should show the numbers of subjects receiving each laboratory test. Also identify and evaluate those subjects who left a trial because of clinical laboratory abnormalities.

4. Summary of Other Safety Assessments

    If there were any special safety examinations performed (e.g., audiometric, electrocardiographic, or ophthalmologic examinations, etc.), these should be summarized here. Include any comparisons with active control drugs and placebo, if available, and the numbers of subjects receiving each test.

5. Overdosage

    Any information available on the treatment of overdosage should be included.

6. Drug Abuse

    If the drug is subject to abuse, provide a summary of the studies or other relevant information. If the drug is not considered to have abuse potential but is a member of a class of drugs known to have abuse potential, and if studies of its abuse potential have not been performed, then the reasons these studies were considered unnecessary should be discussed.

Discussion of Benefit/Risk Relationship and Proposed Postmarketing Studies

Benefit/risk relationship should be included in the Clinical Overview [Module 2, Section 2.5] and this is an extremely important part of a new product submission and must receive particular attention. On the basis of the results of effectiveness trials and the toxicity of the drug in human and animal studies, a benefit-to-risk assessment of the drug should be formulated and presented. The assessment should consider the risks and benefits of alternative treatment(s) for the target population identified in the labeling. In some instances the product may have high risk, however, the benefit can, at times, outweigh the risk.

A reference to the Benefit/Risk detailed in Section 2.5 of the CTD should reflect any proposed postmarketing clinical studies and the reasons for doing such studies, for example, to study further a suspected adverse reaction, or studies in children if there is a potential for use in this group.

SUMMARY AND CRITIQUE

The topics discussed above are considerations to be used as a guide for data submitted in a new product application using a CTD format. The specific details that must go into the Technical Sections of a CTD are fully described in the CTD and eCTD chapter. Special attention is given to the parts of the CTD that address Nonclinical Drug Development (chap. 7) and Chemistry, Manufacturing Controls (CMC) (chap. 13). The old format used to submit a NDA in the United States, at times, resulted in delays in approval due to topics or issues that were not covered in the data application. With the event of the CTD format and its specific details of how and what data is to be submitted in each Module, the new product approval process should move along at a faster pace. The fact that the same data can be submitted internationally will hopefully expedite product approvals globally. There are areas that the CTD format does not address and areas the U.S. NDA format does not address; eventually these will be resolved in future revisions of the ICH guidelines. Listed below are some differences between the CTD items and the U.S. NDA items that need to be addressed in a CTD submission.

Item	CTD	NDA
Numbering selection	Definite	Not addressed
Organization	Definite	Not definite
Amendments	Not addressed (in eCTD)	Allowed
Supplements	Not addressed (in eCTD)	As referenced in the CFRs
Substance and product development	Detailed	Not detailed
Colors by discipline	Not addressed	Definite
Pharmacology and toxicology reports	Text addressed	Text addressed
Tabular summaries	Tabular reports requested	Recommended
Section headings	Defined	Necessary but not defined
Pharmacology	4 sections (primary and secondary pharmacodynamics, safety pharmacology, and pharmacodynamic drug interaction)	Single section
Human biomaterial and in vitro study summaries	Requested in efficacy section	Not required
Subpopulation comparisons	Requested in Efficacy section	Required but not defined in detail
Clinical trial summaries	Requested using CSR synopses	Required but not defined in detail
Analytical chemistry validation reports	1 copy	1 copy in archival and 3 copies in review
Postapproval stability protocols for drug substance and drug product	Requested	Requested but not defined
Quality process validation	Yes	No
Executed batch records translated	No	Yes
Specifications for drug product	Yes	Not specified
DMF TSE/BSE	Certificate	
Pharm development	Yes	Not specified
Method validation	(1 copy)	(3 copies)
Efficacy-Module 5 doses in vitro	Yes	No

This chapter is a guide to be used in the preparation of a New Product Application for global submissions. All Sponsors and applicants must become familiar with the ICH guidelines as they relate to the CTD formats and eCTD specifications. In the United States and countries that follow the ICH guidelines, new product applications now follow the CTD/eCTD format. These new product applications

consist of detailed and complex documents that are organized by highly qualified technical personnel. It takes the collective efforts of many talented people in
a pharmaceutical or consulting company to compile the data necessary to fulfill the
requirements of regulatory agencies throughout the world. The key to the success of
having a product approved for market is to present the data in a package that can be
reviewed with ease and understanding. In addition, the information must contain
validated safety and efficacy data to convince the agencies that the proposed drug
product will benefit the subject population for which it is intended. It is hoped that
the CTD format presented in the ICH guidelines, delineating format requirements
of new product applications, will help produce more consistent and high-quality
documents that will expedite new product approvals globally.

CTD REVIEW GUIDE
1. General Information
    The name of the drug and the associated descriptive features, especially if
    changes occurred during the investigational process.
2. Chemistry, Manufacturing, and Controls or Quality
    Review any problems with clinical implications, especially if a variety of
    dosage forms and/or strengths were used.
3. Nonclinical or Safety
    Pharmacodynamic, pharmacokinetic, and toxicology results should be
    reviewed thoroughly, especially where equivocal results occurred. Do not for-
    get the ICH M4S–requested pharmacology, pharmacokinetic, and toxicology
    tabulated summaries.
4. Clinical Background
    *   Prior history of similar human studies and results
    *   Literature references (pertinent to the drug studied)
    *   Related INDs and NDAs
5. Clinical Studies or Efficacy
    *   Controlled studies
    *   Review trials for objective of the study—rationale for the study
    *   Experimental design, especially designs that may be considered novel or
        unusual
    *   Procedures
    *   Safety considerations (and comparative safety considerations)
    *   Efficacy considerations (and comparative efficacy considerations)
    *   Results of statistical consultation
    *   Results of the study
6. Scientific Conclusions
    *   What will the studies support?
    *   What claims for labeling and advertising?
    *   What are the deficiencies/problems in any study that may need to be
        reflected in the labeling?
7. Regulatory Conclusions
    *   Impact on proposal labeling, especially comparative claims
    *   Adverse effects
    *   Alert reports
    *   Adverse experiences; comparison to placebo or competitive products
    *   Warnings; any severe or life-threatening (boxed)

- Uncontrolled studies; safety data
- An accounting for investigators
- Need for postmarketing surveillance studies—for duration, for specialty groups (e.g., children or elderly)
- Labeling review with a careful evaluation of each section for basic content, clarity, and full disclosure (review 21 CFR 201.56 and 201.57).

REFERENCES

1. ICH CTD and eCTD Guidelines www.ich.org.
2. ICH Quality, Safety, and Efficacy Guidelines www.ich.org.
3. FDA/Center for Drug Evaluation and Research, Last updated: December 28, 2007, Originator: OTCOM/DML, HTML by SJW.
4. FDA Guidance for Industry: Providing Regulatory Submissions in Electronic format—Human Pharmaceutical Product Applications and Related Submissions Using the eCTD Specifications (2006) and FDA eCTD Module 1 Specification Version 1.2 (2006).
5. FDA Form 356 h: www.fdaforms.
6. FDA FDAMA: www.fda.gov/cder/fdama/default.htm.

10 Abbreviated and Supplemental New Drug Applications (ANDAs and SNDAs)

Richard A. Guarino

Oxford Pharmaceutical Resources, Inc., Totowa, New Jersey, U.S.A.

ABBREVIATED NEW DRUG APPLICATION

An abbreviated new drug application (ANDA) is specifically designed for an approval of a generic drug product. When data within an ANDA are submitted to the Food and Drug Administration's Center for Drug Evaluation and Research (CDER), Office of Generic Drugs at 7500 Standish Place, Rockville, Maryland, U.S., the applications are reviewed and approved from that division. On approval of the application, the applicant may manufacture and market the generic drug product with the purpose of providing the American consumer with a safe, effective, and low-cost alternative of a brand name drug.

To nominate a generic drug, it must be a drug product that is comparable to an innovator drug product in dosage form, strength, route of administration, quality, performance characteristic, and intended use.

Background History

The Waxman–Hatch Act also known as the "Drug Price Competition and Patent Term Restoration Act of 1984" established bioequivalence as the basis for approving generic copies of drug products. This Act permits FDA to approve ANDAs submitted to market generic versions of brand name drugs without conducting costly and duplicative preclinical (animal) and clinical (human) trials to establish safety and efficacy. To access additional information on the bioequivalence review of generic products, the Office of Generic Drugs provides a home page to generic drug developers including an interactive flowchart presentation of an ANDA focusing on how CDER determines safety and bioequivalence of generic drug products prior to an approval for marketing.

ANDA CONTENT

General

The term abbreviated is used in generic drug applications because, as stated above, they are usually not required to include preclinical and clinical data to establish safety and efficacy. However, a sponsor of a generic drug must scientifically demonstrate that their product is bioequivalent. Bioequivalent, for the purpose of this submission, refers to having the generic product perform in the same manner as the innovator or reference drug. Bioequivalence measures the time it takes the generic drug to reach the bloodstream as compared to the reference drug in healthy volunteers. The rate of absorption is determined by the bioavailability of

166

the generic drug that then can be compared to the innovator drug. It must be shown that the generic drug version must deliver the same amount of active ingredients into a subject's bloodstream in the same amount of time as the innovative drug. (see Bioavailability and Pharmacokinetics Studies in Chapter 12).

Legal Requirements and Guidance Documents

Guidance documents are prepared for FDA review staff and applicants or sponsors to provide guidelines for the processing, content, evaluation, and approval of an application. In addition, they also provide design, production, manufacturing, and testing of regulated products. The policies emanating from these guidelines are intended to achieve consistency in FDA's regulatory approach and establish inspection and enforcement procedures. It must be remembered that guidance documents are not regulations or laws and, as a result, are not enforceable either through administrative actions or through the courts. However, it is prudent for the applicant to consider these guidelines and review them before the final submission of each ANDA.

The detailed components referred to in chapter 9 on the format of the NDA also detail how the content of the ANDA might be approached. With the exception of the preclinical and nonclinical sections and the clinical section, an ANDA may follow the same items referred to in the NDA. Notwithstanding the guidance documents that have been developed by the FDA to assist applicants in preparing ANDAs, which are listed together on CDER's Guidance Document Index Web page, it would be more prudent for a sponsor of an ANDA to submit the ANDA following the checklist for CTD or an eCTD format. For completeness and acceptability of an application for filing an ANDA, the outline below can be used as a guideline for future submissions.

ANDA CHECKLIST FOR CTD or eCTD FORMAT
FOR COMPLETENESS and ACCEPTABILITY of an APPLICATION
FOR FILING

For More Information on Submission of an ANDA in Electronic Common Technical Document (eCTD) Format please go to: http://www.fda.gov/cder/regulatory/ersr/ectd.htm
*For a Comprehensive Table of Contents Headings and Hierarchy please go to:
http://www.fda.gov/cder/regulatory/ersr/5640CTOC-v1.2.pdf
** For more CTD and eCTD informational links see the final page of the ANDA Checklist
*** A model Quality Overall Summary for an immediate release tablet and an extended release capsule can be found on the OGD webpage http://www.fda.gov/cder/ogd/

ANDA #:   FIRM NAME:
PIV: ELECTRONIC OR PAPER SUBMISSION:

RELATED APPLICATION(S):

First Generic Product Received?

DRUG NAME:
DOSAGE FORM:

Bio Assignments:		☐ Micro Review
☐ BPH	☐ BCE	
☐ BST	☐ BDI	

Random Queue:

Chem Team Leader: PM: Labeling Reviewer:

Letter Date:	**Received Date**:
Comments:	**On Cards:**
Therapeutic Code:	

Archival copy: **Sections**
Review copy: E-Media Disposition:
Not applicable to electronic sections
PART 3 Combination Product Category
(Must be completed for ALL Original Applications)   Refer to the Part 3 Combination Algorithm

Reg. Support Reviewer	Recommendation: ☐ **FILE** ☐ **REFUSE to RECEIVE**
ADDITIONAL COMMENTS REGARDING THE ANDA:	

MODULE 1
ADMINISTRATIVE   ACCEPTABLE

1.1	**1.1.2 Signed and Completed Application Form (356h) (original signature)** (Check Rx/OTC Status)	☐
1.2	**Cover Letter**	☐
*	**Table of Contents (paper submission only)**	☐
1.3.2	**Field Copy Certification** (original signature) **(N/A for E-Submissions)**	☐
1.3.3	**Debarment Certification-GDEA (Generic Drug Enforcement Act)/Other:** 1. Debarment Certification (original signature) 2. List of Convictions statement (original signature)	☐
1.3.4	**Financial Certifications** Bioavailability/Bioequivalence Financial Certification (Form FDA 3454) Disclosure Statement (Form FDA 3455, submit copy to Regulatory Branch Chief)	☐
1.3.5	**1.3.5.1 Patent Information** Patents listed for the RLD in the Electronic Orange Book Approved Drug Products with Therapeutic Equivalence Evaluations **1.3.5.2 Patent Certification** 1. Patent number(s) 2. Paragraph: (Check all certifications that apply) MOU PI PII PIII PIV (Statement of Notification) 3. Expiration of Patent(s): a. Pediatric exclusivity submitted? b. Expiration of Pediatric Exclusivity? 4. Exclusivity Statement:	☐

1.4.1	**References**
	Letters of Authorization
	1. DMF letters of authorization
	    a. Type II DMF authorization letter(s) or synthesis for Active Pharmaceutical Ingredient
	    b. Type III DMF authorization letter(s) for container closure
	2. US Agent Letter of Authorization (U.S. Agent [if needed, countersignature on 356h])
		☐

1.12.11	**Basis for Submission** NDA# : Ref Listed Drug: Firm: ANDA suitability petition required? If Yes, then is change subject to PREA (change in dosage form, route or active ingredient) see section 1.9.1	☐
1.12.12	**Comparison between Generic Drug and RLD-505(j)(2)(A)** 1. Conditions of use 2. Active ingredients 3. Inactive ingredients 4. Route of administration 5. Dosage Form 6 Strength	☐
1.12.14	**Environmental Impact Analysis Statement**	☐
1.12.15	**Request for Waiver** Request for Waiver of In-Vivo BA/BE Study(ies):	☐

1.14.1	**Draft Labeling (Multi Copies N/A for E-Submissions)**
	1.14.1.1
	    4 copies of draft (each strength and container)
	1.14.1.2
	    1 side by side labeling comparison of containers and carton with all differences annotated and explained
	1.14.1.3
	    1 package insert (content of labeling) submitted electronically
	    ***Was a proprietary name request submitted?
	    (If yes, send email to Labeling Reviewer indicating such)
		☐

1.14.3	**Listed Drug Labeling**
	1.14.3.1
	    1 side by side labeling (package and patient insert) comparison with all differences annotated and explained
	1.14.3.3
	    1 RLD label and 1 RLD container label
		☐

MODULE 2
SUMMARIES   ACCEPTABLE

2.3	**Quality Overall Summary (QOS)** **E-Submission: PDF** **Word Processed e.g., MS Word** A model Quality Overall Summary for an immediate release tablet and an extended release capsule can be found on the OGD webpage http://www.fda.gov/cder/ogd/	☐

Question based Review (QbR)

2.3.S

    Drug Substance (Active Pharmaceutical Ingredient)
        2.3.S.1 General Information
        2.3.S.2 Manufacture
        2.3.S.3 Characterization
        2.3.S.4 Control of Drug Substance
        2.3.S.5 Reference Standards or Materials
        2.3.S.6 Container Closure System
        2.3.S.7 Stability

2.3.P

    Drug Product
        2.3.P.1 Description and Composition of the Drug Product
        2.3.P.2 Pharmaceutical Development
            2.3.P.2.1 Components of the Drug Product
                2.3.P.2.1.1 Drug Substance
                2.3.P.2.1.2 Excipients
            2.3.P.2.2 Drug Product
            2.3.P.2.3 Manufacturing Process Development
            2.3.P.2.4 Container Closure System
        2.3.P.3 Manufacture
        2.3.P.4 Control of Excipients
        2.3.P.5 Control of Drug Product
        2.3.P.6 Reference Standards or Materials
        2.3.P.7 Container Closure System
        2.3.P.8 Stability

2.7	**Clinical Summary (Bioequivalence)**

Model Bioequivalence Data Summary Tables □
    E-Submission: PDF
        Word Processed e.g., MS Word
2.7.1 Summary of Biopharmaceutic Studies and Associated Analytical Methods
    2.7.1.1 Background and Overview
        Table 1. Submission Summary
        Table 4. Bioanalytical Method Validation
        Table 6. Formulation Data
    2.7.1.2 Summary of Results of Individual Studies
        Table 5. Summary of In Vitro Dissolution
    2.7.1.3 Comparison and Analyses of Results Across Studies
        Table 2. Summary of Bioavailability (BA) Studies
        Table 3. Statistical Summary of the Comparative BA Data
    2.7.1.4 Appendix
        2.7.4.1.3 Demographic and Other Characteristics of Study Population
        Table 7. Demographic Profile of Subjects Completing the Bioequivalence Study
    2.7.4.2.1.1 Common Adverse Events
        Table 8. Incidence of Adverse Events in Individual Studies

MODULE 3

3.2.S DRUG SUBSTANCE ACCEPTABLE

3.2.S.1	**General Information** **3.2.S.1.1 Nomenclature** **3.2.S.1.2 Structure** **3.2.S.1.3 General Properties**	☐

3.2.S.2	**Manufacturer**
	3.2.S.2.1
	    Manufacturer(s) (This section includes contract manufacturers and testing labs)
	    Drug Substance (Active Pharmaceutical Ingredient)
	    1. Name and Full Address(es) of the Facility(ies)
	    2. Function or Responsibility
	    3. Type II DMF number for API
	    4. CFN or FEI numbers
		☐

3.2.S.3	**Characterization**	☐

3.2.S.4	**Control of Drug Substance (Active Pharmaceutical Ingredient)**
	3.2.S.4.1 Specification
	    Testing specifications and data from drug substance manufacturer(s)
	3.2.S.4.2 Analytical Procedures
	3.2.S.4.3 Validation of Analytical Procedures
	    1. Spectra and chromatograms for reference standards and test samples
	    2. Samples-Statement of Availability and Identification of:
	        a. Drug Substance
	        b. Same lot number(s)
	3.2.S.4.4 Batch Analysis
	    1. COA(s) specifications and test results from drug substance mfgr(s)
	    2. Applicant certificate of analysis
	3.2.S.4.5 Justification of Specification
		☐

3.2.S.5	**Reference Standards or Materials**	☐
3.2.S.6	**Container Closure Systems**	☐
3.2.S.7	**Stability**	☐

MODULE 3

3.2.P DRUG PRODUCT ACCEPTABLE

3.2.P.1	**Description and Composition of the Drug Product**
	    1. Unit composition
	    2. Inactive ingredients and amounts are appropriate per IIG
		☐

3.2.P.2	**Pharmaceutical Development** Pharmaceutical Development Report	☐

3.2.P.3	**Manufacture**
	3.2.P.3.1 Manufacture(s) (Finished Dosage Manufacturer and Outside Contract Testing Laboratories)
	    1. Name and Full Address(es) of the Facility (ies)
	    2. CGMP Certification:
	    3. Function or Responsibility
	    4. CFN or FEI numbers
		☐

	3.2.P.3.2 Batch Formula **3.2.P.3.3 Description of Manufacturing Process and Process Controls** 1. Description of the Manufacturing Process 2. Master Production Batch Record(s) for largest intended production runs (no more than 10x pilot batch) with equipment specified 3. If sterile product: Aseptic fill / Terminal sterilization 4. Reprocessing Statement **3.2.P.3.4 Controls of Critical Steps and Intermediates** **3.2.P.3.5 Process Validation and/or Evaluation** 1. Microbiological sterilization validation 2. Filter validation (if aseptic fill)	

3.2.P.4	**Controls of Excipients (Inactive Ingredients)** Source of inactive ingredients identified **3.2.P.4.1 Specifications** 1. Testing specifications (including identification and characterization) 2. Suppliers' COA (specifications and test results) **3.2.P.4.2 Analytical Procedures** **3.2.P.4.3 Validation of Analytical Procedures** **3.2.P.4.4 Justification of Specifications** Applicant COA	☐
3.2.P.5	**Controls of Drug Product** **3.2.P.5.1 Specification(s)** **3.2.P.5.2 Analytical Procedures** **3.2.P.5.3 Validation of Analytical Procedures** Samples – Statement of Availability and Identification of: 1. Finished Dosage Form 2. Same lot numbers **3.2.P.5.4 Batch Analysis** Certificate of Analysis for Finished Dosage Form **3.2.P.5.5 Characterization of Impurities** **3.2.P.5.6 Justification of Specifications**	☐
3.2.P.7	**Container Closure System** 1. Summary of Container/Closure System (if new resin, provide data) 2. Components Specification and Test Data 3. Packaging Configuration and Sizes 4. Container/Closure Testing 5. Source of supply and suppliers address	☐
3.2.P.8	**3.2.P.8.1 Stability (Finished Dosage Form)** 1. Stability Protocol submitted 2. Expiration Dating Period **3.2.P.8.2 Post-approval Stability and Conclusion** Post Approval Stability Protocol and Commitments **3.2.P.8.3 Stability Data** 1. 3 month accelerated stability data 2. Batch numbers on stability records the same as the test batch	☐

MODULE 3 3.2.R Regional Information   ACCEPTABLE

3.2.R (Drug Substance)	3.2.R.1.S Executed Batch Records for drug substance (if available) 3.2.R.2.S Comparability Protocols 3.2.R.3.S Methods Validation Package Methods Validation Package (3 copies) (Multi Copies N/A for E-Submissions) (Required for Non-USP drugs)	☐

3.2.R (Drug Product)	3.2.R.1.P.1 **Executed Batch Records**
	
	Copy of Executed Batch Record with Equipment Specified, including Packaging Records
	(Packaging and Labeling Procedures)
	Batch Reconciliation and Label Reconciliation
	    Theoretical Yield
	    Actual Yield
	    Packaged Yield
	3.2.R.1.P.2 Information on Components
	3.2.R.2.P Comparability Protocols
	3.2.R.3.P Methods Validation Package
	Methods Validation Package (3 copies) (Multi Copies N/A for E-Submissions)
	(Required for Non-USP drugs)
		☐

MODULE 5
CLINICAL STUDY REPORTS   ACCEPTABLE

5.2	**Tabular Listing of Clinical Studies**	☐

5.3.1 (complete study data)	**Bioavailability/Bioequivalence**
	1. Formulation data same?
	    a. Comparison of all Strengths (check proportionality of multiple strengths)
	    b. Parenterals, Ophthalmics, Otics and Topicals
	    per 21 CFR 314.94 (a)(9)(iii)–(v)
	2. Lot Numbers of Products used in BE Study(ies):
	3. Study Type: (Continue with the appropriate study type box below)
		☐

	5.3.1.2 Comparative BA/BE Study Reports
	    1. Study(ies) meets BE criteria (90% CI of 80–125, C max, AUC)
	    2. Summary Bioequivalence tables:
	        Table 10. Study Information
	        Table 12. Dropout Information
	        Table 13. Protocol Deviations
	5.3.1.3
	In-Vitro–In-Vivo Correlation Study Reports
	    1. Summary Bioequivalence tables:
	        Table 11. Product Information
	        Table 16. Composition of Meal Used in Fed Bioequivalence Study
		☐

	5.3.1.4
	Reports of Bioanalytical and Analytical Methods for Human Studies
	    1. Summary Bioequivalence table:
	        Table 9. Reanalysis of Study Samples
	        Table 14. Summary of Standard Curve and QC Data for
	        Bioequivalence Sample Analyses
	        Table 15. SOPs Dealing with Bioanalytical Repeats of Study
	        Samples
	5.3.7
	Case Report Forms and Individual Patient Listing	

5.4	**Literature References**	☐
	Possible Study Types:	
Study Type	**IN-VIVO BE STUDY(IES) with PK ENDPOINTS** (i.e., fasting/fed/sprinkle) 1. Study(ies) meets BE criteria (90% CI of 80–125, C max, AUC) 2. EDR Email: Data Files Submitted: YES SENT TO EDR 3. In-Vitro Dissolution:	☐
Study Type	**IN-VIVO BE STUDY with CLINICAL ENDPOINTS** 1. Properly defined BE endpoints (eval. by Clinical Team) 2. Summary results meet BE criteria: 90% CI of the proportional difference in success rate between test and reference must be within (−0.20, +0.20) for a binary/dichotomous endpoint. For a continuous endpoint, the test/reference ratio of the mean result must be within (0.80, 1.25). 3. Summary results indicate superiority of active treatments (test & reference) over vehicle/placebo (p<0.05) (eval. by Clinical Team) 4. EDR Email: Data Files Submitted	☐
Study Type	**IN-VITRO BE STUDY(IES)** (i.e., in vitro binding assays) 1. Study(ies) meets BE criteria (90% CI of 80–125) 2. EDR Email: Data Files Submitted: 3. In-Vitro Dissolution:	☐

Study Type	**NASALLY ADMINISTERED DRUG PRODUCTS**
	1. <u>Solutions</u> (Q1/Q2 sameness):
	        a. In-Vitro Studies (Dose/Spray Content Uniformity, Droplet/Drug Particle Size
	            Distrib., Spray Pattern, Plume Geometry, Priming & Repriming)
	2. <u>Suspensions</u> (Q1/Q2 sameness):
	        a. In-Vivo PK Study
	            1. Study(ies) meets BE Criteria (90% CI of 80–125, C max, AUC)
	            2. EDR Email: Data Files Submitted
	        b. In-Vivo BE Study with Clinical End Points
	            1. Properly defined BE endpoints (eval. by Clinical Team)
	            2. Summary results meet BE criteria (90% CI within +/− 20% of 80–125)
	            3. Summary results indicate superiority of active treatments (test & reference) over vehicle/placebo (p<0.05) (eval. by Clinical Team)
	            4. EDR Email: Data Files Submitted
	        c. In-Vitro Studies (Dose/Spray Content Uniformity, Droplet/Drug Particle Size
	            Distrib., Spray Pattern, Plume Geometry, Priming & Repriming)
		☐

Study Type	IN-VIVO BE STUDY(IES) with PD ENDPOINTS (e.g., topical corticosteroid vasoconstrictor studies) 1. Pilot Study (determination of ED50) 2. Pivotal Study (study meets BE criteria 90%CI of 80–125)	☐

Study Type	TRANSDERMAL DELIVERY SYSTEMS
	1. In-Vivo PK Study
	    1. Study(ies) meet BE Criteria (90% CI of 80–125, C max, AUC)
	    2. In-Vitro Dissolution
	    3. EDR Email: Data Files Submitted
	2. Adhesion Study
	3. Skin Irritation/Sensitization Study
		☐

ADDITIONAL COMMENTS REGARDING THE ANDA

Each component and section of the checklist should be carefully reviewed for content and completeness. Every precaution must be taken so that the applicant does not receive a letter from the FDA that clarifies CDER's decision of why they cannot approve the ANDA application. Based on the new regulations, if the ANDA is not approved, CDER will send the sponsor a "complete response" letter that will have specific reasons of what part of the submission is not accepted. They will address any issues that must be resolved or clarified before the product is approved.

When an ANDA is submitted in the eCTD format, specific copies as outlined in the NDA paper submission are not necessary. However, it would behoove the sponsor to ask if a copy of the electronic submission should be sent to the field. Field copies of all NDA, ANDA, and SNDA submissions will expedite the review of all manufacturing/quality modules of a CTD.

Within 180 days of receipt of an ANDA, the FDA will review the application and send the applicant a complete response letter.

Amendments to an Unapproved ANDA

An applicant of an ANDA can amend an ANDA that is not yet approved. For example, an amendment containing significant data constitutes an agreement between the FDA and the applicant to extend the review period only for the time necessary to review the information and for no more than 180 days. These amendments may contain significant data to resolve deficiencies in the application as set forth in a letter from the FDA division reviewing the ANDA. If the amendment pertains to manufacturing, the applicant should be sure that the information goes to the field district office assigned to review the ANDA. If this procedure is used, the applicant should send a statement to the FDA division certifying that a field copy of the amendment has been sent to the applicant's home FDA district office.

Postmarketing Reports

Each applicant having an approved ANDA shall comply with the requirements regarding the reporting and record keeping of adverse drug experiences in the same way as those applicants holding an NDA. These adverse experiences are sent to

MedWatch
FDA Safety Information and Adverse Event Reporting Program
Food and Drug Administration
5600 Fishers Lane

Rockville, Maryland 20852-9787, U.S. (see chap. 19).

Annual or any supplemental reports are sent to the same address as stated for the ANDA submission.

Summary

ANDAs are specifically designed to facilitate the manufacturers of generic drug products to rapidly provide these products to the American consumer at lower cost than those of brand name drug products. The sponsors of these applicants must prepare these applications with the mission of the FDA in the forefront, TO ENFORCE LAWS ENACTED BY THE U.S. CONGRESS AND REGULATIONS ESTABLISHED BY THE AGENCY TO PROTECT THE CONSUMER'S HEALTH, SAFETY, AND POCKETBOOK. They must assure consumers that generic drugs and devices are safe and effective for their intended uses and that all labeling and packaging are truthful, informative, and not deceptive. Bearing this in mind, the preparation of an ANDA and the review of the same will be as intensively examined and scrutinized as if it were a new drug, device, or biologic product.

SUPPLEMENTAL NEW DRUG APPLICATIONS

A supplemental new drug application (SNDA) is for the most part submitted to the FDA for any changes to an approved new drug application or an ANDA. These submissions usually occur post approval of NDAs and ANDAs. As an approved NDA/ANDA fully describes the chemistry and manufacturing of a drug and its direction for use, if any changes occur in any of these areas, for whatever reason, approval must be requested in a SNDA/ANDA so that these submissions on file reflect these modifications. Approval of most supplements is mandatory before certain changes may be implemented. Failure to do so may be a cause for withdrawal of the original application's approval. Depending on the type of change, the applicant shall submit the changes in a SNDA or in an annual report. The most frequently submitted supplements usually fall in one of the following categories:

- Components and composition of products.
- Manufacturing site changes including a different contract laboratory or labeler: to manufacture, process, or pack the drug product.
- *Manufacturing process changes*: For example, new regulatory analytical methods, deletion of a specification or regulatory analytical method, a change in the synthesis of the drug substance including a change in solvents and a change in the route of synthesis, adding or deleting an ingredient in the drug product, and so on.
- *Specification changes in drug products*: For example, relaxing the limits for a specification and to delete a specification or regulatory analytical method of a drug product.
- *Packaging changes*: Container and closure system for a drug product, change in the size of the container, and so on.
- *Labeling changes*: Adding a code imprint by printing with ink on a solid oral dosage for drug product, adding a code imprint by embossing, debossing, or engraving on a modified release solid oral dosage form drug product, and any change in labeling or to a medication guide.
- *Miscellaneous changes*: Extending the expiration date of the drug product based on data obtained under a new or revised stability testing protocol that has not

been approved in the application, to establish a new procedure for reprocessing a batch of the drug product that fails to meet specifications, and so on.
* *Multiple related changes*: Any combination of the described changes that relate to a change in drug substance and product.

SNDAs fall into one of the following three categories:

1. Major changes
    * These are the changes that may have a substantial effect on adverse experiences and may reflect a change related to identity, strength, quality, purity, and potency. As these changes may relate to the safety or effectiveness of the product, an expedited review might be requested. Another incidence where an expedited review is requested may be when the change described would impose an extraordinary hardship on the applicant or on the consumer, for example, a delay in an approval of a new batch of product or approval of a new expiration date of a marketed product. If so, the FDA will give this type of supplement immediate attention. Submission in this category of a supplement is usually labeled.

SUPPLEMENT—EXPEDITED REVIEW REQUESTED

---

2. Moderate changes
    * A moderate change supplemental request is often based on the potential of the product to cause an adverse experience. This type of change may also reflect a change in identity, strength, quality, purity, and potency of a product. As these changes may relate to safety or efficacy but may not require immediate attention, they are placed into two categories:

CBE "SUPPLEMENT—CHANGES BEING EFFECTED"
SNDAs for certain moderate changes for which distribution can occur when FDA receives the supplement.

CBE-30 "SUPPLEMENT—CHANGES BEING EFFECTED IN 30 DAYS
SNDAs for certain moderate changes for which FDA receives the information at least 30 days before the distribution of the product is made using the change.

---

3. Minor changes
    * These SNDAs are considered to be minor changes and are categorized as having a minimal potential to cause any adverse experience. This type also reflects a change in identity, strength, quality, purity, and potency of a product. However, as these changes have a minimal effect on the safety or efficacy of the subject, they are described in the next annual report. These may include the following:
        * Revisions made to comply with an official compendium (e.g., USP/NF).

- Revision in the package insert concerning the Description section, or the How Supplied section, that do not involve a change in dosage strength and/or form, or minor editorial changes in these and other sections.
- Deletion of a colorant from the drug product.
- Extension of the expiration dating based on data obtained using a protocol approved in the application.
- A switch to another container/closure system where the materials used are the same general type as previously approved based upon a showing of their equivalency by a testing protocol either approved in the application or published in an official compendium.
- In the case of solid dosage forms, a change in the container size without a change in the container/closure system.

In some instances, there may be supplements submitted proposing to add a new use of an approved drug to the product labeling. This type of supplemental submission can be categorized as a

---

STANDARD EFFICACY SUPPLEMENT OR AS A PRIORITY SUPPLEMENT

Under the Food and Drug Administration Modernization Act of 1997, the FDA is required to publish in the Federal Register standards for the prompt review of supplemental applications submitted for approved articles. This legislative act indicated that this provision was directed at certain types of efficacy supplements. Supplement applications are proposing to add a new use of an approved drug to the product labeling. According to the statistics reported since 1998, Standard Efficacy Supplements under the Modernization Act can take an average of 10 to 12 months to review. The supplements falling under the PRIORITY REVIEW are taking six months to review. A supplement eligible for PRIORITY REVIEW for the CDER and the Center for Biologics Evaluation and Research (CBER) would fall in the category that "would be a significant improvement, compared to marketed products, including nondrug products and therapies in the treatment diagnosis, or prevention of a disease."

SNDAs must be done with careful consideration as to the type of supplement, the importance of it and the urgency for approval. Caution must be given to each submission as the Prescription Drug User Fee Act (PDUFA) (see chap. 25, page 446) is applicable for certain SNDAs.

SNDA/SANDA Checklist
This checklist represents major points that can cause problems and create delays in the agencies review of supplemental applications.

- Make all submissions in duplicate, including cover letters. Assure that the division you are filing your supplement with is aware when you send a copy of the supplement to the field office.
- In the cover letter, there should be a brief description of what the supplement contains, including the objective heading: "Supplement—Expedited Review Requested," "Special Supplement—Changes Being Effected," and so on.

- Wherever possible, make a side-by-side comparison of current versus proposed conditions.
- Use reference numbers for the NDA/ANDA and the supplement if it is an additional submission.
- Describe in detail all aspects of the change. If referring to parts of the NDA/ANDA, describe them; do not assume that the reviewer is as conversant with the NDA as you are.
- Use dates when referring to the previous submissions of FDA letters so that the reviewer can easily retrieve and evaluate prior communications.
- If not submitted electronically, make sure that all copies are clear and legible.
- When referring to drug master files (DMFs), confirm that they are up to date.
- Make sure that all submissions concerning SNDAs/SANDAs are submitted to the appropriate office and division of the FDA.

SUMMARY

SNDAs have and are becoming increasingly important and popular for a number of reasons. When a new drug is developed, it is difficult enough to complete the research required so that the drug can be marketed for a single indication. If multiple claims are researched simultaneously, an NDA may never be submitted. Once an NDA is approved for a specific indication, SNDAs in a CTD format may be presented to the agencies for approval of additional therapeutic uses for the same drug. Recently, there has been a surge by researchers to reexamine data from marketed drugs to look for surrogate end points that might lead to new indications of NDA-approved products.

BIBLIOGRAPHY

Code of Federal Regulations. CFR Title 21 Food and Drugs, Part 314—Applications for FDA Approval to Market a New Drug Subpart C and D

11 The CTD and eCTD for the Registration of Pharmaceuticals for Human Use

Duane B. Lakings

Drug Safety Evaluation Consulting, Inc., Elgin, Texas, U.S.A.

INTRODUCTION

The year is 1999. You, a pharmaceutical or biotechnology company sponsor or a sponsor's agent or a CRO under contract by the sponsor, have all the drug discovery reports and/or publications, nonclinical study reports, clinical study reports, and other clinical documents, and the chemistry, manufacturing, and control (CMC) information and documentation on a drug candidate necessary for the preparation of a regulatory agency submission for a marketing application. Your charge is to prepare the necessary summaries to "tell the story" of the discovery and development of a drug candidate and to integrate the information in the appropriate formats for submissions to each of the countries where marketing approval is being sought. To complete this endeavor, you need to know the marketing application submission requirements for each of these countries. These requirements vary substantially from country to country and often require the preparation of different summaries to be presented in a different order for each country. In addition, each country has some differences in formatting (e.g., binding and binder size and color, paper and page size, font and font size, heading and subheading type and style) stipulations. Thus, you end up preparing multiple submissions, probably one for each country. The process takes substantial time and resources, sometimes from six months (if everything goes smoothly and according to plan) to a year (or longer if unexpected "surprises" are encountered). After the submissions are made, you start to receive questions and queries from the regulatory agencies in various countries. Each question has to be carefully considered, in light of the information in the submission to that country, and appropriately answered. These activities, both the time necessary to prepare the submissions and to give response to queries from the various regulatory agencies, shorten the time of marketing exclusivity after approvals are received, causing a reduction in revenue. Possibly a substantial reduction if the delays in approval are long (sometimes because additional research studies are necessary to effectively respond to a query from a regulatory agency), and the drug candidate has a projected fifth year sales of $365,000,000 or one million dollars a day.

Fast forward to early 2000. The International Conference on Harmonisation (ICH) has prepared a guideline on the organization of a common technical document for registration of pharmaceuticals for human use or a CTD. This ICH guideline, designated M4, has been published and is thus available for use by the three ICH regions [European Agency for the Evaluation of Medicinal Products for the European Union (EMEA), the Pharmaceutical and Medical Safety Bureau for Japan (MHW), and the Federal Drug Administration for the United States (FDA)]. Since most nonsignatory countries also follow ICH guidelines, the ICH CTD guideline provides a format for the preparation of a marketing application submission that is acceptable to most, if not all, countries in which a sponsor wishes to obtain marketing approval. Thus, the scenario described above for 1999 and before is no longer applicable, and sponsors submitting a marketing application prepared according to the ICH CTD guideline recommendations should be able to obtain quicker marketing approvals with fewer questions and queries from regulatory agencies.

Move forward to 2004. The ICH has issued another guideline; this one is on the specifications and requirements for submission of a marketing application in electronic form or the eCTD, which has a designation of ICH M2. In addition to providing an interface for industry to agency transfer of regulatory information, the eCTD also provides information on the creation, review, life cycle management, and archival of an electronic submission. The specification for the eCTD is based on the content defined within the CTD, which describes the organization of the various modules, sections, and documents. While the eCTD does not list the local requirements necessary for a marketing submission, the guideline provides a backbone to allow transfer of the regional information to be included in a regulatory dossier.

Now, the year is 2008. On January 1, 2008, the FDA indicated that all marketing application submissions were to be submitted electronically in eCTD format. In the European Union and Japan, the ICH guidelines are closely followed and are considered as regulations. Thus, each of the ICH regions now expects marketing applications to be submitted in eCTD format.

This chapter provides summary information on the recommendations listed in the ICH CTD guideline. Readers who desire more details on the information in this ICH M4 guideline should obtain a copy of the document, which is available electronically at various Internet sites, including the ICH Web site (1). The chapter also discusses the eCTD specifications and format requirements and provides summary information on where the regional information is to be placed in the eCTD.

CTD OVERVIEW

The ICH M4 guideline provides the agreed-upon common format for the preparation of a well-constructed CTD that will be submitted to regulatory authorities for marketing approval. The goals of using a common format for the technical documentation are

1. to significantly reduce the time and resources needed to compile applications for the registration of human pharmaceuticals;
2. to ease the preparation of electronic submissions (to be discussed in the section on the eCTD);
3. to facilitate regulatory agency reviews and communications with the sponsor;
4. to simplify exchange of regulatory information between regulatory agencies.

Important points for sponsors to know (and to remember) include the following:

1. The ICH CTD guideline addresses the organization of the information to be presented in registration applications for new pharmaceuticals, including biotechnology-derived products.
2. The ICH CTD guideline does not indicate which research studies are required to support an application or how research studies are to be designed and conducted.

3. The overall organization of a CTD, as outlined in the guideline, should not be modified by the sponsor.
4. The display of information in a CTD is to be unambiguous and transparent in order to facilitate review of the basic data and to assist reviewers in becoming quickly oriented to the application's contents.
5. Text, tables, and figures should be prepared using margins that allow the document to be printed using paper employed by the various ICH regions.
6. Example templates for various tables recommended for inclusion in a marketing application are given in the ICH CTD guideline and these templates, or appropriate modifications of the templates, should be employed for summary presentations of results. A designation of Example Template Available (ETA) will be used throughout this chapter to alert sponsors that recommended table formats are available for their consideration.
7. The left-hand margin should be sufficiently large so that information is not obscured by the method of binding.
8. Font sizes (Times New Roman, 12-point font or equivalent) for text and tables should be large enough to be easily legible, even after photocopying.
9. Every page should be numbered, with the first page of each module designated as page 1.
10. Acronyms and abbreviations should be defined the first time they are used in each module, and in the opinion of this author, these should be uniform among the various modules.
11. References should be cited in accordance with the 1979 Vancouver Declaration on Uniform Requirements for Manuscripts Submitted to Biomedical Journals or equivalent.

The most important point above, in this author's opinion, is the second. The sponsor is responsible for determining which research studies are necessary for characterizing and developing a drug candidate, when these studies should be conducted in relation to other experiments, how these studies are designed, where the studies are conducted, and how the results are interpreted. The sponsor is also responsible for preparing, or having prepared, the study reports that document the studies and the generated results. The ICH CTD guideline only provides a common template for the order of presentation of the summaries describing completed research studies and the individual study reports or other documentation.

A CTD is to be organized in five modules. Module 1 is region specific and should contain documents, such as application forms and proposed label for use, specific to the region. More information on where in Module 1 these region-specific documents are to be located is provided in the section on the eCTD. Modules 2, 3, 4, and 5 are intended to be common for all regions and each of these modules will be discussed in more detail in the following sections. Much of the discussion in this chapter was paraphrased from the text in the ICH CTD guideline and thus should provide the reader with an overview of the material provided in more detail in ICH M4. Module 2 provides summary information on the detailed data and results presented in Module 3 for Quality or CMC information, Module 4 for Nonclinical Study Reports, and Module 5 for Clinical Study Reports and other clinical documentation.

MODULE 2: COMMON TECHNICAL DOCUMENT SUMMARIES

From the standpoint of "telling the story" of the discovery and development of a drug candidate and integrating the results from the various research studies conducted to define manufacturing processes and to characterize the physiochemical properties, pharmacology or efficacy, pharmacokinetics and metabolism, and toxicology or safety of the drug candidate in animal models and in humans, Module 2 is by far the most important module of a CTD. This module provides summary information on all aspects of the discovery and development processes, including CMC information and nonclinical and clinical evaluations. The writers of each of these summaries need to have a good understanding of the "overall story" so that each author can compare, contrast, and integrate the results in his or her summaries with the information in the summaries prepared by other authors.

Most large pharmaceutical corporations have trained and experienced scientific and medical writing groups who have as one of their primary functions the drafting of these quality, nonclinical, and clinical summaries for regulatory agency submissions. Smaller pharmaceutical firms and some larger biotechnology companies may have a few science writers on staff, and when the time comes to prepare a marketing application, these writers may be asked to draft summaries both inside and outside their areas of expertise. Most small biotechnology firms do not have the resources to have an independent scientific writing staff and frequently rely on partners (i.e., large pharmaceutical companies who have licensed or are codeveloping a drug candidate with the discoverer) to perform these important aspects of the drug development process. Whatever the size of the sponsor, resources may not, at times, be available to complete the task within the desired time frame. When that is the case, sponsors may contract with a CRO, a medical writing service organization, or independent science writers to draft the CTD-recommended summaries. Many independent science writers belong to the American Medical Writers Association (AMWA) and information on their background and qualifications can be found on the AMWA Web site (2). The sponsor should carefully assign or select the scientific and medical writers, whether in-house or contract, to ensure that the summaries are appropriately prepared and reviewed. For example, having an expert in clinical or CMC aspects of drug development prepare the nonclinical summaries may result in incomplete or inaccurate descriptions of preclinical and nonclinical study results. However, having the clinical or CMC experts review the nonclinical summaries is highly desirable so that the information shared is effectively integrated with the summaries from the other areas.

Whoever prepares the summaries to be included in Module 2 of a CTD, the information should be presented using the order of presentation described in the ICH CTD guideline. Module 2 should begin with a short (not to exceed one page) general introduction on a drug candidate and is to include the pharmacological class, the mode of action, and the proposed clinical use. The Introduction is to be followed by the Quality Overall Summary (QOS), then the Nonclinical Overview and the Clinical Overview. Following the QOS and overviews are the Nonclinical Written and Tabulated Summaries and the Clinical Summary.

Quality Overall Summary

QOS is a summary that follows the scope and outline of Module 3 and should not include information, data, and/or justifications that are not included in Module 3 or in another part of a CTD. The primary purpose of a QOS is to provide sufficient information so that a reviewer is given an overview of the data in Module 3. A QOS should emphasize key parameters of a drug substance (or a drug candidate as a compound under development is commonly referred to in nonclinical and clinical research efforts; both designations are utilized throughout this chapter) and a proposed drug product and should include discussions of issues that integrate information from sections in Module 3 with supporting information from Modules 4 and 5. The length of a QOS (excluding tables and figures) should generally not exceed 40 pages of text. However, for most biotechnology drug candidates and for candidates manufactured using more complex processes, a QOS may be longer but should not exceed 80 pages of text.

The recommended order of presentation for a QOS in Module 2 and the more detailed Quality information in Module 3 is described in Table 1, where "S" designates drug substance and "P" denotes drug product. A QOS is to start with an introduction that includes the proprietary name, nonproprietary name, and/or common name of a drug substance; company or sponsor name; dosage form(s), strength(s), and route(s) of administration; and proposed indication(s). After the introduction, summary information on a drug substance and then a proposed drug product are provided. Following the summaries and primarily for biotechnology-derived drug candidates, appendices on facilities and equipment and appendices on safety evaluations for adventitious agents are provided. Finally, selected regional information, which is not included in Module 1, is documented.

In the "General Information of the Drug Substance" section, the nomenclature, structure, and general properties of a drug substance are to be provided. Nomenclature could include the recommended international nonproprietary name, compendia name, chemical name(s), sponsor code, other nonproprietary name(s), and/or Chemical Abstracts Service (CAS) registry number. For small organic molecules or NCEs, the structural formula, including relative and absolute stereochemistry (if relevant), the molecular formula, and the relative molecular mass are to be provided. If a drug substance is chiral, information is to be provided on the specific stereoisomer or mixture of stereoisomers (i.e., a racemic mixture) used in nonclinical and clinical studies and the stereoisomer(s) that is (are) to be used in the final drug product intended for marketing. For protein or polypeptide macromolecules, the schematic amino acid sequence with glycosylation sites and/or other posttranslational modifications identified and the relative molecular mass are to be given. For other macromolecules, such as nucleic acids or carbohydrates, sufficient structural information should be provided to describe the chemical structure and the interactions between the various moieties or subgroups. Information on general properties is to include summaries of the physiochemical and other relevant characteristics of a drug substance, including biological activity for macromolecules.

The manufacture section is to include the name, address, and responsibility (e.g., production or testing facility) of each manufacturer, including contractors. A brief description of a drug substance's manufacturing process to adequately describe the synthesis and process control is included. The use of a flow diagram for NCEs and macromolecules prepared by synthetic procedures is recommended. The diagram should include molecular formulas, weights, yield ranges, and chemical structures of starting materials, intermediates, and drug substance (reflecting stereochemistry, if relevant) and should identify operating conditions (pH, temperature, pressure, and time), catalysts, and solvents. The diagram is to be explained using a sequential procedural narrative that includes information on the quantities of raw

TABLE 1 Order of Presentation for Quality Overall Summary (Module 2) and Quality (Module 3)

Material			Module	
S	P	Sequence of presentation	2	3
		Table of contents		3.1
		Body of data		3.2
		Introduction	2.3.I	
S		General information on drug substance	2.3.S.1	3.2.S.1
S		Nomenclature		3.2.S.1.1
S		Structure		3.2.S.1.2
S		General properties		3.2.S.1.3
S		Manufacture of drug substance	2.3.S.2	3.2.S.2
S		Manufacturer(s)		3.2.S.2.1
S		Description of manufacturing process and controls		3.2.S.2.2
S		Control of materials		3.2.S.2.3
S		Control of critical steps and intermediates		3.2.S.2.4
S		Process validation and/or evaluation		3.2.S.2.5
S		Manufacturing process development		3.2.S.2.6
S		Characterization of drug substance	2.3.S.3	3.2.S.3
S		Elucidation of structure and other characteristics		3.2.S.3.1
S		Impurities		3.2.S.3.2
S		Control of drug substance	2.3.S.4	3.2.S.4
S		Specification		3.2.S.4.1
S		Analytical procedures		3.2.S.4.2
S		Validation of analytical procedures		3.2.S.4.3
S		Batch analyses		3.2.S.4.4
S		Justification of specification		3.2.S.4.5
S		Reference standards or materials	2.3.S.5	3.2.S.5
S		Container closure system	2.3.S.6	3.2.S.6
S		Stability of drug substance	2.3.S.7	3.2.S.7
S		Stability summary and conclusions		3.2.S.7.1
S		Postapproval stability protocol and commitment		3.2.S.7.2
S		Stability data		3.2.S.7.3
	P	Description and composition of drug product	2.3.P.1	3,2.P.1
	P	Pharmaceutical development	2.3.P.2	3.2.P.2
	P	Components of the drug product (drug substance and excipients)		3.2.P.2.1
	P	Drug product (formulation development, overages, physicochemical and biological properties)		3.2.P.2.2
	P	Manufacturing process development		3.2.P.2.3
	P	Container closure system		3.2.P.2.4
	P	Microbiological attributes		3.2.P.2.5
	P	Compatibility		3.2.P.2.6
	P	Manufacture of drug product	2.3.P.3	3.2.P.3
	P	Manufacturer(s)		3.2.P.3.1
	P	Batch formula		3.2.P.3.2
	P	Description of manufacturing process and controls		3.2.P.3.3
	P	Control of critical steps and intermediates		3.2.P.3.4
	P	Process validation and/or evaluation		3.2.P.3.5
	P	Control of excipients	2.3.P.4	3.2.P.4
	P	Specifications		3.2.P.4.1
	P	Analytical procedures		3.2.P.4.2
	P	Validation of analytical procedures		3.2.P.4.3
	P	Justification of specifications		3.2.P.4.4
	P	Excipients of human or animal origin		3.2.P.4.5

(Continued)

TABLE 1 Order of Presentation for Quality Overall Summary (Module 2) and Quality (Module 3) (*Continued*)

| Material | | | Module | |
S	P	Sequence of presentation	2	3
	P	Novel excipients		3.2.P.4.6
	P	Control of drug product	2.3.P.5	3.2.P.5
	P	Specification(s)		3.2.P.5.1
	P	Analytical procedures		3.2.P.5.2
	P	Validation of analytical procedures		3.2.P.5.3
	P	Batch analyses		3.2.P.5.4
	P	Characterization of impurities		3.2.P.5.5
	P	Justification of specification(s)		3/2.P.5.6
	P	Reference standards or materials	2.3.P.6	3.2.P.6
	P	Container closure system	2.3.P.7	3.2.P.7
	P	Stability of drug product	2.3.P.8	3.2.P.8
	P	Stability summary and conclusion		3.2.P.8.1
	P	Postapproval stability protocol and commitment		3.2.P.8.2
	P	Stability data		3.2.P.8.3
		Appendix on facilities and equipment	2.3.A.1	3.2.A.1
		Appendix on adventitious agents safety evaluation	2.3.A.2	3.2.A.2
		Appendix on excipients	2.3.A.3	
		Regional information	2.3.R	3.2.R
		Key literature references		3.3

Abbreviations: S, drug substance; P, proposed drug product.

materials, solvents, catalysts, and reagents that identifies critical steps, process controls, equipment, and operating conditions.

For protein macromolecules, a manufacturing process usually starts with a vial(s) of the cell bank and includes cell culture, harvest(s), purification and modification reactions, and storage and shipping conditions. Again, a flow diagram is recommended to illustrate the manufacturing route from the original inoculum to the last harvesting operation. Relevant information (e.g., population doubling levels, cell concentration, volumes, pH, cultivation times, holding times, and temperature) is to be included, and critical steps and intermediates are to be identified. A brief text description of each process step in the flow diagram is to be provided and should include summary information on scale, culture media and other additives, major equipment, and process controls (e.g., in-process tests and operational parameters, process steps, equipment, and intermediates with acceptance criteria). Another flow diagram along with a brief text description is to be provided to illustrate the purification steps and is to include all steps, intermediates, and relevant information for each stage with critical steps for which specifications are established identified. Reprocessing procedures with criteria for reprocessing of any intermediate or a drug substance are to be summarized. Procedures used to transfer material between steps, equipment, areas, and buildings are to be listed. A description of the filling procedure for a drug substance, process controls, and acceptance criteria is to be provided. The container closure system for storage of a drug substance and storage and shipping conditions for a drug substance are to be delineated. Where appropriate, tabulated summaries and graphs should be employed.

All materials (e.g., raw materials, starting materials, solvents, reagents, and catalysts) used in the manufacture of a drug substance must be controlled and a list identifying where each material is used in the process should be provided. Information demonstrating that materials meet standards appropriate for their intended use is to be included.

Test and acceptance criteria performed at critical steps of the manufacturing process are to be summarized to ensure that the process is controlled. For intermediates isolated during the process, information on their quality and control is to be listed. For protein macromolecules, stability data to support storage conditions are recommended.

Process validation and/or evaluation studies for aseptic processing and sterilization are to be briefly described and should contain sufficient information to demonstrate that the manufacturing process is suitable for its intended purpose and to substantiate selection of critical process controls and their limits.

A brief description and discussion of the manufacturing process development history of the drug substance is recommended and should provide summary information on significant changes made to the process or site used in the production of nonclinical, clinical, scale-up, pilot, and production scale (if available) batches. Where appropriate, the significance of the change(s) should be addressed to describe the potential impact of the change(s) on the quality of a drug substance.

Characterization of a drug substance is to include elucidation of structure. For NCEs, confirmation of structure can be provided by spectral analysis techniques and should include summary information on the potential for isomerism, the identification of stereochemistry, and/or the potential for forming polymorphs. For protein macromolecules, structural details should include information on primary, secondary, and higher-order structure, posttranslational forms, biological activity, purity, and immunochemical properties (when relevant).

Information on impurities, including their structure, acceptance limits, and control, is to be briefly described.

For control of a drug substance, specifications, including justifications, and analytical procedures, including validation information, used for testing are to be summarized. Data on reference standards or reference materials used for drug substance testing are to be provided. Information on batches and the results of batch analyses are to be described.

A brief description and discussion of the container closure system for a drug substance is to include the identity of and specification for materials of construction of each primary packaging component. The suitability of each component should be summarized.

A summary, including tabular and graphic presentations of results, of the stability studies undertaken on a drug substance is to include information on testing conditions, batches, and analytical procedures and a discussion of the results and conclusions. Also to be included are the proposed storage conditions, retest dates, or shelf life (where relevant) and a summary of the postapproval stability protocol(s).

The description and composition of a proposed drug product is to be summarized and is to include a description of the dosage form, a list of all components and their amounts on a per-unit basis, the function of the components, and a reference to their quality standards. If more than one proposed drug product is included in a marketing application, the sponsor is to prepare separate drug product or "P" sections for each proposed dosage form. If appropriate, a brief description of accompanying reconstitution diluent(s) is to be provided. Information on the type of container and closure used for a drug product and accompanying diluent(s) is to be summarized.

Using tables and graphs as appropriate, the pharmaceutical development history for a proposed drug product is to be summarized. Information to be shared should include development studies conducted to establish that the dosage form, the formulation, the manufacturing process, container closure system, microbiological attributes, and usage instructions are appropriate for the intended purpose. In addition, a summary should be provided to identify and describe critical formulation and process parameters that might influence batch reproducibility, drug product performance, and drug product quality.

The name, address, and responsibility of each manufacture, including contractors, and each proposed production site or facility involved in manufacturing a proposed drug product are to be provided. A flow diagram is recommended to present the steps of a drug product manufacturing process and should indicate where materials enter the process. The critical steps where process controls, intermediate tests, and final drug product controls are conducted are to be identified. Also to be included is a brief description of the manufacturing process and the controls, including process validation and/or evaluations, that are intended to result in the routine and consistent production of drug product of appropriate quality.

A brief summary on the quality of excipients is to include information on specifications and their justification, analytical procedures and their validation, excipients of human or animal origin, and novel excipients.

Using tables and graphs as appropriate, control of a drug product should be briefly described and should include information on specifications and their justification, analytical procedures and their validation and characterization of impurities. Also, information on reference standards or materials used for control of a drug product should be provided.

A brief description of the drug product container closure systems is to include the identity of materials of construction for each primary packaging component and their specifications. Where appropriate, noncompendia methods and their validation should be summarized.

Summary information on the stability studies conducted on a drug product are to include conditions tested, batches analyzed, and analytical procedures used. A brief discussion of the results and conclusions, with respect to storage conditions and shelf life, from drug product stability studies and an analysis of the data is to be provided. Tables and graphs should be used where appropriate to describe stability data. A brief description of the postapproval stability protocol for each proposed drug product in a marketing application is to be included.

For a macromolecule drug candidate, appendices to QOS are to include a summary of facility information for the production of a drug substance and a proposed drug product and a discussion of measures implemented to control endogenous and adventitious agents during production. A diagram is recommended to illustrate the manufacturing flow, including movement of raw materials, personnel, waste, and intermediate(s) into and out of the manufacturing areas. A tabulated summary of the reduction factors for viral clearance is desirable.

The last section of a QOS is to be a brief discussion, when appropriate, of the information specific for the region for which marketing approval is being sought and which is not included in Module 1 of the application.

Nonclinical Overview

A Nonclinical Overview is to present an integrated and critical assessment of the pharmacological, pharmacokinetic, and toxicological evaluations of a drug candidate in in vitro systems and animal models and it should not exceed about 30 pages of text. Where relevant guidelines (e.g., ICH Safety guidelines) on the conduct of nonclinical studies exist, these guidelines are to be taken into consideration and any deviations are to be discussed and justified. In addition, the nonclinical testing strategy (i.e., the nonclinical drug development plan) should be discussed and justified, and comments included on the status of compliance with Good Laboratory Practice (GLP) Regulations for the research studies being submitted. Where appropriate, any association between nonclinical findings and the quality characteristics of a drug candidate, the results from clinical trials, and/or the effects seen with related drug products are to be described.

Except for macromolecules, an assessment of the pharmacological and toxicological effects of the impurities and degradants present in a drug substance and a drug product is to be included. This assessment should form part of the justification for proposed impurity limits and should be appropriately cross-referenced with the Quality documentation in the QOS and Module 3. The implications of any differences in the chirality, chemical form, and/or impurity profile between the compound evaluated in nonclinical studies and a drug substance in a proposed drug product to be marketed is to be discussed. For a macromolecule, comparability of material used in nonclinical studies, clinical trials, and proposed for marketing is to be addressed. If a drug product contains a novel excipient, an assessment of the information on this material's safety (including safety pharmacology, pharmacokinetics, and toxicology) is to be included.

If references of published scientific literature are to be used in place of nonclinical studies conducted by a sponsor, the information in these citations are to be supported by a detailed justification that reviews the design of the studies, including the quality of the drug substance, the GLP compliance of the study, and documenting any deviations from available guidelines.

The recommended sequence for the Nonclinical Overview is as follows:

1. Overview of the nonclinical testing strategy or nonclinical drug development logic plan
2. Pharmacology
3. Pharmacokinetics
4. Toxicology
5. Integrated overview and conclusions
6. List of literature citations

The material summarized in each section of a Nonclinical Overview should contain appropriate references (i.e., Table X.X, Study/Report Number) to the Nonclinical Tabulated Summaries.

In vitro and animal studies conducted to evaluate and establish the pharmacodynamic effects, the mode of action, and potential adverse effects are to be evaluated with consideration given to the significance of any issues that are noted. In addition and in this author's opinion, any animal model developed or utilized to evaluate the pharmacological activity of a drug candidate should be fully summarized and when available, information on the relevance and predictability of the animal model to the human disease or disorder for which a marketing approval is being sought should be provided.

Assessments of nonclinical pharmacokinetic (PK), toxicokinetic (TK), and drug metabolism (DM) results should address the relevance of the bioanalytical chemistry (BAC) methods and the PK models and derived PK or TK parameters. Where appropriate, cross-referencing may be necessary to the more detailed information on certain issues (e.g., impact of disease state, changes in physiology, antidrug candidate antibodies, and cross-species considerations) within the pharmacology and toxicology studies and any inconsistencies in the data should be discussed. Interspecies comparisons, including that of humans, of metabolism (both extent and metabolite profile) and systemic exposure comparisons in animals and humans are to be described and the limitations and utility of the nonclinical results for prediction of potential adverse effects in humans delineated.

For animal species evaluated in toxicology studies, the toxic effects (onset, severity, and duration) and their dose dependency and degree of reversibility or irreversibility and species- and/or gender-related differences are to be evaluated. Important aspects are to be discussed with regard to (*i*) pharmacodynamics, (*ii*) toxic signs, (*iii*) causes of death, (*iv*) gross pathology and histopathological findings, (*v*) genotoxic activity, (*vi*) carcinogenic potential and risk to humans, (*vii*) fertility, embryo-fetal development, pre- and postnatal toxicity, (*viii*) studies in juvenile animals, (*ix*) the potential consequences of use before and during pregnancy, during lactation, and during pediatric development, (*x*) local tolerance, and (*xi*) studies conducted to clarify special problems.

An overview evaluation of toxicology studies is to be arranged in a logical order to allow all relevant data for describing a given adverse effect to be discussed together. Extrapolation of toxicity data from animals to humans are to be considered with relation to (*i*) animal species evaluated, (*ii*) number of animals studied, (*iii*) routes of administration employed, (*iv*) dosages evaluated, (*v*) duration of treatment, (*vi*) systemic exposure in the toxicology animal species at the no-observed-adverse-effect-levels (NOAEL) and at doses that produce a toxic effect in relation to the human systemic exposure at the maximum recommended human dose, and (*vii*) the toxic effects of a drug candidate observed in animal models to those expected or observed in humans. Tables and figures are recommended for summarizing these extrapolations.

If alternatives to whole-animal experimentation are employed to evaluate the pharmacology, pharmacokinetics, and/or toxicology of a drug candidate, the scientific validity of the alternatives are to be discussed.

An integrated overview and conclusions of nonclinical results are to clearly define the characteristics of a drug candidate as demonstrated by the results of the nonclinical research studies and are to arrive at logical, well-argued conclusions supporting the safety of a drug candidate for the intended clinical use. Using the pharmacology, PK, and toxicology results, the implications of the nonclinical findings for the safe human use of a drug candidate are to be discussed.

Clinical Overview

A Clinical Overview is to provide a critical analysis of the clinical data generated during the development of a drug candidate and to appropriately reference this information in the more detailed Clinical Summary and in the individual clinical study reports presented in Module 5 and in any other relevant study reports. The primary purpose of this overview is to present the conclusions and implications of the clinical results and to provide a succinct discussion and interpretation of these findings in conjunction with other relevant information, such as nonclinical data or quality issues that may have clinical implications. While primarily intended for use by regulatory agencies in the review of the clinical section of a drug candidate's marketing application, the Clinical Overview can also be a useful summary of the clinical findings for reviewers to reference to other sections of a CTD. The overview should include

1. a description and explanation of the overall clinical development plan approach for the drug candidate and include critical clinical study design decisions;
2. an assessment of the quality of the design and performance of the clinical studies and include a statement regarding compliance with Good Clinical Practice (GCP) Regulations;
3. a brief summary of the clinical findings, including important limitations (e.g., absence of data on some patient populations, on pertinent end points, or on use in combination therapy; lack of comparisons with relevant active comparators);
4. a discussion and evaluation of the risks and benefits based on the conclusions of the pivotal clinical trials, including interpretations of how human safety and efficacy results support the proposed dose(s) and target indication(s), and an evaluation of how prescribing information will optimize benefits and manage potential risks;
5. particular human safety and efficacy issues encountered during clinical development and how these issues were evaluated and resolved;
6. any unresolved issues, discuss why these issues are not considered as barriers for approval, and present plans to resolve the issues;
7. a discussion of the basis for important or unusual aspects of prescribing information.

A Clinical Overview will generally be relatively a short document of approximately 30 pages. The length will depend on the complexity of the clinical development program. The use of in-text tables and figures to facilitate understanding of key clinical information is encouraged. Cross-referencing information to the more detailed results provided in the Clinical Summary or in the clinical study reports in Module 5.

The recommended organization and order of presentation for a Clinical Overview is as follows:

1. Product development rationale
2. Overview of biopharmaceutics
3. Overview of clinical pharmacology
4. Overview of efficacy
5. Overview of safety
6. Risks and benefits conclusions
7. References

A discussion of the clinical development rationale for a drug candidate is to (*i*) identify the pharmacological class of the candidate, (*ii*) describe the target indication (i.e., the particular clinical or pathophysiological condition that a drug candidate is intended to treat, prevent, or diagnose), (*iii*) summarize the scientific background that supported the investigation of a drug candidate for the indication(s) studied, (*iv*) briefly describe the clinical development program for a drug candidate and include information on ongoing and planned clinical studies and the basis for submitting the marketing application at this point in the program, and (*v*) briefly describe plans for the use of foreign clinical data to support the application. In addition, this rationale should note and explain concordance or lack of concordance with current standard research approaches (i.e., GCP Regulations) regarding the design, conduct, and analysis of the clinical studies. Published literature is to be referenced. Non–region-specific regulatory guidance and advice is to be identified, and formal advice documents (e.g., official meeting minutes, official guidance, and letters from regulatory authorities) are to be referenced with complete copies included in the reference section of Module 5. Region-specific regulatory guidance and advice is to be included in Module 1.

The purpose of an Overview of Biopharmaceutics subsection is to present an analysis of any important issues related to the bioavailability of a drug candidate that might affect the safety and/or efficacy of a proposed drug product for marketing. These issues could include dosage form and strength proportionality, differences between a proposed drug product and the formulation(s) of a drug candidate evaluated in clinical trials, and the influence of food and the time of eating on the extent and duration of exposure.

An Overview of Clinical Pharmacology subsection is to present an analysis of PK, pharmacodynamic (PD), and related in vitro human data. This analysis will consider all relevant data, discuss how and why the data support the conclusions drawn, and emphasize unusual results and known or potential problems. Items to be addressed in this subsection include the following:

1. Pharmacokinetics including, but not limited to, comparative pharmacokinetics in healthy subjects, patients, and special populations; pharmacokinetics related to intrinsic factors (e.g., age, gender, and race) and extrinsic factors (e.g., environmental factors, diet); rate and extent of absorption; distribution; metabolism and the pharmacological and/or toxicological activity of formed metabolites; rate(s) and route(s) of excretion; stereochemistry issues; clinically relevant drug–drug and drug–food interactions.
2. Pharmacodynamics including, but not limited to, information on the mechanism of action; favorable or unfavorable PD effect on plasma concentration of a drug candidate and/or active metabolite(s) (i.e., PK/PD relationships); PD support for proposed dose, dosing interval, and dosing duration; possible genetic differences in PD response.
3. Interpretation and implication of immunogenicity and clinical microbiology studies.

A critical analysis and evaluation of the clinical data pertinent to the efficacy of a drug candidate in the intended patient population is presented in an Overview of Efficacy subsection. If a sponsor plans to submit a marketing application for more than one disease indication or disorder for a proposed drug product, separate Overview of Efficacy subsections are to be prepared for each indication. All relevant data, both positive and negative, are to be considered with discussions on why and how these data support the proposed indication and prescribing information. Studies considered relevant for the evaluation of efficacy are to be identified and the reasons of why any adequate and well-controlled studies are not being considered should be discussed. Issues that should be considered in this overview include, but are not limited to

1. relevant features of the patient population (e.g., demographics, disease stage, important but excluded patient populations, and participation of children and elderly);
2. implications of the study design(s) and justification of any surrogate end points employed;
3. statistical methods and any issues that might affect the interpretation of study results;
4. similarities and/or differences in results among studies and in different patient subgroups within studies;
5. observed relationships between efficacy, dose, and dosage regimen for each indication in both the overall patient population and different patient subgroups or special populations;
6. for a proposed drug product intended for long-term use, findings pertinent to the maintenance of long-term efficacy, the determination of long-term dosage regimen, and the potential for developing tolerance;
7. data suggestive that treatment may be improved by drug candidate plasma concentration monitoring and the optimal plasma concentration range;
8. the clinical relevance of the magnitude of the observed efficacy.

An Overview of Safety will present a critical analysis of the safety data and indicate how the safety results support and justify the proposed prescribing information. Topics that should be considered in this analysis of human safety include the following:

1. Adverse experiences (AEs) considered characteristic of the pharmacological class.
2. Approaches employed for monitoring of particular AEs (e.g., QT interval prolongation, ophthalmic changes).
3. Findings in relevant animal toxicology and/or drug substance and drug product quality information that affect or could affect the evaluation of clinical safety.
4. The nature of the patient population and the extent of exposure for both a drug candidate and any control treatment(s) evaluated. Limitations of the human safety database as related to inclusion and exclusion criteria and subject/patient demographics are to be considered and discussed.
5. Common and nonserious AEs with reference to the tabular presentations of AEs in the Clinical Summary.
6. Serious adverse experiences (SAEs) (with appropriate cross-reference to tabular presentations in the Clinical Summary) with a discussion on absolute numbers and frequency of SAEs, including deaths, and other significant AEs for a drug candidate and control treatments. Any conclusions regarding causal relationship, or the lack thereof, to a proposed drug product should be provided. Laboratory findings that reflect actual or possible serious medical effects are to be discussed.
7. Similarities and/or differences in human safety results among clinical studies and how these observations affect the interpretation of the safety data.

8. Any differences in the rates of AEs or SAEs in population subgroups or special populations.
9. Possible relation of AEs to dose, dosage regimen, and dose duration.
10. Methods to prevent or manage AEs.
11. Reactions due to overdose and the potential for dependence, rebound phenomena, and abuse or the lack of data on these issues.
12. Worldwide marketing experience and, where appropriate, support for the applicability to the new region of data generated in another region.

A "Risks and Benefits Conclusions" subsection should integrate all the conclusions reached in the other subsections of the Clinical Overview and provide an overall assessment of the risks and benefits of the use of a drug product in clinical practice. Also, the implications of any deviations from regulatory advice, regulations, or guidelines and any important limitations in the available data are to be discussed. An analysis of risks and benefits is expected to be quite brief but should identify the most important conclusions and issues concerning

1. the efficacy of a proposed drug product for each proposed indication;
2. significant human safety findings;
3. dose–response and dose–toxicity relationships and optimal dose ranges and dosage regimens;
4. efficacy and safety in subgroups and special populations;
5. if applicable, results in children of different age groups;
6. risks to patients for known and/or potential drug–drug and drug–food interactions.

A list of references cited in a Clinical Overview is to be included with copies of all relevant references provided in Module 5.

Nonclinical Written and Tabulated Summaries

The information presented in the Nonclinical Written and Tabulated Summaries section of the ICH CTD guideline is intended to assist sponsors and authors in the preparation of nonclinical pharmacology, PK, and toxicology summaries in a format acceptable to the various ICH regions and is not intended to indicate what nonclinical research studies are required or how these studies are to be designed or conducted. Since no guideline can cover all possibilities, a sponsor can modify, if needed, the format to provide the optimal presentation of the generated nonclinical results in order to facilitate the understanding and evaluation of the information. General points to be considered by a sponsor and authors for inclusion in these summaries include that

1. age-related and gender-related effects in animal models are to be discussed;
2. relevant findings on stereoisomers and/or drug candidate metabolites, as appropriate, are to be included;
3. consistent use of units throughout the nonclinical summaries (and in this author's opinion, throughout the quality and clinical sections of a marketing application) will facilitate review and, if needed, a table for converting units may be useful;
4. during discussions, information is to be integrated across studies and across species, and exposure in the animal models is to be related to exposure in humans given the maximum intended dose;
5. when available, results from in vitro studies should precede results from in vivo studies;

TABLE 2 Presentation Order for Species and Routes of Administration for Nonclinical Studies

Species order	Route of administration order
Mouse	Intended route for human use
Rat	Oral
Hamster	Intravenous
Other rodent	Intramuscular
Rabbit	Intraperitoneal
Dog	Subcutaneous
Nonhuman primate	Inhalation
Other nonrodent mammal	Topical
Nonmammals	Other

6. when multiple studies of the same type (e.g., subchronic toxicology studies) are to be summarized, the studies are to be ordered by species, by route, and then by duration with the shortest duration first;
7. species and routes of administration are to be ordered as shown in Table 2;
8. when considered desirable to more effectively display results, tables and figures may be used within the text or grouped together at the end of each subsection;
9. references to citations in the Tabulated Summaries are to be included throughout the text and are to be in the following format: Table X.X, Study/Report Number.

In general, the total length of the three nonclinical written summaries should not exceed 100 to 150 pages.

The order of presentation recommended for the Nonclinical Written and Tabulated Summaries in Module 2 and the Nonclinical Study Reports in Module 4 is presented in Table 3.

The aim of an Introduction is to introduce a reviewer to a drug candidate and the proposed clinical use. This introduction should contain brief information on a drug candidate's structure and pharmacological properties and on the proposed clinical indication, dose, and duration of use.

For a Pharmacology Written Summary, a brief summary of approximately 2 to 3 pages should describe the principal findings from the in vitro and animal pharmacology studies. This summary should include a short discussion of the pharmacological data package and should point out any notable aspects (such as the lack of a relevant animal model or the potential predictability of an animal model to a human disease or disorder).

A subsection on Primary Pharmacodynamics (i.e., studies on the mode of action and/or effects of a drug candidate in relation to the desired therapeutic target) should, when possible, relate the pharmacology of a drug candidate to available data (e.g., selectivity, safety, and potency) on other drugs in the pharmacological class. Where appropriate, secondary PD results (i.e., studies on the mode of action and/or effects of a drug candidate not related to the desired therapeutic target) should be summarized by organ system. The results from conducted safety pharmacology evaluations (i.e., studies conducted to investigate the potential undesirable PD effects of a drug candidate on physiological functions in relation to exposure within and above the therapeutic range) should be summarized and evaluated. For most NCEs and macromolecules, a standard battery of cardiovascular, CNS, and respiratory safety pharmacology studies is recommended, and for some drug

TABLE 3 Order of Presentation for Nonclinical Written and Tabulated Summaries (Module 2) and Nonclinical Study Reports (Module 4)

Sequence of presentation	Module 2	Module 4
Table of contents		4.2
Introduction	2.6.1	
Pharmacology written summary	2.6.2	
Brief summary of pharmacology	2.6.2.1	
Primary pharmacodynamics	2.6.2.2	4.2.1.1
Secondary pharmacodynamics	2.6.2.3	4.2.1.2
Safety pharmacology	2.6.2.4	4.2.1.3
Pharmacodynamic drug interactions	2.6.2.5	4.2.1.4
Discussion and conclusions	2.6.2.6	
Tables and figures	2.6.2.7	
Pharmacology tabulated summary	2.6.3	
Pharmacology: overview	2.6.3.1	
Primary pharmacodynamics	2.6.3.2	
Secondary pharmacodynamics	2.6.3.3	
Safety pharmacology	2.6.3.4	
Pharmacodynamic drug interactions	2.6.3.5	
Pharmacokinetic written summary	2.6.4	
Brief summary of pharmacokinetics	2.6.4.1	
Methods of analysis	2.6.4.2	4.2.2.1
Absorption	2.6.4.3	4.2.2.2
Distribution	2.6.4.4	4.2.2.3
Metabolism	2.6.4.5	4.2.2.4
Excretion	2.6.4.6	4.2.2.5
Pharmacokinetic drug interactions	2.6.4.7	4.2.2.6
Other pharmacokinetic studies	2.6.4.8	4.2.2.7
Discussion and conclusions	2.6.4.9	
Tables and figures	2.6.4.10	
Pharmacokinetics tabulated summary	2.6.5	
Pharmacokinetics: overview	2.6.5.1	
Bioanalytical methods and validation reports	2.6.5.2	
Pharmacokinetics: absorption after a single dose	2.6.5.3	
Pharmacokinetics: absorption after repeated doses	2.6.5.4	
Pharmacokinetics: organ distribution	2.6.5.5	
Pharmacokinetics: plasma protein binding	2.6.5.6	
Pharmacokinetics: studies in pregnant or nursing animals	2.6.5.7	
Pharmacokinetics: other distribution studies	2.6.5.8	
Pharmacokinetics: metabolism in vivo	2.6.5.9	
Pharmacokinetics: metabolism in vitro	2.6.5.10	
Pharmacokinetics: possible metabolic pathways	2.6.5.11	
Pharmacokinetics: induction/inhibition of drug metabolizing enzymes	2.6.5.12	
Pharmacokinetics: excretion	2.6.5.13	
Pharmacokinetics: excretion into bile	2.6.5.14	
Pharmacokinetics: drug–drug interactions	2.6.5.15	
Pharmacokinetics: other	2.6.5.16	
Toxicology written summary	2.6.6	
Brief summary of toxicology	2.6.6.1	
Single-dose toxicity	2.6.6.2	4.2.3.1
Repeat-dose toxicity	2.6.6.3	4.2.3.2

(Continued)

TABLE 3 Order of Presentation for Nonclinical Written and Tabulated Summaries (Module 2) and Nonclinical Study Reports (Module 4) (*Continued*)

Sequence of presentation	Module 2	Module 4
Genotoxicity	2.6.6.4	4.2.3.3
Carcinogenicity	2.6.6.5	4.2.3.4
Reproductive and developmental toxicity (including studies in juvenile animals)	2.6.6.6	4.2.3.5
Local tolerance	2.6.6.7	4.2.3.6
Other toxicity studies	2.6.6.8	4.2.4.7
Discussion and conclusions	2.6.6.9	
Tables and figures	2.6.6.10	
Toxicology tabulated summary	2.6.7	
Toxicology: overview	2.6.7.1	
Toxicokinetics: overview of toxicokinetic studies	2.6.7.2	
Toxicokinetics: overview of toxicokinetic data	2.6.7.3	
Toxicology: drug substance lots used in toxicology studies	2.6.7.4	
Single-dose toxicity	2.6.7.5	
Repeat-dose toxicity: nonpivotal studies	2.6.7.6	
Repeat-dose toxicity: pivotal studies	2.6.7.7	
Genotoxicity: in vitro	2.6.7.8	
Genotoxicity: in vivo	2.6.7.9	
Carcinogenicity	2.6.7.10	
Reproductive and developmental toxicity: nonpivotal studies	2.6.7.11	
Reproductive and developmental toxicity—fertility and early embryonic development to implantation (pivotal)	2.6.7.12	
Reproductive and developmental toxicity—effects on embryo-fetal development (pivotal)	2.6.7.13	
Reproductive and developmental toxicity—effects on pre- and postnatal development, including maternal function (pivotal)	2.6.7.14	
Studies in juvenile animals	2.6.7.15	
Local tolerance	2.6.7.16	
Other toxicity studies (antigenicity, immunotoxicity, mechanistic studies, dependence, metabolites, impurities, and other)	2.6.7.17	
Key literature references		4.3

candidates (depending on their route of administration and potential toxicological profile), some of the secondary battery (renal/kidney system, autonomic nervous system, GI tract, and other system) of safety pharmacology studies may be necessary. For drug candidates with potential risk (such as QT interval prolongation) to the cardiovascular system, additional evaluations may be necessary to further define and characterize the observed adverse effect. Since the results of some secondary PD studies may predict or assess potential adverse effects in humans and thus may contribute to the safety evaluations on a drug candidate, these results should be considered along with the data from safety pharmacology studies. If performed, drug interaction studies on PD effects (i.e., synergy or antagonism of the pharmacological response when two or more compounds are concurrently administered) should be summarized.

A discussion and conclusion subsection allows a sponsor to explain the results from the nonclinical pharmacology evaluations and to consider the significance of any issues that were noted or uncovered.

A Tabulated Summary of Pharmacology should provide, in the same order as the written text and by study with in vitro studies preceding in vivo studies, brief descriptions of (*i*) the type of study, (*ii*) testing facility, (*iii*) an indication of GLP compliance, (*iv*) indication tested, (*v*) the study design, (*vi*) study numbers (i.e., animals/sex/group), (*vii*) the dose levels, method of administration, and frequency and duration of dosing, (*viii*) a synopsis of results, (*ix*) reference to publication citation and/or study report number, and (*x*) any other information that might assist a reviewer in better understanding the results from a given study. Recommended pharmacology tables (ETA) include a pharmacology overview, primary and secondary pharmacodynamics, safety pharmacology, and PD drug interactions.

The recommend order of presentation for a Pharmacokinetic Written Summary is given in Table 3. A brief summary of approximately 2 to 3 pages should provide information on the scope of the nonclinical PK evaluations and should indicate whether the animal species and strains studied where the same as those employed in animal pharmacology and toxicology experiments and whether the formulations tested were similar to or different from the formulations employed in other animal studies. As with the nonclinical pharmacology section, in-text tables and figures can be used, as appropriate, throughout the PK section or can be grouped at the end of the section.

An introductory summary is to be followed by a brief description of the BAC methods employed for the quantification of a drug candidate and its known metabolites in physiological matrices (e.g., plasma, serum, urine, and bile). Where appropriate, method validation results for each species and each matrix, including limits of quantification and stability in physiological specimens, should be summarized. While not listed in the ICH CTD guideline, a recommendation to include in this section information on the synthesis of any radiolabeled compound used to evaluate the pharmacokinetics and DM, including mass balance and tissue distribution, of a drug candidate should be considered. Information on the site of radiolabel in the chemical structure of a drug candidate and on the chemical and metabolic stability of the radiolabeled material should be included as well as a summary of any developed metabolic profiling assay.

A subsection on absorption should discuss available data on the extent and rate of absorption as determined from in vivo and in situ studies and on relative bioavailability animal studies conducted to evaluate changes in formulation or to bridge studies using different routes of administration. This subsection can also summarize the available PK and TK results from each animal species evaluated and compare the generated PK parameter estimates among the various species. These comparisons should include human PK results at the maximum human dose evaluated during clinical trials on a drug candidate and any summary information on extent of exposure after single and multiple dose administration, absorption and disposition kinetics, possible gender effects, and dose linearity and/or proportionality over the evaluated dose range. A distribution subsection to summarize results from protein binding and distribution into blood cells experiments using human and animal physiological samples, single- and repeat-dose (if conducted) tissue distribution studies in rodents, and placental transfer studies conducted to support reproductive and developmental toxicology studies. A primary purpose of conducting metabolism studies is to determine if the metabolic profile (number and amount of metabolites) of a drug candidate is similar or dissimilar in the animal models used for pharmacology and toxicology studies when compared to those found in humans. This interspecies comparison to be presented in a subsection on nonclinical metabolism should include information on the chemical structures and quantities of metabolites in physiological specimens from each species evaluated. The possible metabolic pathways for a drug candidate in each species, including humans, should be described using figures, as appropriate. For a drug candidate to be administered orally, information on the extent of presystemic metabolism (i.e., metabolism in the GI tract or first-pass metabolism by the liver) should be included. Any in vitro metabolism studies conducted to identify the enzyme systems (i.e., CYP450 isozymes) or individual enzymes (i.e., glucuronidases, esterases) responsible for metabolism of a drug candidate should be discussed and any information on metabolizing enzyme induction and inhibition should be included. Research studies conducted to evaluate the rate and extent of excretion of a drug candidate and metabolites or mass balance studies in rodent and nonrodent animal models are to be summarized. In addition and if available, information on the extent of excretion in milk (i.e., lacteal secretion) should be provided as supportive data for completed reproductive and developmental toxicology studies.

If performed, the results from nonclinical PK drug–drug interaction studies should be summarized. The results from any other conducted nonclinical PK studies (i.e., drug–food and drug–drug interaction studies, renally impaired animals, juvenile, and/or aged animal evaluations) should be briefly discussed.

Using a discussion and conclusion subsection, a sponsor-designated author, either in-house or contracted, should discuss any nonclinical PK issues and consider the significance of these findings to the overall development of a drug candidate.

The Pharmacokinetic Written Summary is to be followed by a Pharmacokinetic Tabulated Summary. This tabulated summary should be ordered the same as the written summary and include an overview of all PK studies conducted on a drug candidate with indication of which of these studies were conducted in compliance with GLP Regulations, the study or report number, and the location of the study report in Module 4 of a marketing application. This overview is to be followed by tabulated summaries (ETA) of each conducted individual PK study, such as (*i*) BAC methods and validation reports, (*ii*) absorption after single and repeat doses, (*iii*) tissue distribution, (*iv*) protein binding, (*v*) study in pregnant and/or nursing animals, (*vi*) metabolism (in vitro and in vivo) and possible metabolic pathways, (*vii*) induction and/or inhibition of drug metabolizing enzymes, (*viii*) excretion (urinary, fecal, biliary, and expired air), (*ix*) drug–drug interactions, and (*x*) other PK studies.

The order of presentation recommended for a Toxicology Written Summary is shown in Table 3. A brief summary of the principal toxicology findings should be described in a few pages, generally not more than six, and should include a discussion in relation to the proposed clinical use. If desired and without including toxicology results, a summary table describing the extent of the toxicological evaluations on a drug candidate and a comment on compliance with GLP Regulations for each study conducted can be provided.

Results from single-dose or acute toxicology studies should be briefly presented by species and by route. Repeat-dose (subchronic and chronic) toxicology studies, with supportive TK evaluations, should be summarized by species, by route, and by duration and should provide summary information on methodology and highlight important findings (e.g., number of deaths, target organs or tissues of toxicity, dose or exposure relationship to toxicity, NOAEL, maximum tolerated dose or MTD, gross pathology, and histopathological findings, etc.). Nonpivotal toxicology studies can be summarized in less detail than pivotal studies, which are the definitive GLP-regulated toxicology studies specified in the ICH M3 guideline.

Genotoxicity studies are to be summarized with in vitro nonmammalian cell system evaluations followed by in vitro mammalian cell system studies and then in vivo mammalian system experiments, which may have supportive TK evaluations. For carcinogenicity studies, with supportive TK results, a brief rationale, including the selection of doses evaluated, should be used to explain the types of studies chosen. The results from individual carcinogenicity studies are to be summarized with long-term or lifetime studies first and then short- or medium-term studies. The studies are to be ordered by species and include dose range-finding studies that cannot be appropriately included under repeat-dose toxicity or PK subheadings.

Reproductive and developmental toxicology studies, with information on dose range-finding studies and supportive TK evaluations, are to be ordered by nonpivotal studies and pivotal studies, which include fertility and early embryonic development to implantation, effects on embryo-fetal development, and effects on pre- and postnatal development including maternal function. If conducted, studies in which juvenile animals are dosed and evaluated are to be included in this section.

If local tolerance studies were conducted (and are considered by this author to be necessary for a drug candidate to be administered by any of a number of routes including, but not limited to, intravenous, intramuscular, subcutaneous, dermal, buccal, nasal, pulmonary, rectal, and vaginal), the results should be summarized by species, by route, and by duration and should provide brief details of methodology and highlight important findings.

If other toxicology studies have been performed to support the development of a drug candidate, the results should be summarized with a rationale for conducting the studies and a brief discussion of the methodology and significant findings. Other toxicology study types include antigenicity, immunotoxicity, mechanistic studies (if not summarized elsewhere in the marketing application), dependence, and metabolite(s) and/or impurity(ies) evaluations.

A discussion and conclusions subsection on the toxicology results allows a sponsor's author to discuss the toxicity findings with reference to the significant issues that were noted or observed. The use of in-text tables and figures for highlighting these findings is recommended.

A Toxicology Tabulated Summary should follow a Toxicology Written Summary. A tabulated summary should be ordered the same as a written summary and start with an overview of all toxicology and TK studies conducted on a drug candidate with indication of which studies were conducted in compliance with GLP Regulations, the study or report number, and the location of the study report in Module 4 of the marketing application. Following this overview are to be overview summaries (ETA) on TK studies and TK data and on drug substance lots used in toxicology studies. The tabulated summaries (ETA) of each individual toxicology study (single- or acute-dose toxicity, repeat-dose toxicity, genotoxicity, carcinogenicity, reproductive and developmental toxicity, studies in juvenile animals, local tolerance, and other toxicity studies) are to be presented.

Clinical Summary

A Clinical Summary should provide a detailed, factual summarization of all the clinical information in a marketing application, including results within clinical study reports, from meta-analyses and/or other cross-study analyses reports, and if appropriate, postmarketing data. The length of a Clinical Summary (excluding tables and figures) should range from 50 to 400 pages. The recommended order of presentation, which corresponds to the Table of Contents, for the various items to be included in a Clinical Summary is provided in Table 4.

A Clinical Summary should start with a subsection on biopharmaceutical studies, and associated analytical and BAC methods, conducted during the clinical development of a drug candidate. The background of the formulation development process is to be briefly provided and include information on in vitro and in vivo dosages form performance and the general approach and rationale for developing the bioavailability (BA), comparative BA, bioequivalence (BE) (for a generic drug product), and in vitro dissolution profile database. Also to be included is a summary of the analytical and BAC methods and the validation characteristics of these methods.

A tabular listing (ETA) of all biopharmaceutical studies conducted is recommended. Brief narrative descriptions (e.g., similar to an abstract for a journal article) are to share relevant features and outcomes of each study that provided important in vitro or in vivo data and information relevant to the BA or comparative BA of a drug candidate. These narratives can be abstracted from clinical study reports (i.e., the synopsis of reports prepared according to ICH guideline E3) and should include reference to the full report. A comparison of results across studies, using both text and tables, is to pay particular attention to differences to in vitro dissolution, BA, and comparative BA results. This comparison is to consider

1. the effects of formulation and manufacturing changes on in vitro dissolution and BA;
2. where appropriate, the effect of food (i.e., meal type and/or timing of the meal in relation to dose administration) on BA;
3. evidence of, or lack of, correlations between in vitro dissolution and BA, including the effect of pH on dissolution and conclusions on dissolution specifications;
4. comparative BA of different dosage form strengths;
5. if appropriate, comparative BA of a drug candidate formulation(s) used in clinical trials and a proposed drug product to be marketed;
6. the source and magnitude of observed inter- and intrasubject variability for each formulation in a comparative BA study.

A Summary of Clinical Pharmacology Studies is to provide reviewers of a marketing application with an overall view of the clinical pharmacology of a drug candidate and should include information on clinical studies conducted to evaluate human pharmacokinetics and pharmacodynamics and information on in vitro studies performed with human cells, tissues, or related material (i.e., human biomaterials) and considered pertinent to PK processes. Types of in vitro studies include permeability assessments (e.g., intestinal absorption, blood brain barrier transport), protein binding, and hepatic metabolism. For a vaccine product, immune response

TABLE 4   Order of Presentation for Clinical Summary (Module 2)

Sequence of presentation for Clinical Summary	Module 2
Table of contents	2.7
Summary of biopharmaceutic studies and associated analytical methods	2.7.1
Background and overview	2.7.1.1
Summary of results of individual studies	2.7.1.2
Comparison and analyses of results across studies	2.7.1.3
Appendix (tables and figures not included in text)	2.7.1 (A)
Summary of clinical pharmacology studies	2.7.2
Background and overview	2.7.2.1
Summary of results of individual studies	2.7.2.2
Comparison and analyses of results across studies	2.7.2.3
Special studies (e.g., immunogenicity, clinical microbiology)	2.7.2.4
Appendix (tables and figures not included in text)	2.7.2 (A)
Summary of clinical efficacy	2.7.3
Background and overview of clinical efficacy	2.7.3.1
Summary of results of individual studies	2.7.3.2
Comparison and analyses of results across studies	2.7.3.3
Study population	2.7.3.3.1
Comparison of efficacy results of all studies	2.7.3.3.2
Comparison of results in subpopulations	2.7.3.3.3
Analysis of clinical information relevant to dosing recommendations	2.7.3.4
Persistence of efficacy and/or toxic effects	2.7.3.5
Appendix (tables and figures not included in text)	2.7.3 (A)
Summary of clinical safety	2.7.4
Exposure to drug candidate	2.7.4.1
Overall safety evaluation plan and narratives of safety studies	2.7.4.1.1
Overall extent of exposure	2.7.4.1.2
Demographic and other characteristics of study population	2.7.4.1.3
Adverse events or experiences (AEs)	2.7.4.2
Analysis of AEs	2.7.4.2.1
Common AEs	2.7.4.2.1.1
Deaths	2.7.4.2.1.2
Other serious AEs (SAEs)	2.7.4.2.1.3
Other significant AEs	2.7.4.2.1.4
Analysis of AEs by organ system or syndrome	2.7.4.2.1.5
Narratives	2.7.4.2.2
Clinical laboratory evaluations	2.7.4.3
Vital signs, physical findings, and other observations related to safety	2.7.4.4
Safety in special groups and situations	2.7.4.5
Intrinsic factors	2.7.4.5.1
Extrinsic factors	2.7.4.5.2
Drug interactions	2.7.4.5.3
Use in pregnancy and lactation	2.7.4.5.4
Overdose	2.7.4.5.5
Drug abuse	2.7.4.5.6
Withdrawal and rebound	2.7.4.5.7
Effects on ability to drive or operate machinery and impairment of mental ability	2.7.4.5.8
Postmarketing data	2.7.4.6
Appendix (tables and figures not included in text)	2.7.4 (A)
References	2.7.5
Synopses of individual studies	2.7.6

data is to be provided to support the selection of dose, dosing schedule, and the formulation of a proposed final drug product. The summary is to start with a brief overview of conducted human biomaterial studies followed by the clinical studies conducted to characterize the pharmacokinetics and pharmacodynamics of a drug candidate, and any PK/PD relationships, in healthy subjects and patients. Critical aspects of study designs and data analysis are to be noted and may include rationale for the choice of single or repeat doses, the study population, the choice of intrinsic and extrinsic factors studied, and the choice of PD end points.

A tabular listing (ETA) of all clinical pharmacology studies is recommended and is to be accompanied by brief narrative descriptions, with appropriate reference to the full reports, of the relevant features and outcomes for each of the critical individual studies. The summary information on individual clinical pharmacology studies is to be followed by a comparison and analyses of results across studies. Using as appropriate tables (ETA), figures, and text, the comparison is to provide a factual presentation of all data pertinent to

1. in vitro DM and in vitro drug–drug interaction studies and possible clinical implications of the results;
2. human PK studies, including estimates of standard PK parameters (such as absorption, distribution, and disposition rate constants and their corresponding half lives, extent of exposure, clearance, and volume of distribution), sources of variability, and evidence supporting dose and/or dose individualization in the target patient population and in special populations;
3. comparison between single and repeated dose PK studies;
4. population PK analyses;
5. dose–response and/or concentration–response relationships;
6. major inconsistencies in the human biomaterial, PK, and/or PD database;
7. PK studies conducted to determine if foreign clinical data might be extrapolated for supporting a marketing application in a new region.

In addition, a clinical pharmacology subsection should include information on research studies that provide special types of data that are relevant to a specific type of drug candidate. These study types may include immunogenicity studies for a protein drug candidate and in vitro assessments to characterize the spectrum of activity for an antimicrobial or antiviral drug candidate. For a vaccine or other type of drug product intended to induce specific immune reactions, immunogenicity data are to be described in the section on efficacy. Similarly, clinical studies that include characterization of the susceptibility of clinical isolates to a drug candidate as part of the efficacy determination are to be included in the section on efficacy.

A Summary of Clinical Efficacy subsection describes the program of controlled clinical studies and other pertinent clinical trials that evaluated efficacy specific to the indication(s) sought. If a marketing application is for more than one indication, separate clinical efficacy sections are to be provided for each indication unless the indications are closely related. The use of tables (ETA) and figures is recommended to enhance the readability of the document and, if appropriate (i.e., due to the length of tables or the size of figures), can be provided in an appendix at the end of the subsection. A clinical efficacy subsection should begin with an overview of the design of the controlled clinical trials (e.g., dose–response, comparative efficacy, long-term efficacy, and efficacy in patient population subgroups) that were conducted to evaluate efficacy. Critical features (e.g., randomization, blinding, choice of control treatment, choice of patient population, study duration, end points, and statistical analysis plan) are to be discussed.

A tabular listing of all clinical studies that provided (or were designed to provide) data relevant to the efficacy of a drug candidate is recommended and is to be accompanied with brief narrative descriptions, with references to the full clinical study reports, of important clinical trials. These narratives can be abstracted from the synopses of reports prepared according to the ICH E3 guideline. Narratives for any bridging study using clinical end points (i.e., clinical trials for extrapolating certain types of foreign clinical data to a marketing application to a new region) are to be included.

A comparison and analysis of efficacy results across clinical studies is to summarize all available data that characterize the efficacy of a drug candidate. This summary should include analyses of all data, irrespective of whether the data support the overall efficacy conclusion, and should discuss the extent to which the results of the relevant clinical studies do or do not reinforce to each other. Major inconsistencies regarding efficacy are to be addressed and any area needing further evaluation is to be identified. Important differences in study design (e.g., end points, control groups, study duration, statistical methods, patient population, dose or dose range, and drug candidate formulation) should be identified. Analyses will generally be of two types: (*i*) comparison of results of individual clinical studies and (*ii*) analysis of data pooled from various clinical studies. Comparisons of efficacy results across studies should primarily focus on prespecified primary end points. Also, important evidence that supports efficacy summarized in a clinical pharmacology section should be cross-referenced.

The demographic and other baseline characteristics of patients across all efficacy studies are to be described and should provide information on

1. the characteristics of the disease (e.g., severity and duration), prior treatment in study patients, and inclusion and exclusion criteria;
2. differences in baseline characteristics of the study population in different studies or groups of studies;
3. any differences between populations included in critical efficacy analyses and the overall patient population who would receive a drug product after marketing approval has been obtained;
4. assessment of the number of patients who dropped or were terminated from the studies, the times of withdrawal, and the reasons for discontinuation.

Overview analyses of efficacy in a specific population should be summarized to demonstrate whether the claimed treatment effects are consistently observed across all relevant population subgroups. Due to the limited sample size in many individual clinical trials, analyses across multiple studies may be necessary to evaluate efficacy effects for major demographic factors and relevant intrinsic and extrinsic factors. Areas of special interest may arise from general concern (e.g., treatment of the elderly) or from specific issues related to the pharmacology of a drug candidate or identified during earlier drug development. Efficacy in a pediatric population should routinely be analyzed in marketing applications for a proposed indication that also occurs in children.

An integrated summary and analysis are to be provided on all data that pertain to dose–response or drug candidate plasma concentration–response relationships of effectiveness that have contributed to dose selection, dosing interval, and dosage duration. Relevant data from nonclinical and clinical studies should be referenced and, where appropriate, summarized to further illustrate and describe these relationships. Any identified deviations (e.g., nonlinearity of pharmacokinetics, delayed effects, tolerance, enzyme induction or inhibition) from relatively simple relationships should be discussed. Also, any evidence of differences in the relationships that result from the age, gender, race, disease status, or other factors of the patients evaluated should be described. How the potential for these deviations and differences was evaluated, even if no differences were found, should be addressed.

Available data on the persistence of efficacy over time should be summarized. The number of patients for whom long-term efficacy data are available and the length of exposure should be provided, and any evidence of tolerance over time should be noted.

A summary of data relevant to human safety in the intended patient population is to integrate the results of individual clinical study reports. Safety-related data are to be displayed at three levels, which are

1. the extent of exposure (e.g., dose, dosing duration, number of patients, type of patients) to determine the degree to which human safety can be assessed from the database;
2. the identification and classification of the occurrence of the more common AEs and changes in laboratory test values;
3. the occurrence of SAEs and other significant AEs with the events examined for frequency over time.

With the appropriate use of tables and figures, the human safety profile of a drug candidate is to be described on the basis of analysis of all clinical safety data and is to be outlined in a detailed, clear, and objective manner.

For the assessment of exposure to a drug candidate, the overall human safety evaluation plan is to be briefly described and should include considerations and observations concerning nonclinical data, any relevant pharmacological class effects, and the sources of the safety data. A tabular listing (ETA) of all clinical studies, grouped appropriately, that provided human safety data is recommended. Narrative descriptions of these studies should be provided, or appropriately cross-referenced, and include sufficient detail to allow reviewers to understand the exposure of study subjects/patients to a drug candidate or control agent(s) and how the human safety data were collected. A table (ETA) and appropriate text should be employed to summarize the overall extent of drug candidate exposure from all phases of the clinical development program. The table should indicate the number of subjects/patients exposed in clinical studies of different types and at various doses, routes of administration, and durations of dosing, which can be grouped in an appropriate manner. Dose-level designations could be the maximum dose received by a subject/patient, the dose with the longest exposure, the mean daily dose, and/or the cumulative dose. Duration of exposure can be summarized by the number of subjects/patients exposed for specific periods of time (e.g., 1 day or less, 2 days–1 week, 1 week–1 month, 1 month–6 months, 6 months–1 year, more than 1 year).

A summary table (ETA) should provide an overview of the demographic characteristics of the population that was exposed to a drug candidate during clinical development, and the choice of age ranges studied should be noted. Additional tables should be used to describe relevant characteristics of the population and the number of subjects/patients with special characteristics, such as (*i*) severity of disease, (*ii*) hospitalization, (*iii*) impaired renal function, (*iv*) concomitant illnesses or diseases, (*v*) concomitant or concurrent use of particular medications, and (*vi*) geographical location. Any imbalance(s) between a drug candidate and placebo and/or comparator(s) regarding demographic characteristics should be discussed, particularly in relation to differences in safety outcomes. Separate demographic tables should be prepared for each indication evaluated, unless the indications are closely related and risks to the study populations are considered to be the same.

Tables (ETA) and text should be used to describe the frequency of AEs. All AEs occurring or worsening after initiation of treatment are to be summarized in tables listing each AE, the number of subjects/patients in whom the AE occurred, and the frequency of occurrence in subjects/patients treated with a drug candidate, comparator drug(s), and placebo. These tables could also present AE results for each drug candidate dose level and could be modified to show AE rates by severity, by time from onset of therapy, or by assessment of causality.

When the human safety data are not concentrated in a small number of clinical studies, grouping the studies and pooling the safety results to improve estimates and sensitivity to differences may be considered. However, while often useful, pooling of human safety data across studies is to be approached with caution since in some cases interpretations can be difficult and may obscure real differences. When pooling safety data, items that should be considered include the following:

1. Combining safety data from clinical studies that are of similar design is often appropriate.
2. A safety evaluation from pooled data is usually less informative if the incidence of a particular AE differs substantially across the clinical studies.
3. An unusual AE pattern for any clinical study is indicative that the safety data for that study should be presented separately.
4. The appropriate extent of analysis is dependent on the seriousness of the AE and the strength of evidence of drug candidate causation.
5. Examination of which subjects/patients experience extreme laboratory abnormalities may be useful in identifying subgroups who are at risk for certain AEs.

When a sponsor decides to pool safety data from several clinical studies, the rationale for selecting the method used for pooling should be described. AEs in pooled studies should use standardized terms to describe events and their frequencies and synonymous terms should be collected under a single preferred term. The use of MedDRA is recommended but other specified dictionaries can be used.

Tables of AE rates are recommended to compare rates in treatment and control groups. Combining the AE severity and causality categories may be helpful in providing a simpler side-by-side comparison of groups. While causality categories, if used, may be reported, the recommended presentation of the human safety data is to include total AEs (whether considered related or unrelated to treatment with a drug candidate) since evaluations of causality are considered to be inherently subjective and may exclude unexpected AEs that are in fact treatment related. Another useful examination is to more closely evaluate the more common AEs that are considered to be drug candidate related (e.g., show an apparent dose–response relationship and/or a clear difference between drug candidate and placebo rates) for possible correlation with relevant factors such as (*i*) dosage, (*ii*) dose level expressed in terms of mg/kg or mg/m^2, (*iii*) dosing regimen, (*iv*) dosing duration, (*v*) total dose administered, (*vi*) demographic characteristics, (*vii*) concomitant medication use, (*viii*) other baseline features, (*ix*) efficacy outcomes, and/or (*x*) drug candidate plasma concentrations (where available). Also possibly useful for the apparently drug candidate–related events is a summary of AEs results based on time of onset and duration of the experience. Rigorous statistical evaluations of the possible relationships of specific AEs to each of the factors mentioned above are often not necessary, particularly when inspections of the safety data show no apparent evidence of a significant relationship between AE rate and a given factor.

A table, usually located in an appendix to a Clinical Safety subsection, should list all deaths occurring while subjects/patients are on study, including deaths that occurred shortly following (e.g., within 30 days) treatment termination. Only deaths that are clearly disease related as described in a clinical study protocol and are not related to the administration of a drug candidate can be excepted from this table. All deaths should be examined for any unexpected patterns between study treatment arms and further analyzed if unexplained differences are noted. Deaths are to be examined individually and analyzed on the basis of rates in individual clinical trials and appropriate pools of trials, considering both total mortality and cause-related deaths. Potential relationships of death to demographic, intrinsic, and extrinsic factors should also be considered.

Summaries of all SAEs, other than death but including SAEs associated with or preceding death, are to be displayed in a table and discussed in text. The display should include major laboratory abnormalities, abnormal vital signs, and abnormal physical observations that are considered to be SAEs. Results of analyses and/or assessments of SAEs across clinical studies should be presented and examined for frequency over time, particularly for a drug candidate projected for chronic clinical use. Potential relationships of SAEs to demographic, intrinsic, and extrinsic factors should also be considered.

Other than those reported as SAEs, marked hematological and other laboratory abnormalities and any experience that led to a substantial intervention (e.g., premature discontinuation of drug candidate treatment, dose reduction, or substantial additional concomitant therapy) should be displayed. Experiences that led to premature discontinuation of drug candidate administration are considered to represent an important safety concern and deserve particular attention in the evaluation of human safety data. AEs leading to treatment discontinuation should be considered as possibly drug candidate related even if the event was thought to represent intercurrent illness. Reasons for discontinuation should be discussed and rates of discontinuation should be compared across clinical studies in relation to rates for placebo and/or active control treatment groups and for potential relationships to demographic, intrinsic, and extrinsic factors.

Assessments of causality of, and risk factor for, death, other SAEs, and other significant AEs are frequently complicated by the fact that these events are uncommon in most clinical development programs. Thus, consideration of related events as a group may be of critical importance in understanding the safety profile of a drug candidate. In addition, summarizing AEs by organ system or syndrome is often useful so that AEs may be considered in the content of potentially related experiences, including laboratory abnormalities.

The locations in a marketing application of individual narratives of subject/patient deaths, other SAEs, and other significant AEs should be referenced. These narratives themselves will normally be a part of the applicable clinical study report. In cases where no clinical study report has been generated, narratives can be placed in an appropriate section of Module 5.

A subsection on clinical laboratory evaluations is to describe changes in patterns of laboratory tests with drug candidate use. As mentioned earlier, marked laboratory abnormalities and those that led to a substantial intervention are to be reported in the subsection on SAEs. The appropriate evaluations of laboratory values will usually be determined by the results observed and should include comparison of the treatment and control groups. Normal laboratory ranges given in standard international units, should be provided for each analyte measured. A brief overview of the major changes in laboratory data (e.g., hematology, clinical chemistry, urinalysis, and other data as appropriate) at each time (e.g., at each clinical visit) over the course of the studies should include information on

1. the central tendency as determined by the group mean and median values;
2. the range of values and the number of subjects/patients with abnormal values or with abnormal values of a predefined certain size;
3. abnormalities, including those that led to discontinuation, considered important for an individual subject/patient.

The technique employed for presenting cross-study observations and comparisons of vital signs (e.g., heart rate, blood pressure, temperature, and respiratory rate), weight, and other data (e.g., ECGs, EEGs, and X-rays) related to safety should be similar to that used for laboratory variables. If an effect is evident, any relationship to a drug candidate or to other variables (e.g., disease, demographics, and concomitant therapy) should be identified and discussed for clinical relevance.

Separate subsections in a Clinical Summary are recommended to summarize safety in special groups and situations. These subsections may include brief overviews of safety data pertinent to individualizing therapy or patient management for

1. intrinsic ethnic factors that may include age, gender, height, weight, lean body mass, genetic polymorphism, body composition, other illness, and organ dysfunction (e.g., renal or hepatic impairment);
2. extrinsic ethnic factors that may include environment (e.g., geographic location), use of tobacco, use of alcohol, use of other drugs, and food habits;
3. the potential impact on safety (e.g., changes in pharmacological effect, AE profile, and/or drug candidate plasma concentrations) for drug–drug and drug–food interactions;
4. use during pregnancy and lactation;
5. overdose including signs and/or symptoms, laboratory findings, therapeutic measures and/or treatments, and antidotes, if available;
6. drug abuse and dependence potential, including particularly susceptible patient populations;
7. withdrawal and rebound effects, including events that may occur, or increase in severity, after discontinuation;
8. effects (e.g., drowsiness) on ability to drive or operate machinery or impairment of mental ability.

If a drug candidate has already been or is being marketed, all relevant post-marketing data (e.g., published and unpublished, including, if available, periodic safety update reports) available to a sponsor of a marketing application should be summarized. Details to be provided include the number of subjects/patients estimated to have been exposed to the drug and categorized, as appropriate, by indication, dosage, treatment duration, and geographic location. A tabulation of SAEs reported after a drug is marketed is recommended and should include information on any potentially serious drug–drug interactions.

A list of references cited in a Clinical Summary should be included and copies of important references provided in Module 5. Any reference not included in Module 5 should be available upon request. It is recommended that all references cited in the Clinical Overview and the Clinical Summary be included in Module 5.

The last section of a Clinical Summary is recommended to contain a table entitled Listing of Clinical Studies (ETA). This table is also to be included in Module 5. Following the table are to be individual clinical study synopses organized in the same sequence as the clinical study reports in Module 5. The ICH E3 guideline on Structure and Content of Clinical Study Reports provides an example of a format for a clinical study report synopsis, which can be used for marketing applications in all ICH regions.

MODULE 3: QUALITY

Information to be presented in Module 3 on Quality is to be an expansion of the summary descriptions provided in a QOS (discussed above). As shown in Table 1, the order of presentation is to be same as utilized for QOS with subsections under the main headings for each item for a drug substance (S) and a proposed drug product (P).

Detailed descriptions, using flow diagrams, figures, and narrative text, of the manufacturing processes for a drug substance and proposed drug product are to be provided under the appropriate headings. Alternate processes, if available, should be explained and described with the same level of detail as the primary process. A detailed development history discussion for both the drug substance and proposed drug product is recommended and should provide information on the significant changes made in the manufacturing process and/or manufacturing site for a drug substance and proposed drug product.

Validation protocols and reports, with acceptance and rejection criteria and specifications and experimental data, for all analytical chemistry methods developed and used for the characterization of a drug substance and proposed drug product are to be included within the designated sections. These methods may include, but are not limited to (*i*) identity assays for a drug substance, intermediates, and excipients; (*ii*) content assays for a drug substance, intermediates, and excipients; (*iii*) impurity profiling and quantification assays for a drug substance and proposed drug product; (*iv*) dissolution assays for a proposed drug product or drug products if more than one is included in the marketing application; and (*v*) stability-indicating assays for a drug substance and proposed drug product.

Descriptions of batches and the results of batch analyses for a drug substance and proposed drug product are to be provided under the appropriate sections.

For both drug substance and proposed drug product, the types of stability studies conducted, the protocols used, and the results are to be included in the designated sections. Study types may include forced degradation, stress conditions, and shelf life conditions. Results from stability studies are to be presented using an appropriate format that includes tables, figures, and narrative text. Conclusions with respect to storage conditions and shelf life are to be provided. A postpproval stability protocol and stability commitment for both the drug substance and the proposed drug product are to be included.

For a macromolecule drug substance and drug product, appendices to Module 3 are to include detailed information on facilities and equipment and safety evaluations on adventitious agents. The flow diagram presented in a QOS for facilities and equipment should be included. In addition, information is to be presented with respect to adjacent areas that may be of concern for maintaining the integrity of a drug substance and proposed drug product. Information on all developmental or approved products manufactured or manipulated in the same areas as a sponsor's drug substance or proposed drug product is to be included. In addition and as appropriate, information on the preparation, cleaning, sterilization, and storage of specified equipment and materials is to be provided. Also to be included is information on procedures (e.g., cleaning and production scheduling) and design features of the facility to prevent contamination or cross-contamination of areas and equipment where operations for the preparation of cell banks and drug substance and drug product manufacturing are performed.

For nonviral adventitious agents, detailed information is to be provided on the avoidance and control of these agents. Examples of information include certification and/or testing of raw materials and excipients and control of production processes for a given agent. For viral adventitious agents, detailed information is to be discussed from viral safety evaluation studies, which demonstrate that the materials used in production are considered safe and that the approaches used for testing, evaluating, and eliminating the potential risks during manufacturing are suitable. Information essential to evaluate the virological safety of materials of animal or human origin is to be provided. For cell lines, data on the selection, testing, and safety assessment for potential viral contamination of cells and viral qualification of cell banks should also be included. The selection of virological tests, including the sensitivity and specificity of the test and the frequency of testing that are performed during manufacturing is to be justified. Test results to confirm that a drug substance and proposed drug product are free from viral contamination at an appropriate stage of manufacture are to be provided. In addition, the rationale and action plan for assessing viral clearance and the results and evaluations of viral clearance studies are to be delineated.

A final section of Module 3 provides additional drug substance and proposed drug product information that is region specific and not included in Module 1. Sponsors need to consult the appropriate regional guidelines and/or regulatory authorities for additional guidance. Examples of region-specific information include

1. executed batch records (United States only),
2. method validation package (United States only),
3. comparability protocols (United States only),
4. process validation scheme for drug product (European Union only).

At the end of Module 3, key quality literature references cited in the text are to be included.

MODULE 4: NONCLINICAL STUDY REPORTS

The organization and order of presentation for the nonclinical study reports in a marketing application prepared in the recommended CTD format is given in Table 3 and is the same as described earlier (Section on "Nonclinical Written and Tabulated Summaries") for a Nonclinical Written Summary. Individual animal results are to be located in the corresponding nonclinical study report or as an appendix to that report. Module 4 of an application should start with a Table of Contents that lists all the nonclinical study reports included and that gives the location of each study report in a submission. The last section in a nonclinical study reports module is to provide copies of key nonclinical literature references that were cited to support the pharmacological, PK, and toxicological characterization and development of a drug candidate.

For some nonclinical studies, primarily drug discovery efforts and pharmacology evaluations conducted in-house by a sponsor, technical reports may not have been prepared but reprints of published journal articles may be available. While this situation is not discussed in the ICH CTD guideline, this author recommends that these publications be included in place of a technical report. If both a publication and report are available, the technical report should be included since a study report should contain all the data generated during the study while the publication may only summarize these results and might only contain those data that are supportive of the conclusions being made by the publication's authors. A copy of the publication, along with copies of other key literature references, should be included in the last section of Module 4.

MODULE 5: CLINICAL STUDY REPORTS

The recommended organization for the placement of clinical study reports and related information in a marketing application is described in Module 5 of the ICH CTD guideline. The placement of the individual clinical study reports is to be determined by the primary objective of a clinical trial and each report is to appear in only one section with appropriate cross-referencing to other sections when a trial has multiple objectives. An explanation, such as "not applicable" or "no study conducted" should be provided when no clinical study report or information is available for inclusion in a given section or subsection. This author recommends that sponsors use a similar practice when information is not available for inclusion in a quality (Module 3) or nonclinical (Module 4) section or subsection. Table 5 provides the recommended order of presentation for clinical study reports and related information. In general, this order of presentation is similar to the order of presentation in a Clinical Summary and is to start with a Table of Contents for Clinical Study Reports and then a Tabular Listing of All Clinical Studies. The tabular listing (ETA) is to be the same listing as utilized at the end of a Clinical Summary.

eCTD

In February 2004, version 3.2 of the ICH M2 eCTD guideline was issued. As described above, ICH M4 defines the CTD and describes the organization of modules, sections, and documents. This CTD structure and level of detail were used as the basis for defining the eCTD specification, including structure and content. ICH M2 defines the specifications, including the criteria that make an electronic submission valid, for the eCTD, which are to serve as an interface for industry to regulatory agency transfer (but not for industry to industry or agency to agency transfer)

TABLE 5   Order of Presentation for Clinical Study Reports and Related Information (Module 5)

Sequence of presentation for clinical study reports	Module 5
Table of contents of clinical study reports	5.A
Tabular listing of all clinical studies	5.B
Clinical study reports	5.C
Reports of biopharmaceutic studies	5.1
Bioavailability (BA) study reports	5.1.1
Comparative BA and bioequivalence (BE) study reports	5.1.2
In vitro and in vivo correlation study reports	5.1.3
Reports on bioanalytical and analytical methods for human studies	5.1.4
Reports of studies pertinent to pharmacokinetics using human biomaterials	5.2
Plasma protein binding study reports	5.2.1
Reports on hepatic metabolism and drug interaction studies	5.2.2
Reports of studies using other human biomaterials	5.2.3
Reports of human pharmacokinetic (PK) studies	5.3
Healthy subject PK and initial tolerability study reports	5.3.1
Patient PK and initial tolerability study reports	5.3.2
Intrinsic factor PK study reports	5.3.3
Extrinsic factor PK study reports	5.3.4
Population PK study reports	5.3.5
Reports of human pharmacodynamic (PD) studies	5.4
Healthy subject PD and PK/PD study reports	5.4.1
Patient PD and PK/PD study reports	5.4.2
Reports of efficacy and safety studies	5.5
Study reports of controlled clinical studies pertinent to the claimed indication	5.5.1
Study reports of uncontrolled clinical studies	5.5.2
Reports of analyses of data from more than one study, including any formal integrated analyses, meta-analyses, and bridging analyses	5.5.3
Other clinical study reports	5.5.4
Reports of postmarketing experience	5.6
Case report forms and individual patient listings	5.7
Copies of references	5.D

of regulatory information while at the same time taking into consideration the facilitation of the creation, review, life cycle management, and archival of an electronic submission. Where appropriate, additional details were developed within the eCTD specification. The philosophy of the eCTD is to use open standards, including proprietary standards that through their widespread use can be considered de facto standards that are deemed to be appropriate in general.

The CTD does not cover the full submission of a marketing application that is to be made to a particular region or regions. The CTD provides information on the format and structure of only Modules 2 to 5, which are common across all regions, and does not describe the content of Module 1, which includes regional administrative information and prescribing information. The CTD also does not describe documents that can be submitted as amendments or variations to the initial marketing application.

Therefore, the specification produced for the eCTD is applicable to all modules of an initial marketing application and for other submissions of information, such as variations and amendments, throughout the life cycle of the product. The eCTD describes the parts of the registration application that are common to all regions and some of the life cycle requirements for products approved for marketing. Those parts of the registration application that are specific to a particular region are still covered by regional guidance for that region.

The eCTD specification is designed to support high-level functional requirements such as the following:

1. Copy and paste.
2. Viewing and printing of documents.
3. Annotation of documentation.
4. Facilitate the exporting of information to databases.
5. Searching within and across applications.
6. Navigation throughout the eCTD and its subsequent amendments/variations.

The specification for the eCTD is expected to change over time. Factors that could affect the content of the eCTD specification include, but are not limited to

1. change in the content of the CTD, either through the amendment of information, at the same level of detail, or by provision of more detailed definition of content and structure;
2. change to the regional requirements for marketing applications that are outside the scope of the CTD;
3. updating standards that are already in use within the eCTD;
4. identification of new standards that provide additional value for the creation and/or usage of the eCTD;
5. identification of new functional requirements that will enhance the utility of the eCTD;
6. experience of use of the eCTD by all parties, both sponsors of marketing applications and regulatory agencies.

The basic principles that drove the design and architecture of the eCTD are defined in the ICH M2 guideline with the primary focus of the eCTD being to provide a data interchange message between sponsors and regulatory agencies. The structure of an electronic submission in terms of organization and navigation is to be consistent with the modular structure of the CTD.

An eCTD submission is to employ a directory structure with files (described below) including reports, data, and other submission information and is to support multilingual and multiregion aspects of a submission. Documents that are provided in the different modules are to be formatted as defined by the CTD. Within each document, sponsors are to provide bookmarks and hypertext links to all tables, figures, publications, and appendices. Sponsors should also provide hypertext links throughout the body of these documents to aid efficient navigation to annotations, related sections, publications, appendices, tables, and figures that are not located on the same page. If a list of references is included at the end of a document, sponsors should provide hypertext links to the appropriate publications that are located in Modules 3, 4, or 5. Sponsors are recommended to generate documents from electronic source documents and not from scanned material, with the exceptions where access to the source electronic file is unavailable or where a signature is required.

The eCTD provides highly recommended folder and file names, as shown in Figure 1. However, applicants may modify these folder and file names, where

```
□ ---- m2
    ---- □  22-intro
    ---- □  23-qos
               ---- □   23-qos-intro
               ---- □   23s- drug-sub
               ---- □   23p-drug-prod
               ---- □   23a-append
               ---- □   23r-reg-info
    ---- □  24-nonclin-over
    ---- □  25-clin-over
    ---- □  26-nonclin-sum
               ---- □   261-intro
               ---- □   262-pharm-writ-sum
               ---- □   263-pharm-tab-sum
               ---- □   264-pk-writ-sum
               ---- □   265-pk-tab-sum
               ---- □   266-tox-writ-sum
               ---- □   267-tox-tab-sum
    ---- □  27-clin-sum
               ---- □   271-biopharm-sum
               ---- □   272-clin-pharm-sum
               ---- □   273-efficacy-sum
               ---- □   274-safety-sum
               ---- □   275-lit-refs
               ---- □   276-syn-indiv-studies


□ ---- m3
    ---- □  32-body-data
    ---- □  32a-app
               ---- □   32a1-fac-equip
               ---- □   32a2-advent-agent
               ---- □   32a3-excip-name-1
    ---- □  32p-drug-product
               ---- □   32p-desc-comp
               ---- □   32p2-pharm-dev
               ---- □   32p3-manuf
               ---- □   32p4-contr-excip
               ---- □   32p5-contr-drug-prod
               ---- □   32p6-ref-std
               ---- □   32p7-cont-closure-sys
               ---- □   32p8-stab
    ---- □  32r-reg-info
    ---- □  32s-substance-1-manufacture-1
               ---- □   32s1-gen-info
               ---- □   32s2-manf
               ---- □   32s3-charac
               ---- □   32s4-contr-drug-sub
               ---- □   32s5-ref-std
               ---- □   32s6-cont-closure-sys
               ---- □   32s7-stab
    ---- □  33-lit-ref
```

FIGURE 1 Recommended file structure and folder designations for eCTD.

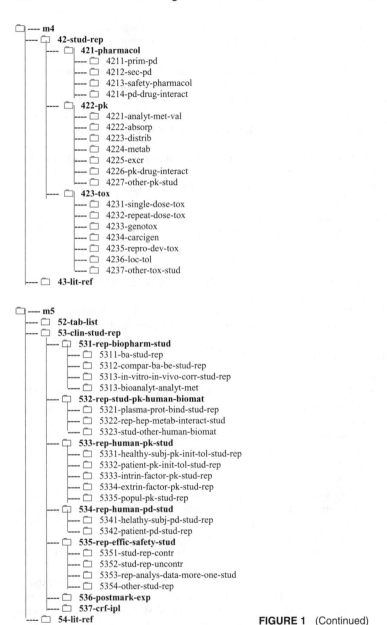

```
---- m4
  ---- 42-stud-rep
    ---- 421-pharmacol
      ---- 4211-prim-pd
      ---- 4212-sec-pd
      ---- 4213-safety-pharmacol
      ---- 4214-pd-drug-interact
    ---- 422-pk
      ---- 4221-analyt-met-val
      ---- 4222-absorp
      ---- 4223-distrib
      ---- 4224-metab
      ---- 4225-excr
      ---- 4226-pk-drug-interact
      ---- 4227-other-pk-stud
    ---- 423-tox
      ---- 4231-single-dose-tox
      ---- 4232-repeat-dose-tox
      ---- 4233-genotox
      ---- 4234-carcigen
      ---- 4235-repro-dev-tox
      ---- 4236-loc-tol
      ---- 4237-other-tox-stud
  ---- 43-lit-ref


---- m5
  ---- 52-tab-list
  ---- 53-clin-stud-rep
    ---- 531-rep-biopharm-stud
      ---- 5311-ba-stud-rep
      ---- 5312-compar-ba-be-stud-rep
      ---- 5313-in-vitro-in-vivo-corr-stud-rep
      ---- 5313-bioanalyt-analyt-met
    ---- 532-rep-stud-pk-human-biomat
      ---- 5321-plasma-prot-bind-stud-rep
      ---- 5322-rep-hep-metab-interact-stud
      ---- 5323-stud-other-human-biomat
    ---- 533-rep-human-pk-stud
      ---- 5331-healthy-subj-pk-init-tol-stud-rep
      ---- 5332-patient-pk-init-tol-stud-rep
      ---- 5333-intrin-factor-pk-stud-rep
      ---- 5334-extrin-factor-pk-stud-rep
      ---- 5335-popul-pk-stud-rep
    ---- 534-rep-human-pd-stud
      ---- 5341-helathy-subj-pd-stud-rep
      ---- 5342-patient-pd-stud-rep
    ---- 535-rep-effic-safety-stud
      ---- 5351-stud-rep-contr
      ---- 5352-stud-rep-uncontr
      ---- 5353-rep-analys-data-more-one-stud
      ---- 5354-other-stud-rep
  ---- 536-postmark-exp
  ---- 537-crf-ipl
  ---- 54-lit-ref
```

FIGURE 1 (Continued)

appropriate and after careful review of the recommended folder and file names to ascertain if they apply or do not apply to the specific marketing application.

The eCTD describes region-specific information for content that is not explicitly included in the CTD and the logistical details appropriate for the transmission and receipt of submissions using the eCTD. Module 1 contains administrative information that is unique for each region and local requirements need to be met for both the content and electronic component of Module 1. However, the eCTD backbone was developed to allow the transfer of the regional information included in a regulatory dossier.

Module 1 includes all administrative documents (e.g., forms and certifications) and labeling, including the documents described in regional guidances. However, not all regionally specific documents are included in Module 1 and sponsors should place technical reports required for a specific region in Modules 3, 4, or 5, using the module most appropriate for the content of the information provided. Each region provides specific guidance on the format and content of the regional requirements of each module.

The design of the eCTD was influenced by many factors, including

1. the submissions need to accommodate full regulatory dossiers, supplements, amendments, and variations;
2. the submissions need to be able to accommodate regional requirements that are represented in regional guidance documents, regulations, and statutes;
3. the technology needs to be extensible so that as technology changes, the new electronic solutions can be accommodated.

The eCTD was designed around the concept of a backbone, with the backbone based on an Extensible Markup Language (XML) Document Type Definition (DTD). XML is an ISO standard for describing structured information in a platform independent manner. The backbone provides the navigation links to the various files and information that make up a marketing application. Regulatory agency reviewers and other readers should be able to directly navigate through the submission at the folder and file level.

The eCTD provides recommendations for the way files are to be constructed and includes file formats that are commonly used in electronic submissions. For font size, sponsors should use, whenever possible, Times New Roman, 12-point font, which is considered adequate for narrative text. Using fonts that are smaller than 12 point in tables, charts, and figures should be avoided, but if necessary, Times New Roman font sizes 9 to 10 are considered acceptable in large, extensive tables but smaller font sizes should not be used.

When providing marketing applications to the FDA in electronic format using the eCTD backbone files, paper copies of the application, including review copies and desk copies, are not required and should not be sent. Sponsors should send a single copy of the electronic portions of a submission to the appropriate central document room facility and copies should not be sent directly to the reviewer or review division. Electronic documents that bypass the controls for electronic files described in 21 CFR 11 regarding electronic signatures are not considered official documents for review. The FDA will provide a sponsor with a number for a sample eCTD submission and the sponsor can then submit a sample submission using the eCTD specification for testing. The FDA will process, but not review, the sample submission to ensure conformation with FDA eCTD guidance and specifications and eCTD guideline. The FDA will provide the sponsor with a report highlighting any errors found. The sponsor should correct all errors and submit the revised sample eCTD submission to the same number. Once the sample eCTD submission is acceptable to the agency, the sponsor can prepare the actual eCTD in the same format with the assurance that the format is acceptable to the agency.

For an EMEA submission, a sponsor has the option of submitting an eCTD alongside the paper CTD. The EMEA advises sponsors that where an eCTD is submitted, the CTD remains the formal submission, and therefore both paper and electronic submissions need to comply fully with the CTD as regards presentation and content of the dossier. Sponsors should liaise with the EMEA if intending to submit an eCTD (two copies are necessary) in addition to the paper CTD.

Sponsors need to be aware of some differences between the CTD and eCTD. The CTD provides information on the format and structure for Modules 2 to 5, each of which needs to have a table of contents. The eCTD provides specifications for Modules 1 to 5 and none of modules have a table of contents. The eCTD follows the CTD format but with slightly different directory names, as shown in the following table:

TABLE

CTD format		eCTD
Section in CTD	Description	Folder name
2.2	Introduction	22-intro
2.3	Quality overall summary	23-qos
2.4	Nonclinical overview	24-nonclin-over
2.5	Clinical overview	25-clin-over
2.6	Nonclinical written and tabulated summaries	26-nonclin-sum
2.7	Clinical summary	27-clin-sum

As documented in FDA Module 1 Specification Version 2.01 that was issued in 2006, the FDA eCTD specified Module 1 folder structure is as follows:

m1-1-forms
m1-2-cover letters
m1-3-administrative information
        m1-3-1-applicant information
        m1-3-2-field copy certification
        m1-3-3-debarment certification
        m1-3-4-financial certification disclosure
        m1-3-5-patent exclusivity
m1-4-references
m1-5-application status
m1-6-meetings
m1-7-fast track
m1-8-special protocol assessment request
m1-9-pediatric administrative information
m1-10-dispute resolution
m1-11-information amendment
m1-12-other correspondence
m1-13-annual report

m1-14-labeling
m1-15-promotional material
m1-16-risk management plans

The information provided above should be of assistance to a sponsor of a marketing application as the submission is being first generated in the recommended CTD format and then converted to an eCTD.

CONCLUSIONS

This chapter has described and discussed the various modules of a CTD as presented in ICH M4 and the eCTD as discussed in ICH M2. A sponsor preparing a marketing application for submission to any of the three ICH regions and to most other regulatory authorities around the world can, and probably should, utilize the recommend orders of presentations outlined in the ICH CTD guideline for quality, nonclinical, and clinical results generated to support the characterization and development of a drug candidate. As recommended by the various regulatory agencies, the sponsor should then compile the generated CTD into an electronic submission as an eCTD.

Using the recommended orders of presentation in the CTD provide a sponsor of a marketing application submission with a number of benefits, which include, but are not limited to

1. the compilation of the generated data and results in an order that is acceptable to various regulatory agencies;
2. easier and more timely evaluation of a marketing application by regulatory agency reviewers since the data and results are presented in a defined order and under the same headings as in other submissions;
3. an indication of missing results (e.g., key research studies not conducted during the drug development process or insufficient information being available to completing describe manufacturing procedures) that may be critical for obtaining marketing approval.

This author recommends that sponsors consider using the CTD-recommended order of presentation for quality, nonclinical, and clinical results as a generic template for the definition of a drug development logic plan (as described in chap. 1). The results from drug discovery efforts, preclinical research experiments, and earlier CMC evaluations can be appropriately summarized and placed in the desired locations of the CTD—recommended format. This compilation of data can then be utilized to support a regulatory agency submission (such as a FDA IND or an EMEA IMPD) for a first-in-human clinical trial. As clinical studies are completed and additional nonclinical and manufacturing information becomes available, the results can be summarized and placed in the appropriate sections or subsections of a CTD. Using this approach and once a sponsor believes that sufficient clinical data on the human safety and efficacy of a drug candidate in the proposed disease indication(s) have been generated, the time needed to prepare a marketing application in eCTD format should be greatly reduced (i.e., a few months versus a year or more).

REFERENCES

1. ICH Web site. Available from http://www.ich.org.
2. AMWA Web site. Available from http://www.amwa.org.

12 The Biologic License Application

Albert A. Ghignone

AAG, Incorporated, Phillipsburg, New Jersey, U.S.A.

INTRODUCTION

The first decade of the twentieth century brought some significant changes to the Center for Biologic Evaluation and Research (CBER). The center was reorganized and the Office of Therapeutic Products, the largest of CBER's review groups, was transferred to the drug center. CBER now had three main review groups—The Office of Blood Research and Review, The Office of Vaccines Research and Review, and The Office of Cellular, Tissue, and Gene Therapies. The first two offices that oversaw blood products and vaccines had been part of the CBER review function for many years. The last office, The Office of Cellular, Tissue, and Gene Therapies was a new office for the CBER review groups. It was an office that would regulate the products generated on the cutting edge of biologic sciences.

The 1990s had brought us the era of FDA regulatory reform. The law, the regulations, and the agency itself had undergone a tremendous change. CBER had undergone some of the most significant changes. As former FDA Commissioner David Kessler, M.D., had wanted, the drug and biologic approval processes have become very similar. Gone forever is the two-license system, the responsible head designation, and all the many other things that had made the biological approval process so unique and distinct and so different from drugs.

All this change has brought us to the new CBER and the single application and single license era. The Biologic License Application (BLA) has replaced the Product License Application (PLA) and the Establishment License Application (ELA). Gone are many CBER regulations, replaced now by CDER regulations. This is not so foreign considering that in the early 1970s, the FDA had declared and defined all biologic products as drugs, thus allowing the FDA to regulate biological products under two laws: the Federal Food, Drug, and Cosmetic Act and the Public Health Service Act.

In the BLA, a biologic product sponsor submits thousands of pages of nonclinical and clinical data, chemical and biologic information, and product manufacturing descriptions. The submission must allow CBER reviewers to make the following three principal determinations:

1. Whether the biologic is safe and effective in its indicated use, and whether the benefits of using the product outweigh the risks.
2. Whether the biologic proposed labeling is appropriate.
3. Whether the methods used in manufacturing and quality control are adequate to preserve the biologic's identity, strength, quality, potency, and purity.

A SHORT HISTORY OF THE LICENSING PROCESS FOR BIOLOGICALS

Given that government regulation of biologics has historically focused on the product manufacturing process, it is not surprising that the ELA has a considerably longer history than the PLA. Congress was first spurred to regulate the biologic industry in 1901, when 10 children died after being treated with diphtheria antitoxin that had been contaminated with tetanus.

But in establishing regulatory controls to prevent the contamination of the biologic products of that day—essentially vaccines and antitoxins—Congress had to work within the limitations of existing scientific knowledge and technology. At that time, it was difficult, and in many cases impossible, to identify the component parts of any biological product or to detect the presence of pathogens and other contaminants. The absence of sensitive assays for identifying, and purification processes for separating, biological contaminants left researchers to use crude immunological and in vivo tests.

This situation was complicated by the fact that the production processes for traditional biologics, usually involving human or animal extracts, were highly susceptible to contamination. The reality that contaminants were often infectious materials or toxins amplified the threat.

At that time, regulating production facilities seemed to be the only mechanism likely to control the quality of biologic products. Consequently, Congress passed the Biological Control Act of 1902, which required that biologics in interstate commerce be manufactured in facilities holding a valid establishment license. Interestingly, the statute failed to mandate government review or sanction of the products themselves, only that the establishments manufacturing and preparing the products meet specific criteria and permit the inspection of their facilities.

Not until 1944, when Congress modified the statute, did federal law require the licensure of products as well. Under the revision, both establishments and products must "meet standards designed to insure the continued safety, purity, and potency of such products, prescribed in regulation."

For the next 52 years, the dual licensure procedure was the centerpiece of biologic regulation in the United States. Because biologic products are difficult to characterize structurally, complete descriptions of the production processes and manufacturing facility have been regarded as essential to the control of product manufacture. Thus, the difficulty in biologic product characterization has been the most important scientific reason for CBER's continuing reliance on the ELA.

In 1994, the FDA began to look for ways to lessen regulatory burdens on industry. Because of this initiative, CBER took steps to modernize its regulatory program to reflect scientific and technological advances. Although these reforms affected virtually every aspect of biologic's regulation, they signaled the end of CBER's dual licensing system.

In 1996, CBER began to consolidate the dual licensing system that had been in place since 1944. Specifically, with a final regulation published in May 1996, CBER established that categories of highly characterized products would require only the submission of a single license application, a BLA, and the granting of a single license for marketing. In justifying this change, CBER stated that "technical advances have greatly increased the ability of manufacturers to control and analyze the manufacture of many biologic/biotechnology–derived products. Methodologies are now available to characterize these products, allowing the product to be more clearly evaluated by end product testing." The end of the dual licensing era had arrived, at least for certain categories of products. For these products, gone forever was the ELA. On November 1997, President Clinton signed the Federal Food, Drug, and Cosmetic Modernization Act of 1997. One section of this law required that all biologic products be licensed under the single licensing system. With his signature, President Clinton put an end to the CBER's dual licensing system. Since the signing of this law, CBER has issued guidances for the submission of the "Chemistry, Manufacturing, and Control Information and Establishment Description" for all categories of biological products. By the end of 1999, the single licensing system was fully implemented. As all these changes were being implemented, CBER was also preparing for the next-phase computerized license applications. Numerous guidance documents already have been issued by CBER to address the computerized format.

INTRODUCTION TO BLAs: CONTENT AND FORMATING REQUIREMENTS
The Center for Biologics Evaluation and Research had established no specific formatting requirements for PLAs. This was in sharp contrast to new drug applications, for which the agency has detailed formatting standards. Although the lack of a uniform PLA format has caused industry concern in the past, significant differences between various license applications, and biologic products themselves, had slowed efforts to standardize PLA formats. However, CBER did make available a series of PLA application forms that identify basic PLA submission requirements for different types of products. Most of these PLA forms applied to blood products, vaccines, and other, more traditional, biologic products.

In most cases, PLA forms identified submission requirements by posing a series of questions that the sponsor had to answer in the application. Essentially, the lack of a standard format was a function of the diversity of questions posed by different PLA forms. Often, applicants based the formats of their applications on the sequence of questions specified in the PLA form.

Given the absence of a standard PLA format and the advent of the new single license system, CBER in 1996 published a new draft BLA form (Form FDA 3439). Subsequent to this, during 1997, CBER and CDER issued the harmonized application form—Form FDA 356(h). This form represented a standard format for all drug, biological, antibiotic, and generic drug products; hence the harmonized form. The form is titled "Application to Market a New Drug, Biologic, or an Antibiotic Drug for Human Use" (see p. 163).

The Form FDA 356(h) is a one-page form that is two sided. The first side is administrative, providing information on the applicant as well as the product. The back side identifies the content requirements for a BLA application. However, because the form is to be used for generic drug and antibiotic products also, not all 20 sections are applicable to BLA's. In addition to the BLA application form, federal regulations, CBER guidelines, and points-to-consider documents developed for specific product classes also offer information on BLA application submission requirements. In general terms, the BLA consists of reports of all investigations sponsored by the applicant, and all other information pertinent to an evaluation of the product's safety, effectiveness, potency, and purity.

THE CONTENTS OF THE BLA
As stated above, the Form 356(h) is a one-page, two-sided document; the front side contains administrative information about the applicant and product, and the back

side includes content and format requirements for the BLA application. In addition to this form, a cover letter should always accompany any FDA submission. Addressed in the following pages are the Form FDA 356(h), the cover letter, and all 20 sections of the BLA application (see p. 163).

Cover letter
Application form—Form FDA 356(h)
Section 1—Index
Section 2—Labeling
Section 3—Summary
Section 4—Chemistry section
Section 4a—Chemistry, manufacturing, and controls information
Section 4b—Samples
Section 4c—Methods validation package
Section 5—Nonclinical pharmacology and toxicology
Section 6—Human pharmacokinetics and bioavailability
Section 7—Clinical microbiology
Section 8—Clinical data section
Section 9—Safety update report
Section 10—Statistical section
Section 11—Case report tabulations
Section 12—Case report forms
Section 13—Patent information
Section 14—Patent certification
Section 15—Establishment description
Section 16—Debarment certification
Section 17—Field copy certification
Section 18—User fee cover sheet
Section 19—Financial information
Section 20—Other

Before each section is addressed individually, it is worth emphasizing the importance of the application form [Form FDA 356(h)], the cover letter, and the first three sections. Applicants frequently overlook their significance, perhaps because they are not technical sections or because they often are not seen as critical. For several reasons, this is unfortunate. First, these items and sections are among the few in the entire application that each member of the BLA licensing committee receives for review. Additionally, because these sections, particularly the cover letter and the summary, provide information in an abridged form, they are also likely to be read thoroughly by each committee member. The sections are also important because they represent, in some ways, the applicant's "opening argument" for its product. In the summary section, for instance, the sponsor is granted what some view as a greater editorial license not available in any of the BLA's other sections. Such views aside, the sponsor must use these sections to frame and build its case for the new biologic's safety and effectiveness.

Cover Letter

Although not required by regulation, the cover letter is requested by the FDA to accompany all FDA submissions. In the cover letter, sponsors often supply the FDA with much of the basic administrative information requested about the BLA application (e.g., sponsor name and address, etc.). The cover letter should provide at least seven types of information:

1. *Name and address of sponsor and others*: The cover letter should provide the name and address of the sponsor. If the sponsor is using outside contractors or manufacturing sites at other locations, the cover letter should provide their addresses and identify their functions.
2. *Product name*: The sponsor should provide the trade and generic names of the product in the cover letter.
3. *Reason for the submission*: The cover letter should identify the type of application being submitted (e.g., original submission, supplement, amendment, etc.).
4. *Information contained in the submission*: In the cover letter, the sponsor should identify what information is contained in the submission. Identify the total number of volumes (disks) being submitted and the contents of each volume (disk) (e.g., volumes 50–150 contain clinical information).
5. *Agreements with the FDA*: If the sponsor has reached any agreements with CBER relevant to the BLA, this information should be included in the cover letter. Given the quantity of applications under review within CBER and the fact that such agreements often are made months in advance, reviewers might not recall the existence or details of such agreements. Reviewer turnover is another factor that makes recounting these agreements good working practice.
6. *Other documents relating to the submission*: To alert CBER reviewers to other documentation that must be referenced during the BLA review, the sponsor should note in the cover letter other documents associated with the application, such as INDs, BLAs, and master files.
7. *Special circumstances*: Alert CBER to any special circumstances surrounding the product. For example, the product may be an orphan drug product. Because of the circumstances relating to the product, CBER may pay special attention to the submission and shepherd it through the licensure process more quickly.
8. *Fast track review*: If your product has been classified for fast track review, remind CBER of the fact in the cover letter.

Application Form FDA 356(h)

The application form [Form FDA 356(h)] serves several functions. First, it is an administrative document providing CBER with information on the applicant, product, and application. Second, it is a legal contract binding the applicant, contractors, suppliers, and physicians to FDA laws and regulations. The applicant is already bound by FDA laws and regulations, but many contractors, suppliers, and physicians are not. Contrary to what many believe, physicians are not regulated by the FDA or FDA laws and regulations. Physicians are licensed by states and controlled in this manner. The Food and Drug Administration will not accept an application unless the application form is signed.

Item 1: Index

Perhaps the single most important factor in a BLA's "user-friendliness" is the speed and ease with which a reviewer can find information during the review process. Because it can influence the speed and efficiency of the review as well, the manner in which the applicant indexes BLA information is of central importance. Applicants can use this format for indexing the BLA:

Item	Description	Volume/page
2	Labeling	1.010

The "Item" column refers to the item number listed on the back of the Form FDA 356(h) application. The "Description" column identifies the subject of the item number listed on the back of Form FDA 356(h). In the "Volume/page" column, the number to the left of the decimal point represents the application's volume number, whereas the number to the right refers to the page within that volume containing the relevant section. In practice, the index is typically far more detailed, with each item broken down into specific subparts. Easier it is for the CBER reviewer to find information, the faster the review and the faster the applicant gets feedback.

Item 2: Labeling Section

This section encompasses the initial draft labeling submitted with the BLA and the final printed labeling that is submitted just prior to licensure. Labeling includes the immediate container label, carton label, insert, and user instructions. The container and package labels should permit accurate identification of the contents, whereas the package insert should summarize the essential information required for the product's safe and effective use. These data should be accurate, balanced, informative, and nonpromotional. When possible, the information should be based on data obtained from the product's use in humans.

Item 3: Summary Section

In many ways, the BLA summary is a condensed version of the entire application. The summary serves as a guide to the full application, explaining the application's intent-to-establish the biologic's safety and effectiveness for a particular indication, and highlighting the studies and evidence supporting the biologic's safety and effectiveness.

The summary's importance cannot be overstated. In this section, the sponsor can state and argue its case for the product's approval. A well-prepared summary includes a straightforward description of the product and its manufacturing technology, testing data, nonclinical data, clinical data, and adverse and beneficial effects.

Such a summary can build CBER's confidence in the applicant, the validity of the BLA's information, and the product itself. In addition, because the summary is one of the few sections reviewed by all members of the BLA licensing committee, it can be pivotal in establishing a foundation for product approval.

The summary, ordinarily 50 to 200 pages in length, provides reviewers in each review area, and other agency officials, with a good general understanding of the product and the application. The summary should discuss all aspects of the application and should be written with about the same level of detail required for publication in refereed scientific and medical journals and should meet the editorial standards generally applied by these journals. To the extent possible, data in the summary should be presented in tabular and graphic forms. The summary should comprehensively present the most important information about the product and the conclusions to be drawn from this information.

The summary should avoid any editorial promotion of the product, that is, it should be a factual summary of safety and effectiveness data and a neutral analysis of these data. The summary should include an annotated copy of the proposed labeling, a discussion of the product's benefits and risks, a description of the foreign marketing history of the drug (if any), and a summary of each technical section.

1. Summary Format
    Description of drug and formulation
    Annotated draft insert
    Product pharmacological class
    Scientific rationale for use of product
    Clinical benefits
    Foreign marketing history
    CMC summary
    7a. Drug substance
    7b. Drug product
    7c. Stability
    7d. Investigational summary (listing of batches used in the clinical studies)
    Nonclinical summary
    8a. Pharmacology
    8b. Toxicology
    Human pharmacokinetics and bioavailability
    Microbiological summary
    Clinical summary
    Benefit/risk relationship

Item 4: Chemistry Section

The BLA's chemistry section is composed of three parts:

1. Chemistry, manufacturing, and controls information;
2. Samples;
3. Methods validation package.

In most aspects, the BLA is essentially a PLA that features a new chemistry section in which the sponsor provides some, but not nearly all, of the data and information previously submitted in the PLA/ELA. The remaining information formerly provided in the PLA/ELA will be reviewed during CBER's preapproval inspection.

The Center for Biologics Evaluation and Research has issued guidance documents identifying the CMC information that will be required in BLAs for each class of product.

Chemistry, Manufacturing, and Controls Information

This section is composed of the following five parts:

1. Drug substance
2. Drug product
3. Investigational formulation
4. Environmental assessment
5. Method validation

Drug Substance

Many of CBER's guidelines address the information required for the drug substance. This indeed does make a lot of sense, because the drug substance is the active moiety, the item that produces the pharmacological response in humans. The information required by CBER for the drug substance is identified below.

Description and characterization. This section should provide a clear description of the physical and chemical properties of the synthetic drug substance, including the chemical structure, primary and subunit structure, molecular weight, and molecular formula. If the product is cellular based, the source of the cell line and all the pertinent physical and chemical properties necessary to characterize the cell line should be listed. The biological name or chemical name, including the USAN name, should also be provided. A description and the results of all the analytical testing performed on the manufacturer's reference standard lot and qualifying lots to characterize the drug substance should be included. The section should provide information from specific tests regarding the identity, purity, stability, and consistency of manufacture of the drug substance. All test methods should be fully described and the results provided.

A description and results of all relevant in vivo and in vitro biological testing performed on the manufacturer's reference standard lot to show the potency and activity of the drug substance should be included. Results of relevant testing performed on lots other than the reference standard lot and that might have been used in establishing the product's biological activity should also be provided.

Manufacturer. The application should include the name, address, FDA registration number, and other pertinent organizational information for each manufacturer performing any portion of the manufacture or testing operations for the drug substance. A brief description of the operations performed at each location, the responsibilities conferred upon each party by the applicant, and a description of how the applicant will ensure that each party fulfills its responsibilities should be included.

For each manufacturing location, the BLA should include a floor diagram that indicates the general facility layout. This diagram need not be a detailed engineering schematic, but should be a simple drawing that depicts the relationship of the subject manufacturing areas, suites, or rooms to one another, and should indicate other uses made of adjacent areas that are not the subject of the application. This diagram should be clear enough to permit the reviewer to visualize the flow of the drug substance's production and to identify areas or room "proximities" that may be of concern for particular operations (e.g., segregation of animal facilities).

This section should provide a comprehensive list of all additional products to be manufactured or manipulated in the areas used for the product. The applicant should indicate the rooms in which the additional products will be introduced and the manufacturing steps that will take place in the room. An explanation should be given as to whether these additional products will be introduced on a campaign basis or concurrently during production of the product under review.

For all areas in which operations for the preparation of cell banks and product manufacturing are performed, including areas for the handling of animals used in production, the following information regarding precautions taken to prevent contamination or cross-contamination should be provided:

Air quality classification of rooms or areas in which an operation is performed, as validated and measured during operations.

A brief narrative description of the procedures and facility design features for the control of contamination, cross-contamination, and containment (air-pressure cascades, segregation of operations and products, etc.).

General equipment design description (e.g., does design represent an open or a closed system or provide for a sterile or nonsterile operation?).

A description of the in-process controls performed to prevent or to identify contamination or cross-contamination.

Method(s) of manufacture. This subsection should include the following information on raw materials and reagents: (*i*) a list of all components used in the manufacture of the drug substance, and their tests and specifications, or a reference to official compendia; (*ii*) a list with tests and specifications of all special reagents and materials used in the manufacture of the drug (e.g., culture media, buffers, sera, antibiotics, monoclonal antibodies, and preservatives); and (*iii*) a description of the tests and specifications for materials of human and animal source that may be contaminated with adventitious agents [mycoplasma, bovine spongiform encephalopathy (BSE) agent for bovine-derived products, and other adventitious agents of human origin].

A complete visual representation of the manufacturing process in flowchart format should be included. This flowchart should indicate the steps in the process, the equipment and materials used, and the room where the operation is performed, and it should provide a complete list of the in-process controls and tests performed on the product at each step. The diagram should also include information, including a descriptive narrative, on the methods used to transfer the product between steps (i.e., sterile, SIP connection, sanitary connection, open transfers under laminar flow units, etc.).

If animals are used in the production process, the subsection should include descriptions of the sources of animals, the method of creating and the genetic stability of transgenic animals, adventitious agent screening and quarantine procedures used to assure that the animals are appropriate for use in manufacturing, animal husbandry procedures, and veterinary oversight. For more guidance, use the appropriate CBER guidelines and "Points to Consider" documents.

For monoclonal antibodies, the submission should include a detailed description of the development of the monoclonal antibody, including characterization of the parent cells, donor history for human cells, immunogen, immortalization procedures, and cell cloning procedures.

For recombinant DNA products, including rDNA-derived monoclonal antibodies produced from cellular sources, the guideline states that the submission should include a detailed description of the host cell and the expression vector systems and their preparation, including the following:

1. *Host cells*: A description of the source, relevant phenotype, and the genotype for the host cell used to construct the biological production system. The results of the characterization of the host cell for phenotypic and genotypic markers, including those that will be monitored for cell stability, purity, and selection, should be included.

2. *Gene construct*: A detailed description of the gene that was introduced into the host cells, including both the cell type and the origin of the source

material, should be provided, along with a description of the methods used to prepare the gene construct and a restriction enzyme digestion map of the construct. The complete nucleotide sequence of the coding region and regulatory elements of the expression construct, with translated amino acid sequence, should be provided, including annotations designating all important sequence features.

3. *Vector*: Detailed information regarding the vector and genetic elements should be provided, including a description of the source and function of the component parts of the vector.

4. *Final gene construct*: A detailed description should be provided of the cloning process that resulted in the final recombinant gene construct.

5. *Cloning and establishment of the recombinant cell lines*: Depending on the methods to be used to transfer a final gene construct or isolated gene fragments into its host, the mechanism of transfer, the copy number, and the physical state of the final construct inside the host cell should be provided. In addition, the amplification of the gene construct, if applicable, the selection of the recombinant cell clone, and the establishment of the seed should be completely described. The method of manufacture section should also include a subsection on the cell seed lot system, which should address three items.

6. *Master cell bank*: In most cases, the cell bank used to manufacture the biological will derive from a larger group of cells called the master cell bank (MCB). A detailed description of its preparation and testing should be provided. The MCB should be described in detail, including the methods, materials, reagents, and media used, date of creation, quantity of the MCB, in-process controls, and storage conditions. This section should also provide the results of the characterization of the MCB for identity and purity using phenotypic markers and the testing of the MCB for endogenous and adventitious agents.

7. *Master working cell bank*: A detailed description of the working cell bank, or WCB, and the cell line used to produce the biological product must be provided. The production of the WCB should be described in detail.

8. *End of production cells*: A detailed description of the end of production cell's (EPC's) characterization that demonstrates that the biological production system is consistent during growth should be included. This section should also include test results showing that the EPC is free from contamination by adventitious agents.

Lastly, the cellular sources subsection of the methods of manufacture section must include a detailed description of the process of inoculation, cell growth, and harvesting. The stages of cell growth should be described carefully, including the selection of the inoculum, scale-up for propagation, and established and proposed (if different) production batch size.

The CMC section of the BLA must also provide details of the purification and downstream processing, including a rationale for the chosen methods. In addition, the precautions taken to ensure the containment and prevention of contamination or cross-contamination should be identified. If applicable, the section should indicate the multiuse nature of areas and equipment (e.g., campaigning vs. concurrent manufacture; dedicated vs. shared equipment) used for these procedures. Finally, the methods of manufacture section must provide a completed (executed) representative batch record of the drug substance's production process.

Process controls. This CMC subsection should provide information in two key areas:

1. *In-process controls*: A description of the methods used for in-process controls (e.g., those involved in fermentation, harvesting, and downstream processing) should be included. A brief description of the sampling procedures and test methods used should be provided. For testing performed at significant phases of production, the criteria for accepting or rejecting an in-process batch should be specified.
2. *Process validation*: A description and documentation of the validation studies should be included. If the process was changed or scaled up for commercial production and this involved changes in the fermentation steps, the revalidation of cell line stability during growth should be described, as in the previous section, and the data and results provided. A description and documentation of the validation studies for the cell growth and harvesting process that identify critical parameters of routine products should be submitted. Similarly, description and documentation of the validation of the purification process should be included. Finally, the subsection should describe and document the validation studies or any processes used for media sterilization and inactivation of cells prior to their release to the environment (if such inactivation is required).
   A summary report, including protocols and results, should be provided for the validation studies of each critical process or factor that affects the drug substance specifications for

   propagation,
   harvest,
   purification,
   inactivation,
   microbiology, and
   aseptic processing.
3. *Reference standard*: If an international reference standard [WHO or compendial reference standard (USP)] is used, the applicant should submit the citation for the standard and a certificate of analysis. If an in-house working reference standard is used, a description of the preparation, characterization, specifications, and testing and results should he provided.
4. *Specifications/analytical methods*: The specifications and tests sufficient to assure the identity, purity, strength, and potency of the drug substance, as well as its lot-to-lot consistency, should be submitted. Certificates of analysis and analytical results for at least three consecutive qualification lots of the drug substance should be provided. Lastly, this subsection should include a discussion of the impurity profiles, with supporting analytical data, as well as profiles of variants of the protein drug substance (e.g., cleaved, aggregated, deamidated, oxidized forms) and non–product-related impurities (e.g., process reagents and cell-culture components).
5. *Container/closure system*: A description of the container and closure system and its compatibility with the drug substance should be submitted. The section should include detailed information concerning the supplier and the results of compatibility, toxicity, and biological tests. Alternatively, a drug master file (DMF) may be referenced for this information.

6. *Drug substance stability*: This subsection should include a description of the storage conditions, study protocols, and results supporting the stability of the drug substance. For more specific information, the FDA guideline "Stability Testing for Drug Substances and Drug Products" should be consulted.

Drug Product

Although less detailed than those for the drug substance, the requirements of the guideline for the drug product are also grouped into eight areas:

1. *Composition*: This subsection should include a tabulated list of all components with their unit dose and batch quantities for the drug product or diluent in accordance with the "Guideline for Submitted Documentation for the Manufacture of and Controls for Drug Products." The compositions of all ancillary products that might be included in the final product should be provided.
2. *Specifications and methods for drug product ingredients*: If the information is not specified in the drug substance section, this section should include a description of tests and specifications for all active ingredients. The specifications for all ancillary products included in the drug product should be provided as well. Information on all excipients, including process gases and water, should be included and should include a list of compendial excipients (and their citations) and tests and specifications for noncompendial excipients.
3. *Manufacturer*: The names and addresses of all manufacturers involved in the manufacture and testing of the drug product, including contractors and a description of their respective responsibilities, should be included. A list of all other products (i.e., research and development, clinical, or approved) made in the same rooms should be provided as well.
4. *Methods of manufacture and packaging*: This subsection should include a complete description of the manufacturing process of the formulated bulk and finished drug product, including a description of sterilization operations, aseptic processing procedures, lyophilization, and packaging procedures. Along with this narrative, the subsection should include a flowchart indicating each production step, the equipment and materials used, the room or area where the operation is performed, and a listing of the in-process controls and tests performed on the product at each step. This flow diagram or narrative should also include information on the methods for transferring the product between steps.
5. *Specifications and test methods for drug product*: This subsection should include the sampling procedures for monitoring a batch of finished drug product. The specifications used for the drug product and a description of all test methods selected to assure the identity, purity, strength, or potency, as well as the lot-to-lot consistency of the finished product, should be provided.
6. *Container/closure system*: A description of the container and closure system and its compatibility with the drug product should be submitted. Detailed information concerning the suppliers, their addresses, and the results of compatibility, toxicity, and biological tests should be included. Alternatively, a DMF can be referenced for this information.
7. *Microbiology*: Information should be submitted as described in the FDA's "Guidance for Industry in the Submission of Documentation for Sterilization Process Validation in Applications for Human and Veterinary Drug Products."

8. *Drug product stability*: A description of the stability protocols and results supporting the product's stability (expiration date and storage condition) should be provided. Stability data supporting the proposed shelf life of reconstituted drug products and for all labeled dilutions should be included. The stability protocol provided should include the following:

Potency
Physiochemical measurements that are potency indicating
Moisture, if applicable
pH, if applicable
Sterility or control of bioburden
Viability of cells
Pyrogenicity
General safety

A plan for an ongoing stability program should be included. This should comprise the protocol to be used, the number of lots to be entered each year, and an indication of how the lots will be selected.

Investigational Product/Formulation
This section should consist of a discussion of any differences in formulation, manufacturing process, or site between the clinical trial materials and commercial production batches of the drug substance and drug product.

Environmental Assessment
If an environmental assessment is required, it should be prepared as outlined in the federal regulations (21 CFR 25). It should include a description of the action being considered and address all components involved in the manufacture and disposal of the product. A statement of exemption under a categorical exclusion may be provided if applicable.

Method Validation
Although the guideline states that the CMC section must include a method validation section, it does not specify submission requirements. Rather, the guideline refers applicants to the FDA's "Guideline for Submitting Samples and Analytical Data for Methods Validation."

As noted above, the CMC subsection is only one of three elements in the BLA's chemistry section. The other two subsections address samples and the methods validation package.

Samples
Before a biological product is marketed, the FDA will want to validate the sponsor's characterization methods for both the biological substance and the finished product. Therefore, at some point during the review process, CBER may request any or all of the following: a biological substance sample, a finished product sample, and the sponsor's reference standards. According to FDA regulations, the sponsor must submit "four representative samples of each sample in sufficient quantity to permit FDA to perform three times each test described in the application to determine whether the drug substance and drug product meet the specifications given in the application."

Methods Validation Package

The methods validation package provides information that allows FDA laboratories to validate all of the analytical methods for both the drug substance and the drug product. Specifically, the package consists of three copies of the analytical methods and related descriptive information in the CMC section for the drug substance and drug product.

According to the FDA's "Guideline for Submitting Samples and Analytical Data for Methods Validation," the methods validation package should include a statement of composition, new drug substance and product specifications, certificates of analysis for each sample submitted, and the regulatory analytical methods. Detailed information in the package should include a tabular listing (lot, identity, etc.) of all samples to be submitted, a listing of all proposed regulatory specifications, information supporting the integrity of the reference standard, a detailed description of each method of analysis, and information supporting the suitability of the methodology for the new drug substance and the dosage form.

Item 5: Nonclinical Pharmacology and Toxicology Section

The BLA must describe all nonclinical pharmacology and toxicology studies conducted on the biologic product. These nonclinical laboratory studies include those submitted in the IND, those submitted during clinical investigations, and new nonclinical studies not previously submitted. The Center for Biologics Evaluation and Research reviews these studies to evaluate their adequacy and comprehensiveness and to ensure that there are no inconsistencies or inadequately characterized toxic effects. The application also should include information on studies not performed by the sponsor but of which the sponsor has become aware (e.g., studies in published literature).

Content requirements for the nonclinical pharmacology and toxicology section of license applications are not defined specifically in CBER regulations or guidelines. As it does in many other instances, the BLA form refers biologic sponsors to regulations for the pharmacology/toxicology section of an NDA. These regulations ask for descriptions, with the aid of graphs and tables, of animal and in vitro studies with the drug, including the following:

1. Studies of the pharmacological actions of the drug in relation to its proposed therapeutic indication and studies that otherwise define the pharmacological properties of the drug or are pertinent to possible adverse effects.
2. Studies of the toxicologic effects of the drug as they relate to the product's intended clinical uses, including, as appropriate, studies assessing the product's acute, subchronic, and chronic toxicity, and studies of toxicities related to the product's particular mode of administration or conditions of use.
3. Studies, as appropriate, of the effects of the drug on reproduction and on the developing fetus.
4. Any studies of the absorption, distribution, metabolism, and excretion of the drug in animals.
5. For each nonclinical laboratory study subject to good laboratory practice (GLP) regulations, a statement that it was conducted in compliance with such regulations or, if not conducted in compliance with those regulations, a brief statement of the reason for the noncompliance.

For each study identified above, the applicant should include a summary, followed by a full report including data and statistical analyses. Summaries assist FDA reviewers in obtaining a brief analysis of the study. Along with the summaries and full reports, the applicant should provide an integrated report. Such a report integrates results from all pharmacology studies in a single, comprehensive analysis. Sponsors should provide a similar report for the toxicology information.

Item 6: Human Pharmacokinetics and Bioavailability Section

Although few biologic products will have bioavailability data, most will have pharmacokinetics data that must be provided in the BLA. As it does for the pharmacology and toxicology section, Form 356(h) refers biologic applicants to the regulatory requirements specified for an NDA human pharmacokinetics and bioavailability section, as follows:

1. A description of each of the bioavailability and pharmacokinetic studies of the drug in humans, including a description of the analytical and statistical methods used in each study and a statement with respect to each study that it either was conducted in compliance with IRB regulations or was not subject to the regulations, and that it was conducted in compliance with the informed consent regulations.
2. If the application describes in the chemistry, manufacturing, and controls section specifications or analytical methods needed to assure the bioavailability of the drug product or drug substance, or both, a statement in this section of the rationale for establishing the specifications or analytical methods including data and information supporting the rationale.
3. A summary discussion and analysis of the pharmacokinetics and metabolism of the active ingredients and the bioavailability or bioequivalence, or both, of the drug product.

More detailed recommendations on the development and presentation of this section are available from CDER's guidelines.

Item 7: Clinical Microbiology

This section is required only for anti-infective products. Because these products affect microbial (rather than clinical, physiology) reports relevant to the product's in vivo and in vitro effects on the target, microorganisms are critical for establishing product effectiveness.

Current regulations require that an application's anti-infective section include microbiology data characterizing (*i*) the biochemical basis of the drug's action on microbial physiology; (*ii*) the antimicrobial spectra of the drug, including the results of in vitro nonclinical studies to demonstrate concentrations of the drug required for effective use; (*iii*) any known mechanisms of resistance to the drug, including the results of any known epidemiological studies to demonstrate prevalence of resistance factors; and (*iv*) clinical microbiology laboratory methods (e.g., in vitro sensitivity discs) needed for effective use of the product.

More specific guidance on developing the microbiology component of the BLA is available from a CDER guideline entitled "Guideline for the Format and Content of the Microbiology Section of an Application."

Item 8: Clinical Data Section

The applicant's clinical data section is a particularly critical element of the filing. Included in this section are the safety and effectiveness data pivotal to the FDA's decision-making process. The clinical data section is also likely to be the applicant's most complex and voluminous section. The clinical data section of a BLA should consist of the following basic elements:

1. A description and analysis of each clinical pharmacology study of the biologic, including a brief comparison of the results of the human studies with the animal pharmacology and toxicology data.
2. A description and analysis of each controlled clinical study pertinent to the biologic's proposed use, including the protocol and a description of the statistical analyses used to evaluate the study. If the study report is an interim analysis, this must be noted and a projected completion date provided. Controlled clinical studies that have not been analyzed in detail for any reason (e.g., because they have been discontinued or are incomplete) should be provided, including a copy of the protocol and a brief description of the results and status of the study.
3. A description of each uncontrolled clinical study, a summary of the results, and a brief statement explaining why the study is classified as uncontrolled.
4. A description and analysis of any other data or information relevant to an evaluation of the product's safety and effectiveness obtained or otherwise received by the applicant from any foreign or domestic source. This should include information derived from clinical investigations (i.e., including controlled and uncontrolled trials of uses of the product other than those proposed in the application), commercial marketing experience, reports in the scientific literature, and unpublished scientific papers.
5. An integrated summary of the data providing substantial evidence of effectiveness for the clinical indications. Evidence is also required to support the dosage and administration section of the labeling, including the dosage and dose interval recommended and modifications for specific subgroups of patients (e.g., pediatrics, geriatrics, and patients with renal failure). See the CBER guideline on Integrated Summary of Effectiveness.
6. An integrated summary of all available information about product safety, including pertinent animal data, demonstrated or potential adverse effects of the drug, clinically significant drug–drug interactions, and other safety considerations, such as data from epidemiological studies of related drugs. This subsection should also include a description of any statistical analyses performed in reviewing safety data, unless it is included elsewhere in the clinical section.
7. If the drug has the potential for abuse, a description and analysis of studies or information related to abuse of the drug, including a proposal for scheduling under the Controlled Substances Act. A description of any studies related to overdosage is also required, including information on dialysis, antidotes, or other treatments, if known.
8. An integrated summary of benefits and risks of the biologic, including a discussion of why the benefits exceed the risks under the conditions stated in the labeling.

9. A statement noting that each human clinical study was conducted in compliance with IRB and informed consent regulations. If the study was not conducted according to these regulations, the applicant must state this fact and the reasons for noncompliance.

10. If a sponsor has transferred any obligations for the conduct of a clinical study to a contract research organization (CRO), a statement providing the name and address of the CRO, identifying the clinical study, and providing a list of the obligations transferred. If all obligations regarding the conduct of the study have been transferred, a general statement of this transfer—in lieu of a listing of the specific obligations transferred—may be submitted.

11. If original subject records were audited or reviewed by the sponsor in the course of monitoring any clinical study to verify the accuracy of the case reports submitted to the sponsor, a list identifying each clinical study so audited or reviewed.

Although there is no required format for the clinical section, I recommend formatting the section in the following manner:

1. Integrated summary of benefits and risks
2. Integrated summary of safety
3. Integrated summary of effectiveness
4. Phase 3 adequate and well-controlled studies used for the determination of product safety and effectiveness
5. All other phase 3 studies
6. Phase 2 studies
7. Human pharmacology studies not included in item 6
8. Other information

This format allows CBER to review the most important information first.

Item 9: Safety Update Report

As implied by its title, the safety update report is not submitted with the original BLA but is submitted in the form of updates at specific points in the application review process. Applicants must submit safety update reports four months after the BLA submission, after receipt of a complete response letter, and at other times requested by CBER. In these reports, the sponsor must update the pending BLA with new safety information learned about the product that may reasonably affect the labeling statements in the contraindications, warnings, precautions, and adverse reactions sections. The updates must include the same types of information from clinical studies, animal studies, and other sources and must be submitted in the same format as the BLA's integrated safety summary. They must also include case report forms for each patient who died during a clinical study or who did not complete the study because of an adverse event.

Item 10: Statistical Section

The statistical section of the BLA is essentially the same as the clinical data section, inasmuch as the clinical reports include all the statistical analyses. With this information, the statisticians can assess the validity of key analyses and evidence supporting the biologic's safety and efficacy.

The statistical section is composed of the following information:

1. A list of investigators supplied with the drug or known to have investigated the drug, INDs under which the drug was studied, and NDAs submitted for the same drug substance
2. An overview of the clinical studies conducted
3. Item 8, the clinical data section
4. Statistics used for the integrated summaries of benefits/risks, safety and effectiveness, and the rationale for the use of such statistical methods

Item 11: Case Report Tabulations Section

During the FDA's most recent revision of its clinical requirements, the agency declared that "an efficient agency review of individual patient data should be based primarily on well-organized, concise data tabulations. Reviews of the more detailed patient case report forms should be reserved for those instances where a more complete review is necessary."

The agency advises sponsors to meet with the FDA to discuss the extent to which tabulations of patient data in clinical studies, data elements within tables, and case report forms are needed. Such discussions can also cover alternative modes of data presentation and the need for special supporting information (e.g., ECGs, X rays, or pathology slides).

According to agency regulations and guidelines, the case report tabulations section must provide

1. tabulations of the data from each adequate and well-controlled study (phases 2 and 3);
2. tabulations of the data from the earliest clinical study;
3. pharmacology studies (phase 1);
4. tabulations of the safety data from all other clinical studies.

Federal regulations add that these tabulations should include the data on each patient in each study, except that the applicant may delete those tabulations that the agency agrees, in advance, are not pertinent to a review of the drug's safety or effectiveness.

Item 12: Case Report Forms (CRFs) Section

As stated above, the FDA does not require the routine submission of patient CRFs. The forms are required only for (*i*) patients who died during a clinical study, and (*ii*) patients who did not complete a study because of any adverse event, whether or not the adverse event is considered drug related by the investigator or the sponsor.

The FDA may request that the sponsor submits additional CRFs that the agency views as important to the drug's review. Typically, the agency will request all CRFs for the pivotal studies. In doing so, the agency's reviewers will attempt to designate the critical studies for which CRFs are required about 30 days after the application's receipt. If a sponsor fails to submit the CRFs within 30 days of the FDA's request, the agency may view the eventual submission as a major amendment and extend the review period as appropriate.

Item 13: Patent Information Section

Applicants must provide information on any patent(s) on the product for which approval is sought or on a method of using the product. Such information is included in the "Orange Book" (*Approved Drug Products with Therapeutic Equivalence Evaluations*). All approved (licensed) drug products are listed in this book.

Item 14: Patent Certification Section

Applicants must provide a patent certification or statement regarding any relevant patents that claim the listed drug or any other drugs on which investigators seeking approval of the application relied, or that claim a use for the listed or other drug. This section is applicable to Generic Drugs only.

Item 15: Establishment Description Section

The CBER guidance documents state that item 15 of the BLA should be composed of three principal sections that provide information describing establishment standards and good manufacturing practices (GMPs) controls in place for the manufacture of the product. The three principal sections are (*i*) General Information, (*ii*) Specific Systems, and (*iii*) Contamination/Cross-Contamination Issues.

General Information

For each manufacturing location, the BLA should include a floor diagram indicating the general production facility layout. Each diagram or accompanying narrative should include product, personnel, equipment, waste, and air flow for production areas; an illustration or indication of which areas are served by each air-handling unit; and air-pressure differentials between adjacent areas.

Specific Systems

Water systems. The BLA should include information for systems used in the production of water for manufacturing and rinsing of product-contact equipment. This subsection should include a general description of water system(s), a validation summary, and information on the routine monitoring program.

Heating, ventilation, and air-conditioning (HVAC) systems. This subsection must also include a general system description, a validation summary, and information on the routine monitoring system.

Computer systems. This section should contain information on computer systems that control critical manufacturing processes. The developer of the system should be identified, and information provided should also include a brief description of procedures for changes to the computer system. This section should also contain a validation summary for each of these systems and a certification that an IQ and an OQ have been completed. As a reminder, any computer system designed to generate records (electronic records) must also be compliant with 21CFR Part 11.

Contamination/Cross-Contamination Issues

For dedicated equipment, the sponsor must provide a brief description of the cleaning procedures and reagents used, as well as certification that cleaning validation for removal of product residuals and cleaning agents has been successfully completed. For shared equipment, including that used for processing the cells of more than one patient, BLA sponsors must provide a description of the cleaning procedures and reagents used, the rationale for the chosen procedures, and a report describing validation procedures, sampling methods, and analytical methods. The section must also provide information on containment features, including segregation and containment procedures for areas, manufacturing operations, personnel, equipment, and waste materials designed to prevent product contamination.

In general, the BLA must provide CBER reviewers with an overview of the manufacturing facility and its operations regarding the product.

Item 16: Debarment Certification Section

Since mid-1992, the FDA has required that all NDAs and BLAs include a certification that the applicant did not and will not use the services of individuals or firms that have been debarred by the FDA. Under the Generic Drug Enforcement Act of 1992, the FDA is authorized to debar individuals convicted of crimes relating to the development, approval, or regulation of drugs or biologics from providing any services to applicants. The statute requires that applications for drug products (including biologic products) include a certification that the applicant did not and will not use in any capacity the services of any person debarred in connection with such application.

Item 17: Field Copy Certification Section

Since 1993, U.S.-based NDA sponsors have been required to submit a "field" copy of the NDA's chemistry, manufacturing, and controls section, application form, and summary directly to the relevant FDA district office for use during the preapproval manufacturing inspection. The applicant has also been required to certify in its NDA that an exact copy of the chemistry, manufacturing, and controls contained in the application has been forwarded to the relevant FDA district office. In the past, CBER itself conducted preapproval biologic inspections, and no such certification was required in the BLA. With the advent of Team Biologics and the introduction of the field force to biologic inspections, it is now advisable to talk to the application division the sponsor is dealing with to get the current requirements.

Item 18: User Fee Cover Sheet Section (Form FDA 3397)

Since January 1994, the FDA has required every new drug application and BLA to include a copy of the User Fee Cover Sheet. This form provides information that permits the FDA to determine whether the application is subject to user fees and, if so, whether the appropriate fee for the application has been submitted. The FDA will not start a review of an application unless verification of receipt of the user fee has been obtained.

Item 19: Financial Information Section

This section certifies that the applicant has paid no investigator in company ownership. That is the applicant has not paid any investigator in

- stock,
- stock options,
- ownership in the company (partner),
- rights to the product,
- paid more money for good clinical results and less money for bad clinical results.

Form FDA 3454 is completed for this purpose.

Item 20: Other
The BLA applicant may provide in this section any other information that may help the agency evaluate the safety and effectiveness of the product.

AMENDING THE LICENSE APPLICATION
During the review of the BLA, the FDA is likely to request additional information to address unresolved issues regarding the original submission. A response to such a request is generally referred to as an amendment. A change to any unapproved application is called an amendment (IND, BLA, and NDA). The content of a BLA amendment will depend on the nature of CBER's information request. The format used in this submission is similar to that used for the original BLA submission. The cover letter for the amendment should be titled "Amendment to BLA_____." In the cover letter, the applicant should clearly identify the purpose of the amendment and the contents of the submission. The amendment should be paginated in a manner that will allow CBER to locate the section of the BLA in which the amendment should be incorporated.

SUPPLEMENT TO THE ORIGINAL BLA
Although amendments are submitted to update or modify an unapproved BLA, supplements are submitted to modify approved license applications. The holder of an approved BLA may seek to change its manufacturing methods, expand the product's indication, or make other changes that reflect new technology or make its product or processes more competitive. Compared with companies holding approved NDAs for drug products, biological licensees traditionally have had considerably less latitude in making minor changes to labeling or manufacturing processes without first obtaining FDA approval through a supplemental application.

In April 1995, however, CBER implemented a new policy creating a three-tier reporting and approval mechanism for postapproval manufacturing and facility changes. Under this policy, only significant changes—those in categories II and III—will require the submission of a supplement. Only category III changes—important proposed changes in manufacturing methods—will require FDA pre-clearance before implementation.

Because category II and III changes can be expected throughout a product's life cycle, supplementing the BLA becomes an ongoing process. Supplement-related activity is particularly high as a company refines, scales up, and streamlines its manufacturing operation. Content requirements for supplemental BLAs will depend on the nature of the proposed change. In general, the applicant provides new data and information sufficient to support the modification.

ASSEMBLING AND SUBMITTING THE BLA
Whether submitting an original BLA, an amendment, or a supplement, the applicant should follow these requirements:

For new BLAs, CBER today will most likely require the Common Technical Document (CTD) format.

The CTD is a five modular format for global use. Now, regulatory can use the same format globally.

1. *Module 1*: Administrative information (region specific). For the United States, included in this section are the Form FDA 356(h), draft labeling, and three integrated summaries.
2. *Module 2*: Summaries and overview.
3. *Module 3*: Information on product quality.
4. *Module 4*: Nonclinical study reports.
5. *Module 5*: Clinical study reports.

For BLA in the paper format, the requirements are as follows:

1. The BLA should be properly indexed and paginated for ease of review. Each volume should be no more than two inches thick, bound on the left side of the page, and printed on standard U.S. paper (8.5 × 11″). The front cover of each volume should specify the name of the applicant, the name of the product, and the BLA number (if known). The lower right-hand corner of each volume should read "This submission: 'Volume _ of _ volumes.'" The upper right-hand corner should read "Volume _."
2. Applicants must submit two copies of the BLA to CBER (most likely the CBER division will ask for additional copies). The copies may be hand-delivered or mailed. If the applicant hand-delivers the BLA, the sponsor should bring an extra copy of the cover letter with the shipment so that the letter may be date-stamped upon delivery to the FDA's Document Control Center. This letter provides evidence that the document was submitted to the FDA. If forwarded by standard mail service, the BLA shipment should include a letter of instructions with a document stating that the BLA submission has been received by the FDA. The FDA document control person will sign the document, place it in a stamped return envelope provided by the sponsor, and return it to the company. This document also serves as proof that the BLA was submitted.

Sponsors mailing the BLA should forward the application and all related submissions to the following address:

Center for Biologics Evaluation and Research Food and Drug Administration
1401 Rockville Pike
Suite 200N, HFM-99
Rockville, Maryland 20852-1448, U.S.

If the applicant forwards the BLA using a commercial overnight service, a return receipt is provided. In this case, the receipt provides evidence of the BLA's delivery.

13 Chemistry, Manufacturing, and Control (ICH Quality Guidelines)

John R. Rapoza

JRRapoza Associates, Inc., Moorestown, New Jersey, U.S.A.

Evan B. Siegel

Ground Zero Pharmaceuticals, Inc., Irvine, California, U.S.A.

INTRODUCTION

With the enactment of the FDA Modernization Act of 1997, Food and Drug Administration Amendments Act 2007, and reauthorization of the Prescription Drug User Fee Act of 2007, the drug approval process by FDA is expected to be streamlined further. The agency is aggressively generating guidance documents to implement the provisions of the statute, so it is up to the drug sponsor to prepare drug submissions that are complete and in a format that will facilitate the review for a rapid approval.

One of the most critical portions of an NDA or ANDA is item 4 of the Form FDA 356(h), the chemistry section. This section, more commonly referred to as CMC, (chemistry, manufacturing, and controls) is actually subdivided into three subsections: the chemistry, manufacturing, and controls information; samples; and methods validation package. Although the chemistry section of a typical application comprises only 5% of a submission, 25% of FDA guidance documents generated refer to CMC issues, making the chemistry section the most highly regulated part of the application.

Nonclinical and clinical studies are usually completed during the investigational phases of drug development. The final formulation(s) for the product, however, along with the associated analytical methodologies and manufacturing procedures, may not be finalized until the latter part of phase 3 clinical trials. Even with no change in the safety, efficacy, and manufacturing process of a drug in the market, the CMC information on a drug filed with FDA is always updated as long as the company manufactures the drug product. Chemistry, manufacturing, and controls issues exist throughout the life cycle of a product.

It is clear that the FDA considers that the CMC section has the potential to significantly decrease NDA review and approval times. In addition to the issuance of guidance documents and CMC initiatives, the regulations permit the submission of item 4 material 90 to 120 days in advance of other sections of the NDA [21 CFR 314.50(d)(iv)] as a further means of expediting the regulatory review process.

Sponsors can help both themselves and the FDA chemistry reviewer by providing sufficient documentation in NDA submissions, particularly regarding the following: (*i*) methods of synthesis, (*ii*) validation of analytical assay methods for both the drug substance and the finished dosage form(s), (*iii*) container/closure systems, and (*iv*) stability testing. Deficiencies in these key areas are also the common causes for the delayed approval of ANDAs. It is important to ensure that the CMC section of an application accurately reflects the actual manufacturing and control

TABLE 1 FDA Manufacturing and Controls Guidelines

1.	Guideline for the format and content of an application summary
2.	Guideline for the format and content of the chemistry, manufacturing, and controls section of an application
3.	Guideline for impurities in drug substances
4.	Guideline for stability studies for human drugs and biologics
5.	Guideline for packaging of human drugs and biologics
6.	Guideline for submitting supporting documentation in drug applications for the manufacture of drug substances
7.	Guideline for submitting supporting documentation for the manufacture of finished dosage forms
8.	Guidelines for drug master files

processes for the batches to be marketed. This will have great impact on the way the FDA conducts a preapproval inspection for the application. In the pages to follow, recommendations as to what information should be provided in both NDAs and ANDAs will be discussed. Appropriate reference(s) to the applicable guideline(s) will be presented throughout, and in Tables 1 and 2, they are listed for convenience. These FDA and International Conference on Harmonization (ICH) guidelines and other pertinent publications issued by FDA can be obtained by mail or e-mail through the FDA Web site (3). Differences in the CMC information needed to be provided for original and abbreviated new drug filings will also be highlighted in this chapter.

In addition to the FDA issued guideline mentioned above, there are a series of quality guidelines issued by the ICH of which the U.S. FDA is a member. These quality guidelines are similar to that issued by FDA and are accepted by international regulatory bodies. In some instances, the ICH guidelines are more detailed and complimentary to the current FDA guidelines; in any event, both are accepted by FDA.

In Table 2 are listed the key ICH guidances with regard to the collection and submission of the technical aspects of data and document format needed in a CMC section of an NDA submission.

The FDA published in August 2001 a guidance document entitled "Submitting Marketing Applications According to the ICH/CTD format—General Considerations." In this document, the FDA describes how to organize new drug applications (NDAs), abbreviated new drug applications (ANDAs), and biological license applications (BLAs) based on the International Conference on Harmonization of Technical Requirements for Registration of Pharmaceuticals for Human Use (ICH)

TABLE 2 ICH Quality Guidelines

1.	Q1A stability testing of new drug substances and products. In addition, to the A suffix guideline, there are a series of other guidelines
2.	Q1B through Q1F, which deal with stability related issues
3.	Q2 validation of analytical procedures: text and methodology
4.	Q3 impurities of new substances, drug products and solvents
5.	Q6A guidance on specifications
6.	Q7A good manufacturing practice guideline for active pharmaceutical ingredients

guidelines on the Common Technical Document (CTD). This CTD consists of five modules:

Module 1	Administrative and prescribing information (region specific)
Module 2	Summary and overview
Module 3	Information on product manufacture and quality
Module 4	Nonclinical study reports
Module 5	Clinical study reports

THE NDA SUMMARY

The FDA regulations published on February 22, 1995 provide for the preparation of a summary of the NDA, including a condensation of the CMC section. (The "Guideline for the Format and Content of an Application Summary" is available to aid in the preparation of this document.) Properly presented, the summary will provide all of the NDA reviewers a general overview of CMC information for both the drug substance and the drug product. It should be written in sufficient detail and in a style that can meet the editorial standards required for publication in refereed scientific journals. The following subsections detail what should be included in the NDA summary regarding CMC information that should be included in summary format for Module 2 and in a detailed format for Module 3 of the CTD document.

The Drug Substance
Names
Include the generic name(s), synonyms, and code designation(s) that have appeared in the published literature or in nonclinical or clinical reports being submitted with the application, the proprietary names (brand name or trademark) if known, identification number [e.g., Chemical Abstracts Service (CAS) registry number], and chemical name(s). List the preferred chemical name first, if available. This information can be found in a reference book called *U.S. Adopted Names Council (USAN) Handbook*, if a generic name for the drug substances has been accepted by the Council.

Physical and Chemical Properties
Describe the physical and chemical properties of the drug substance. Include, as applicable, appearance, odor, taste, physical form, solubility profile, melting point, boiling range, molecular weight, structural and molecular formulas (Wisswesser line notation), isomers, polymorphs, pK_a pK_b, and pH. A description of the data obtained to elucidate the structure (e.g., spectroscopic characteristics) should also be included.

Stability
The results of studies conducted on the drug substance should be summarized and related to the anticipated storage conditions and container/closure system, as well as the retest plan to be used by the sponsor. Statements on whether additional studies are ongoing or planned for the future should be included. Also, provide a

statement regarding the suitability of the methods used (see the section below on specifications and analytical methods).

Manufacture
The name(s) and address(es) of the manufacturer(s), that is, entity(ies) performing the manufacturing, processing, packaging, labeling, and control operations of the drug substance, must be listed. Include a description of the responsibilities of each manufacturer listed, if more than one is used.

Method of Manufacture
Information concerning the method of manufacture may be presented in the form of a flowchart. Supply a brief description of the methods of isolation [e.g., synthetic process, fermentation, extraction, and recombinant deoxyribonucleic acid (DNA) procedure] and purification (solvent recrystallization, column chromatography, and distillation). Include all synthetic pathways that have been adequately characterized during the investigational stages of drug development.

Process Controls
Provide a brief description of the control checks performed at each stage of manufacturing and packaging of the drug substance.

Specifications and Analytical Methods
Describe the acceptance criteria and the test methods used to assure the identity, strength, quality, particle size and polymorphic integrity, and purity of the drug substance. The guidelines also recommend that applicable information be provided regarding actual or potential impurities in the drug substance (e.g., by-products, degradation products, antigenic substances, viral contaminants, isomeric components, heavy metal contaminants, extraction solvents, etc.). As the summary may also be used by the FDA as a reference document in the preparation of the SBA for the product, releasable to the public under the FOI regulations, the information included in the summary regarding impurities should be well considered.

Container/Closure System
Describe the characteristics of, and test methods used for the container, the closure, and other component parts. In addition, highlight stability data and any other information that support their suitability for packaging the drug substance.

The Drug Product
Composition of the Dosage Form
A quantitative composition, including the name and amount of each active and inactive ingredient contained in the drug product, should be provided. In addition, an overall description of the dosage form should be included. This should be in sufficient detail to characterize it fully with regard to its type, release properties (i.e., immediate vs. sustained or controlled release), and physical characteristics such as shape, color, type of coating, hardness, scoring, and identification marks.

Manufacturer
The information provided for the manufacturer is analogous to that provided for the drug substance. In this case, however, there are likely to be more facilities listed.

Contract packagers, for example, are used frequently for preparing samples or unit dose presentations such as blister packages.

Method of Manufacture
Briefly describe the manufacturing and packaging process for the finished dosage form(s) of the product (e.g., wet granulation, direct compression, and lyophilization).

Specifications and Analytical Methods
Detail the regulatory specifications and test methods used to assure the identity, strength, quality, purity, and bioavailability of the drug product. The emphasis lies in the assay methodology(ies) used to quantitate the presence of degradation products that assure stability of the drug product.

Container/Closure System
A description of all the container/closure system configurations for the drug to be marketed should be presented. In addition, stability data and any other information that support the suitability of the container/closure components, including specifications and test methods, should be indicated.

Stability
The proposed expiration-dating period and storage conditions for the product, along with justifications for them based on data obtained from stability studies should be stated.

Test Formulations
Provide quantitative compositions and lot numbers of each finished dosage form used in nonclinical safety studies, clinical studies, and stability during the investigational phases of development for the drug product. In addition, formulation differences should be explained, and each formulation should be cross-referenced to the study or studies in which it was used.

   If these points are clearly and concisely presented, FDA reviewers should have a general understanding of the data and information submitted in the CMC section.

CHEMISTRY, MANUFACTURING, AND CONTROLS INFORMATION
This part of an application, which in the CTD format is Module 3, contains a precise description of the composition, methods of manufacture, specifications, and control procedures for the drug substance and the drug product. It also includes an environmental impact analysis statement for the manufacturing process and the ultimate use of the drug. [Refer to the "Guideline for the Format and Content of the Chemistry, Manufacturing, and Controls Section of an Application" and 21 CFR 314.50(d)(3), which set forth specific data requirements for this section.]

   In preparation of the documents for the CMC section, one of the first items to consider is the selection of a representative batch of the drug substance and the drug product for the NDA. Ideally, the representative drug substance batch selected was used to manufacture the representative drug product batch. This will provide a good and consistent data flow in the CMC section.

The Drug Substance
Names
Include the established (generic) and proprietary (trade) name(s), synonyms (e.g., different names being used for the same drug in other countries), CAS registry number, and code number(s). Most drugs early in their investigation are referred to by some alphanumeric code number until a generic name has been officially approved by the USAN and/or by the WHO as an INN.

Structural Formula and Chemical Name(s)
The chemical structure(s), molecular formula(s), molecular weight(s), and chemical name(s) should be shown. List all chemical names by which the drug was referred to during its development, and highlight the preferred names assigned by USAN or WHO at the time a generic name was approved.

Physical and Chemical Properties
The description provided in this section should include, as applicable, information on the following: (*i*) organoleptic properties (e.g., appearance, odor, and taste); (*ii*) solid-state form (i.e., the preferred crystalline polymorph); (*iii*) solubility profile (limit data to aqueous solubility, pH effect, and at most one or two organic solvents); (*iv*) pH, pKa, or pKb; (*v*) melting and boiling range; (*vi*) specific gravity or bulk density; (*vii*) spectroscopical characteristics such as a specific rotation, refractive index, and fluorescence; and (*viii*) isomeric composition.

Proof of Structure
A reference standard batch of the drug substance is used to conduct structure elucidation and confirmation studies.

The elucidation and confirmation of structure should include physical and chemical information derived from applicable analyses, such as (*i*) elemental analysis; (*ii*) functional group analysis using spectroscopic methods (i.e., mass spectrometry, nuclear magnetic resonance); (*iii*) molecular weight determinations; (*iv*) degradation studies; (*v*) complex formation determinations; (*vi*) chromatographic studies methods using HPLC, GC, TLC, and GLC; (*vii*) infrared spectroscopy; (*viii*) ultraviolet spectroscopy; (*ix*) stereochemistry; and (*x*) others, such as optical rotatory dispersion (ORD) or X-ray diffraction.

Stability
The results from studies conducted to evaluate the stability of the new drug substance should be described fully. In addition, on the basis of these results, recommendations for the storage conditions and retesting period should be discussed. Data should be submitted from studies of the product stored in open and closed containers analogous to the container in which the drug substance is to be stored and marketed. Generally, manufacturers do these studies in 1- to 5-kg containers fabricated from the same materials used for bulk manufacturing storage.

Other studies, conducted at accelerated storage conditions such as effects of temperatures (freezing, 5°C, 40–50°C or higher), humidity (75% or greater), and exposure to light should be submitted. These studies generally help define what handling precautions are necessary for bulk storage and during manufacture of the dosage form. The FDA also recommends that studies be conducted on solutions or suspensions of the drug substance to evaluate the effects of acid and alkaline pH, high oxygen and nitrogen atmospheres, and the presence of added substances, including chelating agents and antioxidants.

Indicate the stability-indicating method(s) used to quantitate the drug substance, its impurities, and its degradation products. Define the possible degradation profile of the drug substance. The availability of samples of these impurities/degradation products permits the validation of assay method(s) used to specifically quantitate their levels in the drug substance. Also, either the same method (preferably) or another method of sufficient sensitivity—at least to 0.1% of active drug—must be used to quantitate levels of degradation products.

To avoid or limit problems in this area after submission of the NDA, the validation of analytical methods and the conduct of stability studies should be planned from the initial phases of clinical research. This will provide the type of data approvable by FDA. The reader is directed to the "Guideline for Stability Studies for Human Drugs and Biologics" and the final "ICH Guideline for the Stability of Drug Substance and Drug Product" for assistance in fulfilling this essential requirement.

Manufacturer

Under this section, the name and address of each facility (including contract testing laboratories) used in the manufacture and control of the drug substance should be provided. Each building involved in the manufacture of the drug substance should be properly identified by street address and, if appropriate, building number. If more than one building is used, state the part of the operation being carried out in each building. The operations that should be covered include manufacturing, processing, packaging, labeling, and control of the drug substance.

For foreign facilities, manufacturing site facilities, operating procedures, and personnel information must be included in this section. This information can also be available as a type I drug master file (DMF); therefore, a letter from the DMF holder to the FDA that authorizes the use of applicable data in conjunction with the review of the sponsor's application is sufficient for this section.

Method of Manufacture
Starting Materials—Specifications and Tests

The starting material(s) used to synthesize the drug substance should comply with FDA's definition of a starting material. For a material to be considered a starting material, it should be (*i*) commercially available; (*ii*) a compound whose name, chemical structure, and chemical and physical properties are generally known; (*iii*) described in the literature; and (*iv*) obtained by commonly known procedures (including starting materials extracted from plant or animal sources, and precursors to semisynthetic antibiotics obtained by fermentation procedures). Most of the time, a material will meet several of these criteria. If it does not meet any of them, it probably is not the starting material.

Describe the analytical controls used to ensure the identity, quality, and purity of each batch of starting material. The source of the starting material need not be specified, but may be requested.

Solvents, Reagents, and Auxiliary Materials

List all reagents, solvents, and auxiliary materials and a statement of the quality of each material (i.e., USP, NF, ACS, and Technical). Describe the specifications and tests used to accept each batch of material. A specific identity test should be included. The need for additional testing depends on the role of the material used in the preparation or isolation of the drug substance.

Drug Substance Synthesis

Provide a full description of the method used in the isolation (e.g., synthesis, extraction, fermentation, and recombinant DNA procedures) and purification of the drug substance.

The description of the isolation of the drug substance should include a diagrammatic flowchart. Such charts should contain (*i*) chemical structures of reactants, molecular weights, and names or code designations; (*ii*) stereochemical configurations, if applicable; (*iii*) structures of intermediates, both in situ and isolated; (*iv*) solvents; (*v*) catalysts; (*vi*) reagents; and (*vii*) significant side products that may interfere with the analytical procedure or that are toxic.

Describe the processes involved in the synthesis of the drug substance. The description synthesis should include information on the following: (*i*) pieces of equipment used; (*ii*) quantities of starting material(s) reagents, solvents, catalysts; (*iii*) workup and isolation procedures; (*iv*) reaction conditions such as temperature, pH, and time; (*v*) purification procedures; (*vi*) manipulative details including addition rate, stirring speed, pressure, and order of addition; and (*vii*) yields (crude and/or purified weight and percent).

The FDA has given approval in the past to the concept of a "pivotal intermediate." This is an analyzed and well-characterized synthetic intermediate that is usually isolated one to two steps before synthesis of the crude final product, but may be obtainable by more than one synthetic route. To obtain approval, material produced by the several routes must be characterized, especially with regard to the identity and level(s) of impurities and the relative qualities of the finished bulk drug substance produced. In addition, a fairly rigorous set of specifications for the intermediate has to be established to assure its ultimate quality by whichever approved route is used in its production (see section on Process Controls below). The benefit to the sponsor is that the level of detail describing the various routes used to make the pivotal intermediate does not have to be as great as normally required. This permits some latitude for implementing modifications to those steps occurring up to the synthesis of the pivotal intermediate without the necessity of receiving prior FDA approval, as long as the quality and impurity profiles of the pivotal intermediate are unaltered from those on file at the FDA.

It should also be noted that FDA may request additional preclinical toxicology studies. This will depend on the degree(s) of difference(s) in the profiles, identities, and the levels of impurities in bulk drug substances produced from the pivotal intermediate made by the various routes of synthesis, and whether the finished drug is intended for short-term or chronic use.

The final steps in the workup, isolation, and purification of the bulk or microencapsulated drug substance should be written in detailed fashion. The description should address the following issues: (*i*) crude product yield (a range should be given); (*ii*) tests performed on the crude product, preferably including at least one purity test appearing in the finished drug substance specifications; (*iii*) the isolation and purification procedures; (*iv*) alternate purification procedures (polymorphic changes should be considered); (*v*) yield of purified product (again it is recommended that a range be provided); and (*vi*) evidence that the purification procedure actually improves purity of the crude product (e.g., chromatographic illustrations).

Any alternate method or permissible variation, such as different starting material, reagent, solvent, or conditions, should be reported with an indication of the circumstances under which it will be used, and comparative analytical data should be provided.

Antibiotics and Other Products Obtained by Fermentation Processes

Similar information is needed for the preparation, isolation, and purification of antibiotics and other drug substances isolated from microbial or cell culture sources. The components of the fermentation media should be defined and specifications established, including, if applicable, a defined degree of purity. The role of each ingredient, if known, should be stated.

Because the specific microorganism cultured is the most critical factor in any antibiotic process, strain identification, including morphologic, cultural, and biochemical characteristics should be performed. The source of the microbial isolate (e.g., soil, air, and water), as well as any genetic engineering or mutation procedures should be documented. Microbial deposition should be reported (e.g., American Type Culture Collection or Type Culture Collection of the U.S. Department of Agriculture).

The stability of the cell culture to repeated transfer should be defined, because numerous transfers lead to strain degradation (attenuation). The factors that should be defined are the number of transfers from individual colonies that do not result in a significant decrease of antibiotic production and the proper method(s) and conditions for maintaining an active culture.

The monitoring and control of the fermentation process should be reported in detail. Parameters to be addressed include the media preparation and sterilization, inoculation procedures, and the fermentation process. Provide a detailed description of the media composition, the method for its sterilization (temperature and duration), and the pH after sterilization. The inoculation stage description should include quantity (by volume percent) and age of the inoculum to be used, as well as information on the morphologic stage of the mycelium, if this parameter is controlled. The fermentation stages should be characterized by duration, temperature, pH, aeration rate (volume of air per volume of medium), concentration of dissolved oxygen, the critical elements regarding agitation, and the pressure in the fermenting vessel. Also cite the name and concentration of any antifoaming agents and precursors or inducers of biosynthesis used. The monitoring of antibiotic concentration in the fermentation broth is one of the most critical parameters in the production process. Therefore, the concentration and the method(s) used for its determination should be reported. If a microbiological method is used, the assay microorganism should be indicated, and information should be provided on the sensitivity and reproducibility of the method along with pertinent literature references. In addition, the microbiological and biochemical methods used to control the fermentation process should be described as well as an indication regarding their frequency of use.

Some antibiotic-related considerations concerning extraction and isolation that should be addressed include (*i*) the presence of impurities and side products, along with their quantitation and the results of tests assessing their immunologic and toxicologic properties; (*ii*) the development of specific analytical techniques capable of differentiating the product from related antibiotics; and (*iii*) identification of minor active components as well as their levels and respective antimicrobial activities.

Drug Substances Isolated from Plant or Animal Sources
For drug substances obtained from plants, the description of their collection and preparation should include the following: (*i*) botanical species and plant section(s); (*ii*) geographical location(s) where plants with acceptable levels of drug substances are found (the same species can have different levels, when harvested from different locales, because of differences in climate and soil constituents); (*iii*) storage and transportation conditions; (*iv*) drying conditions; (*v*) grinding procedures; (*vi*) testing procedures to identify and assay crude material, as well as a listing of typical results; and (*vii*) extraction and isolation procedures, where applicable (see also the previous discussion of antibiotics).

The description of drug substances isolated from animal (including human) sources should contain (*i*) species and organ(s) or tissue(s) used; (*ii*) statement(s) demonstrating compliance with USDA or other applicable requirements; and (*iii*) information corresponding to items c to g for plant-derived drug substances described above.

Process Controls
A brief description of the control checks performed at each stage of the manufacturing process and packaging of the drug substance should be provided. The controls applied to the intermediates should be adequate to assure the correct operation of synthetic and purification procedures, as well as the production of the desired products with the necessary purity. The tests should include identifying the material using at least one physical property (e.g., melting or boiling range, refractive index, and optical rotation), detecting impurity/contaminant levels, and monitoring yield. Testing for pivotal and key/critical intermediates should address all of these criteria.

For a pivotal intermediate (one that can be prepared by several different routes), specifications should be rigid and methodologies used should minimize the possibility of the presence of previously undetected or vagrant impurities. The number of steps between the pivotal intermediate and the penultimate intermediate determines the extent of detail and degree of purity required (i.e., the closer they are, the greater the detail and degree of purity required). It should be noted that the pivotal intermediate and the penultimate intermediate can be one and the same.

For a key/critical intermediate [defined as one in which an essential molecular characteristic(s) is first introduced], specifications and test methodologies should be used that assure that the molecular architecture intended to be conferred (e.g., chirality, stereospecificity) has occurred in the expected yield and required purity. At least one test methodology should be used that can quantitate levels of undesired impurities, such as isomers, reaction by-products, or starting materials. For other intermediates, controls may not have to be as extensive. One or more tests monitoring the progress of the synthesis may be all that is necessary.

Reprocessing
It is expected that operating conditions during the manufacture of the drug substance may occasionally deviate from the synthesis description. If a standard reprocessing procedure has been developed and validated and is expected to be used routinely in the synthesis of the drug substance, include this information in this section.

Reference Standard Preparation

Describe how the reference standard used to perform the proof-of-structure studies was prepared and how new lots of reference standards will be qualified. If the method of synthesis is the same as that of the drug substance, a statement referencing this fact is sufficient, along with a detailed description of any additional purification procedures performed. These procedures (e.g., recrystallization) should be repeated until important parameters, including assay and levels of impurities, remain unchanged after two successive purification procedures as demonstrated by appropriate tests (e.g., chromatography).

The primary reference standard is normally prepared on a laboratory scale using pure starting materials, reagents, and solvents and should be of the highest purity that reasonably can be obtained. The synthetic procedure used to make it and the method(s) used for its purification should also be provided. (If applicable, the method of manufacture section can be referenced.) The purification procedure is normally performed until little or no change is observed through two consecutive cycles in assay purity and levels of impurities.

An analytical reference standard or working standard usually derived from a production batch is normally established as the comparative standard for routine analyses of the bulk drug substance for release purposes. It should be characterized against the primary standard.

Specifications and Analytical Methods

The regulatory specifications and analytical methods used to assure the identity, potency, quality, and purity of the drug substance should be submitted. The following are examples of attributes that should be monitored:

1. *Appearance/description*: Color, taste, odor, crystalline form(s), and feel.
2. *Physical properties*: Melting or boiling range, pH, specific rotation, refractive index, dissolution characteristics in various solvents (including water), and crystallinity (type, such as orthorhombic, cubic, amorphous, and the like).
3. *Specific identity tests*: At least one specific identity test that is capable of distinguishing the drug substance from related compounds must be included. Spectrometric tests are usually used, such as ultraviolet, infrared, nuclear magnetic resonance, and mass spectroscopy. Retention times or factors derived from thin-layer, gas-liquid, and HPLC are also used as identification tests to verify a more specific spectral identity test.
4. *Impurity profile*: Because it requires many hours of work by synthetic and analytical chemists, deficiencies in this area are rather frequent. Impurities should be identified, and at least the major ones should be characterized. Other impurities, when possible, should also be elucidated structurally. Specifications should include limits for each major impurity, as well as a limit for the total level of all impurities. These limits should be based on the known or anticipated toxicologic properties of each impurity, referencing, if necessary, the toxicologic profiles of similar compounds. They should also be based on a review of levels in batches used in longer-term toxicology and clinical studies and demonstrated in these studies to be safe. The reader is referred to the "Guideline for Industry on Impurities in New Drug Substances."
5. *Assay*: The methods for the drug substance and the impurities should be stability indicating. If the identity test is specific and impurities are adequately

controlled by other methods, a less specific method to assay the drug substance may be used. If possible, the same procedure should be used to measure both the overall purity of the drug substance and the levels of impurities or degradation products. The limits for purity should be established on the basis of scientific review of the impurity profile of the drug substance and review of results obtained from individual batches.

6. *Other*: Most drug substances used to manufacture dosage forms are solids. It is therefore necessary to consider other properties that may affect the bioavailability with the possibility of eliciting adverse reactions. These parameters, which should be adequately addressed both in the specifications and in the characterization/structure elucidation section, include the nature and extent of solvation, the possibility of different polymorphs, and particle size.

   The extent of solvation is routinely monitored by LOD testing conducted at a temperature previously defined by TGA. Either the basis for concluding the existence of only one solvated form or information comparing the respective solubilities, dissolution rates, and physical/chemical stability of the different solvates should be provided.

   Polymorphism is customarily monitored by melting point or infrared spectral analysis. However, other methods, such as X-ray diffraction, thermal analytical, and solid-state Raman spectroscopy, can also be used. It is expected that the sponsor will conduct a diligent search by evaluating the drug substance recrystallized from various solvents with different properties. Either the basis for concluding that only one crystalline form exists, or comparative information regarding the respective solubilities, dissolution rates, and physical/chemical stability of each crystalline form should be provided.

   Particle size determination may not be important if (*i*) the drug substance demonstrates good water solubility; (*ii*) particle size reduction or compaction is performed as part of the dosage form manufacture; or (*iii*) the drug substance is intended to be administered in solution (not suspended). However, the sponsor should be prepared to address with the FDA reviewer why it is not important. The appropriate part of the dosage form manufacturing section, where the data are to be found, should be cross-referenced.

7. *Reference standard*: Characterization and structure elucidation data are typically derived from tests conducted on the primary reference standard. Its suitability must be documented by information much more extensive than prescribed in the specifications. In addition to the prescribed analyses—especially levels of impurities—other tests normally conducted include elemental analysis and ultraviolet, infrared, nuclear magnetic resonance, and mass spectrometry, along with reviews of each providing assignments of the important features supporting the structure(s) of the drug substance. Other tests such as optical rotation, refractive index, X-ray crystallography, phase solubility analysis, and differential scanning calorimetry may be provided as well to support its purity and elucidate its structure. Finally, some compounds may require bioassays for full characterization.

Container/Closure System

Provide explicit information regarding the characteristics of, and quality control test methods used by both the manufacturer and the sponsor for, the container, closure, and any other component parts (e.g., desiccant bags) to assure suitability for their intended use. If this information is on file at FDA in the form of a DMF, provide a copy of the letter from the holder of the DMF to FDA authorizing the use of applicable data in conjunction with the review of the sponsor's application. Whenever possible, a similar letter from the fabricator(s) should be obtained and included. In addition, stability data supporting the use of the components should be cross-referenced. Detailed information concerning this subject can be found in the "Guideline for Packaging of Human Drugs and Biologics."

If most of the CMC information drug substance is covered by a DMF, the sponsor needs a letter of authorization to this DMF. The sponsor has to indicate in this section how the drug substance is accepted, maintained, and qualified in its facilities prior to use in the production of the drug product.

Further guidance regarding the required information to be included in support of the manufacture and control sections of the new drug substance can be found in the "Guideline for Submitting Supporting Documentation in Drug Applications for the Manufacture of Drug Substance."

DRUG PRODUCT

Components

Provide a list of all substances used in producing the finished dosage form intended for commercial distribution, regardless of whether they are ultimately contained in the product. This includes excipients as well as in-process materials, such as water or other solvents used in the granulation process and later removed by drying. The quality specifications or grade (ACS, USP, or NF) should be indicated for each substance.

If proprietary mixtures (colorants, coating mixtures, flavors, controlled-release matrices, and imprinting inks) are used as components, information on their compositions should be provided. Any alternatives that have been evaluated and determined to be interchangeable may also be included. The sponsor should be prepared either to delete the alternative from the application or to generate further information, including effects in the bioequivalency, in support of retaining the alternative if FDA initially does not accept it.

Composition

The statement of composition for each active or inactive ingredient per unit of dosage form (e.g., tablet, capsule, ml) should be provided. In addition, include a batch formula that is representative of the scale of manufacture to be used. Besides the name, strength, and type of dosage form, the name and weight of each active ingredient and the identification of all components should be given. This should include their grades in the same manner as defined under Components. Information to be included will usually consist of the weights and measures of each component using the same weight system, any calculated excesses, and the theoretical weight and number of doses to be obtained. Reasonable variations in the amounts of inactive components (e.g., +10%) are usually permitted and are generally indicated on the quantitative composition. Dosage forms, however, must be formulated to contain 100% of the desired potency. Whereas the allowable range for the potency of a drug might be 90% to 110% of its labeled potency during its labeled shelf life period, a sponsor cannot change the formulation to achieve 95% of the labeled potency in an effort to reduce the cost of manufacturing.

Specifications and Analytical Methods for Inactive Components

Inactive components are sometimes referred to as inactive ingredients, ingredients, or excipients. These are all the items in the listing of components used to manufacture the drug product except the drug substance(s). If an inactive component is USP/NF grade, it is acceptable to just reference the current monograph for that component. If the inactive ingredient is non-USP/NF but belongs to a foreign compendium, provide a copy of the actual monograph for this inactive component. The FDA will at times accept the specifications and test methods indicated in the foreign compendium but can ask for validation data for the assay method. Acceptable food or color additives are indicated in the 21 CFR, and batch certifications are needed for some of the color additives before they can be released for production. A batch certificate for the NDA batch should be included.

Indicate which tests will be performed routinely by the sponsor on each lot received. Most sponsors will perform all tests specified in the monograph for the first few batches until comparative data are achieved with the manufacturer's Certificate of Analysis; then, they rely on Certificates of Analysis and perform an identity test for each batch.

In the case of noncompendial materials, specifications and complete descriptions of the test methodologies to be used for quality control release purposes by the sponsor should be included. In addition, it may be necessary for the sponsor to obtain a letter authorizing reference to a DMF from the supplier concerning the manufacturing and controls procedures used to make these materials, such as mixtures of colorants or flavors. It may be necessary to obtain toxicity data if the mixture or component has little or no history of human use (e.g., new polymers). If it is anticipated that an "untried" component will be used, it is recommended that discussions should be initiated with the FDA's reviewing chemist and pharmacologist. These sessions should be scheduled as soon as possible to minimize the possibility of delays in NDA approval caused by inadequate information to support use of the material.

Manufacturer

The names(s) and address(es) of all manufacturers, (type II) contract packagers, and contract analytical laboratories used for testing raw materials or the drug product should be given. If the manufacturing site is in the United States, a general description of site facilities and operations should be incorporated because information on these facilities is available in the FDA District Offices. If the manufacturing site is in a foreign country, letters authorizing FDA reference to site DMFs on behalf of the sponsor should be included. If a DMF is not available, then information that is needed to prepare a type II DMF should be obtained by the sponsor from the manufacturer. This information is then placed in this section. Refer to the "Guideline for Drug Master Files." In addition, Foreign Drug Establishments who import drugs now have to register with the FDA in accordance with 21 CFR 207.40 with an annual reregistration.

Method of Manufacture, Packaging Procedure, and In-Process Control

In this section, include a general description of the manufacturing procedure, including all processing alternatives previously validated as producing acceptable product. The FDA also wants copies of the proposed or actual master production and control record, as well as a copy of a completed production and control record for a typical batch. It is also helpful to provide a schematic diagram for the flow of materials, the production process, and an indication of the equipment to be used.

For other than manual operations (e.g., computerized automated plants), the schematics are more critical to assure that the FDA reviewer understands the process. The description should also indicate the various points of sampling.

The piece(s) of equipment that renders the batch homogeneous before packaging should be identified, with both the useful working and total capacities noted.

Regarding reprocessing operations, adequate information should be submitted to permit approval of such procedures, for bulk, in-process, or finished drug products that do not conform to established specifications. The original application may include proposals for such steps that cover foreseeable deviations, such as unacceptable weight variation, content uniformity, and tablet coating. Deviations not covered in the original application should be covered by a supplemental application and must receive approval before commercial distribution of such reprocessed product. All proposals should include a description of the material that includes a statement of the deviations(s), a detailed description of the reprocessing procedure, including additional controls to be used over and above those established for routine production, and information on the maximum allowable time between initial manufacture and initiation of reprocessing operations, along with the applicable storage conditions to be used during this interval.

A sample packaging record(s) that describes the packaging and label operations should also be included with the manufacturing and control record and the completed production and control record for a typical batch.

Regulatory Specifications and Analytical Methods for Drug Product

Consistency in the quality of the drug product batches is controlled by the specifications and analytical methods set for that product. This means that when the drug is taken by a patient, the expected clinical response will occur. Specifications and analytical methods evolve throughout the investigational phases of drug development. By NDA time, a sponsor has learned much about the nature of the drug product and the critical parameters that have to be monitored to provide maximum assurance of its safety and efficacy. It is at this point that the regulatory specifications and analytical methods are determined for the drug product. These are established to assure the safety and efficacy of every batch of drug product up to the date of its expiration. The NDA should also include appropriate information on in-process controls and a listing of the number or amount of drug product needed to perform each of the regulatory analytical methods.

Regulatory specifications may differ from product release specifications. Regulatory specifications assure acceptable product potency until the labeled expiration date or shelf life. In general, in-house release specifications are tighter than regulatory specifications.

Refer to the "Guideline for Submission of Supportive Analytical Data for Methods Validation in the New Drug Application."

The following items should also be considered.

(a) Tablets, capsules, and other dosage forms
    1. Weight variation.
    2. Content uniformity for tablets, capsules, sterile solids, and sterile suspensions. A common deficiency is the use of different analytical methodologies

for uniformity and for assay purposes without supporting their equivalency or adequately defining correction factors.

3. Dissolution rate tests for tablets, capsules, suspensions, suppositories, or
   other dosage forms. Controlled-release dosage forms or drug delivery systems should also be monitored by appropriate testing methodology.
4. Moisture content. In some formulations of relatively water-insoluble drug
   substances containing anhydrous lactose, storage under high-humidity
   conditions (75% or higher) has been shown to adversely affect dissolution
   rates.
5. Loss on drying, where applicable.
6. Physical characteristics such as color, appearance, odor, shape, hardness,
   thickness, friability, and coating. Fading and brittleness (powdering) are
   common problems.
7. Softening or melting points and particle size distribution of suspended
   drug (suppositories).
8. Assay(s) for the active drug substance in the drug product, for impurities,
   and for degradation products.
9. Residual solvents testing is necessary if a solvent is found in the inactive
   ingredients and if used in manufacture of the drug product and is to be
   tested in accordance with recent revision of USP/NF chapter <467>, effective July 1, 2008.

(b) Solutions and suspensions
1. Clarity, limit for the presence of particulate matter, preservative effectiveness, and assay, isotonicity (ophthalmics and injectables), and pH.
2. Sterility of ophthalmics.
3. Sterility, apyrogenicity, and container fill of injectables.
4. Leakage test for ampules, vials, sachets, aerosols, strips, tubes, and so forth.
5. Spray pattern and container pressure for aerosol products; for a metered
   dose product, reproducibility of actuated dose and defined limits for dose
   administered per actuation.
6. Particle size specifications for the active component; resuspendability, viscosity, sedimentations rates, caking, and syringeability of suspensions.
7. Completeness and clarity of constituted solutions.

(c) Plastic devices containing active drugs
1. In vitro rates and identity testing of all plastic components. If applicable,
   determine sterility and measure levels of residual ethylene oxide and its
   decomposition products.
2. Additional physical tests, such as frame memory, resiliency, tensile
   strength, and seal integrity.

(d) Diluent solution
1. Full specifications and analytical methods, including preservative
   levels.

Container/Closure System(s)

Describe all the packaging configurations to be used for the drug product. List the
components that comprise each container/closure system to be used.

Provide a detailed description of the physical, chemical, and if applicable, biological characteristics of the container, closure, or other component parts of the drug
product package to assure suitability for its intended use. Acceptance specifications

and test methods performed by the drug product manufacturer for each packaging component should be spelled out.

The "Guideline for Packaging of Human Drugs and Biologics" includes specific recommendations for the format and content of this section. Some points need to be emphasized, however, to help the sponsor avoid delays in NDA approval because of deficiencies in container/closure information.

When more than one plastic resin is used to fabricate bottles, it is necessary to demonstrate the equivalency of the container produced using the different resins. In addition, comparative data derived from light transmission, chemical resistance, extractables, and moisture permeation/vapor transmission tests described in the USP should be provided as applicable to the type of product. (For example, moisture permeation for an aqueous dosage form would not be necessary.) Whereas the compendia discuss these tests only in the context of polyethylene, the guideline makes no distinction as to the resin used. It should also be verified that copies of letters authorizing FDA reference to appropriate DMFs from manufacturers of the resins used to fabricate bottles and from the bottle fabricator(s), if available, are included. Although most resin suppliers include information on extractables data in their DMFs, it should be pointed out that fabricators may have to add release agents or other additives not covered by extractables data in the DMF of the resin supplier.

Manufacturers of glass components, in most cases, do not have DMFs. It is recommended that letters should be obtained from fabricators certifying that the glass used will meet appropriate compendial requirements (i.e., U.S. type I or type II glass).

For closures, compatibility of the drug product with the inner liner/contact surface should be evaluated. This is usually done as part of stability studies conducted on a product stored inverted. If available, appropriate DMF authorization letters should be obtained to support suitability of the closure and liner.

Provide information on any adhesives used for blistered packages. Defect classification data should be considered. Permeation and leaching/migration testing should be conducted and reported. (Information in a DMF or data from studies conducted by the fabricator may be sufficient.)

For elastomers (e.g., stoppers), leaching of components is a concern, as is the possibility that components, especially active drug substance from the formulation, will migrate into the closure. Therefore, test data should be provided that demonstrate drug product/closure compatibility. A letter from the closure manufacturer authorizing FDA reference to their DMF should be obtained and included.

Finally, for any unusual or uncommon containers and closures, sufficient information about the materials of fabrication, design performance, and other information that conclusively demonstrates their suitability for use with dosage form should be provided.

Stability

This section, as previously discussed, frequently poses problems leading to delays in NDA approval. Particular attention should be paid to the development of adequate data from studies conducted with commercial formulations packaged in container/closure system(s) to be marketed. It is critical that adequately validated analytical methods should be used as early as possible in the investigational phases of drug development—no later than the initiation of phase 3 studies. Common defects in stability studies submitted to FDA reflect the lack of acceptable long-term or short-term accelerated stability data to support the approval of an expiration date for the product. Another common problem occurs when studies are conducted using only one container size, yet the sponsor is applying to market two or more sizes. As a general rule, FDA wishes to see data from studies conducted on at least the smallest and largest sizes to be marketed (e.g., 100- and 500-tablet bottles or 2- and 32-ounce bottles). Blister packs are generally exceptions to the rule because each dosage unit is individually packaged.

With drug products containing preservatives, the stability protocol should include preservative efficacy testing. Microbial challenge testing should be conducted at appropriate intervals—at least once a year unless significant losses are observed earlier as a result of assay procedures.

Other items worth considering in the design of a stability protocol are the effects of heat, humidity, freezing (for solutions, emulsions, and semisolids), and light. These data are needed to support the recommended storage conditions required to be on the product labeling. The information also helps answer the inevitable questions from the field (e.g., the product has been stored in a warehouse whose air-conditioning unit broke, and the customer wants to know if the product is still good after storage for a month at 110°F). Simulated use tests are also recommended, in which the same bottles are opened and closed a number of times and the data are compared with the stability of drugs stored in unopened containers.

For products intended to be reconstituted, it is necessary to conduct stability studies on the final product form to determine the maximum allowable storage time after reconstitution. Data from these studies, usually conducted over a period of a week or less, support recommendations required to be on the labeling for storage time and conditions after reconstitution [e.g., "Administer within three hours after reconstitution. Store until use under refrigeration (2–8°C or 35–45°F)"]. If previous studies have demonstrated light or heat sensitivity, these conditions should be considered in designing studies of the reconstituted product.

In addition to potency, other design considerations that may need to be incorporated in the stability protocol for various dosage forms include the following:

Tablets: Appearance, friability, hardness, color, odor, moisture, and special emphasis on dissolution rates.

Capsules: Moisture, color, appearance, shape, brittleness, and especially dissolution rates.

Emulsions: Appearance (particularly with regard to phase separation and color), odor, pH, viscosity, and the effects of heating and cooling.

Oral solutions and suspensions: Appearance (clarity, the presence of a precipitate, and cloudiness), pH, color, odor, redispersibility (suspensions), and storage both in upright and inverted positions to determine if the closure or liner adversely affect stability.

Oral powders: Appearance, color, odor, moisture content of powder, and, if intended for reconstitution, appearance, pH, and dispersibility/dissolution properties.

Metered-dose inhalation aerosols: Quantity of delivered dose, total number of acceptable doses delivered, color, solvate formation with propellant, particle size distribution, weight loss of canister (i.e., loss of propellant), pressure, valve corrosion, and storage in both upright and inverted positions.

Topical and ophthalmic preparations: Appearance (clarity, color, and especially homogeneity), odor, pH, resuspendability, consistency, particle size, weight loss (is of more importance if plastic containers are used). Sterility and preservative levels must also be considered if the product is intended for ophthalmic administration.

Small-volume parenterals (SVPs): Appearance, color, clarity (particulates), pH, and sterility checks at reasonable intervals are minimum standards. Powders for reconstitution should also include residual moisture and stability checks after reconstitution. Except for ampules, upright and inverted storage of final product should also be evaluated.

Large-volume parenterals (LVPs): Similar evaluations as described for SVPs should be conducted. In addition, if plastic containers are used, volume and extractables data should be evaluated. Another important parameter to consider, if applicable, is the maintenance of adequate preservative levels over the expiration-dating period.

Suppositories: Appearance, melting range, dissolution at 37°C, body temperature, and aging with respect to hardening and polymorphic transformation.

Drug additive: Compatibility of admixture, appearance over 24 hours including evaluations of both drug and additive for assay, pH, color and clarity, and interaction with the container at the time of mixing (time 0) and 2–3, 6–8, 12, 24, and 48 hours after mixing. Some intervals may be deleted or the time intervals adjusted as considered appropriate or cost effective.

Statistical analyses: The statistical analyses of data submitted to support a proposed expiration date should be described fully. In addition, as part of the stability protocol, provide detailed plans for such analyses of future batches.

Stability reports: These reports are frequently deemed incomplete because adequate information for each lot of product is missing. Data must be provided describing formulation; batch number; scale of manufacture including designation as to whether a laboratory, pilot, or production lot; site(s) of manufacture; and the analytical methodology(ies) used, reflecting changes, if any, made during the course of the investigation. Notations regarding the status of each lot (whether it is terminated or continuing on stability) should also appear on each table of data.

Stability protocol: A postapproval stability protocol should be submitted documenting future plans. It should include information on time points and storage conditions to be evaluated, and indicate whether extensions of expiration dating are intended based on sponsor evaluation of data obtained following the protocol. These data will still have to be submitted, as well as the details of the extensions of expiration dating being implemented, in the annual reports filed with FDA. Also indicate how many batches of drug product will be placed on stability in a year. This postapproval stability protocol is the basis on which any new drug product expiration dating is established.

Environmental Assessment

The format and content of this section for NDAs and ANDAs can be found under 21 CFR 25 Subpart C. In addition, FDA generated a guidance document that provides a more in-depth description and clarification of items to include in this section. This document is entitled "Guidance for Industry on the Environmental Assessment in Human Drug and Biologics Applications, July, 1998."

SAMPLES
Identify all samples being set aside for FDA validation. The samples should include drug substance, drug product, major impurities, degradation products being controlled for, references standard, and internal standard (the latter is not required if commercially available but is recommended to facilitate FDA laboratory work). If appropriate, blanks and any other materials not commercially available but specified in the analytical procedures should be provided. The samples are to be maintained by the sponsor until the FDA's reviewing chemist provides instructions as to where they should be forwarded. The total quantities and the manner of their subdivision (e.g., 400 tablets, 4 × 100 tablets/bottle) should be indicated. The amounts provided should be adequate to permit at least three separate determinations, excluding sterility, by two different laboratories.

METHODS VALIDATION PACKAGE
Unlike the full NDA, which is submitted in duplicate, this section must be provided in triplicate because copies are forwarded to two FDA laboratories. These laboratories will assess the validation data and test the drug substance and drug product to verify the validity of the regulatory specifications and test methods indicated in the NDA. Documents in this package that were taken from the CMC section should retain the original pagination in the CMC section. Intended to expedite the NDA review and FDA laboratory validation of proposed regulatory methods, it is recommended that the submission include the following items.

Test Methods and Specifications
Copies of regulatory specifications and analytical methods for the drug substance and drug product should be provided. These documents should retain the original pagination they had in the CMC section.

Supporting Data
Validation information to support the suitability of the regulatory analytical method(s) is shown by providing data on accuracy, specificity, sensitivity, precision, ruggedness, and linearity over the range of interest. The emphasis for analyzing drug substances is the control of the presence of impurities. With drug products, it is more important to quantify the active drug substance and level of degradation products throughout the expected shelf life of the product. (Levels of impurities that are not degradation products are adequately controlled in the bulk drug substance-release testing.)

Documentation (or lack thereof) provided in support of specificity, sensitivity, and ruggedness are frequent sources of FDA comment and delays in NDA approval.

Specificity. It is not advisable to rely on drug substance assay results (and assay specificity demonstrated only with respect to impurities) on the assumption that degradation products behave similarly. Specific studies to determine degradation pathways must be conducted. These should include exposing the drug substance to acid(s), base(s), heat, light, oxidizers, reductants, and combinations of the above, as appropriate. In the absence of suitably designed degradation studies, it is not possible to know the intrinsic stability of the drug substance, or to determine in future studies whether any given peak on a chromatogram is an artifact or a real degradation product. It may also be difficult to establish whether the chromatogram is run long enough to permit the observation of peaks from degradation products. In addition, excipients in the dosage form may interfere with one or more peaks of interest. The specificity of the method(s) should be evaluated by treating the formulation minus the active ingredient(s) in similar fashion to the dosage form before injecting or spotting. It is strongly recommended that the methods include retention information for all degradation products known or still in the process of being identified to facilitate their monitoring by different analytical chemists during the course of the stability studies.

Sensitivity. This can be a source of FDA comment, when information is not included in the validation documentation on the sensitivity(ies) of the method(s) to detect and quantitate the drug substance and the degradation products. In addition, the methodology description should include the appropriate mathematical formula(s) to be used for calculating their respective levels. Even if the sponsor uses a computerized system that provides the number directly, these formulas should still be provided to facilitate manual calculations.

Ruggedness. This is also an important consideration, because it is directly linked with the probability of success for the FDA laboratories validating the methods internally (i.e., analyst-to-analyst, lab-to-lab reproducibility results). It is recommended that the sponsor have a second laboratory to perform the method using a different instrument and column, if possible. By following this recommendation, potential misunderstandings regarding the performance of the various operations and manipulations can be identified and rewritten for clarity to facilitate use of the selected method. In addition, in the case of chromatographic systems (HPLC or GC), the appropriate peaks and their minimum resolution (separation) factor can be determined and noted in the method of description as the parameters to be monitored by the analyst to assess the suitability and effectiveness of the operating system before conducting the assay. This assessment should be performed routinely and is commonly referred to as "system suitability testing."

Other areas. Those that can lead to approval delays include the following: (*i*) use of instrumentation not commercially available and the absence of a detailed description of the components and assembly, (*ii*) use of single source specifications to permit duplication, (*iii*) use of specialized tools or equipment not available to the FDA chemists for sample preparation, (*iv*) use of an in-house standard or other noncommercial reagent, and (*v*) failure to provide a system suitability test on chromatographic procedures.

Data from these and similar sources should not be submitted unless it can be demonstrated that no acceptable alternatives are available.

Include documentation supporting the integrity of the reference standard.

For additional information, the reader is directed to the "Guideline for Stability Studies for Human Drugs and Biologics," and the "Guideline for Submission of Supportive Analytical Data for Method Validation in New Drug Applications."

Test Results

Provide the certificates of analysis for drug substance, drug product, and reference standard for the lots where the samples were obtained.

In support of samples of impurities, degradation products, and internal standards, it is recommended that copies of relevant spectra and other supportive analyses used to elucidate or verify their structures should be included.

ABBREVIATED NEW DRUG APPLICATION

There are distinct differences and some unique problems likely to be encountered in the preparation of manufacturing and controls sections for ANDA submissions. Some of them are highlighted below.

Summary

A summary is not required by the FDA.

In lieu of a summary, the FDA's Office of Generic Drugs (OGD) requests a question-based review (QBR) for CMC evaluations in an ANDA submission. The QBR has transformed the CMC review into a modern, science, and risk-based approach to pharmaceutical quality assessment. The QBR properly presented will provide the basic information on the development of the drug product. The QBR is designed so that ANDA applications would be organized according to the CTD, a formal submission format adopted by FDA and multiple regulatory bodies. It is recommended that an original ANDA be submitted to FDA in the CTD or electronic CTD format to facilitate the implementation of the QBR and to avoid undue review delays.

Moreover, the FDA has developed an ANDA checklist for CTD or eCTD format for filing applications. This checklist identifies the sections in CTD application that are applicable to the ANDA review process. The sections that are applicable to the CMC review include Modules 2 and 3 of the CTD format.

In the following paragraphs are additional key points that will help assure a complete and prompt OGD review on data/document presentation.

Drug Substance Sources

Drug substances or active pharmaceutical ingredients (APIs) that are used in the manufacture of drug products for subject of ANDAs are usually obtained from one or more external manufacturers, frequently located overseas, and imported into the United States. If the supplier has been previously inspected by FDA, an Establishment Inspection Report (EIR) can be obtained under Freedom of Information (FOI) regulations. This document should be reviewed by the sponsor to assess the likelihood of the supplier's acceptability to FDA as a manufacturer. In addition, the supplier should have a DMF available at FDA for reference purposes. This will describe the facilities, personnel, equipment, and manufacturing and controls procedures used at the site(s) where the bulk drug substance is made. The ANDA sponsor can then submit a much simplified drug substance section because the letter of reference to the DMF serves in place of providing specific details regarding the manufacturing procedures, controls, stability data, and identification of impurities. These and other relevant issues should be assessed by direct discussion with the drug substance manufacturer and, if necessary, arrange to have the manufacturer update the DMF. A letter of authorization from the manufacture through the U.S. agent will be necessary as part of the ANDA filing to allow for FDA cross-reference of the DMF.

Specifications

This subject is usually not a problem, if compendial (USP) monographs exist. Analytical methodology, however, can be a troublesome item. This is especially true with older drugs where assay methodology specified in the monograph is not sufficiently specific and in the case of drugs for which there are no published compendial monographs.

It is prudent to evaluate impurity peaks observed in a supplier's bulk substance and compare them with those observed in the drug product. The extent that the peaks differ may determine the need to obtain further information, including toxicity. Samples of impurities/degradation products methods should be appropriately validated by the ANDA sponsor for their sensitivities and specificities. It is also recommended that the sponsor of an ANDA set up and maintain a stability program for the bulk drug substance. It is important those in setting drug substance and drug product specifications to review the OGD guidance ANDA documents "Impurities in Drug Substances and Impurities in Drug Products." These documents provide information on the setting of specifications and the applicable testing, if any, to support the proposed levels.

Drug Product Requirements

Drug product requirements are similar to those described previously for the NDA. The extent of stability data submitted, however, is much less than that usually available for an NDA. Specifications are usually defined by a published compendial monograph. It must be emphasized that analytical methodologies for many older drugs, as set forth in their monographs, may not be sufficiently specific to be accepted by FDA as "stability indicating." Adequate validation studies should be carried out to verify the accuracy, precision, specificity, recovery, and sensitivity of the method(s) conducted by the sponsor's own laboratory or contact facility. It is also important to compare the release characteristics of the sponsor's product with those obtained with the original brand name product using the same methodology. For example, data comparing the dissolution characteristics and performance of the sponsor's and the brand name tablet or capsule products at several different time points (as applicable to obtain 95% or more of drug in solution)—otherwise referred to as a comparative dissolution profiling—should be obtained. The FDA's OGD does have on its Web site a list of drug product dissolution methodologies that are acceptable to the Office.

ANDA Expiration Dates

Generally, the FDA will tentatively approve a two-year expiration date for a product if satisfactory data reflecting at least three months storage under accelerated conditions are submitted. The sponsor is also expected to provide a commitment to continue to monitor the controlled room temperature stability of the product, to periodically report the results to FDA, and to remove from the market any batches failing to meet specifications prior to the product's labeled expiration period. Final approval for the expiration date is obtained when acceptable shelf life data for two years or more than one production lot is made available to FDA. In contrast to NDAs for which the extended term data are frequently available prior to approval, the importance of the stability protocol describing future plans, including the basis that the sponsor deems appropriate to support an extension of a product's expiration dating, is magnified for an ANDA. In fact, an ANDA will not be approved without the inclusion of a postapproval stability protocol.

CONCLUSION

In the context of the guidance documents issued by the FDA, this chapter has explored the various issues, and described a number of recommendations, concerning the documentation requirements for NDA and ANDA submissions. It is anticipated that as industry representatives become more familiar with these guidance documents, the quality of CMC documentation will be improved, and it is hoped that the frequency and extent of deficiencies will diminish. One of the most positive contributions will be the economical one, because reproducible manufacture of new drugs in well-designed dosage forms can be prescribed by physicians with confidence. The careful preparation of the manufacturing and controls section in an NDA or ANDA can facilitate FDA processing, review, and approval procedures. The result is potentially faster commercialization of new products benefiting both pharmaceutical manufacturers and the patients they ultimately serve.

BIBLIOGRAPHY

ANDA Checklist for CTD or eCTD Format for Completeness and Acceptability of an Application for Filing, FDA Office of Generic Drugs. Available from http://www.fda.gov/cder/ogd.

Cook J, Prunella P, Stringer S, Yacura M (1980). Approvals and non-approvals of new drug applications during the 1970s. OPE Study 57, PB 81-14865. Rockville, Maryland: U.S. Food and Drug Administration.

FDA Web site. Available from http:/www/FDA.gov.

FDA Letter to Industry (October 14, 1994). FDA letter describing efforts by CDER and ORA to clarify responsibilities of CDER chemistry review scientists and ORA field investigators in the new and abbreviated drug approval process in order to reduce duplication and redundancy.

Federal Food, Drug and Cosmetic Act, as Amended, Superintendent of Documents (November 1997). Washington, D.C.: U.S. Government Printing Office.

Federal Register (February 22, 1985). 50 (36):7452–7519.

Food and Drug Administration Modernization and Accountability Act of 1997.

Food and Drug Administration (1971). Guidelines: Manufacturing and Controls for INDs and NDAs. FDA Papers 5, 4–14.

Food and Drug Administration (1979). Requirements of Laws and Regulations Enforced by the U.S. Food and Drug Administration. U.S. Department of Health, Education, and Welfare, Public Health Service, HEW Publication (FDA) 79–1042.

Fry EM (September 22–24, 1981). The role of the inspection in pre-market approval for drug products. Paper presented at the Pharm Tech Conference, Sheraton Centre Hotel, New York.

Generic Drug Office, Guidance Documents. Available from http://www.fda.gov/cder/ogd.

Hyman, Phelps & McNamara PC (HP&M) (1997). The Food and Drug Modernization Act of 1997: A Summary.

Karlton P (October 1996). Meeting the challenge of FDA's CMC initiatives. J Pharm Tech.

Kumkumian CS (November 14, 1978). Manufacturing and controls guidelines for INDs and NDAs—1978. Paper Presented at the 25th National Meeting of the Academy of Pharmaceutical Sciences, Hollywood, Florida.

Kumkumian CS (September 22–24, 1981). New Drugs: filing the manufacturing and controls sections of INDs and NDAs. Paper Presented at the Pharm Tech Conference, Sheraton Centre Hotel, New York.

Kumkumian C (June 1992). New Drug Application Chemistry Review. Format and Content Guide.

McDermaid R (September 22–24, 1981). FDA's foreign inspection program. Paper Presented at the Pharm Tech Conference, Sheraton Centre Hotel, New York.

Personeus GR, Ascione P (1981). Preparation and use of drug master files in the pharmaceutical industry. J Parenter Sci Technol 35, 63–69.

Question-Based Review for CMC Evaluations of ANDA's, FDA Office of Generic Drugs. Available from http://www.fda.gov/cder/ogd.

Schultz RC (November 1, 1978). New drug stability guidelines. Paper Presented at the 11th Annual Industrial Pharmacy Management Conference, Concourse Hotel, Madison, Wisconsin.

The United States Pharmacopeia/National Formulary (USP/NF). United States Pharmacopeial Convention, Inc., Rockville, Maryland. (Edition updated every year with two supplements published yearly.)

US Code of Federal Regulations Title 21, Section 314, part 314.50 Content and format of an New Drug Application and part 314.92 Application Content and format of an Abbreviated New Drug Application.

14 New Medical Device Approval Process in the United States

Max Sherman

Sherman Consulting Services, Inc., Warsaw, Indiana, U.S.A.

BACKGROUND AND HISTORY

There is the long-standing belief that the approval process for medical devices is much faster than the IND/NDA drug method. This is certainly true for Class I, Class II, and some pre-enactment Class III devices—products that can be cleared through premarket notification or 510(k) submissions. Such products are often approved for commercialization in 90 days or less. However, the difference in time is less apparent for manufacturers of new Class III products, where preclinical studies, clinical trials, and the premarket approval process are required. Statistics with respect to time of inception through time to market for new Class III devices is not readily available, but in the author's opinion, it would be similar to that required for a new drug.

A medical device is defined as an instrument, apparatus, implement, machine, contrivance, implant, in vitro reagent, or other similar or related article, including a component, part, or accessory, which is recognized in the official National Formulary, or the U.S. Pharmacopeia, or any supplement to them, intended for the use in the diagnosis of disease or other conditions, or in the cure, mitigation, treatment or prevention of disease, in man or other animals, or intended to affect the structure or any function of the body of man or other animals, and which does not achieve any of its primary intended purposes through chemical action within or on the body of man or other animals and which is not dependent upon being metabolized for the achievement of any of its primary intended purposes. The primary difference between drugs and devices relates to whether there is a chemical action or metabolism to achieve the intended purpose.

Medical devices were included in the 1938 Federal Food, Drug, and Cosmetic Act (1) (the Act), but only in terms of prohibited acts related to adulteration or misbranding. Following passage of the Medical Device Amendments on May 28, 1976, a host of new provisions were added (2). Included among others were regulations pertaining to registration, device listing, classification, performance standards, labeling, good manufacturing practices, premarket notification, and premarket approval. Classification is unique to medical devices—it provides a risk-based system for regulating these products. There are three categories of regulatory control. Class I represents products of lowest risk; they are subject only to general control provisions. Class II devices are subject to general and special controls. The latter can include performance standards, postmarket surveillance, patient registries, certain guidelines (including guidelines for the submission of clinical data), and other information such as special labeling. Class III devices cannot be adequately regulated under either Class I or II; they have the potential for higher risk. They are thus subjected to the strictest type of regulatory requirement. Manufacturers of Class III products must submit a premarket approval application (PMA) containing valid scientific evidence of their safety and efficacy. To understand today's requirements for marketing medical devices that require clinical studies, it would be prudent to review a capsuled history of device legislation. The provisions listed below in most part are limited to those required to achieve product approvals.

1976—The Medical Device Amendments passed on May 28 (*i*) to assure safety and effectiveness of medical devices, including certain diagnostic and laboratory products, and (*ii*) to upgrade the regulatory authority over such devices. In addition, the amendments required classification of all devices with graded regulatory requirements, establishment registration, device listing, premarket notification or 510(k), PMA, investigational device exemptions (IDEs), good manufacturing practice regulations, records and reporting requirements, performance standards, and preemption of state and local regulation of devices.

1990—The Safe Medical Devices Act (SMDA), signed into law on November 28, amended the Federal Food, Drug, and Cosmetic Act to add new requirements and provisions concerning the regulations of medical devices (3). Some provisions went into effect upon enactment of the SMDA, while others had different effective dates or required implementing regulations. New provisions included user facility reporting, distributor reports, Medical Device Reports (MDRs), certification, device tracking, reports of removals and corrective actions, postmarket surveillance, civil penalties, recall authority, temporary suspension of PMA, design validation, new provisions related to 510(k)s, use of PMA data, reclassification of Class III preamendment devices, transitional devices, Class II redefinition, humanitarian device exemptions, combination products, repair, replacement or refund, and establishment of the Office of International Relations.

1992—Medical Device Amendments of 1992 signed into law on June 16 included changes to some of the provisions of the SMDA (4). The amendments (*i*) provided for a broader definition of "serious injury" for MDR reports, (*ii*) deemed failure to comply with postmarket surveillance requirements as misbranding under the FD&C Act, and (*iii*) changed the provision for repair, replacement, and refund. Prior to passage of the 1992 Amendments for FDA to issue an order under Section 518 of the Act, FDA would have to show, among other things, that the device was not "designed *and* manufactured" in accordance with the state of the art at the time of design and manufacture. Under the 1992 Amendments, FDA would only have to show that the device was not "designed *or* manufactured in accordance with the state of the art at that time."

1997—The FDA Modernization Act (FDAMA) was signed into law on November 21 (5). With certain provisions noted in the Act itself, most of the law's provisions became effective on February 19, 1998. The Act complemented and built on FDA's measures to focus its resources on medical devices that present the greatest risks to patients. FDAMA also added a number of provisions affecting clinical studies and PMA. Under Section 201, sponsors who intend to perform clinical studies of any Class III or implantable devices were given an opportunity to have their investigational plan discussed with FDA to reach an agreement on its contents before applying for an IDE. A written request to FDA is required prior to FDA review. The request shall include a detailed description of the device, proposed conditions of use, and a proposed investigational plan (including the clinical protocol). FDA has 30 days to meet with the sponsor after receipt of the written request. An official record is made of any agreement reached between the sponsor and FDA. Agreements reached at these pre-IDE meetings are binding and not subject to change except (*i*) with written agreement of the sponsor; or (*ii*) if the sponsor has been notified by FDA that a substantial scientific issue essential to determining the safety or effectiveness of the device involved has been identified.

Under Section 205 of FDAMA, sponsors planning to submit a PMA can submit a written request to FDA for a meeting to determine the type of information (valid scientific evidence) that is necessary to support the effectiveness of their device. The request must include a detailed description of the device, proposed conditions of use, an investigational plan, and, if available, information regarding the device's expected performance. FDA must meet with the requester and communicate the agency's determination of the type of data that will be necessary to demonstrate effectiveness in writing within 30 days after the meeting. When making this determination, FDA must assure that both the information they have specified are necessary to provide a reasonable assurance that the device is effective and that the agency has considered the method of evaluation that is least burdensome. FDA's decision will be binding and not subject to change unless the agency determines that the decision could be contrary to the public health.

Section 209(b) of FDAMA states that FDA must, upon written request of the applicant, meet with that party within 100 days of receipt of the filed PMA application to discuss the review status of the application. Prior to this meeting, FDA must inform the applicant in writing of any identified deficiencies and what information is required to correct these deficiencies. FDA must also promptly notify the applicant if FDA identifies additional deficiencies or any additional information required to complete agency review. Sections 201(a), 205(a), and 209(b) provide early collaboration and allow for frequent interaction between the applicant and FDA to address deficiencies.

Section 205(c) deals with labeling claims for PMAs. FDA must rely solely on the conditions of use submitted as proposed labeling in the PMA application, so long as the proposed labeling is neither false nor misleading. In this determination, FDA shall fairly evaluate all material facts pertinent to the proposed labeling.

There are a host of other provisions incorporated into FDAMA, many reflect the agency's new philosophical approach that redefines and broadens FDA's original character as a self-reliant public health law enforcement agency (6).

2002—The Medical Device User Fee and Modernization Act (MDUFMA) amended the Federal Food, Drug, and Cosmetic Act to provide FDA important new responsibilities, resources, and challenges (7). MDUFMA has three significant provisions:

1. *User fees for premarket reviews*: PMAs, product development protocols (PDPs), biological license applications (BLAs), certain supplements, and 510(k)s are now subject to fees.
2. Establishment inspections may be conducted by accredited persons (third parties), under carefully prescribed conditions.
3. There are now new regulatory requirements for reprocessed single-use devices.

The standard fee for PMAs, PDPs, BLAs, premarket reports, panel track supplements, and efficacy supplements is $185,000 for FY 2008, rising to $256,384 in 2012. The fee for 510(k)s is $3404 for 2008 rising to $4717 in FY 2012.

2007—Food and Drug Administration Amendments Act of 2007 (FDAAA). Key provisions related to medical devices included amendments to MDUFMA that reauthorized the user fee program for medical devices for an additional five years through fiscal year 2012. The new law restructures the fee schedule to provide manufacturers with more predictability and stability in the payment of fees. The law defines three additional types of applications: (*i*) a "30-day notice" for manufacturing changes to a device subject to a PMA; (*ii*) a "request for classification information" made under Section 513(g) of the Act; and (*iii*) an "annual fee" for a periodic report to a Class III device, commonly referred to as the PMA annual report. The law also defines three types of device establishments that are subject to a registration fee: a manufacturer, a single-use device reprocessor, and a specification developer. The new law reduces the following fee reductions for small businesses: (*i*) 25% reduction for a PMA, a premarket report, a supplement, or periodic (annual) report under and PMA; and (*ii*) a 50% reduction for a 510(k), a 30-day notice, or a request for classification information. The new amendments also extend authority for third party review of 510(k)s, requires FDA to require the label of medical devices to bear a unique identifier, and adds a number of provisions to the Pediatric Medical Device Safety and Improvement Act. Administrative changes related to 510(k)s include the requirement to complete Form FDA 3674 (a Standards Data Report). This form applies to all firms that choose to use a standard in the review of any new 510(k), whether traditional, abbreviated, or special. Device manufacturers who conduct clinical studies should also be aware of new information that must be submitted to FDA's clinical trials data bank. Certification will be required for PMAs, humanitarian device exemptions, and certain 510(k) application with clinical data.

PREMARKET NOTIFICATION (510k)

Premarket notification or a 510(k) is required before a manufacturer can commercialize a nonexempt Class I, a Class II, or a preamendment Class III device. (Preamendment refers to the period before May 28, 1976.) A 510(k) submission is a marketing application submitted to FDA to demonstrate that a medical device is as safe and as effective or substantially equivalent to a legally marketed device that was or is currently on the U.S. market and that does not require PMA. The premarket notification requirements are found in 21 CFR Part 807, Subpart E. A device is substantially equivalent if in comparison to a legally marketed device it has the same intended use, and has the same technological characteristics as the legally marketed device or has different technological characteristics, and submitted information does not raise new questions of safety and effectiveness, and demonstrates that the device is as safe and as effective as the legally marketed device. All 510(k) applications must include descriptive information, labeling, and may require performance and effectiveness testing depending upon the technological characteristics of the device and the risks associated with its application. Performance and effectiveness information may include mechanical bench testing, biocompatibility, animal testing, and clinical evaluation. (Clinical data are required in less than 10% of all 510(k) submissions.) Devices in contact with the human body must be biocompatible (8) and most implanted and life-supporting devices require clinical evaluation in support of a 510(k) application. If the FDA determines the device to be substantially equivalent (SE), it can be marketed. If FDA determines the device is not substantially equivalent (NSE), the manufacturer may resubmit another 510(k) with new data, file a petition to reclassify the device, or submit a PMA. The agency has issued guidance on premarket notification review times to improve and facilitate the clearance process. (See FDA and Industry Actions on premarket notification [510(k)]. Submissions: Effect on FDA Review Clock and Performance Assessment issued May 21, 2004.)

To streamline the evaluation of premarket notifications for certain Class I devices, Class II devices subject to premarket notification, and preamendments Class III devices for which FDA has not yet called for PMAs, the agency has developed "The New 510(k) Paradigm." The new paradigm presents device manufacturers with two new optional approaches for obtaining marketing clearance for devices subject to 510(k) requirements. While the new paradigm maintains the traditional method of demonstrating substantial equivalence, it also presents the "Special 510(k) Device Modification" option, which utilizes certain aspects of the Quality System Regulation, and the "Abbreviated 510(k)" option, which relies on the use of guidance documents, special controls, and recognized standards to facilitate 510(k) review. (See The New 510(k) Paradigm: Alternate Approaches to Demonstrating Substantial Equivalence in Premarket Notifications, Issued March 20, 1998.)

The FDA has issued a guidance document to assist manufacturers who file traditional and abbreviated 510(k)s. (See Format for Traditional and Abbreviated 510(k)s, CDRH, Office of Device Evaluation, Document issued on August 12, 2005. A traditional 510(k) is the most common type, the submitter provides descriptive information about the indications for use and technology and, if not identical to the predicate device, results of performance testing to demonstrate substantial equivalence. An abbreviated 510(k) provides an effective means of streamlining the review of data in a 510(k) through reliance on one or more FDA-recognized consensus standards, special controls established by regulation, or FDA guidance documents. The FDA has also issued guidance for manufacturers who incorporate software components as part of their devices or when devices are composed solely of software. (See Guidance for the Content of Premarket Submissions for Software Contained in Medical Devices issued on May 11, 2005.)

The PMA process must, in most cases, begin with a clinical trial and its requirements are included in the following sections on IDEs. The IDE/PMA process is not a trivial undertaking. It will likely take three to five years to complete (Fig. 1).

CLINICAL DATA

Clinical data are required in all PMAs. The PMA applicant must provide a cogent demonstration of the safety and effectiveness for all diagnostic and/or therapeutic medical claims for the device based on laboratory, animal, and clinical data.

Regardless of the type of marketing application, the clinical data must be based on sound scientific principles to demonstrate the end point of substantial equivalence or safety and effectiveness. These principles consist of a proper study design, including controls and the adequate number of patients, monitoring of the study to assure the protocol is followed by the investigators, and proper analysis of results.

A PMA based solely on foreign clinical data and otherwise meeting the criteria for approval may be approved if the foreign data are applicable to the U.S. population, medical practice, and the requirements for informed consent in conformance with the Declaration of Helsinki; the studies have been performed by clinical investigators of recognized competence; and the data may be considered valid with the

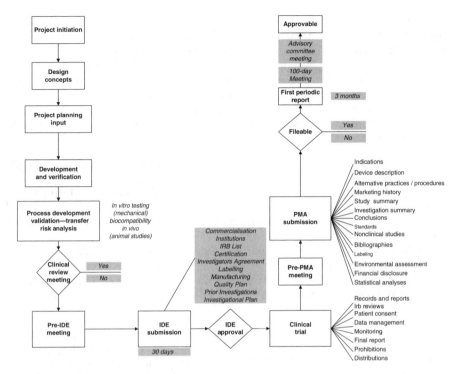

FIGURE 1 IDE/PMA flowchart.

need for an on-site inspection by FDA, or, if FDA considers such an inspection to be necessary, FDA can validate the data through an on-site inspection or other appropriate means. Applicants who seek approval based solely on foreign data should meet with FDA officials in a "presubmission" meeting.

All clinical studies performed in the United States in support of a 510(k) or PMA must be conducted in accordance with the IDE regulation. (21 CFR Part 812.)

INVESTIGATIONAL DEVICE EXEMPTIONS

The IDE regulation was published in 1976 and last updated in 1997. Devices being evaluated under IDEs were exempted from the original current good manufacturing practices regulations (cGMPs) because it was believed that it was not reasonable to expect sponsors of clinical investigations to ensure compliance with cGMPs for devices that may never be approved for commercial distribution. However, sponsors of IDE studies were required to ensure that investigational devices were manufactured under a state of control. When the new Quality System Regulation was passed, the Commissioner made it clear that investigational devices must follow design control procedures found in Section 820.30 (9). To allow device manufacturers intended solely for investigational use to ship devices for use on human subjects, the Act authorizes FDA to exempt these devices from certain requirements of the Act that would apply to devices in commercial distribution. Clinical evaluation of devices not cleared for marketing, unless exempt, requires an approved IDE either by an institutional review board (IRB) or an IRB and FDA, informed consent for all patients adequate monitoring and necessary records and reports. The exemptions from the Act include misbranding under Section 502, registration, listing, and premarket notification under Section 510, performance standards under Section 514, PMA under Section 515, banned devices under Section 516, records and reports under Section 519, restricted device requirements under Section 520(e), current good manufacturing practice requirements with the exception of Design Controls, and color additive requirements under Section 721.

The five primary regulations regarding clinical studies included in the Code of Federal Regulations, Title 21 (21CFR 21), are as follows:

- Part 812, which provides the procedures for the conduct of clinical studies with medical devices.
- Part 50, which provides the requirements and general elements of informed consent.
- Part 54, which provides the requirements for financial disclosure by clinical investigators.
- Part 56, which provides the procedures and responsibilities for IRB.
- *Part 11 Electronic Records and Signatures*: This has become an integral element in all FDA inspections. An excellent paper that excels in demystifying the records process and compliance issues with Part 11 should be reviewed prior to initiating a clinical study (10).

There are other regulations that affect clinical research. These relate to patient privacy, and are included in 45 CFR Parts 160 and 164. They set forth guidelines for the protection of patient health information. 45 CFR Part 142 provides guidance for the security of such information. The regulations are collectively referred to as HIPAA or Health Insurance Portability and Accountability Act (11). HIPAA has definitions for the organizations it covers. These organizations are termed Covered Entities and Business Associates. HIPAA defines Covered Entities as Health Care Providers, Health Care Plans, and Health Care Clearinghouses. These organizations are required to comply with the regulations. However, there is another type of relation entitled Business Associates that covers organizations with access to protected health information (PHI) for legitimate reasons. Business Associates must have legal contacts in place in order to receive PHI. These agreements cover the Business Associate's responsibilities when receiving PHI. Organizations participating in clinical research must have HIPAA compliant informed patient consents and/or data use agreement for any research study. Specific language must inform the patients that they have the following rights:

- The purpose for collecting patient information.
- Who will see the information?
- How and how long the information will be used?
- The patient's ability to cancel permission to use the information.

For specific language and details concerning the informed patient consent and data use agreement, sponsors should review the information available from the Department of Health and Human Services Centers for Medicare and Medicaid Services or their privacy officers (12). Another useful link to a guidance document specifically related to research under the HIPAA privacy regulations can be accessed (see Ref. 13 for link).

All clinical investigations for devices must have an approved IDE or be exempt from the IDE regulations. Exemptions are listed in 21CFR 812(c), which include

(1) exceptions for devices, other than transitional devices, in commercial distribution before May 28, 1976, when used or investigated in accordance with the labeling in effect at that time;

(2) exceptions for diagnostic devices if the testing is noninvasive, does not require an invasive sampling procedure that presents significant risk, does not by design or by intention introduce energy into a subject, and is not used as a diagnostic procedure without confirmation of the diagnosis by another medically established diagnostic product or procedure;

(3) a device undergoing consumer preference testing, testing of a modification, or testing of a combination of two or more devices in commercial distribution, if the testing is not for purpose of determining safety or effectiveness and does not put subjects at risk;

(4) a device intended solely for veterinary use;

(5) a device shipped solely for research on, or with laboratory animals and specially labeled [812.5(c)]; and

(6) exceptions for custom devices, unless the device is being used to determine safety or effectiveness for commercial distribution.

Investigations that are not exempt from the IDE regulation are subject to differing levels of regulatory control depending on the level of risk. The IDE regulation distinguishes between *significant risk* (SR) and *nonsignificant risk* (NSR) device studies and the procedures for obtaining an IDE differ accordingly. The determination of whether a study presents an SR is initially made by the sponsor of the device. A proposed study is then submitted to an IRB for review. If the IRB agrees with the sponsor that the device study presents an NSR, no IDE submission to FDA is necessary. A sponsor of an SR study must obtain both IRB and FDA approval before starting a study. An SR device study is defined [21 CFR 812.3(m)] as a study of a device that presents a potential for serious risk to the health, safety, or welfare of a subject and (*i*) is an implant; or (*ii*) is used in supporting or sustaining human life; or (*iii*) is of substantial importance in diagnosing, curing, mitigating, or treating disease, or otherwise prevents impairment to human health; or (*iv*) otherwise presents a potential for serious risk to the health, safety, or welfare of a subject. An NSR device investigation is one that does not meet the definition of an SR study. (There is a blue book memorandum or FDA Information Sheet #D86-1 that further clarifies the difference between significant and NSR medical device studies.)

AN IDE SUBMISSION

In order to conduct an SR device study, a sponsor must

- submit the investigational plan and report of prior investigations to an IRB for review and approval;
- submit a complete IDE application to FDA for review (see application section below) and obtain FDA approval of the IDE; and
- select qualified investigators, provide them with necessary information (information brochure) on the investigational plan and report of prior investigations, and obtain signed agreements from them.

The following information must be included in an IDE application for an SR device investigation. A sponsor cannot begin a study until FDA and IRB approval are granted. Three copies of a signed application are required and the application shall include

- name and address of sponsor;
- a complete report of prior investigations;
- an accurate summary or a complete investigational plan;
- a description of the methods, facilities, and controls used for the manufacture, processing, packing, storage, and installation of the device;
- an example of the agreements to be signed by the investigators and a list of the names and addresses of all investigators;
- certification that all investigators have signed the agreement, that the list of investigators includes all investigators participating in the study, and that new investigators will sign the agreement before being added to the study;
- a list of the names, addresses, and chairpersons of all IRBs that have or will be asked to review the investigation and a certification of IRB action concerning the investigation;
- the name of address of any institution (other than those above) where a part of the investigation may be conducted;
- the amount, if any, charged for the device and an explanation of why sale does not constitute commercialization;
- a claim for categorical exclusion (e.g., by stating "Devices shipped under the IDE are intended to be used for clinical studies in which waste will be controlled or the amount of waste expected to enter the environment may reasonably be expected to be nontoxic") or provide an environmental assessment, as provided for in 21 CFR 25.31;
- copies of all labeling for the device;
- copies of all informed consent forms and all related information materials to be provided to subjects;
- any other relevant information that FDA requests for review of the IDE application.

An investigational plan shall include the following items and in the following order:

1. Purpose (the name and intended use of the device and the objectives and duration of the investigation).
2. Protocol (a written protocol describing the methodology to be used and an analysis of the protocol demonstrating its scientific soundness).
3. Risk analysis (a description and analysis of all increased risks to the research subjects and how these risks will be minimized; a justification for the investigation; and a description of the patient population including the number, age, sex, and condition).
4. Description of this device (a description of each important component, ingredient, property, and principle of operation of the device and any anticipated changes in the device during the investigation).
5. Monitoring procedures (the sponsor's written procedures for monitoring the investigation and the name and address of each monitor).
6. Labeling (copies of all labeling for the device).

7. Consent materials (copies of all forms and materials given to subjects to obtain informed consents).
8. IRB information (a list of the names, addresses, and chairpersons of all IRBs that will review the investigation and a certification of any action taken by them).
9. Other institutions (the name and address of any other institution not previously identified at which a part of the investigation may be conducted).
10. Additional records and reports (a description of any records or reports of the investigation other than those required in Subpart G of the IDE regulation).

As mentioned above under the FDAMA of 1997, a manufacture should schedule a pre-IDE meeting to discuss its proposed investigational plan prior to submitting an IDE.

A report of prior investigations is also required in an IDE application. It must include reports of all prior clinical, animal, and laboratory testing of the device. It should be comprehensive and adequate to justify the proposed investigation. Specific contents of the report must include:

• a bibliography of all publications, whether adverse or supportive, that are relevant to an evaluation of the safety and effectiveness of the device;
• copies of all published and unpublished adverse information;
• copies of other significant publications if requested by an IRB or by FDA;
• a summary of all other unpublished information (whether adverse or supportive) that is relevant to an evaluation of the safety and effectiveness of the device; and
• if nonclinical laboratory data are provided, a statement that such studies have been conducted in compliance with the good laboratory practice (GLP) regulation in 21 CFR Part 58. If the study was not conducted in compliance with GLPs, include a brief statement of the reason(s) for noncompliance.

SUBMITTING AN IDE

There are no preprinted forms for an IDE application; however, an IDE application must include all of the information described in 21 CFR 812.20(b). FDA will not review an incomplete submission. The sponsor must demonstrate that there is reason to believe that the risks to human subjects from the proposed investigation are outweighed by the anticipated benefits to subjects and the importance of the knowledge to be gained, that the investigation is scientifically sound, and that there is reason to believe that the device as proposed for use will be effective. A suggested format and checklist for preparing IDE applications is included in HHS Publication FDA 96-4159 IDEs Manual available on the FDA's Web site (14). Sponsors can also receive information from the Division of Small Manufacturers Assistance (DSMA) by calling toll free 800-638-2041 or by fax 301-443-8818. All submissions, in triplicate, should be addressed to Food and Drug Administration, Center for Devices and Radiological Health, IDE Document Mail Center (HFZ-401), 9200 Corporate Boulevard, Rockville, Maryland 20850, U.S.

FDA ACTION ON APPLICATIONS

FDA will notify the sponsor in writing of the date it receives an IDE. FDA may approve, approve with modification, or disapprove. An investigation may not begin until 30 days after FDA receives the IDE application for the investigation of a device unless FDA notifies the sponsor that the investigation may not begin, or until FDA approves by order an IDE for the investigation. FDA may disapprove or withdraw approval of an IDE if FDA finds the following:

- The sponsor has not complied with the applicable requirements of the IDE regulation, other applicable regulations, statutes, or any condition of approval imposed by an IRB or FDA.
- The application or report contains untrue statements or omits required material or information.
- The sponsor fails to respond to a request for additional information with the time prescribed by FDA.
- There is reason to believe that the risks to the research subjects are not out-weighed by the anticipated benefits or the importance of knowledge to be gained; that the informed consent is inadequate; that the investigation is scientifically unsound; or that the device as used is ineffective.
- It is unreasonable to begin or continue the investigation because of the way the device is used, or the inadequacy of the investigational plans; the reports of prior investigations; the methods, facilities, and controls used for the manufacturing, processing, packaging, storage, and installation of the device; or the monitoring and review of the investigation.

If FDA disapproves an IDE application or proposes to withdraw approval, it will notify the sponsor in writing. A disapproval order will contain a complete statement of the reasons for disapproval and will advice the sponsor of the right to request a regulatory hearing under 21 CFR Part 16. FDA will provide an opportunity for a hearing before withdrawal or approval unless FDA determines that there is an unreasonable risk to the public health if testing continues.

When FDA grants approval, the sponsor will be notified and the study can commence with due consideration to a host of responsibilities. The study will be granted a unique identifier beginning with the letter G, that is, G08XXXX. The number 08 is used for 2008, the XXXX is a sequential number supplied by Document Management. FDA often grants conditional approval, allowing the study to start, pending correction of minor deficiencies. FDA considers the existence of an IDE as confidential and it will not disclose the existence unless FDA determines that the information had been previously disclosed to the public, or that FDA approves a PMA for a device subject to an IDE or the device has in effect a PDP notice of completion.

Note: PDPs will not be included in this section as they have been rarely employed.

RESPONSIBILITIES OF SPONSORS

Sponsors are responsible for selecting qualified investigators and providing them with the information they need to properly conduct an investigation. Proper monitoring of the investigation, ensuring IRB review and approval, and informing the IRB and FDA promptly of any significant new information that occurs during the device research. Sponsors must ensure that investigators are qualified by training and experience. Control of the device is of critical importance. A sponsor shall ship investigational devices only to qualified investigators participating in the investigation. Sponsors should review 21 CFR 812.43 to ascertain all of the requirements for an investigator's agreement and sponsors should supply all investigators with copies of the investigational plan and the report of prior investigations of the device.

A sponsor who discovers that an investigator is not complying with the signed agreement, the investigational plan, the requirements of Part 812 or other applicable FDA regulations, or any conditions of approval imposed by the reviewing IRB or FDA shall promptly either secure compliance, or discontinue shipments of the device to the investigator and terminate the investigator's participation. A sponsor shall also require that an investigator dispose of or return the device, unless this action would jeopardize the rights, safety, or welfare of a subject.

Once the study begins, sponsors shall immediately conduct an evaluation of any unanticipated adverse device effect. An unanticipated adverse device effect means any serious adverse effect on health or safety or any life-threatening problem or death caused by, or associated with, a device, if that effect, problem, or death was not previously identified in nature, severity, or degree of incidence in the investigational plan or application, or any other anticipated serious problem associated with a device that relates to the rights, safety, or welfare of subjects. On a practical note, adverse effects that appear in a study that are not included in the package insert may be considered "unanticipated."

To further demonstrate that IDE studies are not trivial matters, there are a number of records and reports sponsors are responsible for. The following records must be maintained:

- all correspondence including required reports;
- records of shipment and disposition;
- signed investigator's agreements;
- records concerning adverse device defects whether anticipated or not;
- any other records that FDA requires to be maintained by regulation or by specific requirement for a particular device or category of devices.

The following reports must also be prepared:

- *Unanticipated adverse device defects*: Within 10 working days after receiving notice of the adverse effect, and submitted to FDA and all reviewing IRBs and investigators.
- *Withdrawal of IRB approval*: Within five working days of receipt of the withdrawal of IRB approval, and submitted to FDA and all reviewing IRBs and participating investigators.
- *Withdrawal of FDA approval*: Within five working days after receipt of the notice of withdrawal of FDA approval, and submitted to all reviewing IRBs and participating investigators.
- *Current list of investigators and addresses*: Every six months, and submitted to FDA for an SR device study.
- *Progress reports*: At regular intervals and at least yearly, and submitted to all reviewing IRBs. For an SR device, the sponsor shall also submit the progress report to FDA.
- *Recalls and device disposition*: Within 30 working days after receipt of a request to return, repair, or dispose of an investigational device, and submitted to FDA and all reviewing IRBs.
- *A final report*: The sponsor shall notify FDA and all reviewing IRBs within 30 working days of the completion or termination of an SR device investigation, and submit a final report to FDA and all reviewing IRBs and participating investigators within six months after the completion or termination of the investigation.

For a nonsignificant risk device, the sponsor must submit a final report to all reviewing IRBs within six months after the completion or termination.

- *Use of a device without informed consent*: Within five working days after receipt of notice of such use, and submitted to FDA.
- *SR device determination*: Within five working days of an IRB determination that the device is an SR device and not an NSR device as proposed, and submitted to FDA.
- *Other reports*: Accurate, complete, and current information about any aspect of the investigation that FDA or the reviewing IRB may request.

RETENTION PERIOD

Sponsors shall maintain the records listed above during the investigation and for a period of two years after the latter of the following two dates: the date on which the investigation is terminated or completed, or the date that the records are no longer required for purposes of supporting a PMA or a notice of completion of a PDP.

INSPECTION

FDA has the authority to inspect facilities at which investigational devices are being held including any establishments where devices are manufactured, packed, installed, used, implanted, or where records of use are kept. Sponsors, IRBs, and investigators are required to permit authorized FDA employees reasonable access at reasonable times to inspect and copy all records of an investigation. Upon notice, FDA may inspect and copy records that identify subjects.

RESPONSIBILITIES OF INVESTIGATORS AND IRBS

Subpart D in Part 812 covers the responsibilities of IRBs as specified in Part 56 (The IRB regulation). Subparts E and G include responsibilities for investigators including compliance, device disposition, informed consent, and records and reports.

IDE GUIDANCE

FDA's Office of Device Evaluation, Center for Devices and Radiological Health, has developed a number of information sheets and guidance policies to help sponsors conduct clinical trials. IDE Memorandum #D94-1 is particularly helpful. It contains an IDE Checklist for Administrative Review that sponsors can use to ensure that their IDE is administratively complete. Another important document is entitled "Implementation of the FDA/HCFA Interagency Agreement Regarding Reimbursement Categorization of Investigational Devices—IDE Memorandum #D95-2." This memo establishes procedures pertaining to the reimbursement of investigational devices. Health Care Financing Administration (HCFA), now the Center for Medicare and Medicaid Services (CMS), governs payment for Medicare and Medicaid Services. Sponsors should be aware of the category their investigational device is assigned to, A or B. Category A is reserved for innovative devices believed to be in Class III for which "absolute risk" of the device type has not been established. Category B includes those device types known to be safe and effective because, for example, other manufacturers have obtained FDA approval/clearance for that device type. For purposes of determining Medicare coverage, medical devices classed as Category B could be viewed as "reasonable and necessary" if they also meet all other Medicare coverage requirements. Companies that consider embarking on clinical trials would be wise to investigate whether there are reimbursement issues to consider including coding, coverage, and payment. Clinical utility should be part of the decision process. The study must demonstrate that the subject device has a beneficial therapeutic effect, or that as a diagnostic tool, it provides information that measurably contributes to a diagnosis of a disease or condition. (See FDA Guidance #P91-1, 5/3/91.)

LABELING
Special labeling is required for investigational devices. (See 21 CFR 812.5.)

An investigational device or its immediate package shall bear a label with the following information: the name and place of business of the manufacturer, packer or distributor, the quantity of contents, if appropriate, and the statement—CAUTION—Investigational Device. Limited by Federal (or United States) law to investigational use. The label or other labeling shall describe all relevant contraindications, hazards, adverse effects, interfering substances or devices, warnings, and precautions.

PROHIBITION OF PROMOTION AND OTHER PRACTICES
A sponsor, investigator, or any person acting for or on behalf of a sponsor or investigator shall not (*i*) promote or test market with an investigational device, until after FDA has approved the device for commercial distribution; (*ii*) commercialize an investigational device by charging the subjects or investigators for a device a price larger than that necessary to recover costs of manufacture, research, development, and handling; (*iii*) unduly prolong an investigation; and (*iv*) represent that an investigational device is safe or effective for the purposes for which it is being investigated. (See 21 CFR 812.7.)

IMPORT AND EXPORT REQUIREMENTS
In addition to complying with other sections of the IDE requirements, a person who *imports* or offers for importation of an investigational device shall be the agent of the foreign exporter with respect to investigations of the device and shall act as the sponsor of the clinical investigation, or ensure that another person acts as the agent of the foreign exporter and the sponsor of the investigation. A person *exporting* an investigational device shall obtain FDA's prior approval, as required by Section 801(e) of the Act or comply with Section 802 of the Act.

PMA
PMA is the FDA process to evaluate the safety and effectiveness of all Class III devices. Due to the level of risk associated with Class III devices, FDA has determined that general and special controls alone are insufficient to assure their safety and effectiveness. Therefore, these devices require a PMA application under Section 515 of the Act, in order to obtain marketing clearance.

Under Section 515 of the Act, all devices placed into Class III are subject to PMA requirements. PMA is the process of scientific and regulatory review to ensure the safety and effectiveness of Class III devices. An approved PMA is, in effect, a private license (some would say a regulatory patent) granted to the applicant for marketing a particular medical device. A Class III device that fails to meet PMA requirements is considered to be adulterated under Section 501(f) of the Act and cannot be marketed. PMA requirements apply differently to preamendment devices, postamendment devices and transitional Class III devices.

Manufacturers of Class III preamendment devices, devices that were in commercial distribution before May 28, 1976, are not required to submit a PMA until 30 months after the promulgation of a final classification regulation or until 90 days after the promulgation of a final regulation requiring the submission of a PMA, whichever period is later. FDA may allow more than 90 days after promulgation of a final rule for submission of a PMA.

A postamendment device is one that was first distributed commercially on or after May 28, 1976. Postamendment devices that FDA determines are SE to preamendment device. Class III devices are subject to the same requirements as the preamendment devices. FDA determines substantial equivalence after reviewing an applicant's premarket notification [510(k)]. Postamendment devices determined by FDA to be NSE to either pre- or postamendment classified into Class I or II are "new" devices and fall automatically into Class III. Before such devices can be marketed, they must have an approved PMA or be reclassified into Class I or II.

Class III transitional devices, that is, devices considered to be a new drug or antibiotic drug before May 28, 1976, and "new" devices are automatically classified into Class III by statute and require PMA by FDA before they may be commercially distributed. Applicants may either submit a PMA or PDP, or they may petition FDA to reclassify the devices into Class I or II. Clinical studies in support of a PMA, PDP, or a reclassification petition are subject to the IDE application.

The PMA requirements are found in 21 CFR Part 814. Not all Class III devices require an approved PMA to be marketed at this time. Class III devices that are SE to devices legally marketed through May 28, 1976, and do not currently require PMA may be marketed through the 510(k) process until FDA publishes a regulation requiring the submission of a PMA application process for those Class III devices.

THE PMA SUBMISSION

Section 515(c) of the Act specifies the required contents of PMA applications to be as follows:

(a) Full reports of all information, published or known to or which should reasonably be known to the applicant, concerning investigations that have been made to show whether or not such device is safe and effective.

(b) A full statement of the components, ingredients, and properties and of the principle or principles of operation, of such device.

(c) A full description of the methods used in, and the facilities and controls used for, the manufacture, processing, and, when relevant, packing and installation of such device.[a]

(d) An identifying reference to any performance standard under Section 514, which would be applicable to any aspect of such device if it were Class II, and either

---

[a] Guidance is available to assist manufacturers in preparing the quality system information required in the PMA application. This is particularly valuable for companies who elect modular review. If the company elects to use this method, FDA suggests that the design control information and manufacturing information be submitted in modules that are separate from other information. (See Quality System Information for Certain Premarket Application Reviews; Guidance for Industry and FDA Staff issued February 3, 2003.)

adequate information to show that such aspect of such device fully meets such performance standard or adequate information to justify any deviation from such standards.

(e) Such samples of such device and components thereof as the Secretary may reasonably require, except that where the submission of such samples is impractical or unduly burdensome, the requirement of this subparagraph may be met by the submission of complete information concerning the location of one or more such devices readily available for examination and testing.

(f) Specimens of the labeling proposed to be used for such device.

(g) Such other information relevant to the subject matter of the application as the Secretary, with the concurrence of the appropriate panel under Section 513, may require.

FORMAT

To facilitate FDA's handling of PMA applications, the following recommendations are offered:

- Use paper with nominal dimensions of $8^1/_2$ by $11''$.
- Use at least a $1^1/_2''$ wide left margin to allow for binding into jackets.
- Use three-holed punched paper.
- If the submission exceeds $2''$ in thickness, separate into volumes and identify volume number.
- Clearly and prominently identify submission as an original PMA application or, for additional submissions to a PMA application, clearly identify the FDA assigned document number (e.g., P080000) and type of submission (amendment, supplement, or report) and the type of submission (e.g., Response to an FDA letter dated _____).
- All copies of each submission must be identical.
- Sequentially number the pages, providing a detailed table of contents, and use tabs to identify each section.
- Send six copies of an original PMA and three copies of amendments and supplements (except as specified below) directly to

  Food and Drug Administration
  Center for Devices and Radiological Health
  PMA Document Mail Center (HFZ-401)
  9200 Corporate Blvd.
  Rockville, Maryland 20850, U.S.

- If an amendment or supplement refers to more than one PMA, three copies of the submission must be submitted for each PMA. If more than one PMA is affected by the submission, the applicant may wish to submit three complete copies to one of the PMAs and cover letters to the other PMAs that incorporate by reference that complete copy and identify all affected PMAs.
- All copies of the first volume of each submission must include a signed and dated cover letter.
- Do not combine PMAs, IDEs, and 510(k)s together. They must be separate submissions.
- Only the PMA applicant on record with FDA may amend, supplement, or submit reports to their PMA, unless the PMA includes the original and not a copy of an appropriate letter of authorization from the applicant permitting another person to submit information on behalf of the applicant.

To facilitate review of a PMA, FDA suggests the following information be submitted in separate volumes.

Manufacturing information. Manufacturing information should be submitted in a separate volume of which only five copies are needed for FDA review. Guidance on Quality System Regulation Information for PMAs was released for comment on August 3, 1999.

Environmental assessment (21 CFR 25.34). If an applicant believes that their device qualifies for an exemption, they must provide information that establishes to FDA's satisfaction that the device meets the criteria for a categorical exclusion (21 CFR 25.24). The majority of PMA applications have been granted categorical exclusion.

Color additives. Applicants may have responsibilities to demonstrate color additives remaining in or on the device are safe. The addition of any additives to the device requires biocompatibility information that includes chemical identification and toxic potential determination for all residues remaining in or on the device. Manufacturers may use color additive regulations in 21 CFR Parts 70 to 82 as a reference to get more information, but toxicity of color additives for food may not be relevant to devices. If a color additive has not been previously listed, manufacturers may need to submit a color additive petition. (See HHS Publication FDA-97-4214—Premarket Approval Manual, January 1998.)

Individual subject report forms. A PMA or PMA supplement, if applicable, is required by 21 CFR 814.20(b)(6)(ii) to include copies of individual case report forms for each subject who died during a clinical investigation or who did not complete the investigation. Before submitting the PMA, the applicant should consult with the Office of Device Evaluation (ODE) reviewing division to determine the information to be included in these report forms, how many copies are required, and whether these forms will be required for other subjects enrolled in the study (e.g., subjects experiencing specified adverse effects or complications).

PMA FILING REVIEW

Once the manufacturer files the PMA application, FDA must make a threshold determination about whether the application is sufficiently complete for the agency to undertake a substantive review. The PMA regulation [21 CFR 814.42(e)] states that FDA may refuse to file a PMA if *any* of the following applies:

1. The PMA is incomplete because it does not on its face contain all of the information required under Section 515(c)(1)(a–g) of the Act.
2. The PMA does not contain each of the items required under Section 814.20 and justification for omission of any item is inadequate.
3. The applicant has a pending premarket notification under Section 510(k) of the Act with respect to the same device, and FDA has not determined whether the device falls within the scope of Section 814.1(c).
4. The PMA contains a false statement of material fact.
5. The PMA is not accompanied by a statement of either certification or disclosure as required by 21 CFR Part 54 Financial Disclosure by clinical investigators.

Section 814.20 of the regulation further specifies that PMAs must include, among other things, *"technical sections which shall contain data and information in sufficient detail to permit FDA to determine whether to approve or deny approval of the application* [21 CFR 814.20(b)(6)]." The key issue here is that the phrase "data and information in sufficient detail" sometimes leads to subjective interpretations. Because of this, CDRH has frequently expressed the need for more specific guidance in applying this regulatory standard to the PMA application filing decision-making process.

PRESUBMISSION INTERACTION

Before submitting a PMA, applicants are encouraged to interact with CDRH review staff. Such presubmission interaction is an important way of improving the quality and completeness of a PMA and, thus, increases the likelihood of fileability. Applicants are also encouraged to meet face-to-face with CDRH staff before preparing the PMA to discuss issues related to their specific device and PMA. CDRH PMA Manual (mentioned earlier) as well as other applicable CDRH device–specific guidance documents provide valuable information for preparing PMAs, all of which are available on the Internet (15). Excellent guidance with regard to filing review is now available on the Internet. The document issued on May 1, 2003 is entitled "Premarket Approval Application Filing Review"; it supersedes PMA Filing Decisions (P-90-2), dated May 18, 1990, and PMA Refuse to File Procedures (P94–1), dated May 2, 1994.

FDA ACTION ON A PMA

FDA must review a PMA within 180 days after receiving an application that is accepted for filing and to which the applicant does not submit a major amendment. FDA will review the PMA and the requirements of 814.39(e) after receiving the recommendation of the appropriate advisory committee, and will send the applicant one of the following: an order approving the PMA, approval letter, a not approvable letter, or an order denying approval. The approvable letter and the not approvable letter will provide an opportunity for the applicant to amend or withdraw the application, or to consider the letter to be a denial of the PMA. The applicant may request administrative review under 515(d)(3) and (g) of the Act.

FDA STEPS IN THE PMA APPLICATION PROCESS

From FDAs perspective, the review of a PMA is time and resource intensive (Fig. 2). The review involves a number of offices and divisions.
The following constitutes all of their responsibilities:

- ODE Filing Review
- Office of Surveillance and Biometrics Statistical Review for Filing
- Office of Compliance (OC) Review of Manufacturing Information for GMP Inspection anytime after PMA filing
- PMA Filing Decision
- GMP Inspection(s) by the Field
- Bioresearch Monitoring (BIMO) Audit of several investigational sites
- Substantive Review Coordination and Completion in Areas such as

    preparation of FDA Summary of Safety and Effectiveness Data (SSED)
    nonclinical studies
    microbiological

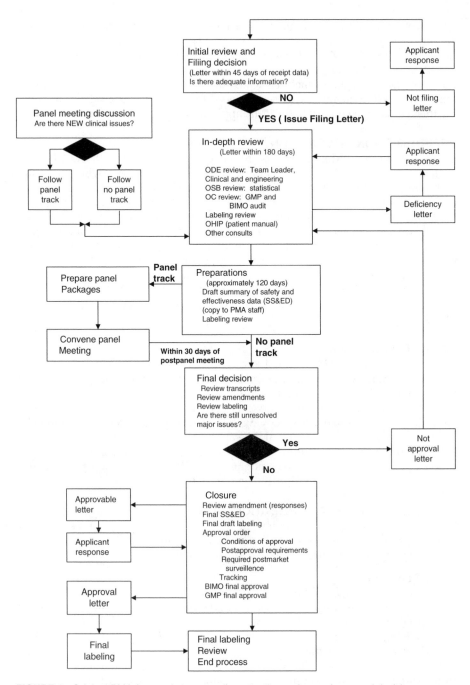

FIGURE 2 Original PMA (premarket approval) application review and approval decision process.

toxicological
immunological
biocompatibility
shelf life
analytical (for in vitro diagnostics)
animal studies
engineering (stress, wear, fatigue testing, etc.)
clinical studies

- Panel Meeting Decision and Mailing (if panel meeting is appropriate)
- Panel Date
- Transcripts Received, Reviewed, and Placed in Administrative Record
- GMP Clearance
- Final Response from OC for GMP/BIMO
- Final ODE Decision Memo
- Approval Package—Action Memo, Approval Order, Federal Register Notice, SSED, Final Draft Labeling

PANEL REVIEW

Unless the device meets the criteria for a "me too" product, panel review will be required. Section 512(c)(2) of the Act requires that a PMA be referred to an appropriate FDA Advisory Panel "for study and for submission . . . of a report and recommendation respecting approval of the application. The definition of a "me too" device can be found in FDA Guidance #P86-6, 7/25/86.

CONDITIONS OF APPROVAL

Whenever the manufacturer has completed all of the requirements for the PMA and FDA has completed its favorable review, the agency will issue standard postapproval conditions. These "conditions of approval" are applicable to all original PMAs and PMA supplements. Applicants should carefully read the conditions of approval enclosed with the FDA approval letter. Conditions of approval include submission of final printed labeling; advertising requirements whereby a brief statement of the intended uses, relevant warnings, precautions, side effects, and contraindications must be provided; supplemental submissions whenever changes are made to the device; postapproval reports; adverse reaction and device defect reporting; and reporting under the Medical Device Reporting (MDR) Regulation.

AVAILABILITY OF SAFETY AND EFFECTIVENESS SUMMARIES FOR PMAS

The FDA publishes a list of PMAs that have been approved. The list is intended to inform the public of the availability of safety and effectiveness summaries of approved PMAs through the Internet and the agency's Dockets Management Branch. Persons with access to the Internet may obtain the documents at the Web site (see Ref. 16 for link) . Copies are also available from the Dockets Management Branch. Submit written requests for copies to the Dockets Management Branch (HFA-305), Food and Drug Administration, 5630 Fishers Lane, Room 1061, Rockville, Maryland 20852, U.S. Cite the appropriate docket number (17).

REFERENCES

1. Public Law No. 75-717, 52 Stat. 1040 (1938).
2. Public Law No. 94-295, 90 Stat. 540 (1976).
3. Public Law No. 101-629, 104 Stat. 4511 (1990).
4. Public Law No. 102-300, 106 Stat. 238 (1992).
5. Public Law No. 105-115, 111 Stat. 2296 (1997).
6. Suydam LA and Kubic MJ (2000). FDA's implementation of FDAMA: an interim balance sheet. Food Drug Law J 56, 131–135.
7. Public Law No. 107-250 (2002).
8. Biological Evaluation of Medical Devices—Use of ISO 10993 (FDA Guidance #G95-1, 5/1/1995).
9. 61 Federal Register 52654 (October 7, 1996).
10. Wood D (Summer 2003). The Management of 21 CFR 11 Compliance in Clinical Trials, Monitor, pp. 39–43.
11. Public Law No. 104-191, 110 Stat. 1936 (1996).
12. http://www.cms.hhs.gov/hipaa.
13. http://www.hhs.gov/ocr/hipaa/guidelines/research.pdf.
14. www.fda.gov/cdrh.
15. http://www.fda.gov/cdrh/guidance.html.
16. http://frwebgate.access.gpo.gov/cgi-bin/leaving.cgi?from=leavingFR.html&log=linklog.
17. 67 Federal Register 67629 (November 6, 2002).

Orphan Drugs

Richard A. Guarino

Oxford Pharmaceutical Resources, Inc., Totowa, New Jersey, U.S.A.

INTRODUCTION

The term "orphan drug" refers to a drug or biologic that treats a rare disease affecting fewer than 200,000 of the US population. Many diseases that fall into this statistic are not treated simply because it is not economically feasible to develop drugs for them. The Federal government had to find a way to make it more attractive for drug manufacturers to develop drugs for this group of diseases. As a result, former President Ronald Reagan signed into law on January 4, 1983, the Orphan Drug Act (ODA). This Act created much needed changes in order to provide resources that would allow the development of products to treat these rare diseases and conditions. The National Institute of Health (NIH) estimates that there are 6000 rare diseases affecting 25 million Americans. As a result, the ODA has become one of the most important pieces of health care legislation today and has had worldwide impact. In Japan, the term orphan drug describes 2.5 cases or less per 10,000 people. The European Union (EU) criterion for establishing an orphan drug is a condition with a population prevalence of five cases or less per 10,000. Orphan drug legislation has been enacted in Japan and has been in force since April 2000, and in the EU via the Committee on Orphan Medicinal Products of the European Medicine Agency (EMEA), aggressive steps in encouraging the development of orphan drugs have been implemented. However, each country makes its own decisions on the pricing and reimbursement of orphan drug products. In late 2007, the FDA and the EMEA had come to an agreement whereby the same application could be used for both agencies, thereby reducing the time and finances required of companies to apply for orphan drug status.[a] There are an estimated 7000 so-called "orphan diseases" identified around the world and they occur in more than one out of ten people. These patients faced very limited treatment for these diseases and most had a poor prognosis. With the ODA in the United States and the implementation of the

---

[a] COMMON EMEA/FDA ORPHAN MEDICINAL PRODUCT/DRUG DESIGNATION. The sponsor of a medicinal product for human use may desire to seek orphan designation of its medicinal product for use to diagnose, treat, or prevent a rare disease or condition from the European Commission in accordance with Regulation (EC) No. 141/2000 of December 16, 1999 and Commission Regulation (EC) No. 847/2000, and from the United States Food and Drug Administration (FDA) in accordance with Section 526 of the Federal Food, Drug, and Cosmetic Act (FDCA) (21 U.S.C. 360bb). In such case, the sponsor may apply for orphan designation of the same medicinal product for the same use in both jurisdictions by using a common application form for its submission to the EMEA and the FDA. The application may be submitted to the EMEA and to the FDA Office of Orphan Products Development. The CFR 21 Part 316 details all the regulations for orphan drugs in the United States.

development of orphan drugs globally, approximately 1800 treatments have entered the research pipeline designated with orphan drug status and more than 300 products have been approved by FDA and other global agencies compared to a mere 10 products developed before 1983 (1).

BENEFITS FOR DEVELOPING ORPHAN DRUGS IN THE UNITED STATES
The ODA provides several development incentives:

1. It provides for the development of drugs for diseases that ordinarily would not generate enough revenue to make it worthwhile for a company, thus benefiting society.
2. It provides tax incentives: a tax credit of 50% of the cost of conducting human clinical trials (2).

Final regulations on the tax credits were published in the Federal Register on October 3, 1988 (53 FR 38708), and the current version of these regulations are in Title 26, Code of Federal Regulations, Section 45c. The Internal Revenue Service administers the tax credit provisions, and specific questions about the interpretation of the law or regulations affecting the applicability of the tax credit provision of the Act should be directed to IRS. If more information on tax credits is needed, contact Pass Through and Special Industries Division, Office of the Chief Counsel, Internal Revenue Service, 1111 Constitution Avenue, NW, Washington, D.C. 20224, U.S.; telephone number is (202) 622-3120.

3. Product exclusivity, a seven-year market exclusivity to sponsors or companies of approved orphan products.

CFR 21 Subpart D 316.31 Orphan Drugs provides a seven-year period of exclusive marketing to the first sponsor who obtains marketing approval for a designated orphan drug or biological product. Exclusivity begins on the date when the marketing application is approved by FDA for the designated orphan drug, and applies only to the indication for which the drug has been designated and approved. A second application for the same drug for a different use could be approved by FDA.

One thing to remember is that although there may be exclusivity to an orphan product granted an NDA, there is no exclusivity to the orphan designation itself; thus, two competitors may be pursuing an NDA for the same indication. If the products are sufficiently similar, the first one with an NDA will be the one with exclusivity. Unless the competitor can show that his product is unique and different from the other product, he will be denied an NDA. If the two products can be shown to be significantly different from each other, both will be granted an NDA, assuming they both pass the government's scrutiny on review.

With regard to the scope of orphan drug exclusivity, FDA notes the following in 21 CFR 316.31—Scope of orphan-drug exclusive approval:

(a) After approval of a sponsor's marketing application for a designated orphan-drug product for treatment of the rare disease or condition concerning which orphan-drug designation was granted, FDA will not approve another sponsor's marketing application for the same drug before the expiration of seven years from the date of such approval as stated in the approval letter from FDA, except that such a marketing application can be approved sooner if, and such time as, any of the following occurs:

          (i)   withdrawal of exclusive approval or revocation of orphan-drug designation by FDA under any provision of this part;

          (ii) withdrawal for any reason of the marketing application for the drug in question;

          (iii) consent by the holder of exclusive approval to permit another marketing application to gain approval

          (iv) failure of the holder of exclusive approval to assure a sufficient quantity of the drug under Section 527 of the Act and Section 316.36.

   (b) If a sponsor's marketing application for a drug product is determined not to be approvable because approval is barred under Section 527 of the Act until the expiration of the period of exclusive marketing of another drug product, FDA will so notify the sponsor in writing.

It should also be noted that if the sponsor receives NDA approval and then is not able to provide sufficient supply, he might lose exclusivity. He can either consent to let other applications be filed, or the director may decide to grant approval to other applications. FDA may withdraw exclusivity even if other applications are not pending. Once withdrawn, exclusive approval may not be reinstated for the drug (3).

4. It provides Federal research grants for clinical testing of new therapies to treat and/or diagnose rare diseases.

The FDA, through Office of Orphan Products Development (OOPD) Grant Program, encourages clinical development of products for use in rare diseases or conditions. The products researched can be drugs, biologics, medical devices, or medical foods. Grant applications are solicited through a Request for Applications (RFA) published in the Federal Register and available on the FDA Web site announcing availability of funds. These announcements are usually published in the Federal Register each year—usually in June. Applications are reviewed by panels of outside experts and are funded by a priority score.

A request for a grant to conduct a clinical trial of safety and effectiveness of an orphan product for a corporate sponsor with limited funds, or an investigator who is conducting research into a disease with an orphan designation or which is eligible for an orphan designation, would file this application. A number of products have been approved from trials given grants.

In keeping with Section 316.40—Treatment use of a designated orphan drug— prospective investigators seeking to obtain treatment use of designated orphan drugs may do so as provided in 21 CFR 312.34.

5. The OOPD coordinates research study design assistance for sponsors of drugs for rare diseases (4).

Often, a sponsor is unable to create appropriate protocols. As mentioned in the incentives, the FDA encourages the sponsor to collaborate with the agency in the development of these special protocols to evaluate the product for the orphan disease. The ODA also provides for formal protocol assistance when requested by the sponsors of drugs for rare diseases or conditions. The formal review of a request for protocol assistance is the direct responsibility of the Center for Drug Evaluation and Research (CDER) or the Center for Biologic Evaluation and Research (CBER), depending on which center has authority for review of the product. The OOPD is responsible for insuring that the request qualifies for consideration under Section 525 of the Federal Food Drug and Cosmetic Act (FFDCA). This includes determining "whether there is reason to believe the sponsor's drug is a drug for a disease or condition that is rare in the United States." A sponsor need not have obtained orphan drug designation to receive protocol assistance.

It should be understood that protocol assistance provided under the Act does not waive the necessity for the submission of an investigational new drug (IND) application by sponsors planning to conduct clinical trials with the product.

6. The OOPD also encourages sponsors to conduct open protocols, allowing patients to be added to ongoing studies. A drug that is not approved for marketing may be under clinical investigation for a serious or immediately life-threatening disease condition in patients for whom no comparable or satisfactory alternative drug or other therapy is available. During the clinical investigation of the drug, it may be appropriate to use the drug in the treatment of patients not in the clinical trials, in accordance with a treatment protocol or treatment IND. The purpose of this section is to facilitate the availability of promising new drugs to desperately ill patients as early in the drug development process as possible, before general marketing begins, and to obtain additional data on the drug's safety and effectiveness.

Criteria: FDA shall permit an investigational drug to be used for a treatment use under a treatment protocol or treatment IND providing (*i*) the drug is intended to treat a serious or immediately life-threatening disease; (*ii*) there is no comparable or satisfactory alternative drug or other therapy available to treat that stage of the disease in the intended patient population; (*iii*) the drug is under investigation in a controlled clinical trial under an IND in effect for the trial, or all clinical trials have been completed; and (*iv*) the sponsor of the controlled clinical trial is actively pursuing marketing approval of the investigational drug with due diligence.

7. Grants companies developing orphan products an exemption from the usual drug application or "user" fees charged by the FDA.
8. Companies may also be eligible for fast track review of their applications for marketing approval if their product treats a life-threatening illness.

Caveats. There are a number of caveats that the FDA adds to the mix when approving drugs for rare diseases or conditions:

1. A designation of a drug shall be subject to the condition that (*i*) if an application was approved for the drug under Section 505(b), a certificate was issued for the drug under Section 507, or a license was issued for the drug under Section 351 of the Public Health Service Act, the manufacturer of the drug will notify the Secretary of any discontinuance of the production of the drug at least one year before discontinuance, and (*ii*) if an application has not been approved for the drug under Section 505(b), and a certificate has not been issued for the drug under Section 507, or a license has not been issued for the drug under Section 351 of the Public Health Service Act and if preclinical investigations or investigations under Section 505(i) are being conducted with the drug, the manufacturer or sponsor of the drug will notify the Secretary of any decision to discontinue active pursuit of approval of an application under Section 505(b) ... or approval of a license under Section 351 of the Public Health Service Act.

2. As stated, one of the key provisions the FDA worked into the regulations was the protection of the holder of the application. For holders of NDAs that have been approved under these provisions, FDA will grant seven years market exclusivity. Section 527 of the Act notes:

    > Except as provided in subsection (b), if the Secretary (*i*) approves an application filed pursuant to Section 505(b); (*ii*) issues a certification under Section 507 (editor note, this was repealed in 1997); (*iii*) issues a license under Section 351 of the Public Health Service Act for a drug designated under Section 526 for a rare disease or condition, the Secretary may not approve another application under Section 505(b) ... or issue another license under Section 351 of the Public Health Service Act for such drug for such disease or condition for a person who is not the holder of such approved application ... or of such license until the expiration of seven years from the date of the approval of the approved application ... or the issuance of the license. Section 505(c)(2) does not apply to the refusal to approve an application under the preceding sentence.

    > The FDA goes on to note that although there is market exclusivity of seven years, if the applicant is unable to meet demand for the product, the Secretary may approve another product to meet such demand. Section 527(b) notes:

3. If an application filed pursuant to Section 505(b) is approved for a drug designated under Section 526 for a rare disease or condition ... or if a license is issued under Section 351 of the Public Health Service Act for such a drug, the Secretary may, during the seven-year period beginning on the date of the application approval ... or of the issuance of the license, approve another application under Section 505(b) ... or issue a license under Section 351 of the Public Health Service Act, for such drug for such disease or condition for a person who is not the holder of such approved application ... or of such license if (*i*) the Secretary finds, after providing the holder notice and opportunity for the submission of views, that in such period the holder of the approved application ... or of the license cannot assure the availability of sufficient quantities of the drug to meet the needs of persons with the disease or condition for which the drug was designated; or (*ii*) such holder provides the Secretary in writing the consent of such holder for the approval of other applications, issuance of other certifications, or the issuance of other licenses before the expiration of such seven-year period.

HOW TO OBTAIN ORPHAN PRODUCT DESIGNATION

It is important to establish before an orphan product development that the product is indeed entitled to an orphan product designation. The government gives one criterion as a *prevalence* of 200,000 individuals in the United States (not *incidence*). Extensive research into the disease must be conducted. There are numerous government sources or national foundations that may be enlisted to help research the disease with appropriate demographic data. All such data should be carefully compiled and tabulated for presentation to the government [21 CFR 316.21(b)].

Careful analysis must be made to assure proper presentation of the specific aspects of the disease and the product itself in relation to the disease. Presentation of the product is very important. Sponsors of orphan products that cannot prove their product's individuality in the treatment of the disease might find themselves competing with another similar product, which has also earned an orphan designation.

Several points should be noted:

1. An orphan designation does not provide any immunity from producing a valid NDA. An orphan drug NDA will be reviewed as rigorously as any NDA.
2. All orphan-designated drugs must be studied under an IND, which will be reviewed as rigorously as any other IND. If the product provides treatment for a life-threatening disease and warrants accelerated development, like any other product under development, it will be treated according to the standards for reviewing such diseases, including review under accelerated development in partnership with the FDA.
3. It also should be noted that often these rare diseases involve such a small population of subjects that they do not require manufacture under the strict requirements as an NDA; rather, these conditions often are treated as stated in the CMC sections submitted in the IND. Filing of such an IND is done with the knowledge of the FDA, and often FDA will note that the IND is granted with their knowledge and acceptance that no new NDA will be filed as a result of the studies performed under the IND. However, this is a unique situation reserved for orphan drugs. Often, there are little resources to pursue the full compliments of an NDA.

Content and format for a request for orphan drug designation can be found in 21 CFR Subpart C 316.20 and content and format of a request for written recommendations of orphan drugs can be referenced to CFR Subpart B 316.10 as outlined on page ____. Any additional data not listed in this section should be added to the request for orphan drug designation.

Once OOPD determines that the proposed compound is for a disease or condition that is rare in the United States, the request will be forwarded to the responsible division for formal review and direct response. OOPD will monitor the review process within the respective CDER/CBER reviewing division and, where possible, assists in resolving specific issues that may arise during the review process.

ORPHAN DRUG APPLICATION

Background and Significance

In order for a sponsor to obtain orphan designation for a drug or biologic product, an application must be submitted to OOPD, and the designation approved. The approval of an application for orphan designation is based upon the information submitted by the sponsor. If the information submitted to OOPD is determined not to contain adequate information on which to base recommendations to proceed with the research for an orphan product, OOPD may deny the application or request additional information. A drug that has obtained orphan designation is said to have an "orphan status." Each designation request must stand on its own merit. The approval of an orphan designation request does not alter the standard regulatory requirements and process for obtaining marketing approval. Safety and efficacy of a compound must be established through adequate and well-controlled studies.

Title 21 of the Code of Federal Regulations, Section 316.20, describes the means by which a company can actually file an application for an orphan drug designation. It is in this section that the government indicates that

> More than one sponsor may receive orphan drug designation of the same drug for the same rare disease or condition, but each sponsor seeking orphan drug designation must file a complete request for designation.

It must also be noted that one may apply for orphan-drug designation at any time in the drug development process prior to the submission of a marketing application for the drug product for the orphan indication. A sponsor may request designation of an already approved drug product for an unapproved use without regard to whether the prior marketing approval was there for an orphan-drug indication.

A sponsor's request for written recommendations from FDA concerning the nonclinical and clinical investigations necessary for approval of a marketing application of an orphan drug shall contain two copies of the following information in the format presented below. However, FDA may require the sponsor to submit additional information if FDA determines that the sponsor's initial request does not contain adequate information on which to base recommendations.

The regulations require that a permanent resident of the United States must act as the sponsor's agent upon whom service of all processes, notices, orders, decisions, requirements, and other communications may be made on behalf of the sponsor. The name of the agent must be provided (5) to

Office of Orphan Products
Development (HF-35), Food and Drug Administration
5600 Fishers Lane
Rockville, Maryland 20857, U.S.

Content and Format of a Request for Written Recommendations of Orphan Drugs (21 CFR Subpart B 316.10) (6)

Two copies or electronic submission (established with OOPD) of a completed, dated, and signed request for written recommendations must contain the following:

1. Sponsor's name and address.
2. Statement requesting written recommendations on orphan-drug development under Section 525 Act.
3. Name, title, address, and telephone number of the sponsor's primary contact person. Where applicable, a statement as to whether the sponsor submitting the request is the real party interested in the development and the intended or actual production and sales of the product. Every foreign sponsor that seeks orphan drug designation shall name a permanent resident of the United States as the sponsor's agent upon whom service of all processes, notices, orders, decisions, requirements, and other communications may be made on behalf of the sponsor. Notifications of changes in such agents or changes of address of agents should preferably be provided in advance, but not later than 60 days after the effective date of such changes. The permanent-resident agent may be an individual, firm, or domestic corporation and may represent any number of sponsors. The name of the permanent-resident agent shall be provided to Office of Orphan Products Development (HF-35), Food and Drug Administration, 5600 Fishers Lane, Rockville, Maryland 20857, United States.
4. Generic name and trade name, if any, of the product, list of the components or description of the product's formulation including chemical and physical properties. Name and address of the source of the drug if it is not manufactured by the sponsor.
5. Proposed dosage form and route of administration.

6. Description of the rare disease or condition being investigated with proposed indications for use of the product for the specific diagnosis. (Note that it is not necessary in this part to deliver volumes of information. The information provided should be factual and concise. Tabulations of statistical data are helpful in describing the subject demographics. The content of the text should be that of a peer-reviewed journal article, about 30 to 40 pages at most. If the volume of data is such that a brief presentation is not thought possible, it is suggested that the agency be contacted to discuss with them the acceptability of providing longer presentations.)

7. Current regulatory and marketing status and history of the product including
    *   whether the product is the subject of an IND or a marketing application;
    *   known marketing experience or investigational status outside the United States;
    *   report on any other similar investigations, if known;
    *   report on any adverse regulatory actions on the product.

8. Basis for concluding that the drug is for a disease or condition that is rare in the United States including
    *   size and demographic characteristics of the patient population including the source of this data;
    *   drugs or biologics that will be used in a population of more than 200,000 must have an explanation that the developing and marketing costs will not be expected to be recovered. An estimated cost and sales data should be provided [21 CFR 316.21(c)].

9. A summary and analysis of available data on the pharmacologic effects of the drug.

10. A summary and analysis of available nonclinical and clinical data on the drug including copies of pertinent published reports. (Note that if there are massive amounts of nonclinical data to be provided, it is wise to discuss the submission of large numbers of volumes to the orphan product review division. Large volumes of information must be submitted with an IND or NDA. Tabular summaries of data, with comprehensive summaries of data, are better suited for the orphan designation application.)

11. An explanation of how the pharmacologic, nonclinical, and clinical data support the rationale for using this product in the rare disease or condition.

12. A description of the population for patient recruitment for this product.

13. A detailed outline of any protocols under which the product has been previously or being investigated. If the sponsor of a drug that is otherwise the same as an already approved orphan drug seeks orphan drug designation for the subsequent drug for the same rare disease or condition, an explanation of why the proposed variation may be clinically superior to the first drug is required. (This is extremely important. The differences alone will not guarantee that the government will grant another application. One must show definitive superiority. Price is not a consideration, unfortunately, in this aspect. Considerable reduction in adverse experiences, superior availability, superior activity, etc., must be considered a part of this process.)

14. An outline of the nonclinical and clinical investigations that the sponsor intends to conduct.

15. Detailed protocols for each proposed U.S. or foreign investigation.

16. Any specific questions to be addressed by the FDA in the development plans.

Recommendations for Submission of an Orphan Drug Designation

The following is a recommended guideline of maximum page limits for the sections outlined above.

Introduction—maximum 3 pages
Research Plan—maximum 25 pages
Biographical Sketch—maximum 4 pages
Project Summary/Abstract—maximum 1 page
Project Narrative—maximum 1 page

Page limits are based on single-spaced pages, with $^1/_2$ inch margins, in unreduced 12 pt. font. Applications may not be accepted for review and may be returned for the following reasons:

1. The applicant organization is ineligible.
2. The application is received after the specified receipt date.
3. The application is incomplete.
4. The application is illegible.
5. The application is not responsive to the (RFA).
6. The material presented in the application is insufficient to permit an adequate review.
7. The dollar amount requested in the application exceeds the recommended threshold stated in the RFA.

Clinical Studies of Safety and Effectiveness of Orphan Products

One way in which orphan products are made available is for the OPD to support clinical research to determine whether the products are safe and effective. All funded studies are subject to the requirements of the FD&C Act and the corresponding Code of Federal Regulations. The goal is the clinical development of products for use in rare diseases or conditions in which either no current therapy exists or current therapy would be improved. Grants that are offered for studies intended to provide data acceptable to the agency should result in or substantially contribute to approval of these products. The FDA asks applicants to keep this in mind. It requires an explanation in the "Background and Significance" section of the application of how their proposed study will either facilitate product approval or provide essential data needed for product development.

Orphan Drug Grant Requests

In fiscal year 2008, grants awarded to support clinical trials on the safety and effectiveness of products for a rare disease or condition were anticipated to be in the range of $14 million, of which $11.2 million will be for noncompeting continuation awards. Grants will be awarded up to $200,000.00 to $400,000.00 in total. Direct and indirect costs per year up to four years, fourth year funding is available only for phases 2 and 3 clinical studies. Note that the dollar limitation will be total costs not direct costs as in previous years. Applications for grants must be submitted electronically (7). The FDA supports studies covered by this notice under Section 301 of the Public Health Service Act. Work plans submitted under the application should comply with "Healthy People 2000," a copy of which may be obtained through the Superintendent of Documents, the Government Printing Office, Washington, D.C. 20402-9325 (Stock no. 017-001-00474-0).

The FDA will consider awarding grants only to support clinical studies for determining whether the products are safe and effective for either premarket approval (devices) or in support of an IND for drugs or biologics.[b] Investigations of approved products to evaluate new orphan indications are also acceptable; however, these are also required to be conducted under an IND or IDE to support a change in official labeling. Studies that are submitted for the larger grants ($400,000) must continue in phase 2 or phase 3 of investigation. Those that are submitted for the smaller grants ($200,000) may be phase 1, 2, or 3. The various phases of clinical investigations are discussed in other chapters in this volume. Annual reports by the holder of an orphan drug designation must be made on an annual financial status report (FSR) (SF-269) form. The original and two copies of this report must be submitted to the grants management officer within 90 days of the budget expiration date.

Applications must propose a clinical trial of one therapy for one indication. The applicant must provide supporting evidence that a sufficient quantity of the product to be investigated is available to the applicant in the form needed for the clinical trial. The applicant must also provide supporting evidence that the subject population has been surveyed and that there is reasonable assurance that the necessary number of eligible subjects are available for the study. In addition, subjects must provide informed consent, and the studies must be conducted in accordance with GCP under the oversight of a duly constituted IRB/IEC.

Applications are accepted at designated times during the year. The announcements for this are published in the *Federal Register*, usually midyear. The most recent version was published in June 2007; another should be published about the same time in 2008.

Application forms are available from, and completed applications should be submitted to the Grants Management Officer, Division of Contracts and Procurement Management (HFA-522), Food and Drug Administration, 5600 Fishers Lane, Park Bldg., Room 2129, Rockville, Maryland 20857, U.S.; telephone no. 301-827-7185. Applications hand carried or commercially delivered should be addressed to 5630 Fishers Lane, rm 2129, Rockville, Maryland 20852, U.S.

Applications will be evaluated for responsiveness to the application requirements; those deemed unresponsive will be returned. Responsiveness will be based on the following criteria:

1. The application must propose a clinical trial intended to provide safety or efficacy data of one therapy for one orphan indication. Additionally, there must be an explanation in the "Background and Significance" section of how the proposed study will either facilitate product approval or provide essential data needed for product development.

---

[b] Beginning October 1, 2003, you are required to have a DUNS number to apply for a Federal grant. This is a nine-digit identification number that uniquely identifies business entities. Obtaining a DUNS number is easy and there is no charge. In order to apply electronically, applicants must have a DUNS number and register in the Central Contractor Registration database at http://www.ccr.gov. To obtain a DUNS number, call 1-866-705-5711; be certain to identify yourself as a Federal grant applicant when you call. Please place this number on the face page of the application.

2. The prevalence, *not incidence*, of population to be served by the product must be fewer than 200,000 individuals in the United States. The applicant should include, in the "Background and Significance" section, a detailed explanation supplemented by authoritative references in support of the prevalence figure. If the product has been designated by FDA as an orphan product for the proposed indication, a statement of that fact will suffice. Diagnostic tests and vaccines will qualify only if the population of intended use is fewer than 200,000 persons per year.

3. The number assigned to the IND/IDE for the proposed study should appear on the front page of the application with the title of the project. Only medical foods not requiring premarket approval are exempt. The IND/IDE must be in active status and in compliance with all regulatory requirements of the FDA at the time of submission of the application. To meet this requirement, the original IND/IDE application, pertinent amendments, and the protocol for the proposed study must have been received by the appropriate FDA reviewing division at least 30 days prior to the due date of the grant application. Studies of already approved products, evaluating new orphan indications also, must have an active IND. Exempt INDs must have their status changed to active to be eligible for this program. If the sponsor of the IND/IDE is other than the principal investigator listed on the application, a letter from the sponsor verifying access to the IND/IDEs required, and both the application's principal investigator and the study protocol must have been submitted to the IND/IDE.

4. The requested budget should be within the limits as stated in the application.

5. Consent and/or assent forms and any additional information to be given to a subject should be included in the grant application.

6. All applicants should follow guidelines specified in the PHS 398 grant application kit (8).

Scientific/Technical Review Criteria

To provide the first level of review, the FDA will convene an ad hoc expert panel. The applicant will be apprised of the makeup of the panel and will have the opportunity to discuss its makeup to assure that there will be no one sitting on the panel with a conflict of interest.

The application will be judged on the following scientific and technical merit criteria:

1. The soundness of the rationale for the proposed study.

2. The quality and appropriateness of the study design, including the rationale for the statistical procedures.

3. The statistical justification for the number of subjects chosen for the trial, based on the proposed outcome measures and the appropriateness of the statistical procedures to be used in analysis of the results.

4. The adequacy of the evidence that the proposed number of eligible subjects can be recruited in the requested time frame.

5. The qualifications of the investigator and support staff, and the resources available to them.

6. The adequacy of the justification for the request for financial support.

7. The adequacy of plans for complying with regulations for protection of human subjects.

8. The ability of the applicant to complete the proposed study within both its budget and the time limitations stated in the RFA.

A priority score will be given based on the scientific and technical review criteria noted above.

FDA Review and Actions

FDA will review the applications and make recommendations as to the completeness of the submission and any additional information that may be needed.

In Section 316.12, providing written recommendations, FDA notes the following:

(a) FDA will provide the sponsor with written recommendations concerning the nonclinical laboratory studies and clinical investigations necessary for approval of a marketing application if none of the reasons described in Section 316.14 (Refusal to provide written recommendations).
(b) When a sponsor seeks written recommendations at a stage of drug development at which advice on any clinical investigations, or on particular investigations, would be premature, FDA's response may be limited to written recommendations concerning only nonclinical laboratory studies, or only certain of the clinical studies. Prior to providing written recommendations for the clinical investigations required to achieve marketing approval, FDA may require that the results of the nonclinical laboratory studies or completed early clinical studies be submitted to FDA for agency review.

FDA may refuse to provide written recommendations concerning nonclinical and clinical investigation for various reasons such as

- incompleteness or absence of required information;
- insufficient information about the product to identify the active moiety and its physical and chemical properties;
- insufficient evidence that the disease warrants orphan designation;
- insufficient data that the product may be useful for treating the rare disease;
- regulatory and marketing history of the product demonstrating that the scope or type of investigation has already been conducted;
- proposed safety and efficacy investigations are insufficient;
- sponsor unclear asking for agency's advice;
- agency determines that the disease in question is not rare;
- agency determines there is inadequate information to permit an investigational use of the product;
- request for information from the agency contains an untrue statement of material fact.

Such refusal will be in writing. The FDA will describe the information or material it requires or the conditions the sponsor must meet for FDA to provide recommendations (9). Within 90 days after the date of a letter from the FDA requesting additional information or material, the sponsor shall provide additional information requested or amend the request or withdraw the request for written recommendations. Failure to respond to FDA with the 90-day deadline will be considered a withdrawal of the request.

Once an orphan designation is granted, it is transferable, provided the owner of the designation informs the FDA in writing of the name of the transferee, and what rights to the designation have been transferred (not all rights need to be transferred). In addition, the new owner must submit a letter accepting orphan drug designation and the date the change is effective, stating that he or she has a complete copy of the request for orphan designation including amendments and supplements and all relevant correspondence. A list of the rights assigned should also be provided. The new owner of the designation should provide a new contact name, including a U.S. agent if the new owner is a foreign company. The FDA notes that no sponsor may relieve itself of responsibilities under the ODA by assigning rights to another without assuring that the sponsor will carry out its responsibilities, or without obtaining prior permission from FDA (10).

Annual Reports

As with other submissions to FDA, the recipient of orphan designation must provide a report to the FDA within 14 months and annually thereafter until marketing approval to indicate progress, stated in 21 CFR 316.30 as follows:

(a) A short account of the progress of drug development including a review of preclinical and clinical studies initiated, ongoing, and completed, and a short summary of the status or results of such studies.
(b) A description of the investigational plan for the coming year, as well as any anticipated difficulties in development, testing, and marketing.
(c) A brief discussion of any changes that may affect the orphan-drug status of the product. For example, for products nearing the end of the approval process, sponsors should discuss any disparity between the probable marketing indication and the designated indication as related to the need for an amendment to the orphan-drug designation pursuant to Section 316.26.

The FDA will not publicly disclose the existence of a request for orphan designation, but there are certain conditions that apply, including whether the sponsor has made it publicly known that he has orphan designation. The FDA will determine whether the disclosure can be made in accordance with confidentiality requirements of INDAs and NDAs. Once public availability eligibility has been determined, FDA will publish a list in accord with Part 20 and Section 314.430 of the CFR and other applicable statutes and regulations (11).

SUMMARY

To receive an orphan drug designation for a product, a sponsor must file an application (two copies) with the FDA, according to the prescribed format in 21 CFR 316.20. If the disease affects fewer than 200,000 persons per year (or, in the case of a vaccine, the administration will be to fewer than 200,000 persons per year), the agency may grant an orphan designation. Once so designated, a proper IND must be filed, which will need to contain a full description of the product, its synthesis and method of manufacture as a drug product, its preclinical pharmacology and toxicology, and clinical protocols for the studies to be conducted. If the sponsor is unable to write the protocols, the FDA will assist in the writing and will even fund the studies if the sponsor has insufficient funds. Orphan designation is assignable, provided the sponsor assures that the new owner will act responsibly in developing the drug. If an NDA is filed and approved, there will be seven years of market exclusivity granted, as well as tax benefits. The biggest benefit is to the subjects who receive much needed help in the treatment of their disease.

It is clear that the ODA, as implemented by existing administrative practices, has significantly increased the rate at which new orphan drugs are marketed. While two or three drugs that might be eligible as orphan drugs were approved annually prior to the ODA, an average of 300 orphan drug products have been approved and marketed since 1983. Thus, the ODA, as implemented since 1983, has provided an effective stimulus for the development and marketing of drugs for diseases or conditions that are rare globally.

In debating the need for orphan drug exclusive marketing, Congress weighed the potential dangers of granting orphan drug exclusive marketing. However, Congress determined that the benefits exceeded the dangers.

Any form of exclusive marketing may have negative consequences, such as noncompetitive pricing. To date, however, there has been insufficient experience with the implementation of the statute to judge whether an optimal benefit–cost balance has been attained. It is clear, nonetheless, that these incentives have been highly successful in contributing to the development and approval of orphan drugs that would not otherwise have been developed.

The Regulatory Flexibility Act requires that the agency considers the impact of the regulation on small entities. FDA believes that these rules benefit, rather than disadvantage, most affected small businesses. Prior to enactment of the ODA, few small businesses could afford to devote resources to the discovery of new treatments for rare diseases, because the small market for such products severely limited the profitability of this research. Subsequent to enactment, the combined stimulus of research grants, tax credits, and exclusive marketing influenced many small firms to develop new products for formerly inaccessible markets. FDA and other global agencies find that the incentives provided for the developing of orphan products have brought new hope to populations suffering from rare diseases and conditions.

REFERENCES

1. Oncology Business Review,March 2008, Pharma Voice April 2008.
2. 26 CFR 1.28–1. (These are the IRS regulations on rare disease research tax credit.)
3. 21 CFR 316.36. Insufficient quantities of orphan drugs.
4. Haffner ME (1998). Orphan drug development—International program and study design issues. Drug Inf J, 32, 93–99.
5. 21 CFR 316.22. Permanent-resident agent for foreign sponsor.
6. 21 CFR 316.10. Content and format of a request for written recommendations.
7. www.grants.gov.
8. http://grants.nih.gov/grants/submitapplication.htm.
9. 21 CFR 316.14. Refusal to provide written recommendations.
10. 21 CFR 316.27. Change in ownership of orphan-drug designation.
11. 21 CFR 316.52. Availability for public disclosure of data and information in requests.

16

Clinical Research Protocols

Richard A. Guarino

Oxford Pharmaceutical Resources, Inc., Totowa, New Jersey, U.S.A.

INTRODUCTION

The clinical development of pharmaceutical products is the most important part of the new drug approval process. It is the part of an NDA/CTD submission that determines whether or not regulatory agencies, throughout the world, will approve the product to be marketed to the public. Clinical research is often the most expensive and time-consuming step in product development. Accomplishing this task requires careful scientific and strategic planning in order to meet the research objective of proving the product is not only safe for human use but also effective.

Writing clinical research protocols that objectively or subjectively evaluate pharmaceutical products is key in assuring the success of bringing products to market. A protocol becomes the "Bible" for each research trial. It must be followed exactly, without deviations, and must be the reference for any questions that arise during the course of clinical investigations. This chapter will give recommendations on the content and how to write clinical protocols for all phases of clinical research. It addresses all necessary regulatory requirements that meet GCP for FDA and EU directives. An organized format for protocol development is recommended based on its successful use in phases of clinical research. The recommendations throughout this chapter are not mandatory but may be used as guidelines and are not always applicable to all clinical programs.

The objective of most clinical trials is to record scientific data concerning the efficacy and safety of a treatment for a specific disease on which valid conclusions can be drawn. The degree of success in achieving this objective depends largely, but not entirely, on the quality of the basic trial design. Faulty execution, due either to sloppiness or (in rare instances) dishonesty, can undermine the validity and usefulness of the data generated from a particular trial site. All investigators and their staffs must be meticulous in observing and reporting their clinical observations. On the other hand, even if a lengthy trial is carried out with the utmost care, the data generated will be useless if the protocol has not been designed intelligently. Overall, it must include all the necessary ingredients so that the eventual clinical results will support IND and NDA submissions.

Because the framework of every clinical research trial relies on a number of interdependent disciplines, the development of a clinical trial protocol is ideally a multidisciplinary task. Teamwork, coordinated by one experienced person in clinical research with good knowledge of the regulatory requirements for new drug development, is essential. The protocol design team should also include input, recommendations, and review by the following:

A chemist who is fully conversant with the physical and chemical properties of the investigational drug.

A pharmacologist and/or toxicologist with a full understanding of the pharmacology and toxicology of the drug in animals and the expected effective dose, therapeutic effects, and possible adverse experiences in humans.

A medical monitor, preferably one who specializes in the condition or illness to be studied, and who is experienced in the logistics and practicalities of clinical trials.

A statistician who will address those aspects of trial design that determine the form the trial data will take for analysis and the types of analyses that will be applied to the data.

A data management person who will be both involved in coding and in charge of data entry.

A potential investigator or consultant who understands the indication of the product to be researched can determine if the objectives of the protocol and procedures are reasonable.

A capable program manager who can coordinate the multidisciplinary effort to form a final protocol, affect practical execution in the clinical setting, ensure data entry and analyses, meet timelines, and coordinate the statistical and clinical reports.

Once the specific objective of the protocol and its components have been established by the team members, an introduction containing a brief overview of the protocol development will give investigators and their staffs a better understanding of the clinical trial. The introduction should contain a summary of the Investigator's Brochure (referencing the Brochure), the purpose of conducting the trial, and the rationale of the inclusion and exclusion criteria.

The following sections of the protocol are recommendations, not requirements. There are no regulations as to what a protocol should contain or in what order the sections should be presented. However, the protocol format presented can be used as a guide in order to ensure that all the essential components of a protocol are addressed.

TRIAL OBJECTIVE

A common fault in trial design is to have too many objectives in a single trial. Objective(s) should be clearly and concisely stated. If a trial has more than one objective, the objectives should be listed in order of priority. The fewer objectives to be evaluated in one trial, the greater the chance that the results will be conclusive. The key to successful clinical trial design is simplicity. One objective per trial is an ideal way to conduct clinical research.

GENERAL CONSIDERATIONS IN PROTOCOL DESIGN

The trial protocol is the end point of research design. It is the blueprint that displays the elements of the trial plan and provides explicit instructions as to how the plan should be executed.

The protocol designers should approach the subject by first organizing a checklist similar to the one presented later in this chapter (see "Elements of a

Protocol: A Checklist"). This list will serve in protocol design much as an outline helps a writer or a speaker touch on all salient points in an article or speech. Judging from the number of NDAs that are returned to their sponsors for more clinical information requested from the FDA, one might assume that there are tricks to the art of a successful filing. No secret ingredients are needed for the successful preparation of a clinical protocol or its presentation within an IND and ultimately the NDA—just logic, completeness, and a practical and meaningful approach in evaluating the disease under investigation.

In drug development, time is of the essence. Clinical protocols should be concise, straightforward, and logical. The demands upon the investigators, their staffs, and the subjects must be reasonable. The FDA's guidelines and other countries requirements for new pharmaceutical product development, by disease, must be considered and reasonably incorporated into the protocols. The objective to remember throughout protocol development, execution and presentation of the clinical data, is to demonstrate safety and efficacy that will fulfill global regulatory requirements.

DIFFERENT TRIAL DESIGNS

Conventionally, phase 1, 2, and 3 trials refer to the successive stages of clinical product investigations while phases 3b and 4 are usually referred to research conducted during or after a product is approved. Although the objectives of all of the phases are different, they are not entirely separate entities because the information obtained from one phase provides the basis for the next. In broad terms, the objective of phase 1 is a demonstration of safety based on dose tolerance usually conducted in normal subjects; phase 2 evaluates dose tolerance and safety balanced with the degree of efficacy in a target subject population (probably the most important phase in clinical research development); phase 3 reconfirms the efficacy and safety of the selected dose established in phase 2 in a larger target subject population; phase 3b is designed for large-scale safety. Phase 4 trials are usually classified as marketing trials and are designed to demonstrate how similar or competitive products may show one having certain advantages over another. The basic principles of good scientific methods of trial design apply equally to all five phases. The major tenets of all scientific experimentation should be regarded as fundamentals of the design: the possibility of coincidence as well as bias should be ruled out, and the results produced by the trial design should yield conclusive data of safety and efficacy as confirmed by statistical reliability and specificity.

CONTROLLED TRIALS

A controlled trial is defined as one that governs and challenges an investigational drug, biologic or at times a device against a placebo or a standard marketed product that has been proven to be safe and effective and accepted in medical practice for the indication under investigation. In order to ensure that bias does not occur, the product and the controls are blinded from the investigator and the subjects; thus the trial is double blinded. Double-blind trials are usually indicated to ensure that there is no bias in data obtained from the clinical trials and the results of the statistical analysis will support the safety and efficacy claims of the investigational product. Because of ethical considerations, however, there are some drugs that cannot be evaluated under double-blinded conditions. In these cases, a sponsor should review the situation with the regulatory agencies and establish the acceptability of data with an alternate trial design. It is not unusual; however, for phase 1 trials to be open label (not blinded), because the objective is to observe the response of the investigational product primarily in terms of safety and tolerance.

Double-blinded, controlled trials that are well designed, yield the most valid results. In the majority of investigations, experimental products are blinded against placebo controls. The FDA's NDA and CTD approvals, in most cases, are based on the following:

- Two well-conducted clinical trials following GCP, proving that the test product evaluated versus placebo or another control shows statistically significant differences of safety and efficacy as compared with the control. These are termed as pivotal trials. Rare exceptions are made, with active products used as controls assumed to demonstrate similar therapeutic conditions.
- Rigid criteria should be well established to preclude investigator or subject bias. Impressions of drug efficacy or lack of the same based on previous evaluations of reported efficacy must be avoided. If the investigator or the subjects are aware of the treatments administered, the preconceptions and prejudices of both toward the treatments can create a significant bias. This extraneous variable of bias can be minimized by suitable double-blinding techniques.

The single-blind method, as the name implies, ensures that only the subject is unaware of the distribution of treatments during the trial. The possibility of investigator bias must be considered if this type of blinding is used. The double-blind method, which is now accepted as the standard blinding procedure in comparative drug trials, ensures that investigators, their staffs, and the subject are unaware of the type of treatments that are being prescribed and administered.

Blinding Techniques

Maintaining double-blind conditions in a clinical trial requires strict attention to a number of details. A product form identical to the experimental product is necessary for double-blind conditions. Pharmaceutical manufacturers usually supply their test agents and placebo in forms that meet these requirements. In some clinical trials, comparative evaluation trials using the double-blind method cannot be done on products with dissimilar formulations, for example, tablets versus syrups, ampules versus suppositories, or liquid concentrates versus capsules. Some comparison of products present additional blinding problems such as variations in physical characteristics including color, taste, texture, viscosity, shape, or size. In these instances, alternative blinding methods should be considered. The double-placebo (double-dummy) method first reported by Guarino in 1971 establishes manifest equality of product characteristics. It consists of simultaneously administering to each subject an active test agent and a placebo of the other active agent that is being evaluated (Table 1).

TABLE 1 Double-Placebo Method

Group 1 subjects	Group 2 subjects
Active drug A (tablets)	Active drug B (liquid)
+	+
Placebo B (liquid)	Placebo A (tablets)

TABLE 2 Delivery of Two Active Agents with Different Administration Regimens

	Group 1 subjects	Group 2 subjects
Time of administration	Drug A (tablets)	Drug B (capsules)
7:30 AM	Drug A placebo + Drug B placebo	Drug A placebo + Drug B active
4:00 PM	Drug A active + Drug B placebo	Drug A placebo + Drug B active
8:00 PM	Drug A active + Drug B placebo	Drug A placebo + Drug B placebo

Inasmuch as the two agents (whatever their forms) are administered simultaneously to each subject at all times during the trial, there is no way of telling the difference between active drug and placebo. In all cases, the assigned placebo is physically identical to the test agent and is administered through an identical route. In addition, the method can be adapted to compare a suppository with a liquid concentrate or syrup with a capsule. Any two drugs with different routes of administration, or different forms, can be effectively blinded in this manner and can satisfy all the rigid requirements of classical, double-blind, clinical research trials.

The procedure can also accommodate the double-blind evaluation of two active agents that must be administered at different times of the day because of their dissimilar modes of actions. Table 2 demonstrates how all subjects receive an active agent and placebo or two placebos at the same time.

Active drug and placebo are administered twice a day to all subjects in both groups: 4:00 PM and 8:00 PM for group 1 subjects, and 7:30 AM and 4:00 PM for group 2 subjects. During each day, subjects in both groups receive a total of two doses of drug A or drug B, but at different times of the day.

The double-placebo method can help overcome the problem of blinding drugs that are dissimilar with regard to color, taste, viscosity, volume, dosage equivalency, or dosage regimen. It can only prove successful under good clinical management conditions and meticulous monitoring of the trial to ensure full compliance. Double-blind, double-placebo techniques depend on reliable research coordinators who consistently check on drug administration and accountability.

No matter how rigorous the enforcement of blinding techniques, circumstances may arise that threaten the integrity of the blindness of a clinical trial. For example, a larger number of adverse reactions in one treatment group compared with another may provide a clue as to which treatment is involved, particularly in placebo-controlled trials. Likewise, different patterns of symptom response in treatment groups may suggest the treatment involved.

Blindness can also be destroyed by accidental breaking of the randomization code. With good design and adequate safeguards, however, this should not occur.

The only circumstance under which the identity of trial materials should be deliberately known is when a subject has a severe adverse reaction to a test product that makes it imperative for the investigator to know which treatment the subject received. However, the method of labeling the trial drugs should allow for this to be done without revealing the randomization code for the entire trial (see "Elements of a Protocol, Labeling of Trial Medications").

UNCONTROLLED TRIALS

Most regulatory agencies, reviewing a new product application, especially for new drugs for clinical use, do not accept the results of uncontrolled trials as stand-alone evidence of safety and efficacy. There are, however, circumstances under which data from uncontrolled trials can provide acceptable evidence of safety as well as efficacy: (*i*) the treatment results demonstrating consistent and clinically significant improvement in a disease with a well-established natural course and remission rate, or (*ii*) the treatment consistently results in significant improvement in all or almost all of the subjects evaluated.

Apart from the limited value of uncontrolled trials for the demonstration of efficacy, they may be helpful in obtaining an early indication of the optimum dose, an adverse reaction profile, and the preferred route of administration of a drug. Open trials are also useful in assessing safety especially when data is gathered on large numbers of subjects who were exposed to the experimental product. As a general rule, it is best to confine clinical trials in phases 1, 2, 3, and 4 to those that use adequate controls and unbiased techniques.

PARALLEL AND CROSSOVER TRIAL DESIGNS

Controlled trials can be conducted under matched pairs, parallel, crossover, group comparisons, or mixed design conditions. Parallel and crossover trial designs each have advantages and disadvantages. Both can be used to compare two or more treatments, one of which may be placebo.

In a crossover trial design, all treatments to be compared are administered to every enrolled subject in a carefully designed and blinded sequence. Subjects first randomized to the test product or control will be evaluated for a time period dictated by the protocol. Subsequently, after undergoing an interim drug washout period, the same subjects will then be rerandomized to either the test product or the control product according to what they were previously administered. Each subject receives all treatments and thus serves as his or her own control.

In trials using a parallel design, subjects are randomly assigned to one of two treatments (one which might be placebo). In spite of adequate selection criteria and random assignment, the treatment groups in a parallel design trial may indeed differ. Parallel design trials consist of comparing two groups of subjects equal in number. One group will receive the active product and the other will be assigned the control product. However, the two products will be randomly assigned in order to prevent bias.

Although the desired duration of exposure to each treatment can be achieved with both designs, there are considerations that must be taken into account before the trial design is selected. Subjects participating in a crossover trial design must be enrolled in the trial for at least twice as long as in a parallel trial design. This makes it especially necessary that investigators have a good rapport with the subjects, therefore demonstrating the ability to maintain a low subject attrition rate, as well as protocol compliance. In addition to this potential source of difficulty, another consideration would be when two active drugs are being compared, all subjects are exposed to the possible safety hazards of both drugs, or in the case of a placebo, the risk of allowing the pathology to go untreated. For the results of a crossover trial to be valid, each subject must be in the same clinical condition at the beginning of the second treatment period as at the initiation of the first treatment period. In practice, this is frequently difficult to achieve because the pharmacologic and psychological effects of the first treatment often have a carryover effect on the response to the second treatment. This is especially true if the drug administered during the first treatment period has a long biological half-life. Theoretically, these objections can be minimized by imposing a sufficiently long washout period between treatments. The theory, however, is often more easily prescribed than achieved.

There are certain obvious caveats concerning the use of the crossover design. It should not be used in drug trials involving self-limiting diseases of short duration, or with treatments that result in rapid relief or cures because of the likelihood of the illness being resolved and symptoms alleviated before the crossover takes place. Parallel group trials are more popular than crossover comparisons because they present fewer problems. The parallel group trial is probably a less complicated and expeditious way to double blind and complete a trial in a much shorter period. The difficulty, at times, using a parallel design is in recruiting the number of subjects. If inclusion and exclusion criteria are extremely difficult to recruit subjects, a parallel design might require a longer overall duration of the trial.

A Guideline for Elements of a Protocol: A Checklist

The following items provide an outline of the components that must be addressed in planning and writing a protocol for all phases of clinical research (including bioavailability trials). Although some of the headings cited below may seem obvious, often they are completely overlooked or not addressed by the protocol design team. The items listed are to be used as a checklist and not as a format. There is no regulatory requirement for protocol format. It is up to the protocol designers to decide on how a protocol should be presented to their regulatory agencies and investigators.

Title Page

Provide the full title of the trial, including, if possible, a precise description of the trial's objective. List the investigator(s) who will conduct the trial and where the investigation will take place. Many protocols are identified by a trial number assigned by the sponsor; this number should be cited throughout the protocol where necessary, particularly if there is the possibility of confusion with similar trials being conducted at the same time and location. It is sound practice to have the sponsor's name and address listed on the title page. More than one sponsor may be using the same teaching hospital or institution to conduct other clinical trials on other drugs. The following is an example of a protocol title page:

A PHASE 2 DOUBLE-BLIND PARALLEL TRIAL OF DOSE TOLERANCE, SAFETY, AND EFFICACY COMPARING DRUG A TO PLACEBO IN CONTROLLING SYMPTOMS OF MILD TO MODERATE HYPERTENSION

Chief Investigator:
Coinvestigator(s):
Address where trial will be conducted:

Trial Number:
Sponsor (Name and Address):
Date:

Table of Contents
An investigator should read the entire protocol to understand how the objective(s) of the trial will be accomplished. However, as protocols can be voluminous and certain sections and subsections of the protocol are more pertinent to other specialists who are participating in the clinical trial, for example, project coordinators, nurses, psychologists, cardiologists, radiologist, and others, a table of contents becomes invaluable. These individuals often have to refer quickly to the protocol to clarify a particular procedure or method, regulatory requirements, and so on, and will be able to do so easily with the aid of a table of contents.

Introduction/Background
The introduction of a protocol should justify the purpose of conducting the clinical investigation. Each clinical trial should have a significant purpose of why the trial is necessary and what is projected to result from the trial. No clinical trial should ever use a target subject population without the potential goal of yielding the product's risks and benefits when used for a specific diagnosis or medical advancement. If this is a single trial and the only one to be conducted using this protocol, it should be stated as such. However, if this trial is part of a multicenter trial then the overall number of subjects that will be enrolled in this multicenter trial should be stated in addition to the number of centers that will participate and the expected overall duration of the research program.

An optional part of the introduction can include all significant past research and literature references, if any, on the product being investigated; this should be carefully reviewed, summarized, and incorporated into the introduction. This section should include the following: all relevant published materials, preclinical information from the Investigator's Brochure, and any previously conducted clinical trials [with appropriate comment on the methods of observation and qualitative evaluations used in the other trials (i.e., design, placebo controls, active controls, and statistical methods)]. Other considerations are identity and potency of the product(s) being investigated, trial setting (nursing homes, psychiatric wards, outpatient clinics, etc.) and the rationale for using that setting. This should not be a repeat of a clinical brochure, but a summary of any knowledge about the drug based on completed evaluations. Many protocol writers consider the clinical brochure an adequate introduction to the protocol and the product being developed. However, it is always a concern that investigators do not always take the time to read voluminous clinical brochures but they will read the introduction of a protocol.

One of the critical areas considered by the FDA in reviewing a clinical protocol is the merit of a clinical research investigation. The introduction should satisfy the reviewer that this trial will attempt to produce a reliable solution to a scientific question about the product being tested.

Bibliography
All interpretive commentary should be referenced in a bibliography, together with all of the citations of previous research. This will assure the investigators and their colleagues about any questions that need more referencing for the experimental product.

Objective
The objective is the goal of a protocol. It should state explicitly the purpose of the clinical research project. One short statement should describe the type of trial

(i.e., open, double-blind, and crossover) and why the trial is being conducted. In addition, a brief description of the products to be used, the indication(s) for safety and effectiveness, and the type of subject population to be evaluated should be included. The objective should be stated succinctly, as in the following example: "This is a controlled, double-blind, parallel trial to evaluate the safety and efficacy of product X versus product Y in subjects (diagnosis of disease or use of the product) as found in an outpatient (or other) population." In one simple statement, the purpose of the trial, the controls, the diagnosis of the subject population, and the setting where these subjects will be observed have been presented. Objectives should reflect the phase or type of clinical research that will be conducted.

A phase 1 trial with safety evaluations based on dose tolerance as its major objective would not necessarily be double-blinded as in most phase 2, 3, and 4 trials; on the other hand, when possible, attempts should be made to use double-blind standards to guard against bias.

General

This optional section usually contains a condensed summary of the protocol. It can prove helpful to personnel charged with recruiting clinical research investigators and their staffs. In many cases, the first contact with a prospective investigator is by telephone. Initial reactions—interest or no interest—can be elicited by a reading of the general section of the protocol. It should offer a brief description of the trial objective, the trial design, the trial duration, how many evaluations will be needed for efficacy and safety, and the estimated amount of the time required from the investigators and their staffs. More importantly, it should answer the question as to whether the investigator has the subject population that meets the inclusion and exclusion criteria of the trial design. The preparation of a succinct general section can save hours of needless conversation describing protocol design and responsibilities of the investigator and staff.

Risks

Whereas risks are always a factor in all medical interventions, the relatively unknown magnitude of risks entailed in the use of a new investigational substance is the focus of much of the FDA's and other agencies' concern. The burden of proof for justifying the experimental use of an investigational product lies with the sponsor. Documentation within the IND or a preclinical submission to regulatory agencies must be presented based on data that justifies the introduction of the investigational product for use in humans. This is heavily based on preclinical research in animals: the pharmacology and toxicology of the investigational drug that affirm that the drug is probably safe at a specified dose in the defined human population. It is sometimes appropriate to weigh the relative risks of untreated disease with the projected risks with use of the investigational product. In any event, the design of the clinical trial should minimize risks to the subjects by governing adequate safety measures so that potentially the benefits will outweigh the risks.

Confidentiality

The doctor–patient relationship has traditionally entailed the right of the subject to complete confidentiality. Enrollment in a clinical trial should not compromise this right. Just as the staff in a physician's office is trained to understand that they must not breach a subject's right to confidentiality, any additional staff working with files of subjects enrolled in clinical trials must also respect this confidentiality.

Procedures by which subjects can be numbered or identified by their initials and site number should be spelled out to ensure that there is no unnecessary disclosure of the identity of the participants in the trial. (See Informed Consent and HIPAA.)

Materials and Methods
This section may include the following:

Subject Sample
Provide a statement describing the total number of subjects expected to complete the trial; this number can include an estimate of treatment failures but should not include administrative dropouts. [If subjects are transferred to other clinics, if they relocate, or if they do not complete the trial for any other reason (not product related), they should not be included in the total.] Establish the number of subjects that must complete the trial and are projected to be in the final statistical analysis. Additional subjects should always be targeted for enrollment to replace those that drop out for administrative reasons. Dropouts due to product failure are not to be replaced and will be entered as part of the statistical analysis. In conjunction with the subject's willingness to participate in the clinical trial, it is prudent to establish that each subject enrolled should be fully eligible according to the protocol criteria. Each subject should also give every clinical and personal indication that he or she can be expected to complete the full course of the investigation otherwise they should not be enrolled. Nothing is more frustrating to a sponsor—or to the designer of a protocol—than to have subjects drop or be dropped from a trial because they do not meet criteria for entry, or they fall into categories that disqualify them from receiving the trial medications, or they simply do not wish to continue in the trial because their obligations for participation in the trial were not clearly spelled out. Obviously, any subject has the right to withdraw from a clinical trial at any time, but it is up to the investigators to select trial subjects they feel are most likely to complete the trial and to avoid entering those with doubt.

Age Range
Include a precise age range for the trial subjects. Do not allow an investigator to amend the age range during the course of the investigations; it should be established before the trial is initiated and strictly adhered to. The age range for subjects should be carefully selected according to the disease being investigated. It would not be advisable, for example, to conduct a trial with schizophrenic subjects aged 65 years or older; nor should mononucleosis be studied in subjects' 40 years of age or older, inasmuch as the disease is more prevalent in younger adults. However, it should be noted that the age range selected in the clinical trials used for a new product submission is the one that will be referred to and included in the product package insert.

Gender
Indicate whether or not males, females, or both sexes will be used in the trial.

Subject Inclusion and Exclusion Criteria
These are the most important parts of protocol design. Every effort must be placed in subject selection. If the right subjects are selected for a clinical trial then the results will yield significant data for the product being investigated. No deviations should be made once the inclusion and exclusion criteria are set down in the protocol

design. If deviations are made, there will be protocol violations and the subject will become invalid for statistical analysis of safety and efficacy of the test product. If changes are to be made in one or the other of these criteria, they must be made after the protocol is amended and approved by the proper authorities. For these reasons, these criteria deserve careful and laborious consideration by experts who understand and have experience in the objective of the protocol.

Subject inclusion criteria. Describe the type of subject to be admitted into the trial. The criteria for selecting subjects must be clearly and accurately stated; the diagnosis must be well established and confirmed by the medical history of the subject. (Regulatory agencies favor a protocol with a specific diagnosis.) For example, if the diagnosis is severe hypertension, and the subject must have had it for a minimum of two years, the medical records must demonstrate that there is a history of severe hypertension for two years. Symptom criteria that will confirm the diagnosis must be carefully thought out. The inclusion criteria must state the specific symptoms that must be present in order to confirm the diagnosis. It is up to the investigator to confirm and document the diagnosis with an accurate account in the medical history and the results of a complete physical and laboratory examinations.

Subject exclusion criteria. Any subject who by every reasonable expectation would be incapable of responding to a trial drug or does not meet inclusion criteria must be ruled out. Subjects with existing ailments that would prevent the trial medication from showing its maximum therapeutic effect must be excluded from participation, as should any subject who is hypersensitive to the medications or products under investigation. The exclusion criteria should also exclude any subject whose medical history, physical condition, abnormal laboratory results nonrelated to the diagnosis, concomitant medications contraindicated with the trial medications, use or history of drug addiction, or personal habits (e.g., smoking) might compromise the integrity of the data evaluating the experimental product.

The protocol designer must pay particular attention to the number of exclusions listed in the protocol; too many can make it extremely difficult to recruit enough subjects in the trial, and too few can compromise the trial results.

Trial Procedures
An explicit explanation of the sequence of events that each subject will be expected to complete during the course of the trial is essential. Screening visits, baseline laboratory evaluations, day 1 of dosing, washout periods, postdosing evaluations, and so on, should all be discussed and mapped out. A table or flowchart of what and when these events are to take place are of key importance. At a glance, the timing of the clinical and laboratory evaluations can be monitored by the investigator and the staff. Posting this flowchart in an assigned area will facilitate all involved in keeping on tract.

Washout, drug free, dry-out, run-in-periods are all terms used to prepare the subjects to meet the inclusion criteria of the protocol especially when they were on a previous product regimen. These periods must be long enough to assure that any previous medications that might interfere or interact with the trial medications will be eliminated from the subject's system before trial medications are administered. Washout periods are critical to the success of a trial. (Placebo responders must also be considered during the predrug evaluation period.)

There are, however, exceptions to the washout period conditions. For example, if a subject exhibits symptoms of sufficient severity to warrant not withholding treatment, this subject may be entered into the trial even though the washout period is less than that specified. If a note to this effect is included in the protocol, the investigator should provide ample justification of why the washout period was not completed in the comments section of the case report form. In the monitoring of a trial, subject records should be carefully checked for validity of the reasons for exemption from the full washout period.

Note: If a pre-experimental product symptom rating falls into the category of mild or moderate and the inclusion criteria states that the symptoms should demonstrate a severe rating, and if the subject is entered into an investigation before the washout period is terminated, this rating will not justify the subject's exemption from the medication-free period unless a valid and acceptable reason is given by the investigator or a provision for this exception is stated in the protocol.

Trial Drugs
Include a complete description of the medications or products used in the protocol, including the lot number, to be used in the trial. The generic as well as the trade name (if available) should be stated. Describe the form of the drug and the placebo or comparative product (i.e., capsules, tablets, injectable, shunt, instrument, etc.). Also provide the methods of preparation, especially for the placebo (e.g., lactose or sucrose fillers). Detail the way the trial medication will be blinded. In addition, the strength of the trial medication must be stated in milligrams, grams, cubic centimeters, and so on. Description of all products must be completely and precisely stated. If marketed products are used, the details that would be stated in a package insert should be provided. If a marketed drug is used as a control, the package insert for that medication should be included as an appendix to the protocol. The dose of each product must be listed (e.g., "capsules containing 10 mg of drug X," description of any other type of product that will be used must be detailed). Ingredients and composition of each product must be listed by name, amounts of each component, and quantity.

Assignment of Trial Products
It is important to do two things for product assignment: (*i*) outline the method of randomization so that the procedure is clear and is set as a standard for all sites (in the case of multicenter trials); and (*ii*) make certain that the method of randomization is shown to be truly random and thus supportive of scientifically valid conclusions and equitable to the subjects.

Prepare an explicit description of the actual assignment of the type or types of product(s) used in the trial. For example, numbers 01 to 100 will be assigned to the trial medication bottles on a random basis, as determined by the use of a table of random numbers. Subjects will then be assigned to bottles 01 to 100 in sequence, that is, the first subject admitted into the trial will be assigned to the bottle marked 01, the second subject to the bottle marked 02, and so on. (Numbers are assigned to bottles, and subjects are assigned to numbered bottles.) When each subject is to receive only one bottle, this should be stated: "Each subject will be assigned one bottle of trial medication. The bottle will contain a total of X capsules (or tablets, cc's, etc.) of trial medication—a quantity sufficient to meet the maximum medication requirement as required by this trial (X days or X weeks, etc.)." If medication is to be administered on a daily or weekly basis, for example, bottle numbers and the quantity in each bottle for that period should be specified. A reference to the type of randomization table used should be made and footnoted. The investigator should be aware of how the medications were randomized, for example, in blocks of 4, 6, 10, and so on, so that he or she will strive to complete a block of subjects. A note should be added stating: "To allow for possible attrition, sufficient drugs will be provided for X subjects, a number beyond that required by the protocol." This point is important to explain, as it may not be immediately obvious why, if 50 subjects are required to complete a trial, the medication will be randomized for 70. This is necessary to allow for circumstantial attrition and subjects dropped for administrative reasons.

Dosage Range (if any)

Describe the dosage range to be used in the trial. If applicable, include daily minimum and maximum dosages. The dosage range, when applicable, usually is established at the end of phase 2, or if the product is marketed, these should reflect recommendations in the manufacturer's package insert.

Be sure to correlate the phase of clinical research that is being conducted and the dosage range recommended; the range used in a phase 1 trial is often much broader than that used in a phase 2. When phase 3, 3b, or 4 trials are conducted, the dosage or dosage range have already been established.

Designed to measure dose tolerance and safety, phase 1 dose ranging should be initiated and augmented very conservatively, usually based on animal toxicology data. During phase 2, the suggested dose range will, for the most part, have been influenced by results derived from the phase 1 trials. The objectives of dose tolerance and safety and efficacy in a phase 2 trial establishes the final dosage(s) to be used and are often concluded by evaluating the lowest noneffective dose and the highest nontolerated dose. The tolerated dose derived from the phase 1 trial often is not the final dose determined in the phase 2 trial. The phase 2 trials reflect responses of diseased subjects in contrast to those observed with normal subjects. Prior to the preparation of a phase 3 protocol, the minimum and maximum dosage(s) will have been determined from the phase 2 program. If not, it is almost invariably a sign that phase 2 clinical trials were not adequately conducted.

Dosage Schedule

This section addresses the question of when and what time of day or week or month the appropriate amounts of drug are to be administered: once daily (q.d.), twice daily (b.i.d.), every four hours (q4h), three times daily (t.i.d.), and so forth. If specific dosages are to be given in the morning or evening, or both, specific instructions should be provided based on the administration of trial medications.

Administration of Trial Medication

A statement should describe how the drug is to be administered to or taken by the subject: with meals, before or after meals, with liquids or dissolved in specific juices, and so on. These directions are extremely important, because different medications effectiveness may be affected by dissolution and absorption rates; some cause gastric upset if not given with food or may interact with certain elements or foods, or effect on sleep, and so on.

Labeling of Trial Medications

Labeling medications for clinical trials is completely different than marketed medication labels. It is essential that the blinding of the trial drugs be protected. Labels printed for trial drugs must be designed so that no one involved in the trial knows which medication is being administered or dispensed. The labels designed for experimental clinical research can come in different forms. Whatever form is chosen, there must be a duplication of the label on the experimental product that can be detached or matched to the identical label that is usually attached to the case report form.

One of the most reliable is the dual-labeled form in which the code is covered by a mercury film that can be scratched off easily by a coin or similar blunt object to reveal the identity of the contents of the medication/product being evaluated. Another effective type is the three-sided envelope: A B C in front and C B A in back. Section C contains the written code and is sealed to part B. If an emergency arises, the detached code label portion is immersed in warm water for two minutes and then peeled apart. If the A B C form is used, the investigator should remove and save the coded portion prior to dispensing the medication, and attach it to the case report form. These labels are to be returned to the sponsor at the conclusion of the trial. If a code label is missing from a subject evaluation form, the sponsor may not accept that subject's data for statistical analysis.

Medication Accountability

An important part of clinical research is ensuring medication accountability. Medications administered during clinical research must be counted precisely before, during, and after the completion of the clinical trial. If medications cannot be accounted for, the results of the research may be invalid. All trial medications distributed by and returned to the sponsor must be recorded. These records are extremely important and should be available upon request during all regulatory inspections in the investigators and sponsor's files. All used and unused trial medications including any unopened bottles should be accounted for by the investigator and the sponsor. While the investigator is responsible for the ultimate accountability of trial medications, it is unwise to rely solely on his or her calculations. It is recommended that the clinical research monitor either perform a medication count on-site or have them returned to the sponsor's clinical pharmacy department for recounting.

Duration of Drug Treatment

During protocol design, it is important to determine how long a medication should be evaluated before it can be determined as safe and effective. This decision is usually based on previous research or a history of clinical experience of the disease under investigation. Medications must be administered, monitored, and evaluated long enough to demonstrate optimum therapeutic response. However, diseases that have a short duration (e.g., a cold, acute headache, etc.) should not be studied longer than necessary. Evaluating a short-acting drug such as an antihistamine for two weeks in treating a cold is impractical (if more than three days are required for this type of drug to show effectiveness, it is pointless to continue treatment). In contrast, the effect of most antidepressants take at least two to three weeks in many patients before an effect can be observed. One of the most crucial determinations of effectiveness of any medication relies on whether it is possible to administer the drug for the predetermined duration and achieve a maximum therapeutic outcome without the occurrence of adverse experiences that would prohibit continuing the use of the medication.

Concomitant Medications

The protocol must list all medications that subjects are allowed to receive simultaneously with the trial medication. Any contraindicated medications or those that are to be excluded during the investigation because they might interfere, interact, or add to the action of the trial medication must be listed. It should be emphasized that subjects who receive any kind of concomitant medication contraindicated in the protocol will be dropped from the trial as a protocol violation and their data will not qualify for inclusion in the final statistical analysis of efficacy.

Regarding other medications allowed during the trial, the following or a similar statement may be useful: "Other medications that are considered necessary for the subject's welfare and that will not interfere with the trial medication may be given at the discretion of the investigator. Administration of all concomitant medications must be recorded in the appropriate section of the case report form." If the investigator administers to a subject any drug that is determined to be similar to the one under investigation, that subject will be considered a protocol violation and will dropped from the trial.

Case Report Forms (CRFs)

All data gathered on an individual subject during the course of a clinical trial are recorded on a subject's CRF. Designing an easy-to-complete, accurate case report form containing all the essential and significant data can be an arduous task. All the data evaluating the safety and efficacy of the product under trial must be recorded on the CRF. Depending on the phase of clinical research, the trial design, the products, the indication(s), the parameters being evaluated, and the duration of the observation and evaluation period, a CRF can be anywhere from five to hundreds of pages in length.

Note: The more complicated the CRF, the more chance of data inconsistency.

The case report form is the vital record of a clinical trial. It is necessary to design the CRF to collect all the data required by the protocol in a precise and orderly manner. Carefully designed CRFs are essential for the following reasons:

- As a means of checking the logistics, design, and practicality of the protocol.
- For processing data entry and statistical analysis and interpretation of the records.
- To evaluate and record safety and efficacy data that is consistent from subject to subject.
- To check for protocol adherence and/or investigator compliance.
- To fulfill regulatory requirements.

The design of the CRF is a collaborative effort of the investigator, trial coordinator, clinical monitor, program manager, statisticians, and data management personnel.

Content of the Case Report Form
1. Ensure that the history and demographic data reflect the protocol and can be verified by the subject's office/hospital records.
2. That the questions on the CRF directly address those defined in the protocol.

3. Provide definitions for terminology and scales to obtain consistency in evaluations from CRF to CRF within a trial, as well as across trials. These definitions should appear directly on the case report forms to make them readily available to the investigator.
4. Do not include additional questions that address ancillary issues. The attempt to collect and record too much information often leads to carelessness and lack of enthusiasm by the trial participants. The more that is asked for, the more variability will occur in the answers.
5. Questions should be asked directly and unambiguously free from jargon.
6. In long-term trials, the CRF may be formatted in sections and used for each visit or group of visits. This helps to decrease the likelihood of ambiguity in recording when an event occurs, as well as to help expedite the flow of data in-house and through data processing.
7. Order the questions on the CRF logically, following the order in which a physician would ordinarily collect data. Separate questions that routinely would be asked by a trial nurse from those that would be asked by the clinical investigator.
8. Be clear on how precise answers should be—should a value be rounded or carried to one or more decimal places? Lack of clarity creates some doubt in the trial recorder's mind; these result in inconsistencies and increase the difficulties for the data processing staff. Collect direct numerical measurements, where possible, rather than broad categorical judgments. This usually improves overall consistency, especially across trials. Do not ask for written text.
9. When questions include comparative terms, use positive terms such as better, bigger, and more, rather than negative terms such as worse, smaller, or less. Research has shown as much as a 20% difference in accuracy when positive terms are used.
10. Use design techniques that make the form easy to read and complete:
    (a) Balance white space with text. Make the form aesthetically pleasing, not cluttered.
    (b) Use check-off blocks (coded responses) wherever possible. Checking a block is less time consuming and error prone than entering a value or term.
    (c) Block sections of the form to make them easy to locate and complete.
    (d) Use variations in size and attributes of type (e.g., bold, italics, and underlining) for headings and for emphasis of important questions.
    (e) Highlight the areas of the form where the investigator is expected to make entries. This decreases the chance that the investigator will overlook a question and helps during the in-house review and processing of the data.
    (f) Keep calculations to a minimum.
    (g) Alphanumeric fields (such as for adverse experiences) should be sized to hold the largest possible response. Include instructions for filling out the CRF (e.g., use black ink, print, etc.).

These suggestions are also applicable to remote data entry. Whether the CRFs are physically completed or the data is entered remotely by filling out the form on the computer, the CRF instructions are applicable in both cases.

Laboratory Assessments
Laboratory assessments and electronic measures are one aspect of determining the safety of an experimental product. At times, laboratory assessments can also be applied to evaluating the efficacy of a product. Laboratories usually provide normal

ranges with appropriate notations to highlight values outside the normal ranges. These are then reviewed to determine whether the abnormality or deviations are clinically significant or severe enough to cause concern for the safety of the subjects in the clinical trial. Safety evaluation criteria can include such determinations as sequential multiple analysis computer (SMAC) tests, CBC, urinalysis, vital sign monitoring, EEGs, ECGs, CAT and PET scans, MRI, and radiologic examinations, including barium enemas and endoscopies. There are many other specialized tests capable of providing objective safety measurements. Expertise in what test to use for safety as well as efficacy evaluations should be examined. These results, coupled with any signs and symptoms attributed to drug reactions will help complete the overall picture of a drug's safety profile. Many of the safety parameters, in most instances, do not reflect the efficacy of a drug. Whereas drugs with a spotless safety profile may be more desirable, therapeutic efficacy, in balance with an acceptable safety profile, is, after all, the more realistic goal.

Safety and efficacy evaluations may be objective or subjective. Objective evaluations are simpler and more realistic to record; they represent true values of a subject's response to the experimental product.

Objective values such as numerical and photographic recordings, and so on, are easily recorded and interpreted. For example, the numbers for blood pressure, pulse rate, cholesterol, and so on, either go up or down. Other objective measurements such as lesions seen on endoscopy, radiographs, ECGs, and so on, are easy to measure the effectiveness of products. In these cases, recordings on CRFs should be easy to enter and interpret.

Subjective evaluations are much more difficult to accurately and consistently measure. Impressions of improvement of symptoms, such as a reduction in pain or assessing psychiatric disorders, measuring and rating cognitive functions, or feelings of well-being are so dependent on a myriad of factors, including investigator and staff assessments and interpretation of the subject's response, the variations of the subject's threshold as a reaction to symptoms, the mood, the day, the weather, and so on. As a result, proper standardization of the symptoms to be evaluated is essential. Although there is some confidence in using certain subjective, validated evaluations to distinguish between improvement and deterioration, it is often difficult to have the results unanimously accepted. One approach to measuring subjective evaluations with unknown scales is to ascertain that there is an acceptable explanation for quantifying the severity or improvement that the investigator is evaluating. For example, if a symptom such as pain is being measured using a seven-point scale [from 0 (absent) to 7 (extremely severe)], the interim points may be designated as very mild, mild, moderate, moderately severe, and severe, each term being precisely defined. As an example, the types of definitions, listed below, are designed to reduce bias (variables) and increase accuracy in scoring the results. In other words, a numeric value is placed on a degree of pain that corresponds to a definition. By using this method to rate subjective symptoms, we gain consistency of data, especially when the trial is multicenter.

1 (=Absent): Feels no pain.
2 (=Very mild): Feels pain once a week.
3 (=Mild): Feels pain three times per week.
4 (=Moderate): Feels pain every day, but not severe enough for medication.
5 (=Moderately severe): Feels pain every day and needs mild pain medicine for relief.

6 (=Severe): Feels pain all the time and needs strong pain medicine for relief.
7 (=Extremely severe): Feels pain all the time and gets no relief from pain
    medication.

Of course, variations in defining degrees of severity for any subjective rating
are totally dependent on the experience of the investigators evaluating the symptoms of the diagnosis under treatment with the product being evaluated. Once this
input is defined, the creator of the scale and the scope of the overall objective of the
trial should be reflected in the final clinical research evaluation form.

Adverse Experiences

The protocol should include an adverse experience statement, such as "All adverse
experiences occurring during the trial must be reported on the drug reaction record
provided in the subject case report forms." The drug reaction record is a complete
questionnaire that covers all pertinent items concerning adverse experiences. (See
chap. 19.)

In addition, there should be a procedure for reporting serious, fatal, and life-
threatening reactions expeditiously to the sponsor or the CRO assigned this responsibility. A qualified physician should be on call during the overall conduct of the
trial. Adverse experiences, whether they result in death, life-threatening situations,
or adverse reactions to the experimental product must be reported on a consistent
basis to the sponsor and the IRB/IEC. This will enable the sponsor and the IRB/IEC
to make any changes in the protocol necessary for safety of the subjects and to
report the applicable adverse experiences within the required time frame following
GCP regulations. This is discussed in chapter "Adverse Reactions and Interactions
of Drugs." Most protocols require that unexpected and severe, life-threatening, or
fatal adverse experiences be reported immediately by telephone to the sponsor or
their designate; a "24-hour" telephone number must be included in every protocol.
The information recorded on the drug reaction record or report should be complete
enough to enable the sponsor to provide the regulatory authorities with the proper
and legal material necessary for reporting these adverse experiences.

Data Entry and Statistical Methodology of Data

No clinical protocol is complete without a statistical methodology sections. The statistical handling section of the protocol must be finalized before an investigational
trial begins. Protocol design should be reviewed and discussed with a biostatistician before it is finalized and presented to clinical investigators. Early input from
a biostatistician is vital in the planning and writing of a protocol and leads to the
success of a clinical research program. The CRFs should be developed and coded
with statisticians before printing; this will facilitate data entry and expedite data
processing. Electronic data entry should be programmed to reject any data that do
not comply with the protocol. Requirements set forth in the protocol require careful planning and adherence to procedures such as numbers of subjects necessary
to achieve statistical significance, time when efficacy and safety evaluations must
be done, and so on. This will generate the type and quantity of scientific data necessary to achieve statistically valid documentation that is expected to confirm the
safety and efficacy of a drug. The statistical handling of the data is an integral part
of the research protocol and is designed in the early planning stages of the trial.
It cannot be an afterthought when a mass of data has already been collected. The

FDA will not accept the clinical data of any phase of a clinical trial if the statistical methodology is not incorporated into the protocol before the initiation of the trial.

Overall Duration of the Trial

The maximum allowable time required by an investigator to complete the evaluations of all subjects entered into the trial should be clearly stated. The agreed-upon schedule should be strictly observed. Be realistic in your expectations. If an investigator estimates that he or she can handle 50 subjects in one year, it may be safe to assume that it may take two years to complete the investigation. Some investigators do not realize how much work is required in completing the CRFs for the number of subjects necessary to conclude a clinical trial successfully. Another area that consistently prolongs a clinical trial, especially in phases 2 and 3, is subject recruitment. The timetable described in the protocol must be reviewed with the investigator so that the time commitment is fully understood. If a flowchart is created, use it to demonstrate how many evaluations have to be completed over a defined period. For example, if a trial calls for the entry of five subjects per week and four or five CRF pages for that subject's entry (e.g., a physical, a history, a laboratory examination, and baseline determinations) and, in subsequent weeks, the trial calls for two or three evaluations per week, by the third week an investigator will have 16 to 21 evaluations. In a 50-subject trial with each subject evaluated for five weeks, by the fifth week, the investigator will have 28 to 37 evaluations. It is apparent, then, that it is more practical for an investigator to enter fewer subjects over a longer period and to persevere in completing the trial in a precise manner rather than be faced with an impossible burden of work, deadline, sloppy data evaluations, and failure. It should be emphasized to the investigator that subjects meeting the criteria of the protocol are not the same as in clinical practice, but scientific research and adherence to the protocol requires a different discipline and a more concentrated effort in recruiting subjects that meet protocol criteria.

Institutional Review Board (IRB) Independent Ethics Committee (IEC)

A formally recognized and certified IRB/IEC must review the proposed clinical research protocol to determine whether the relative safety and anticipated benefits to subjects are adequately and fairly represented in the protocol design. If the research is to be done at a large hospital or teaching institution, it is likely that there is an affiliated IRB/IEC. Independent certified IRBs/IECs are used for investigator sites that conduct clinical research that do not require an affiliation with a hospital or institution. A protocol designed for a multicenter trial must be reviewed by an IRB/IEC for every site requiring that the investigator obtain their institutions review before conducting a clinical research trial. Providing that the investigator is not obligated to do this, a central IRB/IEC may give permission to investigators to conduct the clinical research. All protocols used in clinical research must have an IRB/IEC approval before subjects may participate in a clinical research trial. (See chap. 21.)

No clinical trial plan is complete unless all the necessary precautions have been taken to protect the safety and rights of the subject. All trials conducted in the United States must be designed and carried out in accordance with Parts 50 and 56 of Title 21 of the Code of Federal Regulations (CFR), the regulations concerning the safety and rights of subjects. For foreign investigations, either ICH guidelines or European Directives must be followed according to the requirements of each country.

It must be remembered that an IRB/IEC will assess the following principal ethical requirements of a clinical research trial before allowing the research program to start:

1. The risks to participants are minimized and are reasonable in relation to the anticipated benefits. That periodic review of the trial's progress will conclude that the benefits outweigh the risks.
2. Selection of subjects is equitable.
3. Appropriately worded and documented informed consent is obtained from each prospective participant or from a legally authorized representative if the participant is considered unable to give such consent.
4. The research plan makes appropriate provisions for monitoring the safety of the participants.
5. The privacy of the participants and confidentiality of the data will be maintained.
6. The protocol objective will conclude a benefit for subjects suffering with the disease under investigation.

Informed Consent (IC)

Some institutions have a preferred format for the IC form to be executed by subjects that will be participating in the clinical trial under the auspices of that institution. The purpose of an IC is to ensure that no clinical experimentation is carried out on people who are unaware or unwilling to participate in an investigational clinical program. As this is a crucial tenet of modern investigational medicine, the protocol must specify that each subject must execute an IC document prior to enrollment in the clinical research trial. This does not mean prior to being administered an experimental product. Specifically, before a subject is entered into a trial the IC must be signed. In the case of a participant who is considered incompetent, a legally authorized representative must execute the document. Children under the age of 18 must have a parent or guardian sign the IC. These consent forms become part of the subject's permanent records and made available upon request for inspections by regulatory agencies. (See chap. 21.)

Monitoring

The following statement should be included in all trial protocols: "At regular intervals throughout the trial, the investigator will allow a representative of the sponsor's monitoring team, or the sponsor's designate, or a representative of the FDA to inspect all case report forms and corresponding portions of an enrolled subject's original office and/or hospital medication records. These inspections are for the purpose of verifying adherence to the protocol, the viability of the data entered on the case report forms, adverse experience reporting, product accountability, and investigator reliability.

The monitor overseeing a clinical trial (typically called a Clinical Research Associate, or CRA, in the pharmaceutical industry) has to confirm that all of the necessary information requested on the CRF has been recorded accurately. During a site visit, the monitor should be alert to the items on the CRF that are key to the trial objectives. In an anxiety–depression trial, for example, the most important symptoms are anxiety, tension, depression, or other anxiety–depression-related symptoms. These must be carefully noted and documented. The CRA should notice any changes recorded during the course of an investigation that indicate trends occurring across the participating subject population, for example, an adverse experience that is consistently reported, an increase in dropout rate, and so on. If there are significant rating changes after a certain number of weeks or after an assumed drug effect, these should be carefully documented and discussed with the investigator. A completed evaluation form for every subject in a clinical trial is of paramount importance.

It is also the monitor's responsibility to account for all concomitant medications. Unfamiliar drugs should be cross-checked in the *PDR* to determine if any component(s) of the medication taken concomitantly with the investigational drug violates the protocol. All brand and generic names of drugs should be legible and identifiable. Monitors must assure that every adverse experience has been reported and documented properly.

Other items, such as dosage titration information, should be examined, recorded, and (when applicable) reported with comments as to the reasons for these changes. Any incomplete item on a CRF must be explained and any data changes must be legible and not erased. All these must be signed and dated, and when needed, a statement from the investigator substantiating the reasons for the incomplete or changed entry must be obtained. Any problems a monitor encounters during a clinical trial should be discussed as soon as possible and expeditiously resolved and reported. (See chap. 21)

Location of Trial
List the investigator(s) name(s), address(es), and telephone number(s) where the trial is to be conducted. If more than one location is involved (institutions, universities, and other medical offices), provide their locations as well.

Location of Laboratory Testing Facilities
List the names, addresses, and telephone numbers for all test laboratories involved in the trial. An investigator must be able to contact laboratory personnel at all times. The protocol must include the information of where laboratory testing is being conducted. The laboratory director's CV and the laboratory's certification number have to be kept on file.

Investigator's Obligations
When agreeing to participate in the sponsor's clinical trial, an investigator is making several contractual agreements that must be clearly understood. The protocol must be adhered to, especially the enrollment criteria, the blinding procedures, and the meticulous and timely record keeping. A realistic estimate of the number of eligible subjects the investigator will be able to enroll and keep in the trial to last evaluation follow-up will help to minimize the difficulties of conducting rigorous clinical investigations. Not baring any unexpected delays, the agreed-upon time frame for completion of the trial should be adhered to. It is also advisable to receive written assurance from the investigator that he or she agrees to conduct the trial according to the protocol design and will adhere to the GCP regulations (21 CFR Part 312). The investigators should also be aware that signing the Form FDA 1572 also obligates them by federal law to follow GCP. When foreign investigators participate in clinical programs that emanate data that will be used in U.S. regulatory submissions, they also should sign a Form 1572.

In addition, the investigators in the United States must complete Financial Disclosure Forms, that is, Form FDA 3454 (no financial interest) or Form FDA 3455 (financial interest). These forms will confirm any or no financial involvement of the investigator with the company or product they are investigating.

Signature Page

Allow space for the investigator's signature and the date the protocol agreement is signed. The sponsor's clinician also should sign off on the protocol.

Amendments and Addenda

Amendments

Amendments to protocols have created a lot of controversy through the years. According to regulation 312.30 in the CFR, any change in phase 1, 2, and 3 protocols that significantly affects the safety or efficacy of subjects, the scope of investigation, or the scientific quality of the trial will require an amendment to the protocol. Some examples of these changes are an increase in drug dosage, an increase in the duration of exposure to an experimental product, beyond that stated in a protocol, or increase of trial population size. Other examples are adding or dropping a control group, adding a new test or procedure or reduce the risk of, adverse experiences or, conversely dropping a test intended to monitor safety. Overall, any significant change in the design of a protocol that may affect the subject's safety requires additional testing of the subject, and will, require an amendment to the protocol.

Any change that would apply to any of the above-stated items must have approval from the FDA, and should be submitted as an amendment to the FDA with written approval from an IRB before its implementation. At the same time, if there is a change in the protocol intended to eliminate an apparent hazard to subject's well-being, it may be implemented immediately, provided that the FDA and the IRB are subsequently notified of a protocol amendment. It is important to remember that all protocol amendments to the FDA should be properly identified and labeled "Protocol Amendment: Change in Protocol." In the case of a change in a protocol, a brief description of the change in reference to the submission that contained the original protocol should be submitted with the amendment. When new investigators are added to the trial, this amendment to the IND can be implemented as soon as the investigator receives IRB approval.

Although amendments can be submitted at any time during the conduct of a clinical investigation, not more than one amendment per month is the rule. Amendments should be very carefully thought out before it is decided to make one. Statistically, it is very difficult to deal with the changes made from the original protocol design in the final statistical analysis. The analysis of these data must reflect the results of the subject's evaluations before and after amendments. In the analysis of the results of all subjects in trials with or without amendments, it is difficult to conclude results based on different protocol designs, such as subjects previously admitted to the trial with no history of hepatic disease and subsequently, through an amendment, allowing subjects into a trial having a hepatic disease one year before entering the trial. It is imperative, therefore, to abide by the initial recommendation of this chapter, that is, whenever possible, do not change a protocol once it has been designed with diligence, intelligence, and expertise to meet the original objectives of the clinical trial plan. It should also be remembered that any amendments that reflect on the subject must be incorporated into the IC and presented to the subjects for their signature of acceptance. Amendments should never be done after 49% of the subjects have entered the trial unless to further guard the safety of the subject.

Addenda
Often when protocol designers speak of addenda, they confuse them with amendments. There is a distinct difference from amendments, which are changes that can affect the safety and efficacy of the subject. Addenda are simply additions to the protocol that do not change the safety and efficacy evaluations of the subjects or the original protocol design. For example, if specific quantities of blood are being drawn from a subject and another laboratory test is added using this same blood sample, this is an addendum. This typical addendum to the protocol does not change any procedures from the original protocol and does not affect the safety of the subject. It is usually an additional test that may be reported in the final statistical analysis and clinical report.

Addenda to the protocol do not have to be submitted to the FDA or IRB committees for approval.

SUMMARY
Many approaches and different styles are useful in the development and preparation of a sound clinical research trial protocol. The foregoing guidelines can be modified, reordered, condensed, or even some sections eliminated to suit the applicant's needs and objectives. No matter which path is mapped out in writing a clinical protocol for phases 1, 2, 3, 3b, or 4, it is imperative that investigators make the commitment to agree and adhere to the final protocol. Strict discipline to a well-designed protocol will result in research trials that will answer the objectives conclusively.

BIBLIOGRAPHY

Armitage P (1984). Controversies and achievements in clinical trials. Control Clin Trials 5, 243–251.

Bradford Hill A (1971). Principles of Medical Statistics, 9th edn. London: The Lancet.

Clinical trials: design and analysis (1981). Semin Oncol 8, 347–477.

Davey P (1984). Comparative clinical trials of antimicrobial drugs. J Antimicrob Chemother 13, 204–208.

Doongaji DR (1983). Some problems in the conduct of psychotropic drug trials (a review). J Postgrad Med 29, 67–74.

Feinstein AR (1984). Current problems and future challenges in randomized clinical trials. Circulation 70, 767–774.

Finkel M (1977). General Considerations for the Clinical Evaluation of Drugs. HEW (FDA) 77–3040. Washington, D.C.: U.S. Government Printing Office.

Fischer-Cornelssen KA (1980). Methods of multicenter trials in psychiatry, part I: a review. Prog Neuropsychopharmacol Biol Psychiatry 4, 545–560.

Friedewald WT (1982). Overview of recent clinical and methodological advances from clinical trials of cardiovascular disease. Control Clin Trials 3, 259–270.

Grahame-Smith DG, Aronson JK, eds. (1984). Oxford Textbook of Clinical Pharmacology and Drug Therapy. London: Oxford University Press.

Guarino RA (1975). Writing protocols for new drugs. Drug Cosmet Indus 117, 50.

Hadler NM (1983). On the design of the phase III drug trial: the example of rheumatoid arthritis. Arthritis Rheum 26, 1354–1361.

Haegerstam G (1982). Placebo in clinical drug trials—a multidisciplinary review. Methods Find Exp Clin Pharmacol 4, 261–278.

Johnson FN, Johnson S, eds. (1971). Clinical Trials. Oxford: Blackwell Scientific Publications.

Johnson FN, Johnson S (1977). Clinical Trials. Oxford: Blackwell Scientific Publications.

Lavori PW, Louis TA, Bailor JC 3rd et al. (1983). Designs for experiments—parallel comparisons of treatment. N Engl J Med 309, 1291–1299.

Linden M (1984). Phase IV clinical research: specifics, objectives and methodology. Pharmacopsychiatry 17, 162–167.

Louis TA (1983). Critical issues in the conduct and interpretation of clinical trials. Annu Rev Public Health 4, 25–46.

Louis TA (1984). Crossover and self-controlled designs in clinical research. N Engl J Med 310, 24–31.

Maxwell C (1973). Clinical Research for All. Cambridge: Cambridge Medical Publications.

Pocock TJ (1985). Current issues in the design and interpretation of clinical trials. Br Med J 290, 39–42.

Pollack AV (1983). Review article: controlled clinical trials. Life Support Syst 1, 7–233.

Proceedings of a Conference on the Recent History of Randomized Clinical Trials (November 1981). Kroc Foundation, Santa Ynez Valley, California,

Rossi AC (1983). Discovery of adverse drug reactions. A comparison of selected phase IV trials with spontaneous reporting methods. JAMA 249, 26–28.

Sachar DB (1984). Placebo-controlled clinical trials in gastroenterology. A position paper of the American College of Gastroenterology. Am J Gastroenterol 79, 913–917.

Sackett DL, Haynes RB, eds. (1976). Compliance with Therapeutic Regimens. Baltimore: Johns Hopkins University Press.

Smith W (1983). Randomization and optimal design. J Chronic Dis 36, 609–615.

Spilker B (1983). Practical considerations in planning clinical trials with investigational or marketed drugs. Clin Neuropharmacol 6, 325–347.

Tallarida RI (1979). A scale for assessing the severity of diseases and adverse drug reactions. Application to drug benefit and risk. Clin Pharmacol Ther 25, 381–390.

Venn RD (1969). Experience with the collection and evaluation of drug adverse reaction data. In: The Proceedings of the European Society for the Trial of Drug Toxicity. Vol. 10. Amsterdam: Excerpta Medica Foundation.

Warrington SJ (1985). Limitations of dose tolerance trials on predictability for phase III. Arzneimittel Forschung 35, 781–783.

Wittenborn JR, ed. (1977). Guidelines for clinical trials of psychotropic drugs. Pharmacol-Psychiatry 10(3), 207–231.

Wittenhorn JR (1972). Reliability, validity and objectivity of symptom-rating scales. J Mental and Nervous Dis 154, 79–87.

Zelen M (1979). A new design for randomized clinical trials. N Engl J Med 300, 1242–1245.

17 Institutional Review Board/Independent Ethics Committee and Informed Consent: Protecting Research Subjects in the U.S. and Foreign Clinical Trials

Rochelle L. Goodson

R. L. Goodson Consulting, Inc., Hewlett, New York, U.S.A.

INTRODUCTION

The increasing globalization of human subjects' research over the last few years has resulted in a corresponding need to develop initiatives that ensure the protection of research subjects on a worldwide basis. The regulatory requirements promulgated by the FDA for U.S.-based trials, as well as foreign trials [including Health and Human Services (HHS) funded research that is subject to FDA regulations], underscores the concept that fostering research standards that reflect international cooperation and harmonizing efforts has become an imperative for sponsors and institutions that conduct clinical research in foreign countries.

The U.S. Food and Drug Administration (FDA) statutes that are published in Title 21 of the Code of Federal Regulations (21 CFR) identify and define the activities involved in the clinical research process. These codified regulations are designed to protect the rights, safety, and welfare of subjects of clinical investigations. An amendment to Title 21, dated July 27, 1981, specifically required that the conduct of clinical investigations would include (*i*) obtaining informed consent of all subjects and (*ii*) approval of all research proposals by Institutional Review Boards (IRBs).

On May 9, 1997, the Department of Health and Human Services, Food and Drug Administration, published the 1996 guideline entitled "Good Clinical Practice: Consolidated Guideline," in the Federal Register (FR) that underscored its relevance to the implementation of clinical research activities. Although the guideline is not perceived by the FDA as a substitute for the codified regulations, the FDA's recognition of this guideline is evidenced by a statement noting it as representative of the agency's current thinking on good clinical practices. The significance of the guideline, "The International Conference on Harmonization (ICH) of Technical Requirements for Registration of Pharmaceuticals for Human Use," is that it supports the concept and implementation of a unified standard for designing, conducting, recording, and reporting trials that involve the participation of human subjects in clinical investigations in the United States, Japan, and the European Union. Informed consent and IRB activities are discussed throughout the document to address how studies are conducted.

Despite federal regulations and established guidelines mandating good clinical practice procedures, the complexity of protecting research participants continues to challenge the research community. As recently as the late 1990s, several tragic and widely reported research-related events, including several deaths, prompted the

DHHS to commission the Institute of Medicine (IOM) to assess the current national system of regulated research. An IOM committee formulated the concept of implementing a human research participant protection program (HRPPP) in all research environments. In its first report (issued in 2001), the committee outlined key elements and activities to ensure protection of every research participant. Most significant, however, was the recommendation of accreditation programs that assess protection activities in a uniform and independent manner, as indicated by the report's title "Preserving Public Trust: Accreditation and Human Research Participant Protection Programs." To date, two independent organizations developed accreditation standards for organizations that review research involving human participants. The National Committee for Quality Assurance (NCQA) was contracted by the Veteran's Administration in April 2000 to develop an accreditation program specifically for VAs, and in 2001, the Association for the Accreditation of Human Research Protection Programs (AAHRPP), under a grant from the IOM, developed an interim accreditation program for broad-based research programs. AAHRPP started its testing of accreditation standards in 2002 and began accrediting organizations the same year. Subsequently, NCQA partnered with the Joint Commission on Accreditation of Healthcare Organization in 2003 and formed the Partnership for Human Research Protections. During the period from early 2003 through to the third quarter of 2005, NCQA accredited 51 Veteran Affairs Medical Centers (VAMCs). However, in 2005, the Department of Veteran Affairs contract expired and AAHRPP was awarded a contract following consideration of the bids submitted by NCQA and AAHRPP. Currently, AAHRPP is the only accreditation program. By the end of the first quarter of 2008, AAHRPP accredited 107 organizations, and the 33 VAMCs that were previously accredited by NCQA will be required to attain AAHRPP accreditation by the end of 2008 or forfeit their accreditation status. Although accreditation remains a voluntary effort, the ongoing debate continues in the research community of whether mandatory accreditation will eventually be a requirement.

Ensuring the protection of human subjects in foreign clinical studies has also been addressed by the FDA as evidenced by the recent publication of a final rule on April 28, 2008, amending the Investigational New Drug (IND) Application regulation (21 CFR Part 312) for acceptance of foreign clinical studies not conducted under an IND application. The amended regulation updates the required standards by requiring that studies have to be conducted in accordance with good clinical practice (GCP), including review and approval by an Independent Ethics Committee (IEC).

BACKGROUND

The National Research Act passed by Congress on July 12, 1974 mandated the establishment of IRBs, which for the first time formalized the review of federally funded research. Also, this Act provided for a National Commission for the Protection of Human Subjects of Biomedical and Behavioral Research and resulted in the publication of The Belmont Report in 1979. Although the Belmont Report was never officially adopted by Congress, it provided a fundamental guideline for the protection of human subjects in research.

Historically, private practitioners conducting clinical research were exempt from the IRB and informed consent regulations required of institutional, that is, university or hospital researchers. The amended regulations on July 27, 1981, requiring IRB review and approval of all research, increased the need to establish IRBs that would review and approve research proposals that might not be affiliated with a major research center, teaching hospital, or university. In the current regulatory environment, all new drug applications (NDAs) submitted to the FDA in support of all drugs, biologics, or medical devices require proof that IRB approval was obtained before implementation of the research. Evidence of continuing review by the IRB throughout the trial must also be demonstrated. The only exemptions from IRB review are investigations that started before July 27, 1981 and that fit categorical descriptions defined in the regulations.

IRB DUTIES

The goal of the IRB (a.k.a. IEC) is the protection of the rights, safety, and welfare of human subjects involved in clinical research investigations. The review board is, therefore, primarily responsible for the evaluation of the proposed research. All evaluations should have the following objectives: (*i*) to determine that the research is properly designed; (*ii*) to determine that the benefit of the intended therapy will outweigh the potential risk; and (*iii*) to determine that the patient will be provided with adequate information to enable him or her to make an informed decision regarding participation in the clinical trial.

If the benefits do not sufficiently outweigh the risks, the IRB may either refuse to award approval of the project/study protocol or require a modification to research that limits the risk/benefit ratio by approving it for a more defined or limited patient population.

Since IRB review/approval and continuing review processes are required for all clinical investigations performed in support of a research application or a marketing permit for FDA-regulated products, it is important to assure that projects are not initiated before these approvals are obtained.

It is also important to note that, although IRBs are subject to codified regulations stipulating their functions and responsibilities, other key players in the clinical research process are intrinsically involved in review processes to ensure the protection of subjects' rights. Specifically, clinical investigators are bound by 21 CFR 312.66 (Assurance of IRB review) to obtain initial and continuing approval reviews, to report changes in research activity, to report unanticipated problems relating to risks to subjects, and to provide study status. In addition, sponsors of clinical trials are bound by 21 CFR 312.53 (Selecting investigators and monitors) to inform the IRB, albeit through the investigator, of these obligations. The sponsor secures the investigator's agreement to fulfill these obligations by obtaining a signed and dated Investigator's Statement before initiating a trial.

IRB MEMBERSHIP AND RESPONSIBILITIES

The composition of an IRB membership is specifically defined by the FDA in Title 21 CFR Part 56 and must include the following basic requirements, which must be adhered to

- members of both sexes at each meeting
- scientific (e.g., physician, research scientist) and nonscientific (lawyers, clergy) members, a minimum of one nonscientific member at each meeting
- a minimum of one member who is unaffiliated with the institution at each meeting

- no member with a conflict of interest
- a minimum of five voting members at each meeting.

Some IRBs have expanded their working policies or standard operating procedures to include the following additional requirements:

- One member representing cultural or ethnic diversity
- One member representing a special interest group, if applicable (e.g., handicapped)
- The considerations of socioeconomic factors and local attitudes
- Financial considerations

Because there are some IRBs with a large membership and all members may not attend every meeting, it is imperative that the basic requirements for constituting an IRB be met by all present and voting members. A standard roster or an IRB membership list should be maintained, which lists the alternative members and indicates that they have equal professional status and meet the basic qualifications.

All IRBs are ultimately responsible for the unbiased determination of whether a proposal for clinical research is acceptable in terms of the standards of professional practice, the institution or individual undertaking the research, and the patient population. Therefore, proposals considered for approval at convened meetings must receive approval of a majority of the members present at that meeting.

If a voting member has a conflicting interest in the review, for example, a member who will be directly involved in the proposal being reviewed for approval, he or she may provide information but must abstain from voting. In addition, individuals with expertise in a specialized area may be invited to assist in reviews at a meeting; however, these individuals will not be permitted to vote.

IRB DOCUMENTATION AND OPERATIONS

IRBs must maintain written procedures of all operations. All activities associated with the following operations must be recorded:

- Conducting initial review and continuing review/approval of research
- Conducting expedited review/approval of research
- Ensuring that changes in research activity are reported
- Ensuring that changes in previously approved research are not implemented without review and approval
- Reporting of serious risks
- Reporting of significant findings

All IRBs are required to maintain records (minutes) of meetings and documents for at least three years after completion of a study. In addition, IRBs are responsible for reporting investigator noncompliance to their institutions, sponsors of clinical research, and the FDA. It is important to note that IRBs have the regulatory authority to suspend or terminate research they previously approved if the research ceases to be conducted in accordance with the IRB's requirements. Research that has been associated with unexpected and/or serious harm to research subjects may be suspended or terminated.

INFORMATION REQUIRED FOR IRB REVIEW

All information submitted to an IRB for review of a research protocol is provided by the clinical investigator seeking approval to conduct the research. The standard documents typically provided are the research protocol, a sample of the intended informed consent, and the Investigator's Brochure or Package Insert. It has become common practice recently to also provide patient information sheets or instruction guides, advertising that will be used to recruit subjects, and any scheduled reimbursements to compensate patients for their time or expenses incurred during participation in a trial. Although the regulations do not require these additional documents, FDA information sheets suggesting that they be provided have served as guidelines or references for common practices that facilitate regulated activities. The regulations require that the Investigator's Brochure be submitted for studies conducted under an IND application in the section defining IND content and format [21 CFR 312.23(a)(5)] and in the section regarding informing investigators [21 CFR 312.55(a)]. In the ICH GCP guideline, it is specifically stated that certain documents be obtained for review, as part of the responsibility of the IRB/IEC (ICH GCP Section 3.1.2).

The review of the protocol ensures that there are adequate selection criteria and procedures to protect vulnerable study populations. In addition, information within the protocol, the informed consent, and the Investigator's Brochure are reviewed to assess safety information that may affect subjects. IRBs are empowered with the authority to approve or disapprove research activities that are covered by regulations, as well as to require modifications to secure approval. Informed consents will be reviewed to assure that all the information provided is in accordance with 21 CFR 50.25; the IRB may also require that additional information be provided to study subjects in a separate format, such as a patient information sheet. If this requirement is waived, a written statement may be given to the subject. If a very short "window of opportunity" exists to dispense a research treatment to avoid a devastating or fatal outcome, a waiver for this requirement may be requested. It is important to note, however, that the sponsor must clearly describe or define the situations that would require testing without administering a written informed consent. Also, provisions that will be made to obtain the consent from family members must be in place. This issue will be discussed in more detail in the section on informed consent. In summary, the following criteria are used by IRBs to approve research:

- Minimal risk
- Risk/benefit ratio
- Equitable patient population
- Informed consent documentation
- Planned study management/monitoring
- Patient privacy and confidentiality
- Rights and welfare of a vulnerable population

The FDA does not prohibit the use of advertising. However, since it has become an increasingly popular tool for increasing the enrollment rate of subjects in clinical studies, the FDA has created an information sheet, Advertising for Study Subjects, to serve as a guideline. This guideline recognizes advertisements as an extension of the informed consent and subject selection process and defines them as a research activity and subject to review, primarily to protect subjects from misleading advertisements. Since advertisements are perceived as a research activity, they should be submitted for review and approval, although the regulations do not specifically require a review.

The information sheet notes what the contents of advertisements should be limited to as follows:

- The name and address of the clinical investigator
- The purpose of the research and, in summary form, the eligibility criteria that will be used to admit subjects into the study
- A straightforward and truthful description of the benefits (e.g., payments for free treatment) to the subject from participation in the study
- The location of the research and the person to contact for further information

Sample advertising submitted to the IRB may be in various media format. Whether or not the advertisement is in the form of newspaper advertisements, posters, brochures, leaflets, radio or television advertisements, and even notices posted on the Internet, they are all subject to the same requirements noted above. All copy, including audio or video scripts or videotape, should be submitted for review and approval before use. All of the requirements for written copy apply to all advertising modes.

The IRB must ensure that advertising does not include misleading information or statements implying that the drug or device is safe or effective for the indication being investigated or that the drug or device is equivalent or superior to any other drug or device. In addition to misleading potential subjects, statements that could be considered to be promotional claims would be in violation of statutes regulating the promotion of investigational drugs or devices.

The issue of subject reimbursement also has to be considered by the IRB to ensure that subjects are not induced to participate in a study because of excessive payments, but rather are remunerated adequately for the time and inconvenience that they experience in order to participate. If subjects participate in studies involving more than one study visit, the amount of reimbursement on a per visit basis should be stated. Visits that require additional time and/or cause inconvenience to the subject and have higher remunerations should be stated when applicable. Conversely, it should be stated if there are visits for which no reimbursement is scheduled. Finally, subjects should be informed when there is a caveat that if the study is not completed, a prorated amount will be reimbursed rather than the total amount indicated for study completion. All of these items should be delineated in the informed consent.

Informed consents, which must be signed by subjects before they participate in a study, reflect payments that will be made and, as mentioned, should include how they will be scheduled. The review of this information falls under the purview of IRB responsibility for two reasons. First, payment is perceived as a benefit, and it is the IRB's responsibility to determine that the benefit does not reflect an unduly coercive amount that may persuade a subject to participate in a study he or she ordinarily would not consider. Second, the IRB is also responsible for evaluating the investigator's responsibilities regarding the submission of this document.

INITIAL APPROVAL AND CONTINUING REVIEW

The critical documents required for approval of research, that is, protocol, informed consent, and Investigator's Brochure, are usually presented to an IRB chairperson by the principal investigator. Copies of the pertinent documents are supplied to the IRB members for thorough review before they vote on the proposed research project. Any and all elements of the project may be deliberated and may result in recommendations to modify any part of the research.

Clinical investigators will be notified, in writing, of all IRB decisions regarding the approval/disapproval of research or modifications to the research that will be required to obtain approval. Approvals will identify the study and include the date of approval and the IRB chairperson's signature. If a decision to disapprove a research proposal is rendered, the notification will include the reasons to provide the investigator with an opportunity to respond in person or in writing. All written documentation between the IRB and the clinical investigator should be accompanied by a transmittal letter to ensure verification after any action or decision. All correspondence should be date-stamped upon receipt, and all study documentation should be stamped with the date of IRB approval. In addition, documentation submitted to the clinical investigator (and the IRB) should be dated to distinguish between final documents and draft versions to avoid accidental approval of a draft document.

Regulations regarding the IRB review of research require the continuing review of protocols at least once per year; however, the intervals are based on the degree of risk to the subject and are usually specified by the IRB at the time of initial approval. Finally, IRBs have the authority to observe or designate a third party to observe the consent process and the research.

EXPEDITED REVIEWS

Expedited reviews are used by IRBs to review and approve minor changes in previously approved research, either because the change is administrative in nature or because the research (or change in the research) involves no more than minimal risk to the subject. This procedure requires only the IRB chairperson's review or review by one or more reviewers designated by the chairperson who are voting members of the IRB. In addition, when and if the expedited procedure is invoked, every member must be advised of all approvals made via this procedure. It is important to note that expedited review procedures are used only under the limited circumstances addressed above and do not replace a full IRB review of research proposals. The original documentation of all IRB reviews and decisions should be maintained by the principal investigator; copies should be maintained by a trial's sponsor.

THE INFORMED CONSENT FORM

Overall, the informed consent regulations (21 CFR, Part 50) apply to all clinical investigations regulated by the Food and Drug Administration, including clinical investigations that support applications for research or marketing permits for products the FDA regulates. The general requirements for informed consent are discussed below.

As mentioned earlier, the clinical investigator is ultimately responsible for assuring that a subject in a clinical investigation is not only fully informed of the project but also apprised of the procedures to be followed and the risks and benefits of the therapeutic regimen proposed in the research. The informed consent process requires that a written consent is obtained from each patient (or his legally authorized representative) to verify that the above-referenced obligations have been satisfied. On November 5, 1996, the FDA published a final rule, that is, a change to an existing regulation, requiring that a consent form signed by the subject or the subject's legally authorized representative be dated by the subject (or legally authorized representative) at the same time it is signed. This ruling became effective on December 5, 1996, enforcing via regulation a GCP procedure that has been routinely implemented by clinical researchers in recent years. In addition, the FDA amended the regulation regarding case histories (21 CFR 312.62) to specify that case histories must document that informed consent was obtained before a subject participated in a study and to clarify what should be included in a case history.

The IRB's oversight responsibility regarding informed consent is highlighted by this amendment, which was enacted to further ensure that an informed consent is obtained before any clinical trial–related procedures are performed.

During the informed consent process, clinical investigators should plan to allot sufficient time for patients to review a consent and ask questions regarding the research. Patients must be permitted to take the form with them while they are considering participation; however, the form must be signed in front of a witness. In addition, the IRB may request that a witness sign the informed consent, as well. The principal investigator may not serve as a witness. A copy of the consent document must be provided to the patient.

Informed consents should be written so that they can be understood by a layperson. In general, the overall document should not contain words or explanations that could not ordinarily be understood by an individual who has completed an eighth-grade level of education. All technical, medical, or legal terminology should be explained to a prospective subject. Patients unable to read English should have the informed consent made available in their native language. The translation of the informed consent should be documented as being completed by a qualified individual. It is recommended that translations be used only in instances where a significant amount of the proposed study population would require a translation.

Finally, informed consents should not contain any coercive language that unfairly persuades or influences a subject's decision to participate. The consent should not contain exculpatory language that either requires or appears to require a subject to waive any legal rights or releases or appears to release an investigator, sponsor, institution, or any other agent of a clinical investigation from liability for negligence. The moral and legal ramifications of this type of language are obvious.

Aside from the general requirements for informed consent that have been discussed, there are basic elements that must be included in all informed consents. Additional elements are to be included only when they are deemed appropriate.

BASIC ELEMENTS OF THE INFORMED CONSENT (21 CFR 50.25)

1. A statement that the study involves research, an explanation of the purposes of the research, the expected duration of the subject's participation, a description of the schedule of events to be followed, and identification of any procedures that are experimental.
2. A description of any reasonable foreseeable risks or discomforts to the subject.
3. A description of any benefits to the subject that reasonably may be expected as a result of the research.
4. A disclosure of appropriate alternative procedures or courses of treatment, if any, that may be advantageous to the subject.
5. A statement describing the extent to which the confidentiality of records identifying the subject will be maintained, including mention of the possibility that the FDA may inspect the records.

6. Since all clinical research investigations entail more than minimal risk, a statement describing compensation (if any) that will be paid and an explanation as to whether any medical treatment is available if an adverse reaction occurs, what the treatment consists of, and/or where further information can be obtained.

7. A list of people to contact in the event of a study-related adverse experience and to answer pertinent questions about the research, including the subject's rights.

8. A statement that participation in the study is voluntary, that refusal to take part in the research will not result in a penalty or loss of benefits to which the subject is otherwise entitled, and that the subject may withdraw from the study at any time without penalty or loss of benefits to which he or she is otherwise entitled.

ADDITIONAL ELEMENTS OF THE INFORMED CONSENT [21 CFR 50.25(B)]

1. A statement that the particular treatment or procedure may involve currently unforeseeable risks to the subject (or embryo or fetus, if the subject is or may become pregnant).

2. Circumstances under which the subject's involvement may be terminated by the investigator without regard to the subject's consent.

3. Additional costs to the subject, if any, that may result from participation in the research.

4. Consequences that may result from the subject's decision to withdraw from the research, and the procedures for an orderly termination of the subject's participation.

5. A statement that, during the course of the study, any significant new findings related to the subject's willingness to continue in the program will be presented and reviewed with him or her.

6. The approximate number of subjects involved in the study.

All consent documents and the entire informed consent process should be designed and implemented to be in compliance with the above-stated regulations, as well as consistent with the principles of the Declaration of Helsinki, World Medical Assembly, Revised 2008, 59th General Assembly, the accepted basis for clinical trial ethics incorporated into the ICH GCP guideline.

The ICH GCP guideline encompasses the procedures involved in the administration of the informed consent process that is included in the U.S. CFR. However, it is worth noting that, in addition to expanded explanations for some of the basic and additional elements of informed consent in the regulation, other items are included.

The guideline's descriptions of the procedures also require that the probability for random assignment for each treatment be included in the discussion. Also, the guideline explicitly states that invasive procedures must be explained when they are part of the treatment. Furthermore, the guideline states that if there are anticipated prorated payments to the subject for participating in the trial, the subject should be informed via the consent form. This is somewhat of a departure from the U.S. regulations, which do not require that this information be stated in the informed consent. However, the FDA information sheets state that payments should not be contingent on study completion and that the proposed schedule should be evaluated by the IRB to determine that payments are reasonable and do not unduly influence a patient to remain in a trial. Since payments are perceived as a benefit, it is suggested that the outline of the payment schedule and the conditions determining the payments be outlined in the informed consent.

The guideline specifically states that an explanation of the subject's responsibilities must be discussed during the informed consent discussion and included in the consent form and any other written information.

GCP procedures dictate that the safety and welfare of clinical subjects are intrinsic to the clinical research process and are an integral responsibility of the clinical investigator, the IRB, and the sponsor; therefore, the importance of a correctly documented informed consent and an adequately implemented consent procedure cannot be stressed enough. In addition to understanding these requirements, one should be equally mindful that there are situations that may deviate from the norm but require equal attention. This includes the necessity of resubmitting an informed consent and obtaining reapproval from an IRB when a consent has been significantly revised or altered, usually because of a protocol amendment. A full explanation of the revisions and any associated changes in the study procedures should be provided to each subject who signed the original consent form, and he or she must be required to re-sign a revised form before any changes in the research are performed. All revised forms must be submitted to the IRB for review and approval. If, during the course of a trial, an informed consent was signed by a legally authorized representative because a subject was incompetent or a minor, the consent should be readministered to obtain the signed/dated signature of the patient who regained competency or reached the age of majority, respectively.

Although the age of majority in most states is 18 years, approximately 10 states permit higher or lower consent ages. Also, some local/state laws permit consent at lower ages dependent on various circumstances, for example, abortion, prevention, treatment, or diagnosis of a sexually transmitted disease (STD), pregnancy, and drug or alcohol abuse.

ORAL CONSENT

A "short-form" written consent document, stating that the elements of informed consent required by 21 CFR 50.25 have been presented orally to the subject or the subject's legally authorized representative, is included in the regulations. However, clinical investigators do not recognize oral consent as a practical or appropriate alternative to obtaining documented informed consent whenever possible. The following requirements are necessary when the use of a short-form informed consent is implemented:

- A witness to the oral presentation must be present.
- The IRB must approve a written summary of what will be said to the subject/representative.
- The short form is to be signed by the subject/representative.
- The short form and summary will be signed by the witness.
- The person administering the consent will sign a copy of the summary.
- Copies of the short form and the summary will be given to the subject/representative.

Any research conducted in the United States must comply with the federal regulations regarding informed consent, despite the type of form or procedure used. It is important for those involved in patient safety and welfare issues to know that there are some state or local laws that may have additional requirements regarding informed consent procedures. The California Research Subjects Bill of Rights is an example of a state law in California that requires all research subjects to be provided with a document entitled "Experimental Subjects Bill of Rights" before they participate in a research trial.

EMERGENCY USE OF INVESTIGATIONAL DRUGS/BIOLOGICS
The regulations include a provision for the emergency use of an investigational drug or biologic when a human subject is (*i*) in a life-threatening situation in which no standard acceptable treatment is available and (*ii*) there is not sufficient time to obtain IRB approval (21 CFR 56.102).

When a human subject does not meet the criteria stipulated in an existing study protocol or if an approved study protocol is not available, the manufacturer of the test article should be contacted to determine if the company will make the test article available for emergency use under the manufacturer's IND. If an emergency occurs before an IND submission and the manufacturer agrees to make the test article available, the FDA would have to authorize shipment.

The specific regulation (21 CFR 56.104) is actually an exemption from prior review and approval by the IRB; however, it can be used only when the specific conditions described in 21 CFR 56.102 are met, and it allows for only one emergency use of the investigational product. The investigator must file a report of its use within five days to comply with the exemption regulation. Also, some institutions require IRB notification before the emergency use. Finally, the manufacturer may require an emergency use approval letter or at least a written statement that the IRB has been informed of the emergency use and acknowledges that the requirements stipulated in the exemption regulation have been met. All subsequent uses of an unapproved test article are subject to usual IRB review and approval procedures.

INFORMED CONSENT DURING EMERGENCY USE
In an emergency use situation where an investigator has determined that there is not sufficient time to obtain informed consent from a subject or legally authorized representative, he or she is required to have the determination reviewed by a physician who is not participating in the clinical investigation and to obtain a written certification of the following informed consent requirements (21 CFR 50.23) before use:

- The subject is confronted by a life-threatening situation necessitating the use of the test article.
- Informed consent cannot be obtained because of an inability to communicate with the subject or obtain legally effective consent from the subject.
- Time is not sufficient to obtain consent from the subject's legal representative.
- No alternative method of approved or generally recognized therapy is available that provides an equal or greater likelihood of saving the subject's life.

Although it is optimal for both the investigator and a physician independent of the clinical trial to determine the necessity for emergency use of an investigational product prior to its use, if this is not possible, the investigator must have the determination of use reviewed, evaluated, and submitted to the IRB within five working days after use of the test article.

HEALTH INSURANCE PORTABILITY AND ACCOUNTABILITY ACT (HIPAA)
In 1996, DHHS passed the HIPAA to facilitate the sharing of information while protecting patient confidentiality (medical records); subsequently, associated privacy

regulations were issued in 2000 (Privacy Rule). Amendments to the Privacy Rule were proposed on March 27, 2002 to address research-related situations and went into effect on April 14, 2003. In essence, the Privacy Rule is the governing law for the use and disclosure of individually identifiable protected health information (PHI) by "covered entities," defined as health care providers, health plans, or health clearing houses. HIPAA-compliant consents that include elements specified in federal regulations (45 CFR 164.508) will have to be provided by "covered entities" that carry out the activities of health care payment, treatment, or operations (PTO). Clinical research-related uses and/or disclosures of PHI beyond PTO will require that a specifically defined authorization be obtained from a research subject. (See chap. 18.)

ASSURING THAT REGULATORY OBLIGATIONS ARE ADEQUATELY IMPLEMENTED

The complexity of clinical research is evidenced by the associated regulatory and clinical documentation required before an IND is filed, throughout the clinical trial process, and ultimately, during the preparation of an NDA filing. A sponsor must ensure that the studies supporting an NDA contain quality data that substantiates claims of safety and efficacy. This process is facilitated when a sponsor evaluates the acceptability of the regulatory obligations and responsibilities required by investigators and sponsors. Thus, the penultimate concern regarding the safety and efficacy claims stated in a submission can be assessed. Although this chapter does not address the auditing and inspectional techniques used to identify potential deficiencies, it is important to understand why these regulations have been established, the type of deficiencies that are identified, and the impact of poorly implemented GCPs.

In 1986, the preamble to the IND Rewrite stated that the detail of an inspection may be based on the knowledge that a sponsor has audited subject records. The preamble further reiterated that "FDA's policy to audit two or more critical studies will continue." These statements regarding FDA's inspectional efforts, as well as the FDA Statement of Enforcement Policy (1990) and recent activities promulgated through the Office of Criminal Investigations, have encouraged sponsors of clinical trials to establish and implement quality assurance departments and programs. Internal clinical quality assurance departments have developed standardized procedures to provide objective, independent assessments of processes that will assure upper management that trials are being conducted according to GCP procedures that include patient protection, safety, and welfare to produce accurate and reliable data. In addition, tools to identify and oversee corrective actions facilitate the speed and quality of submissions and provide opportunities for training in monitoring and the continuing improvement of standard operating procedures used in the oversight of clinical research. The ability to identify, correct, and prevent inadequacies that could result in disciplinary regulatory actions or, in the worst case, delay or prevent an approval underscores the benefit of this proactive approach. Optimally, quality assurance personnel can facilitate the inspection process by helping to identify the appropriate staff in the functional area being inspected. Furthermore, a quality assurance presence can be helpful in advising functional personnel regarding study documents that are provided to the FDA, providing a scribe to generate minutes, facilitating daily debriefing meetings, and advising management of inspection findings and corrective actions. The importance of the IRB and IC regulations has also been highlighted by FDA's recognition of the ICH GCP guideline, which underscores these elements in the regulations.

AUDITS VERSUS INSPECTIONS

The focus of both audits and inspections is to review clinical research–related activities and associated documentation, to determine the adequacy of the conduction of the activities, and to determine the accuracy and reliability of the data reported. Historically, clinical research nomenclature commonly refers to audits as internally generated processes and inspections as official reviews by a government authority, for example, the FDA. Both audits and/or inspections are actually assessments of the clinical research process and share the goal of identifying deficiencies for corrective action. The essential difference is that an audit initiated as an independent review by a company is often conducted proactively to identify and correct inadequate procedures and/or to verify the accuracy and reliability of data being collected for submission. Inspections are routinely conducted by regulatory authorities to protect the public safety and welfare, as well as to respond to potentially illegal or inappropriate research activities that have been exposed. Regulatory authorities can also impose punitive actions or pursue legal sanctions to promote correction of inadequate or illegal clinical research activities.

Irrespective of whether audits are initiated by the IRB, a sponsor, or the FDA, a number of commonly identified deficiencies have been noted and are addressed below. It is important to note that investigational sites, sponsors, and IRBs are all subject to FDA-issued warning letters or repeat inspections to verify that deficiencies have been adequately corrected.

COMMON AUDITING/INSPECTIONAL FINDINGS: IRBS

Clinical investigators routinely submit protocols and informed consent documents to IRBs to obtain an independent evaluation of the risk/benefit ratio of a study in order to meet their obligation to protect patients' safety and welfare. The Institutional Review Branch of the FDA's Division of Scientific Investigations conducts inspections of the IRBs that review and approve investigational studies for biologics, drugs, medical devices, and food additives. Although the regulations specifically outline the IRB requirements and responsibilities in this review process, inspectional findings from routine surveillance, as well as directed inspections, have revealed seven commonly cited deficiencies that have resulted in regulatory or administrative actions:

1. A lack of sufficiently documented standard operating procedures describing an IRB's procedural responsibilities and activities.
2. Meeting minutes that do not fully detail actions taken or voting conducted at a meeting. Examples of insufficiently documented minutes may include inadequate reporting of voting on protocols or amendments to protocols, the basis for disapproving a protocol, or summaries of relevant discussions or issues.
3. Documentation that is not available to verify that a quorum was present at convened meetings to review proposed research and that a majority of those members present at the meeting approved the proposal.
4. Lack of documentation to verify that the IRB provided continuing review of research activities that it initially approved at intervals of no less than one year, but appropriate to the level of risk to the subject.

5. IRB membership lists or rosters that are not consistent with the elements required in 21 CFR 56 (see section on IRB MEMBERSHIP AND RESPONSIBILITIES).
6. IRB records that do not adequately track or log research documents that have been submitted by the clinical investigator, including protocols, amendments, consent forms, Investigator's Brochures, IND safety reports, advertisements, patient information sheets, and correspondence between the investigator and the IRB.
7. A lack of approval notifications, approval notifications that do not adequately identify the research document (or the version of the research document) that has been approved, and/or missing dates of approvals.

COMMON AUDITING/INSPECTIONAL FINDINGS: INFORMED CONSENT

Informed consent issues rank among one of the most commonly cited deficiencies reported by FDA inspectors. Findings can include deficiencies in the actual content of the informed consent, as well as the actual informed consent administration process. Most frequently noted are the following inadequacies:

1. All the basic elements of the informed consent (according to 21 CFR 50.25) are not included.
2. The content of the informed consent is inadequate.
3. IRB approval of the consent or revised consent(s) has not been obtained.
4. The informed consent has not been properly administered to the subject of the clinical investigation or a legal guardian.

To limit inspectional findings related to informed consent deficiencies, auditor reviews of informed consents can be conducted proactively, that is, before being submitted to IRBs for review and approval. Inadequacies regarding the lack of required content, the use of technical rather than lay language, readability above an eighth-grade level, and consents that are culturally and linguistically inappropriate for the anticipated population are examples of problem areas that are frequently overlooked. Also, it is important to assure that subjects of clinical trials are provided with the most recent version of an IRB-approved informed consent. It is recommended that informed consents include the version number, date, and page number on the bottom of each page of the consent form that has been either signed or initialed and dated. In addition to a correctly signed/dated informed consent, it is often beneficial to provide patient information sheets or subject instruction sheets to clarify and/or reiterate the study procedures.

Once the regulatory compliance issues regarding informed consent have been satisfied, it is essential to ascertain the subject's comprehension of the informed consent. Documentation of the administration and comprehension of the informed consent by the subject should be a routine component of the process.

SAFETY AND WELFARE CONSIDERATIONS FOR SUBJECTS IN FOREIGN TRIALS

Regulatory protections for human subjects, often referred to as the Common Rule (45 Code of Federal Regulations, Part 46), is a federal policy that governs all human subject research in the United States that is federally funded; in addition, it applies to federally funded research conducted in foreign countries. Although research in countries outside the United States is covered by this policy, the country-specific procedures that are followed to protect research subjects may differ; therefore, OHRP has had to determine if alternate procedures provide protections that are equivalent to the Common Rule. Office of Human Research Protection (OHRP) has not provided criteria used to determine equivalency; therefore, a notice was published in the FR on March 25, 2005 entitled "Protection of Human Subjects, Proposed Criteria for Determinations of Equivalent Protections," following recommendations made to the (OHRP), by a working group of representatives from various HHS agencies. In addition to determine the equivalency of the protection in the foreign procedures to those in the Common Rule, it is further recommended that the institution in a foreign country offer a formal assurance that the procedures that are substituted will be followed for research that is federally funded by the United States. Furthermore, if the FDA accepts foreign data that support a marketing application and the study has not been conducted under an IND application or investigational device exemption (IDE), the FDA must be able to ensure that subject protections are compliant with the Declaration of Helsinki or country-specific regulations, that is, whichever affords the subjects greater protection.

Most recently, the FDA published a final ruling on April 28, 2008 (effective October 27, 2008) to address an amendment to the regulations on the acceptance of foreign clinical studies not conducted under an IND in support of an IND or marketing application for a drug or biological product. The FDA specifically stated in its notice, "The final rule replaces the requirement that these studies be conducted in accordance with ethical principles stated in the Declaration of Helsinki (Declaration) issued by the World Medical Association (WMA), specifically the 1989 version (1989 Declaration), with a requirement that the studies be conducted in accordance with GCP, including review and approval by an IEC." The FDA explains their decision to relinquish adherence to the 1989 Declaration, as originally required in the proposal for the ruling on June 10, 2004, by reiterating the FDA's decision (in 1997) to adopt the GCPs Consolidated Guideline that includes a definition of GCP that is consistent with many of the ethical principles stated in the 1989 Declaration. Also cited was that the detail and enumeration of specific responsibilities outlined in the ICH GCP guideline permitted enough flexibility to accommodate the way in which various countries regulate the conduct of clinical research and obtain informed consent. For example, since May 2004, the implementation of the European Directive required Member States to be subject to an approval of an Investigational Medicine Product Dossier (IMPD) approved by the competent authorities and the IECs of the Member States where the investigation will be conducted. The IMPD must present sufficient animal safety and manufacturing data to allow products to be introduced in humans.

BIBLIOGRAPHY

Advertising for Study Subjects, FDA Information Sheet (February 1989). Rockville, Maryland: Public Health Service, Department of Health and Human Services, Food and Drug Administration.

Association for the Accreditation of Human Research Protection Programs (AHRPP) Press Release (March 2008).

Clinical Investigator Information Sheets, Food and Drug Administration (1989).

Code of Federal Regulations, Food and Drugs. Title 21, Part 50.

Code of Federal Regulations, Food and Drugs. Title 21, Part 56.

Code of Federal Regulations, Title 45, Part 46.

Declaration of Helsinki, Code of ethics on human experimentation, Helsinki, Finland (1964). Amended in 1975, 1983, 1989, 1996, 2000, 2002, 2004, 2008 (59th World Medical Association General Assembly)

Federal Register (March 25, 2005). Protection of Human Subjects, Proposed Criteria for Determinations of Equivalent Protections. Volume 70.

Federal Register (April 28, 2008). Department of Health and Human Services, Food and Drug Administration (21 CFR Part 312); Human Subject Protection; Foreign Clinical Studies Not Conducted Under an Investigational New Drug Application. Volume 73, Number 82.

Federal Register (June 10, 2004) (69 FR32, 467). Human Subject Protection: Foreign Clinical Studies Not Conducted Under an Investigational New Drug Application.

Institute of Medicine Committee on Assessing the System for Protecting Human Research Participants Report (2001). Preserving Public Trust: Accreditation and Human Research Participant Protection Programs.

International Conference on Harmonisation of Technical Requirements for Registration of Pharmaceuticals for Human Use (ICH): E6 Good Clinical Practice: Consolidated Guideline, April 1996.

IRB Information Sheets, Food and Drug Administration (1989).

IRB & Clinical Investigator Information Sheets, Food and Drug Administration (1995).

Standards for Privacy of Individually Identifiable Health Information, 45 CFR, Parts 160 and 164.

The National Commission for the Protection of Human Subjects of Biomedical and Behavioral Research (1978). The Belmont Report: Ethical Principles and Guidelines for the Protection of Human Subjects of Research. Washington: DHEW Publication No. (OS) 78–0012.

18

HIPAA: A New Requirement to the Clinical Study Process

Glenn D. Watt and Earl W. Hulihan

Medidata Solutions Worldwide, New York, New York, U.S.A.

Richard A. Guarino

Oxford Pharmaceutical Resources, Inc., Totowa, New Jersey, U.S.A.

INTRODUCTION

HIPAA is the acronym for The Health Insurance Portability and Accountability Act of 1996. HIPAA's roots start in the early 1990s when the Bush Administration called health care leaders together to discuss how to reduce the cost of health care administration. The answer was electronic data interchange (EDI). As the group sharpened its focus on EDI, it became known as the Workgroup for Electronic Data Interchange (WEDI).

WEDI discovered that at the time there were more than four hundred different formats for transmitting health information. The cost nonstandardization was enormous. By comparison, WEDI published white papers that estimated a standardized EDI would save nine billion dollars annually. With savings of this magnitude, it didn't take long for Congress to recommended federal legislation.

WEDI's recommendations were incorporated as the Kennedy–Kassenbaum bill, an outgrowth of the Clinton administration's attempt to revamp the health care system. The result in HIPAA was an effort to streamline and standardize the health care system and to establish the privacy of subject information. The result of this effort was the issuance of the final HIPAA rules in August 2002 that establishes the requirements that prevent the disclosure of individually identifiable health information (privacy rule) without authorization from the subject. An accidental posting of individual's health records and fraudulent use of medical records precipitated the passage of HIPAA.

Case 1. A Michigan-based health care system accidentally posted the medical records of thousands of subjects on the Internet (references: The Ann Arbor News, February 10, 1999). A speculator bid $4000 for the subject records of a family practice in South Carolina and then used them to sell them back to the former subjects (The New York Times, August 14, 1991).

Case 2. A Nevada woman who purchased a used computer discovered that the previous owner of the computer left a database with the names, addresses, Social Security numbers, and a list of all prescriptions received by the individual (The New York Times April 4, 1997 and April 12, 1997).

HIPAA has some important provisions affecting research that are included in the Administration Simplification Provision under which the privacy rule evolved. In addition, it provided another provision with respect to the fraud and abuse rule that provided certain restrictions for inducement to subjects. With the implementation of HIPAA, subjects can now find out how their health information may be used. It also limits the release of information to a minimum time reasonably needed for the purpose of disclosure. In addition, it gives subjects the right to examine and obtain a copy of their health records giving them an opportunity to request corrections. Most important, it allows individuals to control certain uses and disclosures of their health information. Subjects generally will have full access rights to their health care information under HIPAA. However, the rights may be waived if their authorization states that their health information will not be available during the clinical trial or the authorization states whether the information will be available at the end of the trial and whether the subject has agreed to these waivers.

HIPAA and the Administration Simplification Provisions cover the electronic transactions and code sets, national identifiers for plans and providers, employers and will include subjects, security, and privacy provisions that were intended to balance the simplification of the transactions and identifiers. The HIPAA privacy regulations are in Title 45 of the Code of Federal Regulations. Those who work in research are familiar with the common rule, Institutional Review Board (IRB), and informed consent (IC) regulations, also in Title 45, part 46. Administrative simplification and privacy rules can be found in Title 45, parts 160 and 164 (2).

HIPAA Basics

Who are the covered entities?

Directly "covered entities" of HIPAA are health care providers who engage in electronic transactions, health care clearinghouses, a kind of billing agencies that some physicians offices use to submit their claims, and health plans. The "covered entities" are responsible for the privacy standards as well as for any other contracted individuals (called "business associates") to perform essential functions. Business associates do not include members of the covered entity's workforce or volunteer medical staff. Among the business associates functions or activities are legal, actuarial, accounting, consulting, clinical research, data analysis, processing or administration, quality assurance, and practice management. Contracts with business associates must be signed between the covered entity and the business associate requiring the business associate to keep protected health information safeguarded. Components of a sample business associate agreement have been included in the HIPAA privacy rules as amended in August 2002.

HIPAA also allows for the creation of "hybrid entities" where certain parts of the entity are not engaged in the covered activities. However, research components of these hybrid entities that function as health care providers and engage in standard electronic transactions are subject to the privacy rule.

Electronic transactions include

1. health care claims,
2. health care eligibility/benefit inquiries,
3. health care eligibility/benefit information,
4. health care services review information,
5. health claim status inquiries,

6. health claim status responses,
7. benefit enrollment and maintenance,
8. claim payment and remittance advice,
9. premium payments,
10. first report of injury,
11. health claim attachments.

Although the HIPAA security rules were designed to protect individually identifiable protected health information (PHI) in electronic transmission, processing, and storage of the data, the actual objective of the HIPAA security rule is to embody the five basic principles of information security, integrity, confidentiality, authenticity, nonrepudiation, and availability.

Throughout the HIPAA security rule, many standards are listed as either "addressable" or "required." "Addressable requirements" allow covered entities flexibility with respect to compliance with the security standards. If within covered entities' organization, the security rule does not really apply, or would be unreasonable to enact, the entity can choose to "address" this rule with an alternative technique, or procedure. The only requirement is that the entity must fully document the decision and any alternative procedures. "Required" rules must be implemented without question.

Who are not covered entities?

Anybody that is not a covered entity; pharmaceutical, biotech, medical device companies, and contract research organizations—typically they will not be covered entities. It is possible that a large organization may have a health clinic, infirmary on-site, there may be doctors there, they may provide services, and those services may be billed to an insurer under those circumstances. It is possible that that portion of a pharmaceutical or a contract research organization could be a covered entity. But for the most part, pharmaceutical companies, medical device companies, and contract research organizations are not health care providers, plans, or clearinghouses.

The HIPAA security rule exists to protect PHI in electronic formats. To accomplish this, the HIPAA security rule establishes administrative safeguards, physical safeguards, and technical safeguards to protect PHI.

Section 164.308—Administrative Safeguards (2)

Administrative safeguards are administrative policies and the associated operational procedures to protect electronic PHI. In general, these safeguards should prevent security violations, and if that fails then detect, contain, and correct security violations. The security procedures implemented to reduce risks and vulnerabilities should undergo a comprehensive risk analysis. The results of this analysis should then be logged in a corrective action plan to mitigate the identified risks.

The risk analysis should explore the potential risks and vulnerabilities to the integrity, confidentiality, authenticity, availability, and nonrepudiation of the electronic PHI. The process of the risk analysis is one of identifying, reviewing, and evaluating existing policies, controls, and procedures in both the covered entity as well as its computer systems. The evaluation generally consists of evaluating the PHI life cycle from creation, access, processing, storage, and destruction in the electronic system. At the conclusion of the analysis, the risk would be determined by calculating the losses, tangible and intangible, if security measures were not in place.

Covered entities are required to identify a security official who is responsible for the development and implementation of the required security policies and procedures. The optimum solution for many organizations is to create a senior c-level position that oversees both information security and data privacy. The minimum requirements are that one individual needs to have accountability for the security procedure of the organization.

To accomplish that accountability requirement, the Information Security and Privacy Officer will be required to monitor user-access activity over computers. The Privacy Officer should implement procedures to collect and to regularly review records of system activity. This would include, but is not limited to, audit logs, access control anomalies, firewall logs, intrusion detection logs, and records of any security incidents.

If a violation is detected during the review of these security logs and the perpetrator is an employee then HIPAA requires that sanctions be applied against the employees. This also applies to employees who fail to comply with the organization's information security policies and procedures. The company can decide the type and severity of the sanction imposed, but some sanction must be imposed. Comprehensive documentation is, of course, required.

At all times, a covered entity must have "positive control" over the PHI they possess. Positive control means that the organization defines what procedures will be used to allow or deny access to the electronic records and that only employees with the appropriate need to know are able to access the data. The procedures must be codified and known and included in HIPAA training to all the employees. HIPAA requires employees to receive training on the organizations security procedures as well as periodic updates on information security and data privacy. If an organization follows these procedures, there should never be an instance when positive control of the PHI is lost.

Another aspect of positive control is maintaining the integrity, confidentiality, authenticity, and the availability of the data. The HIPAA security rules require organizations to specifically prevent, detect, and report malicious attacks. These attacks could come in the form of viruses or worms, or they could be manifested as malicious attacks from hackers attempting to steal or alter information. The first form can be easily managed with commercial-off-the-shelf virus scanners, while the second form will require more sophisticated intrusion detection devices and reviews of the detection logs.

Should an actual intrusion or some other disaster occur, HIPAA requires then a plan to be established to deal with the situation. The plan should address everything from containment of a virus or malicious attack to continuing operations in the event of a natural disaster, to recovering data from a safe archiving location.

In summary, HIPAA requires an organization to evaluate its own security program and determine the information security weaknesses and vulnerabilities. By identifying and mitigating these weaknesses, an organization can achieve compliance with the HIPAA security rules.

Section 164.310—Physical Safeguards (2)

In addition to the administrative safeguard, HIPAA also has physical safeguard requirements. Physical safeguards are security measures to protect a covered entity's electronic information systems as well as the related buildings and equipment from natural disasters and unauthorized physical intrusion. To maintain the physical security of facilities that house PHI information, HIPAA requires that an organization develops a "facility security plan," develops a "disaster recovery plan" for unexpected occurrences, and then standard operating procedures for access to a facility.

HIPAAs Impact on Clinical Research

HIPAA requirements for subject privacy are increasing the amount of documentation needed for the initiation of a clinical trial. Besides the requirement for IC that has evolved from the Declaration of Helsinki, there is now an additional need for authorization from the subject for release of the "individually identifiable health information" that the drug sponsor must enter into their data bank for statistical analysis to comply with the requirements necessary for new product approvals. However, HIPAA does not include data needed for adverse experience reporting assessments for clinical trials.

Covered and Not Covered Entities

Who are the covered entities?

Directly "covered entities" of HIPAA are health care providers who engage in electronic transactions, health care clearinghouses, a kind of billing agencies that some physicians offices use to submit their claims and health plans. The "covered entities" are responsible for the privacy standards as well as for any other contracted individuals (called "business associates") to perform essential functions. Business associates do not include members of the covered entity's workforce or volunteer medical staff. Among the business associates functions or activities are legal, actuarial, accounting, consulting, clinical research, data analysis, processing or administration, quality assurance, and practice management. Contracts with business associates must be signed between the covered entity and the business associate requiring the business associate to keep PHI safeguarded. Components of a sample business associate agreement have been included in the HIPAA privacy rules as amended in August 2002.

HIPAA also allows for the creation of "hybrid entities" where certain parts of the entity are not engaged in the covered activities. However, research components of these hybrid entities that function as health care providers and engage in standard electronic transactions are subject to the privacy rule.

Who are not covered entities?

Anybody that is not a covered entity; pharmaceutical, biotech, medical device companies, and contract research organizations—typically they will not be covered entities. It is possible that a large organization may have a health clinic, infirmary on-site, there may be doctors there, they may provide services, and those services may be billed to an insurer under those circumstances. It is possible that that portion of a pharmaceutical or a contract research organization could be a covered entity. But for the most part, pharmaceutical companies, medical device companies, and contract research organizations are not health care providers, plans, or clearinghouses.

Applicability

HIPAA applies to the use or disclosure of health information. The following listings are among the items considered to be part of the privacy rule:

- *Individual identification*: Identification includes name, birth date, admission date, treatment date, telephone number, Social Security number, photo, and vehicle identification numbers. Among the other items that are considered to make the subject "identifiable" are medical record numbers, health plan numbers, and device identifiers/ serial numbers. Even zip codes with more than the first three numbers (except in some cases) will be considered as subject identifiers.
- Information relating to the individual's health, health care treatment, or health care payment.
- Information maintained or disclosed in electronic format, or in hard copy. All information that is created or received by a provider, plan, clearinghouse, or employer relating to past, present, or future physical or mental health or condition, provision of health care, or past, present, or future payment for the provision of health care that identifies the individual or reasonably could be used to identify the individual and it is transmitted in any form. Any information relating to the condition, care, or payment that could identify the individual.

HIPAA Syntax
Reasonable is the HIPAA catch phrase when deciding how to comply with HIPAA standards.

PHI Authorization for Clinical Trials
Background
Investigators participating in clinical research must obtain from each subject authorization that accurately describes the uses and potential disclosure of PHI. The authorization may be presented as part of the IC. In any event, authorization for access to PHI generated prior to research must be obtained from the subject (e.g., past medical history, previous treatments, hospitalizations, etc.). The authorization will state who will have access to the PHI and detail the specific duration of the use of the PHI; for example, the expiration of use can be referred to a specific event such as an FDA approval. If data will be used as a research database then an expiration of "none" might be acceptable to the subjects. The authorization must disclose whether there is compensation to the researcher from a third party and the use or disclosure of the PHI; however, the amount of compensation is not required. If the subject revokes the PHI authorization, information already obtained under the authorization may still be used to preserve the integrity of the clinical trial such as marketing application, ADR reporting, and so on. If this is the case, no new PHI on that subject may be collected or disclosed.

Enforcement of HIPAA
While enforcement authority for ICs exists in FDA and other non-U.S. national and regional health authorities, the enforcement agency responsible for HIPAA in the United States is the Office of Civil Rights (OCR) within the Department of Health and Human Services (HHS). Monitoring of HIPAA will likely occur by the Office of the Inspector General.

There are civil and criminal penalties that exist for violating the HIPAA. An individual who knowingly and wrongfully discloses or obtains individually identifiable health information faces fines of up to $50,000 and a year in prison. Individuals who disclose information with the intent to sell the data face a maximum $250,000 fine and 1 to 10 years imprisonment. It is important to understand that the OCR recognizes that this is a complex set of rules. They themselves are spending a fair amount of time trying to understand it. They have issued several guidances to help comprehend the application of HIPAA. So one should not be in fear that we cannot do anymore research because now there is a statute governing this and you will go to jail. Certainly, if one is in good faith trying to comply with these rules, it is unlikely that there would be any serious challenge.

Individuals bound by the HIPAA privacy requirements may be more reticent in releasing the needed information to the drug sponsors. Assurance of an adequate authorization statement from the clinical subject will be needed to overcome this concern. To ensure that this information, that is, to access drug efficacy and safety data, is made available for use and review by the product sponsors, the sponsors may need to include, in addition to the IC, a written authorization from the subject's participation in a clinical trial that allows the sponsor to use the subject information in any future data analysis. A provision within the authorization should include that if the authorization is withdrawn, it may constitute grounds for removal of subjects from specified clinical trials.

Authorization for Clinical Trials

How is the HIPAA framework applicable for clinical research? There are several different ways to disclose and use information for research including database research. There is nothing in HIPAA and its application to research that is specific for databases. Each type of database research whether it is in the creation of the database, the type of study using the database, the analysis, future analysis, and so on, must be assessed with the same HIPAA privacy rules that apply to research and the question must be asked, "How would this apply to this database and what is the best mechanism in order to be able to disclose the information for research purposes?"

The most effective way to gain authorization from the trial subjects is to obtain the consent/acknowledgment and written authorization from the subjects permitting the disclosure and access to use the clinical trial data.

A single consolidated authorization for the subject, which includes needed authorization for access to data for the clinical trial, can be included with the covered entities authorization's for subject privacy, according to the HIPAA regulations. However, the drug sponsor's access to the needed data is best handled by a separate authorization from each subject for each clinical trial. In addition, a special authorization for subjects is needed for the release of records that involve psychotherapy notes. Drug sponsors should be sure that a special authorization is available for the drug sponsor's access to psychotherapy notes to successfully complete the trial.

The authorization needed to access the subject privacy must include the information that will be used for treatment, payment, or health care operations. Authorizations must be clearly written so that the subject can fully understand the document.

Authorization must include the following:

- Description of the subject information that will be reviewed.
- Persons authorized to make the requested use or disclosure of this information. The drug sponsor should assure that this disclosure extends to all authorized parties involved in the clinical trial assessment including clinical research associates, clinical research organizations, other consultants, and so on.

- *Expiration date of the authorization*: The best choice is for the use of "none" as the expiration date so that review of records can continue to be accessible for future reviews. Although one suggested expiration date was the "end of research," the uncertain time frame may raise questions that will require additional resources.
- Statement that the individual's access rights to inspect and obtain copies of their health records relative to the trial are suspended while the clinical trial is in progress and will be reinstated when the clinical trial is concluded.
- In addition to the required elements, the authorization has to include a statement that the subject has the right to revoke the authorization. There are limitations about the right of the subject to revoke the use of the research information. For example, if the data are already entered in the database and the subject then revokes the authorization, does that mean that all of their information has to be edited out of the results? The privacy rules make it clear that in so far as information has already been disclosed, and that the information has been relied upon, then there is no requirement that that information be removed. However, you would not be able to continue to put in further information on that particular subject into the database. If the removal of the information would have an impact on the results, you might have to do an analysis with and without the information to justify why it should stay in. In other words, if you can demonstrate how the analysis would be greatly affected by removing these data and therefore affect the integrity and impact of the final results, you can justify keeping in those data. The privacy rules do allow for these exceptions.

Relationship to IC

The HIPAA authorization can be included with the IC document or it can be separated from the IC. The required information that must be included in the IC along with the other data comprising the IC, as it pertains to the investigational product, must contain specific and a meaningful description of the information to be disclosed including

- name of the person or class of persons authorized to make the disclosure, for example, principal investigator, subinvestigators, research coordinators, and so on;
- name of the person or class of persons that will receive the disclosed information, for example, sponsor, monitors, CROs, statisticians, and so on;
- statement that communicates that information received by the users may be used for future studies or statistics;
- expiration date or expiration event as to when authorities may disclose the information;
- statement containing a subject's right to revoke their authorization for disclosure;
- statement documenting the ability to condition enrollment on IC/authorization;
- statement documenting the possibility that the information may be redisclosed by the recipient (e.g., to FDA);
- signature of subject and date of the signing of the HIPAA agreement;
- document should be written in a language understood by the subject and a copy of the document must be given to the subject.

It should be noted that the HIPAA privacy rules, in the final form where research has obtained valid consent or waiver of consent from an IRB prior to the enforcement date of April 14, 2003, the research may continue without requiring a HIPAA authorization. Therefore, if subjects who are in a clinical trial and they gave their informed valid consent prior to that date, the data can be continued to be collected and analyzed after the compliance enforcement date without needing an authorized waiver. On the other hand, if subjects that were enrolled in a trial prior to April 14, 2003 and new subjects will then be enrolled after that date, authorization or a waiver or creation of a limited data set must be obtained from these subjects.

IRBs
Where HIPAA requirements are combined with the IC requirements, the entire document needs to be reviewed by the IRB. The OCR as well as FDA's General Counsel as of April 7, 2003 had confirmed that IRB approval of subject authorization for use or disclosure of PHI required by the HIPAA privacy rule is only required if the authorization language is going to be part of the IRB-approved IC document for human subjects' review (1).

IRBs are also permitted to waive authorization requirements for a drug sponsor using expedited review procedures permitted by the Common Rule. Expedited review is permitted for each ongoing research protocol when the only addition is that of the subject authorization for the use or disclosure of PHI. This waiver may be permitted to a researcher when the research is not possible without the waiver. The IRB must assure that an adequate plan is available to protect identifiers and to be sure that at the earliest possible date the identifiers are destroyed.

Privacy Boards
In cases where IRBs are not responsible to review the HIPAA authorization, Privacy Board may be formed to undertake this task. Members of Privacy Boards should have varying backgrounds and appropriate professional competency. At least one member must not be affiliated with the covered entity or research sponsor. Similar to the IRB, there can be no conflicts of interest based on a case-by-case basis. A quorum consists of a majority of members. Expedited review by the chairperson or designees is allowed for the waiver of authorization.

IRB or Privacy Waivers of Authorization
Three criteria must be met for the IRB or Privacy Board to waive authorization for research:

- The use or disclosure of PHI involves no more than a minimal risk to the privacy of the individual.
- The research could not be practicably done without the waiver.
- The research could not be practicably conducted without access to and use of the PHI.
- The research will not adversely affect privacy rights or welfare.
- The privacy risks are reasonable in relation to anticipated benefits and the importance of the knowledge of the clinical results.

Before initiating the clinical trial, the drug sponsors need to have documentation of the waiver in their files. The identification of the IRB or Privacy Board should be included. The date of approval of the waiver, a statement that relevant waiver criteria have been met, a description of the information, and the statement of whether the action was taken under normal or expedited review procedures must be stated clearly.

Waiver of a Research Database

A research database using PHI may be created by a noncovered entity without an individuals' authorizations. Documentation must be obtained from the IRB or the Privacy Board that the specified waiver criteria were satisfied. This database could then be used or disclosed for future research studies as permitted by the privacy rule. Specifically, the database can be used as the basis for future research in which individual authorization has been obtained or where the IRB or Privacy Board grants a waiver.

Similarly, existing databases or repositories created prior to the April 14, 2003 compliance data can be disclosed for research either with individual authorizations or with a waiver from either the IRB or Privacy Board. Approval from both the IRB and Privacy Board is not required for the covered entity.

Study Recruitment

The covered entity's workforce can use PHI to identify and contact prospective research subjects. The covered entity's health care provider can discuss the enrollment in a clinical trial with a potential subject before authorization is completed or there has been an IRB or Privacy Board waiver of authorization. A clinician may use or disclose the PHI if such information is being used to treat the subject or using an experimental treatment that may benefit a subject. However, at no time can the research health care provider remove the protected data from the covered entity's site according to the HIPAA requirements.

If a researcher is not employed by the covered entity, the researcher can still have access to the protected information as a result of a partial waiver of individual authorization by an IRB or Privacy Board. These exceptions are rare.

Limited Data Sets

HIPAA provides for the creation of limited data sets that can be provided to a researcher without obtaining the IRB or Privacy Board's waiver of authorization. All of the direct identifiers of the individual or of relatives, employers, or household members of the individual are required to be deidentified with the following exceptions: admission, discharge and service dates, date of death, age, and five-digit zip code.

Deidentification requires the covered entity to retain individual(s) who have experience using methods with generally accepted statistical and scientific principles and methods that mask identifying characteristics of information to assure that the information is not individually identifiable; for example, statisticians who use scientific principles and methodology in statistical analysis.

Limited data sets must take into consideration the following direct identifiers of the individual or of their relatives, employees, and household members that would be a violation of the HIPAA data use agreement:

- Names
- Postal address
- Telephone/fax numbers
- Electronic mail addresses

- Social Security numbers
- Medical record numbers
- Health plan beneficiary numbers
- Account numbers
- Certificates/license numbers
- Vehicle identifiers
- Device identifiers/serial numbers
- Web universal resource locators (WURLs)
- Internet protocol (IP) address numbers
- Biometric identifiers (including finger and voice prints)
- Full face photographic images and any comparable images

The privacy to subject information that HIPAA commands is not totally unjustified especially in the world of telecommunication we live in. However, it places a great deal of burden on investigators and sponsors who conduct clinical research in the process of new product development. This could possibly delay the research progress to bring new and innovative products in the pharmaceutical field to market. One of the biggest obstacles in completing clinical research in a timely manner stems from the difficulty of adequate subject recruitment. HIPAA is another obstacle that could interfere with this essential step in conducting clinical research.

Possible solutions in overcoming this could be a two-step authorization:

1. Giving initial authorization to permit investigators to use PHI to identify potential subjects that would meet the selection criteria as stated in a clinical protocol.
2. Giving authorization to allow study sponsors or others to disclose PHI. This information could be specifically directed in order to allow subjects to be enrolled in a clinical trial.

In summary, HIPAA is here to stay and the most efficient way to enact on it would be to create a HIPAA questionnaire that could be used on its own or incorporated into an IC.

REFERENCES

1. HIPAA Informed Consent/Authorization Form. Available from http://www.fda.gov.
2. Privacy Regulation. Available from http://www.hhs.gov/ocr/hipaa/.

BIBLIOGRAPHY

Available from www.urac.org.
DHHS Fact Sheet "Protecting the Privacy of Subjects' Health Information." Available from http://www.fda.gov.
Office of Civil Rights guidance "Standards for Privacy of Individually Identifiable Health Information." Available from http://www.fda.gov.
Privacy Rule guidance posted on the website for the NIH which was approved by the Office of Civil Rights. Available from http://www1.od.nih.gov/osp/ospp/hipaa/faq.asp and FDA April 7 response to the International Pharmaceutical Privacy Consortium.
Subscribe for updates on HIPAA documents and events. Available from http://www.fda.gov.

19

Adverse Events and Reactions: Etiology, Drug Interactions, Collection, and Reporting

Richard A. Guarino

Oxford Pharmaceutical Resources, Inc., Totowa, New Jersey, U.S.A.

INTRODUCTION

There is an old but nonetheless true dictum in pharmacology: no drug has a single action. Unfortunately, multiple actions of therapeutic drugs are not always in the best interest of the patient. In addition to the primary therapeutic event for which a drug is prescribed, the likelihood exists for the emergence of concurrent or delayed, unwanted, and potentially harmful adverse events that may be due to other known pharmacologic or toxic events of a drug. Such reactions also may be attributed to some idiosyncrasies in certain individuals. Any active drug, therefore, may be a double-edged sword, doing good on one hand and perhaps harm on the other.

With the recent impressive advances in pharmacology and the ability to synthesize new, complex, and more potent drugs without commensurate knowledge of how and under what conditions they act in humans, the question of adverse events (AEs) and the interactions of drugs has become an increasingly serious aspect of modern therapeutics. It is not surprising, therefore, that drug legislation in most countries is concerned as much with the safety of drugs and devices as with their efficacy. As a result, this aspect of drug evaluation is demanding more and more attention from those involved in drug, device, and biologic or gene research and development, particularly with respect to unwanted or toxic events.

According to the International Committee on Harmonization and Good Clinical Practice guidelines (ICH/GCP) in the preapproval clinical experience with a new medicinal product or its new usages, particularly as the therapeutic dose may not be established, all noxious and unintended responses to a medicinal product related to any dose should be considered AEs. The phrase "responses to a medicinal product" means that a causal relationship between a medicinal product and an AE is at least a reasonable possibility (i.e., the relationship cannot be immediately ruled out). Regarding marketed medicinal products, an AE is a response to a drug that is noxious and unintended and that occurs at doses normally used in humans for prophylaxis, diagnosis, or therapy of diseases or for modification of one or more physiologic functions (1). Once an AE is proven to be caused by the pharmacologic product in question, it can be named an adverse reaction.

Because of the difficulty in obtaining accurate records, the true incidence of AEs to drugs in the population at large is unknown. In the April 15, 1998, issue of the *Journal of the American Medical Association,* Lazarou and colleagues (2) attempted to assess the incidence of serious and fatal AEs in hospitalized subjects by searching through four electronic databases and selecting 39 prospective studies from hospitals in the United States. The overall incidence of serious AEs was 6.7% and of fatal AEs 0.32%. Indeed, serious AEs were between the fourth and sixth leading cause of death in hospitalized subjects. The incidence of AEs of all severities (including serious and nonserious) was 10.9%. Although the authors recommend that the results be reviewed with circumspection because of heterogenicity among studies and small biases in the samples, they concluded that AEs represent an important clinical issue.

The necessity of a clear understanding of the total pharmacology of therapeutic drugs, particularly of their potential for inducing AEs either alone or in concert with other drugs, needs no further emphasis. It has become a major concern for those responsible for developing, prescribing, and dispensing therapeutic agents.

CLASSIFICATION OF ADVERSE DRUG REACTIONS

In general, AEs occurring from a drug may be either dose dependent or independent. Although both types may be produced to a greater or lesser extent by the same drug, dose dependency is a convenient and satisfactory method for classification.

Dose-Dependent AEs

If an active drug is administered in sufficiently large doses, eventually all individuals will manifest AEs. The dosage levels at which the AEs occur, however, may vary considerably from individual to individual. Dose-dependent AEs are usually specific for the drug concerned. They can be categorized as follows: (*i*) known for unwanted pharmacologic events (e.g., the anticholinergic events of the phenothiazine tranquilizers); or (*ii*) exaggerated therapeutic events (e.g., orthostatic hypotension with antihypertensive drugs such as clonidine and guanethidine when these agents are taken at higher than usual doses); or (*iii*) AEs unrelated to the therapeutic events (e.g., ototoxicity produced by excessive doses of streptomycin).

Dose-dependent AEs are influenced by a number of physiologic and pathologic factors that have little or no bearing on dose-independent events. Prominent among these factors are liver and kidney disease, enzyme abnormalities, and drug interactions that may affect absorption or involve competition for transport binding sites of action, certain physiologic conditions altering drug excretion and age. Dose-dependent AEs are often more prominent at the chronologic extremes of life. The fetus, the newborn infant, and the aged are more susceptible than young adults and the middle aged to the AEs of many drugs.

Precautions of Drug Use in Pregnant Women

The fetus is particularly susceptible to the toxic effects of certain drugs that pass the placental barrier. The ill effects of such drugs may vary according to the stage of pregnancy at which they are administered. Drugs with teratogenic properties, for example, given during the first trimester—the period of fetal organogenesis— may cause congenital abnormalities. Moreover, susceptibility of particular organs to drug-induced malformation depends on the time the drug is given during the first trimester. The critical teratogenic period for the nervous system is from gestation days 20 to 40, for the limbs, gestation days 24 to 36, and for the eye, gestation days 24 to 40. Drugs given to the mother after the first trimester may affect the growth or function of normally formed fetal tissues or organs (3). The classic example of a drug with teratogenic activity in humans is thalidomide that is associated with phocomelia; this stimulated the drug regulatory bodies in many countries, including the United States, to adopt more stringent controls on new drug development.

Antineoplastic drugs such as 6-mercaptopurine, methotrexate, cyclophosphamide, and aminopterin administered in early pregnancy have produced various congenital malformations. Cytotoxic drugs also have induced fetal malformation and early abortion of malformed fetuses (4–6).

Corticosteroids administered during the period of fetal organogenesis have been associated with anencephaly (7) and carry a high risk of inducing cleft palate. Lysergic acid diethylamide (LSD), among other hallucinogenic drugs, has been shown to produce chromosomal damage; on less certain evidence, its use during pregnancy may result in congenital anomalies.

The more frequently prescribed drugs that have been reported to affect growth and function of organs when given to the mother after the period of fetal organogenesis, or to the newborn infant, are discussed below.

Antibacterial and Antibiotic Drugs

Sulfonamides are extensively protein bound. If these drugs are administered to mothers immediately before delivery or to the premature or full-term infant while there is physiologic hyperbilirubinemia, they may displace bilirubin from plasma protein causing severe jaundice or kernicterus (8).

Chloramphenicol is not adequately detoxified and excreted by the fetus or the premature infant. Administration of this antibiotic to the mother shortly before parturition may produce gray coloration of the infant's skin with associated muscle hypotonia and circulatory collapse, known as "the gray baby syndrome" (9). (This side event is more noted in premature infants.)

Anticoagulants

Coumarin and indandione derivatives given during pregnancy cross the placental barrier. Even though the maternal prothrombin times remain normal, the use of these anticoagulant compounds may result in fetal death owing to hemorrhage in utero (10) or to intracranial bleeding caused by birth trauma (11).

Antithyroid Drugs

Congenital goiter and neonatal hypothyroidism may occur if thiouracil drugs are administered during pregnancy (12).

Oral Hypoglycemia Drugs

Intrauterine fetal death and prolonged symptomatic neonatal hypoglycemia have been reported after treatment of the mother with sulfonylurea drugs (13,14).

Cardiovascular Drugs

In general, cardiovascular drugs have the same but exaggerated events on the fetus as on the mother. Beta-receptor stimulants (e.g., isoproterenol) and beta-receptor–blocking agents, such as propranolol, may respectively cause significant fetal tachycardia or bradycardia. Norepinephrine and other alpha-receptor stimulants given during pregnancy may induce constriction of the uterine vessels, and thus indirectly result in fetal asphyxia.

Anesthetics, Analgesics, and Hypnotics

If anesthetics, analgesics, and hypnotics are given during labor, they can adversely affect the newborn child by inducing respiratory depression and neonatal asphyxia.

The appearance of typical withdrawal symptoms in the newborn infant of an opiate-addicted mother has been well documented.

So that the aforementioned teratogenic events can be avoided, pregnant women should, in general, be excluded from clinical trials in which the drug is not intended for use in pregnancy. Before the inclusion of pregnant women in clinical trials, all the reproductive toxicity studies (15,16) and the standard battery of genotoxicity tests (17) should be conducted. In addition, safety data from previous human exposure are usually needed. If a subject becomes pregnant during administration of the drug, treatment should generally be discontinued if this can be done safely. For clinical trials of a medicinal product for use during pregnancy, follow-up studies of the pregnancy, the fetus, and the child are important.

Nursing Women
In investigations allowing nursing women, excretion of the drug or its metabolites into human milk should be examined where applicable. When nursing mothers are enrolled in clinical studies, their infants should be monitored for the effects of the drug.

Women of Childbearing Potential
The subjects included in clinical studies should, in general, reflect the population that will receive the drug when it is marketed. For most drugs, therefore, representatives of both sexes should be included in clinical trials in numbers adequate to allow detection of clinically significant sex-related differences in drug response.

Appropriate precautions should be taken in clinical studies to guard against inadvertent exposure of fetuses to potentially toxic agents and to inform subjects and subjects of potential risk the need for precautions. In all cases, the informed consent document and the Investigator's Brochure should include all available information regarding the potential risk of fetal toxicity.

In general, it is expected that reproductive toxicity studies will be completed before there is large-scale exposure of women of childbearing potential (i.e., usually by the end of phase 2 and before any expanded access program is implemented).

Except in the case of trials intended for study of drug events during pregnancy, during investigational clinical research, clinical protocols should include measures that will minimize the possibility of fetal exposure to the investigational drug. These would ordinarily include provisions for the use of a reliable method of contraception (or abstinence) for the duration of drug exposure (which may exceed the length of the study) and the use of pregnancy testing [beta human chorionic gonadotropin (HCG)] to detect unsuspected pregnancy before study treatment begins.

Geriatric Population
The geriatric population is arbitrarily defined as comprising subjects 65 years or older (although this should readily be changed due to the increased longevity reported in modern statistics). The older the population likely to use the drug, the more important it is to include the older age range, 75 years and older. For drugs used to treat diseases not unique to, but present in the elderly, a minimum of 100 subjects usually would allow detection of clinically important differences between the elderly and younger subjects with respect to efficacy as well as AEs reactions.

Elderly individuals often develop AEs to drugs at dosage levels well tolerated by younger persons. These events reactions may be due to an age-related increase in sensitivity to drugs or impairment of detoxification (metabolism) and excretion functions.

Sedating, hypnotic, tranquilizing, and tricyclic antidepressant drugs are prone to precipitate confusional states in the elderly, particularly if there is preexisting evidence of impairment of cognitive function (18–21). Extrapyramidal symptoms such as akathisia and parkinsonism are more common in the elderly than in younger subjects treated with phenothiazine tranquilizers, particularly piperazine derivatives, butyrophenones, and tricyclic antidepressants (22). Furthermore, these psychotropic agents and other drugs with anti-intestinal motility events in the elderly result in troublesome constipation, fecal impaction, and occasionally paralytic ileus (23,24).

Digitalis toxicity is not infrequently encountered in geriatric subjects given digitalizing doses considered normal for younger subjects. The elderly also are more likely to develop hypokalemia with the potassium-wasting diuretics. If these drugs are given concurrently with digitalis, the therapeutic regimen further increases the risk of digitalis toxicity.

It has also been reported that heparin administered to women older than age 60 renders them approximately 50% more susceptible to bleeding complications than men similarly treated (25).

Pediatric Population

The pediatric population consists of four pediatric subgroups: neonates (birth up to 1 month), infants (1 month to 2 years), children (2–12 years), and adolescents (13–16 years).

Many drugs labeled only for adult use are in fact widely used in pediatric subjects for the same indications. Less than half the drugs approved for treatment of HIV infection carry any pediatric safety or effectiveness information. Almost no information on use in subjects younger than two years of age is available for most drug classes (26).

Some AEs occur in children because of inadvertent drug overdoses or other drug administration problems, such as inadequate treatment, that could have been avoided with better information on appropriate pediatric use. This is of particular concern in infants and neonates, because correct pediatric dosing cannot necessarily be extrapolated from adult dosing information using an equivalence based either on weight (mg/kg) or body surface area (mg/m^2). Potentially significant differences in pharmacokinetics may alter a drug's event in pediatric subjects. The events of growth and maturation of various organs, maturation of the immune system, alterations in metabolism throughout infancy and childhood, changes in body proportions, and other developmental changes may result in significant differences in the doses needed by pediatric subjects and adults.

One of the earliest cases in which serious AEs were observed in neonates after administration of a drug that had not been adequately studied in pediatric subjects was the development of "gray baby syndrome" from chloramphenicol, an antibiotic (27). After an initial report of five deaths and a subsequent report of 18 deaths in neonates, it was learned that the immature livers of these infants were unable to clear chloramphenicol from the body allowing toxic doses of the drug to accumulate. Other cases in which inadequately studied drugs have resulted in serious AEs in pediatric subjects include teeth staining from tetracycline, kernicterus from sulfa drugs, withdrawal symptoms after prolonged administration of fentanyl in infants and small children, seizures and cardiac arrest caused by bupivacaine toxicity, development of colonic strictures in pediatric cystic fibrosis subjects after exposure to high-dose pancreatic enzymes, and hazardous interactions between erythromycin and midazolam (26–37). Many such AEs could be avoided if pediatric studies were conducted before drugs were widely used in pediatric subjects.

The absence of adequate pediatric labeling could pose significant risks to pediatric subjects. The FDA will require pediatric studies if the drug product will be widely used in the claimed indication. Clinical studies will also be required if the drug product is indicated for a very significant or life-threatening illnesses.

Enzyme Abnormalities

Enzyme abnormalities may be inherited or acquired. Some of the more important inherited enzyme abnormalities are discussed below. The acquired conditions are dealt with later in this chapter under Drug Interactions.

Inherited Enzyme Abnormalities

It is becoming increasingly evident that a number of AEs to drugs are due to genetically transmitted inborn enzyme abnormalities or deficiencies. The best known example of this category is the hereditary relative deficiency of the enzyme glucose-6-phosphate-dehydrogenase (G-6-PD), which occurs in 5% to 10% of Mediterranean littoral races, blacks, Pakistanis, and Sephardic Jews. This condition renders affected individuals susceptible to acute hemolytic anemia when they are exposed to drugs such as primaquine, phenacetin, aspirin, chloramphenicol, nitrofurantoin, and sulfonamides, and to the fava bean.

Other hereditary enzyme deficiencies that may result in AEs to certain drugs are comparatively rare, often familial, and of worldwide distribution. Examples of these conditions are pseudocholinesterase deficiencies in certain people who, when given succinylcholine or suxamethonium, develop a profound, general neuromuscular blockade with apnea (38).

Tuberculosis subjects lacking in liver N-acetyl transferase who are treated with isoniazid are likely to develop polyneuritis (39). An enzyme abnormality is also responsible for the precipitation of acute intermittent porphyria by the barbiturate drugs (40). Likewise, the rare hereditary resistance to coumadin anticoagulant drugs is thought to be due to an enzyme deficiency (41).

Liver Diseases and Functions

Biotransformation of most drugs takes place in the liver. Any disease of this organ may affect liver function, and may impair the metabolism and inactivation of drugs. This will increase the degree and duration of action of a drug to the extent that exaggerated therapeutic effects and AEs may occur at normal therapeutic dose levels. The list of therapeutic agents so affected is long and varied. It includes widely used drug groups such as phenothiazines, barbiturates, narcotic analgesics, corticosteroids, and oral anticoagulants. Also, subjects with markedly reduced liver function are especially prone to develop hepatic encephalopathy when given potassium-wasting diuretics, narcotic analgesics, and central depressant medications.

Drugs on the other hand may also be the cause of impaired liver function. Direct hepatotoxicity is induced by known hepatotoxins that produce fatty infiltration, degeneration, and widespread necrosis of the liver cells. Carbon tetrachloride, arsenic, gold, mercury, iron, phosphorus, some insecticides, and industrial solvents all have a dose-dependent, direct toxic event on the liver. Fortunately, except perhaps when taken in massive overdoses for suicidal purposes (such as acetaminophen), direct hepatotoxicity with therapeutic drugs is rare. This sinister potential of hepatotoxicity is usually detected in preclinical animal studies, and the drug candidate is then rejected on this account. A dose-dependent form of drug-induced hepatitis, clinically similar to viral hepatitis, may be produced by halothane anesthesia, particularly after multiple exposures (42). Cholestatic jaundice, the most common manifestation of drug-induced liver dysfunction, is essentially an allergic-type phenomenon and is discussed under dose-dependent events.

Renal Function
If renal function is sufficiently impaired, unchanged drugs and their metabolites that are primarily excreted in the urine can be retained in the circulation to a greater or lesser degree. As a result, the therapeutic or AEs of the unchanged portion of the drug may be exaggerated and prolonged; additional AEs due to accumulating metabolites may also appear. Impaired renal function markedly increases the likelihood of ototoxicity due to the administration of the aminoglycosides streptomycin, kanamycin, and gentamicin. The likelihood of toxic effects of normal doses of digitalis preparations on the heart is greatly increased in subjects with renal insufficiency.

Dose-Independent AEs
Occurring less frequently than dose-dependent AEs, dose-independent incidents are largely confined to allergic reactions in persons sensitized by previous administration of the same drug, or by another drug with cross-antigenicity with the original medication. Allergic responses also may occur in individuals who are uniquely susceptible to relatively weak antigens or who develop sensitivity on the first use of a drug—the so-called idiosyncratic reaction.

Allergic responses to drugs are mediated by the release of histamine or histamine-like substances, and they commonly present as skin rashes, particularly urticaria. More serious hypersensitivity responses include bronchospasm or the acute, explosive anaphylactic reaction with cyanosis and cardiovascular collapse. A delayed reaction known as serum sickness, although more often associated with such drugs as the penicillins and cephalosporins rather than with serum, manifests clinically 7 to 10 days after receiving the drug or serum as fever, malaise, joint pains, and urticarial skin rashes.

Blood dyscrasias, mostly dose independent, are among the most important allergic-type AEs to drugs. Aplastic anemia is a serious but rare (presumably) idiosyncratic reaction. It has been reported in association with chloramphenicol, quinacrine, phenylbutazone, mephenytoin, gold compounds, and potassium chlorate. Hemolytic anemia, thrombocytopenia, and agranulocytosis may result from an unusual, acquired sensitivity to a variety of widely used drugs including aminopyrine, phenylbutazone, phenothiazines, propylthiouracil, diphenylhydantoin, penicillins, chloramphenicol, sulfisoxazole, and tolbutamide.

Certain collagen-like diseases are caused by hypersensitivity reactions to drugs. Hydralazine, and particularly procainamide, may produce a clinical picture similar to systemic lupus erythematosus (43). A number of cases of polyarteritis nodosa have developed during treatment with guanethidine and after repeated exposure to the sulfonamides, penicillin, and iodides (44). Nephropathy has been reported following high doses of methicillin and benzylpenicillin (45).

Dose-independent, drug-induced liver dysfunction (cholestatic jaundice) is not an unusual AE. Caused by a number of different, commonly used drugs, cholestasis is a hypersensitivity reaction that primarily affects the biliary canaliculi, causing an intrahepatic obstructive jaundice. An alteration in bile secretion by the hepatocytes, however, may also be involved (46). Among the drugs known to be responsible for the development of cholestatic jaundice are the phenothiazines, the tricyclic antidepressants, the benzodiazepines, phenylbutazone, erythromycin, chlorpropamide, methyltestosterone (dose dependent), and the oral contraceptives containing estrogens and progestins.

DRUG INTERACTIONS

Surveys in the United States and now in some international hospitals have revealed the discomforting fact that subjects on the average receive as many as 10 to 14 different medications during hospitalization. This regrettable trend, in most incidences, toward unnecessary "polypharmacy" has greatly increased the likelihood of drug interactions and has become a new and important professional responsibility for the pharmacist, as well as physicians (47).

The number of documented adverse drug interactions is formidable. They should, however, be viewed in perspective. The prescribing physician needs to be aware of all serious drug interactions that may occur within the range of drugs prescribed. Many drug interactions, though of academic interest, may not be of sufficient clinical significance to justify withholding a drug's use. A number of drugs may offer therapeutic benefits in spite of adverse interactions with other medication.

No attempt will be made to list the major drug interactions. These are readily available in a large number of texts devoted to this subject. The general principles and typical samples of various types of drug interactions, however, which may be of interest in clinical drug research, are discussed below.

Mechanisms of Drug Interactions

The various factors that influence responses to single-drug therapy, including age, race, and physiologic and pathologic states, play an equally important role in drug interactions. The concurrent or close sequential administration of two or more drugs adds further dimension to the mechanisms of action and the possible outcome of the therapeutic program. Two or more drugs may act independently, interact directly with one another, or interact indirectly with one another; one drug acting on an intermediate endogenous substrate that in turn modifies the events of the other drug. Whichever mechanism is involved, the therapeutic event of one or both drugs may be either increased (additive or synergistic) or decreased (antagonistic), and a new and unexpected adverse reaction may emerge. Drugs also may interact with other therapeutic devices or their containers, including disposable plastic syringes, rubber stoppers, and plastic bottles (48,49). This aspect of interaction is outside the scope and intent of this chapter.

Pharmacokinetic Pathways and Drug Interactions

Interactions may occur at one or more of the various states in the pharmacokinetic pathways of drugs in the body [i.e., during absorption, distribution, biotransformation (metabolism), sites of action, and excretion]. Each of these states is considered separately.

Absorption

The extent and rate of absorption of drugs from the gastrointestinal tract is dependent on a number of factors such as bacterial flora, pH, motility, and the transport system involved in the absorptive process. Interaction of therapeutic agents in the gut may seriously impede absorption. Elevation of the pH of the stomach contents by antacids, for example, greatly delays absorption of acidic drugs such as aspirin and phenobarbital. Interaction of drugs forming poorly absorbed complexes, which occurs with tetracycline and antacids containing calcium, aluminum, and magnesium salts, may significantly decrease blood levels of the antibiotic (50).

Distribution Competition for Transport Sites

The distribution of drugs is affected by the circulating plasma that transports them to sites of action, metabolism, and excretion. After absorption, most drugs are partially or almost totally bound to plasma and tissue proteins. The portion that is protein bound is pharmacologically inactive. It serves as a reservoir from which the usually much smaller unbound active fraction can be replenished as the free drug is metabolized and excreted (51).

When two drugs compete for a limited number of binding sites, the drug with the greater affinity for protein binding will displace a portion of the other drug. This increases the unbound active fraction of the other drug, thereby enhancing its pharmacologic event. Sodium warfarin, for example, is about 98% bound to plasma protein and 2% free. If phenylbutazone, which has a greater affinity for protein binding, is given concurrently, it displaces warfarin from its binding sites. As a result, the bound portion of warfarin may drop to 96%, thereby increasing the active unbound fraction to 4%. Consequently, there is twice the amount of active warfarin available, and evidence of overdosage, such as spontaneous hemorrhage, may result (52).

It is evident that displacement of even small amounts of extensively protein-bound drugs can result in a relatively large increase in the active fraction. This commensurate rise in the therapeutic effect often leads to an undesirable or even dangerous level. Competition for protein-binding sites is an example of one drug acting on an intermediate endogenous substrate, thus affecting the activity of another medication.

Interference with Drug Metabolism

Biotransformation or metabolic inactivation of drugs occurs mainly in the liver and, to a lesser extent, in the plasma, kidney, and other tissues, depending on the enzyme system involved. In the liver, microsomal enzymes catalyze many of the metabolic processes involved in the biotransformation of drugs. These metabolic processes may involve nonsynthetic reactions such as oxidation, reduction, or hydrolysis, or synthetic reactions, including conjugation, whereby the drug is coupled with an endogenous substrate (53).

A number of different drugs, especially phenobarbital, have the capacity for enhancing synthesis and activity in the liver microsomes—a process known as enzyme induction. The increased amount of metabolizing enzymes induced by one drug results in the accelerated metabolism of a number of other drugs with metabolic inactivation pathways similar to that of the enzyme-inducing drug. Subjects receiving phenobarbital, for example, metabolize coumarin anticoagulants, steroid hormones, antihistamines, analgesics, anti-inflammatory agents, diphenylhydantoin, and many hypnotic drugs at a greater-than-normal rate. They consequently experience diminished therapeutic activity and duration of action (54).

Some drugs, such as glutethimide, phenylbutazone, probenecid, and tolbutamide, stimulate only their own metabolizing enzymes. This may explain the increasing tolerance to these drugs that often develops after prolonged administration. On the other hand, there are drugs that can slow down or even arrest the metabolism of other drugs, resulting in their prolonged and intensified action, presumably by enzyme inhibition. Diphenylhydantoin intoxication, for example, may occur if either bishydroxycoumarin or isoniazid is given concurrently, as both the latter drugs inhibit the metabolic inactivation of the former. Also, allopurinol, a xanthine oxidase inhibitor, is used to reduce the synthesis of uric acid in gout. Xanthine oxidase is also the enzyme responsible for the deactivation of two potentially toxic antileukemic and immunosuppressant drugs, mercaptopurine and azathioprine. Concomitant medication with allopurinol will therefore elevate the plasma levels of these two cytostatic drugs and greatly increase the risk of serious bone marrow depression (55). More recently, cimetidine has been shown to inhibit the hepatic metabolism of theophylline, resulting in significant increases in serum concentrations of this drug (56). Cimetidine also interacts with, and produces significant increases in, the bioavailability of propranolol, oral anticoagulants, and diazepam, probably by the same mechanism (57–59).

Modification of Drug Event at Sites of Action

Apart from drug interactions that result in increasing or decreasing the amount of drug available to the target organs, there are many interactions that can directly or indirectly alter the response of the receptors in the target organs. A classic example of this type of interaction is the hypertensive crisis produced in subjects concurrently receiving monoamine oxidase (MAO) inhibitors and an indirectly acting amine such as amphetamine or tyramine (found in aged cheeses and some fermented foods). The MAO inhibitors reduce the intraneuronal breakdown of norepinephrine, whereas the amines stimulate release of the excess of norepinephrine from the adrenergic neurons, thus inducing the crisis. Subjects who respond well to MAO inhibitors must be cautioned about this AE that may occur when ingesting foods with a high content of tyramine.

An altered response of one drug on its target organ may be affected by the action of a concurrently administered drug on another organ. The hypokalemia produced by potassium-wasting diuretics, for example, may potentiate the action of digitalis on the heart to the point of toxicity.

Excretion

The kidney is the prime organ for excretion of drugs. Drugs may be eliminated from the body either unchanged or as metabolites of the parent drug. Excretion of one drug through the kidney may be affected by concurrent administration of another and may result in an increased or reduced rate of excretion of either one or both drugs. This mechanism of action can be used to therapeutic advantage. The blood level of penicillin, for example, can be maintained at a higher level for longer periods by the concomitant administration of probenecid, which inhibits the penicillin transport system. On the other hand, quinidine reduces the renal clearance of digoxin. It also may displace digoxin from tissue-binding sites, increasing the serum level of digoxin and enhancing the risk of digoxin cardiotoxicity (60).

Drugs that alter the pH of urine can significantly affect the renal excretion of other drugs. Acid urine increases the eventiveness of mercurial diuretics. It also accelerates the excretion of basic drugs such as meperidine, tricyclic antidepressants, amphetamines, and antihistamines. Acidic drugs, such as aspirin, streptomycin, phenobarbital, sulfonamides, nalidixic acid, and nitrofurantoin, have been shown to increase renal clearance in alkaline urine (61). The possible effects of urine pH on the renal excretion of drugs have been illustrated by the observation that if urine is rendered sufficiently alkaline, the excretion of amphetamine is markedly delayed, and effective blood levels, after a single dose, can be maintained for several days (62).

The Beneficial Effects of Drug Interactions

It is customary, and indeed prudent, to emphasize the possible hazards of drug interactions. However, a number of drug interactions have demonstrated beneficial therapeutic effects and have been used to an advantage in clinical practice for many years. Well-known examples of these include the chelating events of calcium disodium edetate, dimercaprol, and penicillamine in chronic poisoning with arsenic, bismuth, gold, and lead. The other examples include simple expedient of alkalinization of the urine to increase renal elimination in poisonings with acidic drugs such as barbiturates and aspirin; the use of protamine sulfate to bind with heparin; forming an inactive complex, thus counteracting the events of overheparinization; and the synergistic antibacterial effects of trimethoprim and sulfamethoxazole in the urine when these drugs are administered together.

Paradoxically, the unpleasant effects of a toxic metabolite produced by a drug interaction can have therapeutic benefits, such as the administration of disulfiram in the treatment of alcoholism. Furthermore, interactions at receptor sites to block the effects of a drug may be used to advantage (e.g., nalorphine in morphine poisoning). It is common practice to use antiparkinsonian drugs such as benztropine to ameliorate extrapyramidal symptoms—the commonly occurring adverse reactions to psychotropic drugs such as the phenothiazines, butyrophenones, and thioxanthenes. Combination therapy with the potassium-wasting diuretics and spironolactone (an aldosterone antagonist) or triamterene can be used to reduce excessive potassium loss and avert hypokalemia.

Whereas these and other beneficial drug interactions are well known and often used in clinical practice, some drug interactions that are currently considered to be adverse may also be applied therapeutically. For example, the analgesic events of meperidine and the opiates are augmented by the concurrent administration of MAO inhibitors. This interaction can be used to increase the desirable effects of the analgesics without having to increase the dose. The regimen may have a place in the relief of severe chronic pain in subjects with terminal malignant disease.

In spite of the well-known AEs and dangers that attend the concomitant administration of many drugs, it is reassuring that the selective use of certain drug interactions has a positive place in pharmacotherapy; "sweet uses of adversity" as Hollister (63) has so aptly phrased it.

COLLECTION, EVALUATION, AND REPORTING OF ADVERSE EVENTS TO DRUGS

Overview

The AE potential of an investigational new pharmaceutical product, to some extent, may be indicated by its molecular structural similarities to other drugs of known actions and by pharmacologic and toxicologic preclinical studies in appropriate species of laboratory animals. The full adverse reaction profile of a drug, however, can only be determined by reports from human experience when the drug has been administered to a relatively large number of subjects of different ages, both sexes and diverse ethnic groups geographically dispersed for extended periods of time.

Phase 1, 2, and 3 clinical research programs required by the FDA and most global regulatory bodies in other countries are sufficient to initially define the more frequently occurring AEs and reactions to establish the safety of an investigational new pharmaceutical product. The safety evaluations observed during clinical product development is not expected to characterize rare AEs—for example, those occurring in less than 1 in 1000 subjects—but it is expected to characterize and quantify the safety profile of a drug over a reasonable duration of time consistent with the intended short- or long-term use of the product. The number of subjects treated for six months at dosage levels intended for clinical use should be adequate to characterize the pattern of AEs over time, usually evaluated in 300 to 600 subjects.

There is always concern although they are likely to be uncommon, some AEs may increase in frequency or severity over time, or that some serious AEs may occur only after drug treatment continues for more than six months. Therefore, when chronic administration of a drug product is intended, some subjects should be observed for 12 months during clinical investigations. In the absence of more information about the relationship of AEs to treatment duration, selection of a specific number of subjects to be monitored for one year is to a large extent a judgment based on the probability of detecting a given AE frequency level and practical considerations. One hundred subjects exposed for a minimum of one year is considered acceptable (64). However, the expected duration of clinical investigations and evaluations for short-term use of drug administration is 3 months and for chronically administered drugs is 12 months.

Once a drug, biologic, or device is approved by a regulatory agency and labeling is established, the expectation from physicians, patients, and other health care professionals is that the medication or device is safe and effective, if used as directed by the package insert. It is well known and generally accepted that there will be some AEs associated with the use of these products, and these AEs are usually described in the labeling. However, the risk/benefit ratio should be considered for the class of drug. Nonetheless, some less frequent and rare AEs will not always be known at the time of approval and marketing (65). As previously addressed, only after a medication or device is prescribed in large numbers of people under circumstances not always observed in controlled clinical trials, could the rare and less frequent AEs be observed. A single rare AE may only be seen with the exposure of about 10,000 subjects. It can be hypothesized that in order to accumulate an adequate number of AEs, many thousands of subjects should be exposed to the medication or device and that is usually accomplished with postmarketing studies of various types. In addition, the AEs that are reported after the product is marketed are reviewed very carefully by the sponsors and regulatory agencies and, if appropriate, will be included in the package inserts.

Collecting AEs—Legal Responsibilities
Since there is a difference between the procedures for investigational and marketed medications and devices, the collection, evaluation, and reporting of AEs are discussed in sequence so that the differences are easily identified.

Investigational Drugs
Reporting AEs from Study Subjects During Clinical Investigations
There are three generally accepted methods by which AEs may be elicited from study subjects:

(a) Systematic questioning using a checklist containing the AEs considered most likely to occur with the particular drug or biologic being studied; often based on animal data.
(b) Direct questioning without the use of a formal checklist. Questions concerning untoward symptoms should be put to subjects in such a way that they do not, by suggestion, lead the subject into giving invalid information.
(c) Recording only those AEs that are volunteered by the subject or observed by the investigator or others involved in the clinical study.

Of the three methods, the first, or checklist technique, has the greatest tendency to make subjects introspective regarding their symptoms. Not surprisingly, this approach elicits the largest number of AE reports. Regardless of the method used, however, it is imperative that the questions be applied in the same way at each subject assessment, preferably by the same person, for the duration of the clinical trial. It is also recommended that subjects be carefully questioned *prior* to administration of the study drug. It is remarkable how many so-called AEs are, in fact, symptoms of other conditions present before the treatment starts and never should be charged to the study medication as an AE.

Postmarketing Reporting
It is only by continued pharmacovigilance and tracking after a medication is available for general clinical administration and under an expanded variety of circumstances that rare, sometimes severe, and even life-threatening adverse drug reactions or drug interactions are detected. Only then can the full adverse reaction spectrum and profile of a drug be finally delineated. Examples of a serious adverse reaction that was discovered postmarketing is the occurrence of serious regurgitant cardiac valvular disease during use of dexfenfluramine, an antiobesity drug, especially when the drug is used in combination with phentermine (FEN/PHEN). It should be noted that use of the combination was not approved by the FDA or other regulatory agencies. Another example is the incidence of Vioxx, a drug effective in millions of people but was taken off the market due to cardiac lesions reported postmarketing.

There are numerous examples of serious adverse reactions identified after a drug has been marketed and used extensively in large numbers of subjects. In some instances, the knowledge of these serious adverse reactions have resulted in the withdrawal of some drugs from the market on the basis of postmarketing experience and others have labeling changes as in specific "Warnings" and "Black Box Warnings."

The collection of AEs for investigational drugs is a standardized and controlled regulated process. The collection of AEs for marketed drugs is more complex since there are many sources, phase 4 clinical trials, physician, pharmacist, and consumer reports.

The Marketing Authorized Holder (MAH)

The company marketing the product or the MAH is responsible for the reporting, updating, and evaluation of the safety profile of their drugs. This applies to MAHs marketing the brand or the generic product. The MAH is responsible to collect information from all sources in addition to the spontaneous AE reports that are generally reported directly to the MAH and from studies performed by the MAH. These additional sources are described below. In turn, the MAH must report all AE reports to the regulatory authorities.

The European Community requires the individual MAHs to submit all received adverse reactions in electronic form (save in exceptional circumstances). The reporting obligations of the various stakeholders are defined in the Community legislation, in particular

- Regulation (EC) No. 726/2004; and
- for human medicines, European Union Directive 2001/83/EC as amended and the EU Directive 2001/20/EC.

Regulatory Agencies Globally

AEs may be reported directly to the health authorities or regulatory agencies by health care professionals or consumers. It is the responsibility of the MAH to be certain that this information from the regulatory agencies is reported to the MAH. If there is a standard procedure or agreement with the regulatory agency to provide these reports to the MAH, these should be regularly reviewed with the regulatory agencies. Information collected by a regulatory authority may be provided to other regulatory authorities of other Member States on a regular basis.

Professional (Physicians and Pharmacists) and Consumers

Reports of AEs are sent to regulatory agencies and/or the MAH by practicing physicians, health care professionals, and consumers. In some countries, physicians are required to submit potential AEs directly to the health authorities.

Literature

Practicing physicians may observe a specific and sometimes serious AE or reaction that may be attributable to the drug and submit an article or letter to a journal describing a specific observation as a potential AE. In addition, publications of study results are published with data from comparative studies of a marketed product. This information could reveal new information about the profile of a specific drug particularly if the study is a very large one. The MAH is responsible to review the literature for reports of new AEs not included in the labeling or a possible change in the known frequency of an AE. Companies performing studies comparing their drug to another marketed drug from another company are required to notify the MAH of the competitive drug about the potential AE.

Postmarketing Surveillance

Postmarketing surveillance programs are large observational studies designed mainly to evaluate safety. There are many designs and purposes for performing postmarketing studies. In some cases, more frequently observed in the United States, a postmarketing study may be part of a commitment from the MAH as a condition for approval of an NDA; if so, the protocol to conduct this study must be discussed with the FDA before the study is initiated. Postmarketing studies may be prospective involving thousands of subjects or AEs may be derived from claims compiled in electronic health databases that capture provider, facility, and pharmacy claims identifying diagnoses of interest from established health care insurance plans such as United health care, Medicaid, and so on. Also, registries are often established to monitor specific AEs for specific drugs. Pharmacoepidemiologic studies may be designed as cohort (prospective or retrospective) case control, nested case control, case-crossover, or using other models. Frequently, these large studies have a medical monitoring or advisory board comprised of experts in the specific areas of interest. A good reference for these studies is the FDA's "Guidance for Industry Good Pharmacovigilance Practices and Pharmacoepidemiologic Assessment," March 2005 (66).

Since there are so many sources for collecting AE data, one of the problems encountered by the MAH and regulatory agencies is duplicate reporting of the same AE. So the MAH and the regulatory agencies are often faced with the task of identifying duplicate reports before evaluating them for a risk assessment.

Evaluation of AEs

Investigational Drugs

Clinical trials for investigational drug products are, for the most part, blinded trials, and the treatment group and the control group are unknown to investigators and subjects participating in the clinical trial. When a serious AE occurs, in many instances, the blind is broken. It is important, however, to monitor AEs by groups (A or B) and to look for emerging trends to access serious AEs by treatment group. It is also important to closely monitor laboratory results, for example, radical changes from normal to abnormal or abnormal to a more pronounced abnormal. Close monitoring is mandatory for any new drug or biologic evaluation. AEs occurring during clinical investigations, if not thoroughly assessed, could cause life-threatening situations and even death.

Completed Clinical Trials

There are standardized tables and approaches to statistical analyses for the evaluation of AEs, ADRs, laboratory and objective electronic recordings, and image readings. The interpretation and the relationship of each of these values must be considered in the overall assessments of any abnormal value in relationship to the disease being evaluated. The risk–benefit considerations must be assessed for every AE reported. A detailed record must be included in each trial summary submitted in the NDA.

Postmarketing Surveillance

Once a drug is marketed, there is greater exposure to patients prescribed the drug and in patients with multiple medical conditions taking the drug with other medications. These subjects may have been excluded from participating in investigational phase 1 to 3 controlled clinical trials. In order to detect rare and unexpected AEs, not generally identified during clinical trials, exposure of a new drug to a larger population will give an expanded safety profile of the drug. Therefore, postmarketing surveillance data are very critical for an appropriate benefit/risk assessment of a drug. This information is collected from individual spontaneous AE reports, and through pharmacovigilance and pharmacoepidemiology studies.

The pharmacovigilance effort in Europe is coordinated by the European Medicines Agency (EMEA) and conducted by the National Competent Medicines Authorities (NCA). The main responsibility of the EMEA is to maintain and develop the pharmacovigilance database consisting of all suspected serious adverse reactions to medicines observed in the European Community. The system is called Eudrac Vigilance and contains separate but similar databases of human and veterinary reactions.

Spontaneous Reports
In pre-NDA approval controlled clinical trials, there is a standardized approach to evaluating individual AEs and monitoring overall safety. In spontaneously reported events, it is difficult to estimate the product-exposed population, and it is well known that there is underreporting. "FDA suggests that sponsors calculate reporting rates by using the total number of spontaneously reported cases in the United States in the numerator and estimates of national subject exposure to product in the denominator" (67).

Observational Studies
Such studies evaluate a drug's use in the "real world." These studies use estimations of the relative risk associated with a drug and some cohort studies can also provide estimates of risk (incidence rate) guidance document (68).

Registries
A "registry" is an organized system for the collection, storage, retrieval, analysis, and dissemination of information on individual persons exposed to a specific medical intervention who have either a particular disease, a condition (e.g., a risk factor) that predisposes them to the occurrence of a health-related event, or prior exposure to substances (or circumstances) known or suspected to cause adverse health events (69).

Reporting Adverse Reactions
Drug safety and adverse reactions are closely related in an inversely proportional manner. In the United States, drug safety is under strict legislative control mandated by the FDA. U.S. Federal regulations require sponsors and investigators (MAH) to report adverse reactions for a drug product at both the investigational and the postmarketing stages. In Europe, drug safety is coordinated by the EMEA and conducted by the NCA.

Investigational Stage
A distinction should be made between an ADR and an AE. An AE is any untoward medical occurrence in a patient or clinical investigation subject who has been given a pharmaceutical product, which does not necessarily have a causal relationship with this treatment. An AE can therefore be any unfavorable and unintended sign (including an abnormal laboratory finding), symptom, or disease temporally associated with the use of medicinal (investigational) product, whether

or not related to the medicinal (investigational) product (1). An adverse drug reaction is one that is proven to be caused by the pharmaceutical product either during the development of the product or after the marketing of the product.

During the clinical investigation of a new drug (phases 1, 2, 3, and 3b) before FDA approval, it is the sponsor's responsibility to notify the FDA of all AEs as described in this chapter and the IND and IMPDs chapter.

The FDA has recently revised the regulations for expedited reporting and assessing AEs and has issued definitions of terms to comply with recent ICH Guidelines (70). These new definitions are the same as those in the CFRs. The difference is this includes global reporting.

Disability: This is defined as a substantial disruption of a person's ability to carry out normal life functions.

Associated with the use of the drug: There is a reasonable possibility that the experience may have been caused by the drug.

Unexpected or serious AEs: An unexpected AE is any reaction, the specificity or severity of which is not consistent with the current Investigator's Brochure. If an Investigator's Brochure is not required or available, the specificity or severity of which is not consistent with the risk information described in the general investigational plan or elsewhere in the current application, as amended. For example, under this definition, hepatic necrosis would be unexpected (by virtue of greater severity) if the Investigator's Brochure referred only to elevated hepatic enzymes or hepatitis. "Unexpected," as used in this definition, refers to an adverse drug experience that has not been previously observed (e.g., included in the Investigator's Brochure or package insert) rather than one that has not been anticipated from the pharmacologic properties of the pharmaceutical product.

When a serious adverse drug experience occurs, the investigator will provide the following information:

- Subject identification number, age, and sex.
- Duration of drug administration (includes dates of drug administration).
- Dose administered (whether or not the code was broken in the case of a double-blind study) and route of administration.
- Indication of drug (diagnosis for use).
- Description of AE, including date and time of onset, as well as the date and time the event subsided. The outcome (recovered, alive with sequelae) should also be stated. Any laboratory evaluations, ECGs, autopsy reports, and so on, that are needed for understanding the AE should be submitted.
- Concomitant medication, including the dose and dates of administration.
- Current disease state, diagnosis, and medical history.
- Dechallenge and rechallenge information.
- Whether the subject was in imminent danger of death at the time of the AE.
- Relationship to study drug. The investigator should state whether there was a reasonable possibility that the AE was caused by the drug/device.
- Whether the AE was unexpected.

In the United States, the investigator should complete and sign the appropriate form as required by the FDA. The FDA Medical Products Reporting Program (MedWatch) FDA Form 3500A allows for use by user facilities, distributors, and manufacturers for "mandatory" reporting of AEs and product problems during the use of drugs, biologics, and devices. Form 3500 is for use by health care professionals and consumers for voluntary reporting. AEs associated with vaccines are reported to the FDA and the CDC using the Vaccine Adverse Event Reporting System (VAERS).

All AEs occurring during clinical investigations must be resolved or justified by the principal investigator during and, if necessary, after the clinical investigation is completed. Each investigational site reporting any AE should be contacted by the sponsor or the sponsors' representative on a regular basis to determine the status of the subject's condition until the AE is resolved.

If the serious adverse experience is unexpected, fatal, or life threatening, and is associated with the use of the drug, then the division of the FDA that is assigned to the product and has the responsibility for review of the IND must be informed by telephone or facsimile transmission as soon as possible and no later than seven calendar days after the first knowledge of the event. The initial notification must be followed by a complete written IND safety report to the FDA within 15 calendar days. In addition, all investigators involved in a multicenter study must be notified in writing of the AE within 15 calendar days. The investigators must apprise the individual IRBs/IECs of the AE report.

Postmarketing Stage

Marketing authorization holders (original as well as generic MAHs) are required to develop written procedures for the surveillance, receipt, evaluation, and reporting of postmarketing AEs to the FDA The definitions of postmarketing adverse experiences and unexpected adverse experiences are as follows (71):

Adverse experience definition: An AE is any event associated with the use of a drug, biologic, or device product in humans, whether or not considered product related, including the following: an AE occurring in the course of the use of a product in professional practice; an AE occurring from overdose of the product, whether accidental or intentional; an AE occurring from abuse of the product; and an AE occurring from withdrawal of the product and any failure of expected pharmacologic action.

Unexpected AE: An unexpected AE is any AE that is not listed in the current labeling for the product. This includes events that may be symptomatically and pathophysiologically related to an event listed in the labeling, but differs from the event because of greater severity or specificity. "Unexpected," as used in this definition, refers to an adverse experience that has not been previously observed (i.e., included in the labeling) rather than one that has not been anticipated from the pharmacologic properties of the pharmaceutical product.

Serious and life-threatening AEs: A serious AE is one that occurs at any dose that results in any of the following outcomes: death, a life-threatening AE, inpatient hospitalization or prolongation of existing hospitalization, a persistent or significant disability/incapacity, or a congenital anomaly/birth defect. Important medical events that may not result in death, but are determined to be life threatening or require hospitalization may also be considered serious AEs. Any AE that may jeopardize the patient's welfare or may require medical or surgical interventions in the view of a physician should be considered a serious AE.

Serious and unexpected AEs: Adverse drug experiences that are both serious and unexpected, whether foreign or domestic, must be reported to the FDA and Member States in the European Union that market the products as soon as possible, but no later than 15 calendar days after initial receipt of the information (15-day Alert Reports). In the U.S. Form 3500A (MedWatch) and in the EU, the International C10MS 1 Form must be used for reporting. Any additional information must be forwarded to the FDA or the competent authority of each MS marketing the product, in a follow-up report.

In addition, the frequency of reports of serious and unexpected AEs and reports of therapeutic failure must be reviewed periodically. An increase of frequency of an AE must be reported to the FDA or the MS within 15 working days of determining the significant increase.

Postmarketing reports: In the United States, postmarketing periodic AE reports are required at quarterly intervals for three years from the date of approval of the NDA and then at annual intervals within the annual report.

The reporting requirements in the EU are slightly different from the United States with respect to the postmarketing periodic reports. The reader is referred to Volume 9A of The Rules Governing Medicinal Products in the European Union—Guidelines on Pharmacovigilance for Medicinal Products for Human Use for the periodicity and description of the Periodic Safety Update Report (PSUR).

Assessment of Adverse Reactions
ICH Guidelines
The most difficult part of AE reporting is the accurate assessment of the causal relationship of a drug to an alleged reaction. The likelihood that a drug contributes to, or is responsible for, an AE with any degree of certainty can be established only if adequate information is available.

The degrees of causal relationship between a drug and a suspected adverse reaction are defined as follows:

1. A remote causal relationship between a drug and an event exists when the temporal association is such that the drug would not have had any reasonable association with the observed event.
2. A possible causal relationship between a drug and an event exists when the reaction (*i*) follows a reasonable temporal sequence from administration of the drug; (*ii*) follows a known response pattern to the suspected drug; or (*iii*) could have been produced by the subject's clinical state or other modes of therapy administered to the subject.
3. A probable causal relationship between a drug and an event exists when the reaction (*i*) follows a known response pattern to the drug; (*ii*) is confirmed by withdrawal of the drug; or (*iii*) cannot be reasonably explained by the known characteristics of the subject's clinical state.
4. A definite causal relationship between a drug and event exists when the reaction (*i*) follows a reasonable temporal sequence from the time of drug administration or from the time the drug level has been established in body fluids or tissues; (*ii*) follows a known response pattern to the suspected drug; or (*iii*) is confirmed by improvement upon withdrawal of the drug (dechallenge) and reappearance of the ADR upon reintroduction of the suspect drug (rechallenge).

Accurate assessment of a causal relationship of a drug to an AE is beset with many difficulties. Most prominent among these are (*i*) incomplete, time-related, drug-related information; (*ii*) multiplicity of drugs administered in most cases; (*iii*) lack of an objective means of demonstrating a direct relationship between a drug and an adverse reaction; and (*iv*) the limited number of reaction patterns of the body to the entire range of physical, chemical, and biological causes of disease.

Because of these and other potential problems, the majority of drug-induced diseases fall into the "possible" category. Very few can unequivocally be labeled as definite.

Adverse Event Disclaimers
General
In assessing an AE, whether it is reported during the clinical development of a product or from a marketed product, the question always arises as to the etiology of the AE. Was it a direct result of being administered the product; was the AE caused by a drug interaction with another product; or was it attributable to other products administered simultaneously with the product in question? These questions have always caused a dilemma in assessing the causality of AEs. Regulations pertaining to the reporting of AEs are well documented in this chapter and command that all AEs must be reported to the regulatory agencies. However, sponsors are allowed to file a disclaimer based on information that the AE does not necessarily reflect a conclusion by the sponsor or FDA, that the report or information constitutes an admission that the product caused or contributed to an AE.

Before a disclaimer is considered, a sponsor should always do causality assessments. These assessments can be categorized as follows:

1. *Definite*: A reaction that follows a reasonable temporal sequence from administration of the medication, follows a known or suspected response pattern of the medication, is confirmed by improvement upon stopping or reducing the dosage of the medicine (*dechallenge*) and reappears upon repeated exposure (*rechallenge*).
2. *Probable*: A reaction that follows a reasonable temporal sequence from administration of the medication, follows a known or suspected response pattern of the medication, is confirmed by improvement upon stopping or reducing the dosage of the medication, and cannot be reasonably explained by the known characteristics of the subject's clinical state.
3. *Possible*: A reaction that follows a reasonable temporal sequence from administration of a medication, follows a known or suspected response pattern of the medication, but that could readily have been produced by a number of other factors.

   OR

   A reaction that follows a reasonable temporal sequence from administration of the medication, is not a known or suspected response pattern, and could be explained by another etiology.
4. *Doubtful*: A reaction that does not follow a reasonable temporal sequence from administration of the medication, does not follow a known or suspected response pattern, and could be explained by another etiology.
5. *Unknown*: Relationships for which insufficient information exists.

6. *Not related*: A reaction for which sufficient information exists to indicate the eti-
    ology is unrelated to the clinical trial medication.

AEs having a causality assessment of possible, doubtful, unknown, or not
related should be questioned and if found not to be caused by the product should
be followed by an AE product disclaimer. The AE reports submitted to the FDA on
products where subsequent information or data prove that the product was not the
cause of the AE reported should have a follow-up letter requesting a disclaimer. The
letter should be submitted to the FDA stating the following:

> Information submitted does not necessarily reflect a conclusion by the sponsor or
> FDA that the report or information on the adverse event constitutes an admission
> that the drug/product caused or contributed the adverse event.

Sponsors need not admit and may deny that adverse reports or information
submitted by the sponsor constitutes an admission that the drug caused or contributed to an AE.

European Guidelines on Collection and Verification of Adverse Reactions

The European Guidance specifically addresses adverse reaction reporting arising
from clinical trials on medicinal products for human use. The assessments of AEs
are basically the same as enumerated on page 367 under "Reporting of Adverse
Reactions." However, there is a slight difference: when investigators in the United
States report an AE, they are obligated by GCPs to report it to the sponsor and
the Institutional Review Board. The sponsor, after assessing the AE, is obligated
to report it to the FDA and notify all investigators of the AE. Based on the severity of the AE, the sponsor reports it to the FDA as a 7- or 15-day report or in the
annual report as detailed on page 369 of this chapter under "Reporting of Adverse
Reactions." Under the European Guidelines, the investigator reports the AE to the
sponsor and the sponsor reports it to the concerned competent authorities and to
the Ethics Committee under the same time constraints as listed above.

SUMMARY AND CONCLUSION

AE assessments, evaluating, and reporting is the most effective way to assess the
safety of all pharmaceutical products during product development and after the
product has been approved for marketing. AEs reported on a drug product do not
necessarily indicate that the product is unsafe; it basically represents that the product is active. However, when the AEs outweigh the benefits of a drug product to the
degree of being life threatening to the point where it commands total withdrawal
of the drug from the subjects, it is usually declared to be unsafe and is removed
from further clinical investigations. In the case of an approved drug, removal from
the market becomes a serious consideration. In situations where significant AEs
are reported and corrective measures effectively protect the subject's safety and the
overall benefits outweigh the risks, the product may be allowed to be administered
with closer safety surveillance.

It is essential for all pharmaceutical product developers to understand the
importance of reporting and tracking every AE. Basic clinical research can only
give limited data of AEs. Only when a product is marketed and prescribed to large
populations, can a true picture of the safety of the product be revealed. Significant

emphasis is being placed on safety especially through pharmacovigilance. It is the responsibility of MAH, physicians, and all health care personnel to continually be alert to observing and reporting of AEs from consumers. It is only through the accumulation of AE reporting that significant conclusions can be drawn about the incidence of AEs and a true assessment of risk versus benefit. Regulations governing the control of AEs may seem overly restrictive. However, the prime interest of the global regulators is to protect the safety and welfare of the population prescribed or consuming these pharmaceutical products. The regulations, guidelines, and recommendations presented in this chapter are a foundation for all persons participating in pharmaceutical product development.

REFERENCES

1. Federal Register (May 9, 1997). Vol. 62, No. 90.
2. Lazarou J, Pomeranz BH, Corey PN (1998). Incidence of adverse drug reactions in hospitalized subjects: a meta-analysis of prospective studies. JAMA 279, 1200.
3. Turner P, Richens A (1973). In: Clinical Pharmacology. Edinburgh: Churchill Livingstone.
4. Nicholson HO (1968). Cytotoxic drugs in pregnancy. J Obstet Gynaecol Br Commonw 75, 307.
5. Shaw EB, Steinbach HL (1968). Aminopterin induced fetal malformation. Am J Dis Child 115, 477.
6. Brandner Nussle M (1969). Foetopathie due a l'aminopterine avec stenose congenitale d l'espace medallaire des os tubulaires longs. Ann Radiol 12, 703.
7. Warrell DW, Taylor R (1968). Outcome for the foetus of mothers receiving prednisolone during pregnancy. Lancet 1, 117.
8. Elmes PC (1972). Antibacterial drugs used in miscellaneous infections. In: Meyler L, Herxheimer A, eds. Side Events of Drugs. Amsterdam: Excerpta Medica.
9. Kouvalainen K, Unnirus V, Wasz-Hockert O (1967). Side events of chloramphenicol in prematurely born infants. Ann Paediatr Fenn 13, 23.
10. Hirsh J, Cade JF, Gallus AS (1965). Fetal events of coumarin administered during pregnancy. Blood 26, 623.
11. Mahairas GH, Weingold AB (1963). Fetal hazard with anti-coagulant therapy. Am J Obstet Gynecol 85, 237.
12. Crooks J (1972). Thyroid and antithyroid drugs. In: Meyler L, Herxheimer A, eds. Side Events of Drugs. Amsterdam: Exerpta Medica.
13. Zucker P, Simon G (1968). Prolonged symptomatic neonatal hypoglycemia associated with maternal chlorpropamide therapy. Pediatrics 42, 824.
14. Hussar A (1970). The hypoglycemic agents—their interactions. J Am Pharm Assoc 100, 169.
15. ICM Harmonized Tripartate Guideline (S5B). "Detection of Toxicity to Reproduction for Medicinal Products."
16. ICM Harmonized Tripartate Guideline (S5B) "Toxicity to Male Fertility."
17. ICM Topic S2B Document "Standard Battery of Genotoxicity Tests."
18. Kramer M (1963). Delirium as a complication of imipramine therapy in the aged. Am J Psychiatry 120, 502.
19. Bender AD (1967). Pharmacodynamic consequences of aging and their implications in the treatment of the elderly subject. Med Ann 36, 267.
20. Gibson JM II (1966). Barbiturate delirium. Practitioner 197, 345.
21. Hamilton LD (1966). Aged brain and the phenothiazines. Geriatrics 21, 131.
22. Ayd FJ Jr (1960). Tranquilizers and the ambulatory geriatric subject. J Am Geriatr Soc 8, 909.
23. Hollister LE (1965). Nervous system reaction to drugs. Ann N Y Acad Sci 123, 342.
24. Ritama V, Vapaatalo HI, Neuvoner PJ (1969). Phenothiazines and intestinal dilatation. Lancet 1, 470.

25. Jick H, Slone D, Borda T (1968). Efficacy and toxicity of heparin in relation to age and sex. N Engl J Med 279, 284.

26. Pina LM (August 15, 1997). Drugs widely used off label in pediatrics, report of the pediatric use survey working group of the pediatric subcommittee. Draft (Federal Register, Vol. 62, No. 158).

27. Powell DA (1982). Chloramphenicol: new perspectives on an old drug. Drug Intell Clin Pharm 16, 295.

28. Oski FA (1994) Principles and Practice of Pediatrics, 2nd ed. Philadelphia: J.B. Lippincott Co., 864.

29. Nathan DG (1993). Hematology of Infancy and Childhood, 4th ed. Philadelphia: W.B. Saunders Co., 92.

30. Kauffman RE (1991). Fentanyl, fads, and folly: who will adopt the therapeutic orphans. J Pediatr 119, 588.

31. McCloskey JJ (1992). Bupivacaine toxicity secondary to continuous caudal epidural infusion in pediatric subjects. Anesth Analg 75, 287.

32. Fisher DM (1983). Neuromuscular events of vecuronium (ORG NC45) in infants and pediatric subjects during N2O halothane anesthesia. Anesthesiology 58, 519.

33. Agarwal R (1992). Seizures occurring in pediatric subjects receiving continuous infusion of bupivacaine. Anesth Analg 75, 284.

34. Mevorach DL (1993). Bupivacaine toxicity secondary to continuous caudal epidural infusion in pediatric subjects. Anesth Analg 77, 1305.

35. Cystic fibrosis and colonic strictures (1995). Editorial. J Clin Gastroenterol 21, 2.

36. Olkkola KT (1993). A potentially hazardous interaction between erythromycin and midazolam. Clin Pharmacol Ther 53, 298.

37. Hiller A, Olkkola KT, Isohanni P et al. (1990). Unconsciousness associated with midazolam and erythromycin. Br J Anaesth 65, 826.

38. Theodore J, Millen JE, Murdaugh HV (1967). Prolonged postoperative apnea with pseudo- cholinesterase deficiency. Am Rev Respir Dis 96, 508.

39. Evans DAP, Manley KA, McKusick VA (1960). Genetic control of isoniazid metabolism in man. BMJ 2, 485.

40. Goldberg A, Remington C (1962). Diseases of Porphyrin Metabolism. Springfield, IL: Thomas.

41. O'Reilly RA, Aggler PM (1965). Studies in coumarin anti-coagulant drugs: hereditary resistance in man. Fed Proc 24, 1266.

42. Trey C, Lipworth L, Davidson CS (1969). Clinical syndrome of halothane hepatitis. Anesth Analg 48, 1033.

43. Siegal M, Lee SL, Peress NS (1967). The epidemiology of drug-induced systemic lupus erythematosus. Arthritis Rheum 10, 407.

44. Dewar HA, Peaston MJT (1964). Three cases resembling polyarteritis nodosa arising during treatment with guanethidine. BMJ 2, 609.

45. Baldwin DS, Levine BB, McCluskey T (1968). Renal failure and interstitial nephritis due to penicillin and methicillin. N Engl J Med 279, 1245.

46. Popper H (1968). Cholestasis. Annu Rev Med 19, 39.

47. Zupko AG (1969). Drug interactions—a new professional responsibility. Pharm Times 33(Sept); 38(Oct).

48. Autian J (1966). Interaction between medicaments and plastics. J Mondial Pharm 316.

49. Cooper J (1966). Interaction between medicaments and containers. J Mondial Pharm 259.

50. Kunin CM, Finland M (1961). Clinical pharmacology of the tetracycline antibiotics. Clin Pharmacol Ther 2, 51.

51. Brodie BB (1965). Clinical events of interaction between drugs. Displacement of one drug by another from carrier or receptor sites. Proc R Soc Med 58, 946.

52. Eisen MJ (1964). Combined event of sodium warfarin and phenylbutazone. JAMA 189, 64.

53. Goodman LS, Gilman A (1980). The Pharmacological Basis of Therapeutics. New York: MacMillan.

54. Burns JJ, Conney AH (1965). Clinical events of interaction between drugs. Enzyme stimulation and inhibition in the metabolism of drugs. Proc R Soc Med 58, 955.
55. Vessle ES, Pasananti GT, Greene FE (1970). Impairment of drug metabolism in man by allopurinol and nortriptyline. N Engl J Med 283, 354.
56. Jackson JE, Powell RJ, Wandell M (1980). Cimetidine–theophylline interaction. Pharmacologist 22, 231.
57. Donovan MA, Heagerty M, Patel L (1981). Cimetidine and the bioavailability of propranolol. Lancet 1, 164.
58. Serlin MJ, Moisman S, Sibeon RG (1979). Cimetidine: interactions with oral anticoagulants in man. Lancet 2, 317.
59. Klotz U, Reiman I (1980). Delayed clearance of diazepam due to cimetidine. N Engl J Med 320, 1012.
60. Doering W (1979). Quinidine–digoxin interaction. N Engl J Med 301, 400.
61. Hartshorn EA (1970). Handbook of Drug Interactions. Cincinnati, Ohio: Donald E Francke.
62. Cadwallader DE (1971). Biopharmaceutics and drug interactions. Nutley, NJ: Roche Laboratories.
63. Hollister LE (January 1972). The beneficial events of drug interactions: sweet uses of adversity. New York, Symposium of Drug Interactions; Drug Information Association.
64. Federal Register (March 1, 1994). Vol. 59, No. 40. pp. 9746–9748. International Conference on Harmonisation; Draft Guideline on the Extent of Population Exposure Required to Assess Clinical Safety for Drugs Intended for Long-Term Treatment of Non-Life Threatening Conditions.
65. Food Drug Cosmetic Law (November 29, 1993). Report No. 1626.
66. Guidance for Industry Good Pharmacovigilance Practices and Pharmacoepidemiologic Assessment (March 2005).
67. Guidance for Industry Good Pharmacovigilance Practices and Pharmacoepidemiologic Assessment (March 2005). pp. 21, ref. 19.
68. Guidance for Industry Good Pharmacovigilance Practices and Pharmacoepidemiologic Assessment (March 2005). pp. 12.
69. Guidance for Industry Good Pharmacovigilance Practices and Pharmacoepidemiologic Assessment (March 2005). pp. 15, ref. 25.
70. Guidance for Industry Good Pharmacovigilance Practices and Pharmacoepidemiologic Assessment (March 2005).
71. Federal Register (October 7, 1997). Vol. 62, No. 194. (21 CFR Parts 20, 310, 312, 314 and 600). Expedited Safety Reporting Requirements for Human Drug and Biological Products.

20 Biostatistics in Pharmaceutical Product Development Facts, Recommendations, and Solutions

Mark Bradshaw

Global Consulting Partners in Medical Biometrics, Princeton, New Jersey, U.S.A.

INTRODUCTION: THE ROLE OF BIOSTATISTICS IN LATE-STAGE PHARMACEUTICAL DEVELOPMENT

The premise of this chapter is that many of today's standard pharmaceutical development practices in experimental design, trial conduct, and statistical analysis are in need of review and revision if the goals of assuring the development and approval of safe, effective pharmaceuticals are to be maintained. The last four decades have confirmed the value of prospective, controlled, blinded, randomized clinical trials in pharmaceutical development. Refinements of experimental designs and statistical analyses, along with global harmonization of regulatory dossiers, have led to our present status where the basic tenets of phase I to III clinical trials are ubiquitous. The current chapter will not cover a great deal of this old ground. However, a sense of complacency with our status quo could lead us to ignore some serious problems with many of the current practices.

The role of the biostatistician in this process is more important than ever, but the statistical community must be challenged to develop better approaches to solving some old limitations, and some new problems. Some of these problems will be explored in this chapter along with recommendations for solutions. The areas selected for review are those that in the author's opinion require the attention of statisticians in both pharmaceutical sponsor organizations and regulatory agencies. Some provocative examples will be highlighted in this introduction, and some will be covered in greater depth.

Alpha = 0.05

Biostatistical analysis of the human clinical trials that are required during the last stages of the pharmaceutical development process has effectively become a hurdle over which every drug, device, and biologic must jump on its way to market. The all-important p-value is often used as a surrogate for comprehensive statistical and medical judgment by scientists and regulators whose job is to take into account a wide variety of information, weigh it all against risks and benefits, and make the difficult decision to either provide a new medical miracle to awaiting subjects or prevent a dangerous product from causing harm.

A cursory review of most introductory statistics texts will usually reveal a section on inferential analysis that explains how one can make a qualified leap from a sample to a population, then dutifully cautions that a p-value should only be viewed as one type of evidence in evaluating that leap of faith. It is designed to be one of many ingredients leading to a rich, deep understanding of the phenomenon under trial, when that phenomenon is surrounded by unexplained variability. Inferential statistics and the p-value are particularly useful when it is not possible to understand or control some of the sources of variability, and this clearly applies to human biological data.

Many texts caution that confidence intervals are more appropriate decision-making tools than an arbitrary gold-standard p-value (alpha) in this context. If a particular alpha level is to be used in decision making, its value should always reflect the circumstances of each different situation, taking into account both the risks of a false positive decision as well as the costs of a false negative. Nonetheless, the pharmaceutical approval process has effectively ignored these elementary cautions. It has instead established a single alpha value of 0.05 as the Procrustean bed into which every potential new product must somehow fit before it can be approved for market.

The Price of Power

With regard to the demonstration of efficacy of a new product, achievement of a p-value ≤ 0.05 comparing the new therapy to the control group is critical as discussed above. However, it is often not well understood that most products with even a modest potential therapeutic benefit can clear this hurdle if the company sponsoring the product is willing to spend enough money and/or time to perform a very large trial. Sample size can overcome the limitations of modest benefits. Hence, the true decision criteria regarding effectiveness can sometimes be more financial than medical or scientific.

Is this the best model for the evaluation and approval of new therapies? Should a product's approval be based in large part on the financial strength of the sponsor, and the value of the product's future revenue potential? These are the very real questions the next generation of statisticians, medical scientists, and regulators must face.

Safety by Design

Safety concerns are the other half of the approval process. Surely, sound statistical criteria should be used to quantify this critical process and ensure public health concerns are addressed appropriately, both before and after approval. Safety is of concern both for the clinical trial participants as well as future subjects if the product is approved. Yet the simple questions, "How much safety data is enough?" and "Where do the greatest risks lie?" are usually answered based on regulatory precedent rather than any statistical modeling of risk or variability.

Precedent may be an adequate societal basis for common law and a good way to price real estate, but the unprecedented types of pharmaceutical products under development today must be evaluated against standards relevant to their unique risks. Historic precedents will be of little help in judging risk in the brave new world of tightly targeted therapies developed through genomics and proteomics.

Signal Detection and EDA (Exploratory Data Analysis)

As clinical trials progress, we are increasingly awash in a continuous flow of raw data, but the early detection of signals amidst the ocean of noise receives very little attention until a signal is made obvious by unfortunate and potentially avoidable human costs. Statistical principles can indeed be applied to build new models to estimate risk and create reasonable monitoring processes and criteria, but to date,

there is very little activity in this direction. Efficacy targets are required to be identified in advance along with analysis methodologies. Based on the results of both
preclinical and phase I clinical trials, it is possible to identify for new drugs those
areas of "reasonably foreseeable risk" for safety concerns.

Once identified biologically, targets for proactive surveillance during the
clinical trials can be used by statisticians to develop highly sensitive monitoring
schemes, trend analyses, and cross-variable signal and syndrome detection. EDA
techniques abound in other industries. However, in pharmaceutical development,
we are far more advanced in real-time data collection technologies than in the use
of statistical techniques for the ongoing analysis of trends and detection of safety
signals that may be present in the real-time flood of bits and bytes. This deficiency
may be responsible in part for the postapproval withdrawal of a number of products from the market in recent years. The question for the biostatistician is whether
a different paradigm for signal detection coupled with a priori targeting of reasonably foreseeable risks might identify safety issues much earlier in the clinical trial
process, and well before approval and broad marketing exposure.

Sources of Bias
Finally, the very data on which safety and effectiveness decisions are made, while
voluminous and scrupulously "cleaned," may be of questionable value due to
the very process by which investigators and subjects are selected (not randomly
sampled) and the data are revised (not simply "cleaned") to fit our preconceived
data models. Regulatory oversight has focused not on the scientific validity of the
sampling frame or the meaningfulness of the data, but rather on adherence to a
set of technical procedures that may assure neither. These three points deserve
clarification.

Sampling
Statistical analysis relies on a clear distinction between random variability and variation in results due to deliberate manipulation of known factors in an experiment.
Treatments are assigned systematically to subjects, while individual subject characteristics contribute to random variability. It is important to understand that studies
are not performed to learn what happened to the participants—they are conducted
to provide a basis for predicting what will likely happen to an entire future subject population if a product is approved and broadly marketed. Inferences from a
sample to a larger population are only possible when certain statistical principles
are followed in the selection of that sample. Those principles are rarely followed
in clinical research today, and inferences to future subject populations are therefore
not generally supported from a statistical standpoint.

Data Refinement
Data begins as clinical information collected from subjects in a trial. Initially, data
reflect some component of "truth" about treatment effects, and some component
of variability or "error." Statistical analysis techniques can estimate the magnitude
of the "error" component, and in turn use that as a metric to estimate the size and
reliability of the "truth" component. But statisticians generally require consistent
and relatively simple clinical assessments to create data tabulations and perform
analyses. "Raw" data often do not meet this expectation. When we engage in data
"cleaning," the resulting altered data consist of three components: truth, error, and

systematic bias. The impact of systematic bias introduced during the cleaning process is not normally assessed statistically, or even widely recognized as a factor. Yet like the Heisenberg uncertainty principle, the act of making the data conform to our preferred measurement systems may obscure the very phenomena we seek to understand.

Regulatory Oversight

As discussed above, the pharmaceutical industry has drifted into a number of subject recruitment and data refinement practices that, though no doubt well intentioned, may at times undermine the very basis for statistical analysis and decision making. Regulators' scrutiny of the processes and the electronic systems for authorizing and tracking data changes, along with the industry's rigorous interpretation and adherence to the letter of those regulations, has effectively pointed the spotlight at the individual trees, missing the forest. Through extensive audit trails and authentication procedures, we know who changed what to what, when they did it, and what reason they gave. But understanding the implications of the process by which investigators are influenced to "refine" data to fit preconceived data collection models is different from simply assuring that investigators have, at the end of the day, formally authorized each of these changes. Our industry appears focused on the latter, not the former.

In summary, the intention of clinical trials is to accurately forecast the benefits and risks of new therapies to the broad population of subjects seeking better therapies, while protecting the safety of those subjects who volunteer to provide the data needed to make that forecast. The design and conduct of the forecasting process in clinical trials is the role of the professional biostatistician. If we view the landscape from the perspective of the theoretical statistician, we would have to conclude that most of the studies performed today reveal little more than the outcomes for the subjects who participated in the trial, and even those outcomes can be clouded or biased by data refinement and categorization practices that are entirely compliant with current regulations and accepted practices. Strictly speaking, inference (forecasting) from such trial results to larger populations is not possible due to the violation of some critical principles of inferential statistics. Subject safety data, though voluminous, precise, and timely, is not monitored in the aggregate with adequate frequency or the best available exploratory analysis tools to assure the early detection of critical safety warning signals that could foreshadow unexpected risks.

It should be clear that the purpose of this chapter is not to review the normal role of the statistician in the pharmaceutical industry today. Instead, this chapter is intended to challenge the status quo and to highlight some critical problems and largely unmet needs that logically intersect both the expertise and sphere of influence of professional statistician in the pharmaceutical industry. In some ways, the intention is to revisit the basic tenets of experimental design and analysis to see where we have drifted away from sound scientific principles, and where we may have unexplored opportunities for the future—a future certain to be different from the past.

The topics are intended to be provocative, but there is no intent to criticize the profession or those individuals who diligently play a critical role in the industry today. As statisticians take up the challenges we face today, an expanded role for statisticians can evolve. This should lead to the ability to take full advantage of the statistical perspective, one that has already helped lead to important advancements in public health, and can address the challenges of the future.

EXPERIMENTAL DESIGN IN CLINICAL TRIALS: THEORY AND PRACTICE

Clinical trials for a new drug, device, or biologic typically are organized in three sequential phases prior to submission of the data to a regulatory agency for approval. To varying degrees, the biostatistician is involved in the design and analysis of clinical trials in each of these phases.

(a) Phase I trials normally involve a small number of volunteers who are not suffering from the medical condition the new entity is intended to treat. (Note that in some disease areas such as oncology, even phase I trials are often conducted using subjects as subjects, due to the experiences caused by some new therapies.) One intention of these studies is to determine the nature and speed with which the new drug is distributed within the body, and then in what way and how quickly it is eliminated. This is the trial of pharmacokinetics. Another is to determine the highest dose in man that is consistent with an acceptable level of experiences.

(b) Phase II comparative trials are usually the first to be conducted in subjects with the medical condition for which the new drug is targeted. The numbers of subjects are greater than in phase I, but still well below the numbers required in phase III. These studies usually provide the first opportunity in man to estimate the degree to which the drug may be effective in its intended therapeutic area, and the type of experiences subjects may experience. Multiple-dose regimens are often studied, and a large number of experimental tests and parameters are evaluated both to assess the effectiveness (efficacy) of the drug and its safety. At the conclusion of phase II, sufficient evidence should be available to choose a specific dosing regimen, a detailed experimental design for proof of efficacy, a small set of pivotal efficacy variables to measure, and a target for the expected magnitude of clinical effect. In other words, a successful phase II program provides encouragement that the drug will be safe and effective, and at the same time sets the stage for the phase III pivotal proof-of-efficacy trials.

(c) Phase III comparative trials are usually large in numbers of clinical investigators and subjects, determined both by regulatory agency requirements and by statistical forecasts based on phase II and other relevant data. The trials are often international in scope and cover multiple years in duration. A few predefined efficacy parameters are measured in a large number of subjects treated in a fashion similar to the intended treatment regimen for the drug, should it be approved for general use. Safety data are also collected in the form of experience reports and (typically) a panel of laboratory analyses of blood samples collected from subjects at various time points during the trial. If the results of these trials demonstrate adequate safety, clinically meaningful efficacy results, and importantly a statistically significant difference benefit of the new drug over a control group, a marketing approval may be granted by the regulatory agency.

Sample Size and Experimental Design

An important role of the biostatistician is to collaborate with medical, regulatory, and data management experts in the design of these studies. Trial design includes the definition of what to measure, how often to measure it, how to select subjects and randomly assign treatments to them, and how to analyze the results. Everything must be prespecified in the clinical protocol including the expected results, all analysis strategies, and the rationale for the number of subjects to be studied. The latter is called the sample size.

Although a statistician should be consulted on all the factors above, in practice the most common reason why a statistician is consulted at the beginning of a trial is to establish the sample size. Fortunately, to answer this single question, all the factors above must be considered, hence one way or another, the statistician usually winds up in a collaboration on experimental design. Because the discussion often starts with sample size, we will also start there.

A clear understanding of the required sample size is particularly critical for phase III trials, due to the requirement for the establishment of statistical significance in the final analyses of phase III trials to support a submission for marketing approval. Even if a new drug seems to show evidence of clinical efficacy, without a statistically significant result, the trial will normally not be accepted as pivotal evidence in support of an approval. Insufficient sample size is one of the leading causes of phase III trial failures for drugs that otherwise appear to have adequate safety and efficacy for approval.

In principle, the results of phase II should provide enough evidence to establish the required sample size for phase III trials. Factors include the expected size of the clinical benefit of the new drug relative to the control group, the nature of the primary efficacy parameter (continuous, discrete, time-to-event, etc.), the variability one can expect to see in the data from the subjects in the trial, the p-value required to establish statistical significance (called the alpha level and normally set equal to or less than 0.050 by the regulatory agency), and the degree of risk the drug's sponsor is willing to take that the trial will fail to achieve the required alpha level even though the drug may in fact have the magnitude of efficacy predicted by the protocol. The last item, when described in a positive way as assurance instead of risk, is called statistical power. It is generally defined as the probability that a statistically significant outcome of a single trial will occur when the drug performs as expected.

This at first sounds quite odd. If a drug performs as expected, why shouldn't the trial always show a statistically significant benefit if the trial was designed correctly? The answer lies in the concept of a sample, and in a biological fact of life called unexplained variability.

We are actually not interested in the treatment results for the subjects in a clinical trial. We are instead very interested in the forecast that a trial allows us to make about the future results of treating an entire population.

Individual biological characteristics of humans along with the many differences in their daily lives plus the limitations of our understanding of biology and pharmacology make it impossible to predict with complete certainty how an individual subject will respond to a drug. This also means that the response of one individual cannot with certainty predict the response of another individual to the same drug. Yet the goal of clinical research is to predict the responses for both efficacy and safety of the entire population of subjects who may receive prescriptions for the drug if it is approved and marketed around the world.

Unpredictable variability in individual responses, coupled with the need to forecast the aggregate responses of an entire population of future subjects, provide the reasons why biostatisticians are involved in clinical trial design and analysis.

Inferential statistics is the discipline of making inferences about populations by analyzing data from samples that were drawn from those populations in a prescribed way. If we could somehow look into a crystal ball and measure the actual future responses to a new drug from the entire population, there would be no need for clinical trials or inferential statistics. However, the best we can do is analyze a sample and understand that the results from that sample are unlikely to exactly match what our crystal ball would show us about the population, due to unexplained individual variability.

If we make an important assumption that the sample was drawn at random from the population, then the larger the sample, the closer the aggregate sample results will come to matching the future response of the overall population. Now, we can answer the paradox raised earlier. A clinical trial may fail to show a significant result even if the drug being studied actually does meet its design criteria. The reason is that the trial is based on a sample. The aggregate results from the sample reflect both the overall population response and some degree of random variability. The larger the sample, the smaller the effect of the variability on the overall results. Inferential statistics allows us to quantify our uncertainty in this regard. Statistical power measures the degree to which the intended sample size can overcome unpredictable variability in subject response, and the degree to which we can be confident that the results of the sample will approximate the future response of the population.

Sensitivity and Cost

To put it simply, increasing sample size in a trial increases the level of assurance that an effective drug will reach statistical significance when the results of the trial are analyzed using the normal statistical techniques. Because every sponsor of a new drug has some financial and time limitations, sample sizes are always a compromise between what is ideal and what is affordable. The biostatistician must be involved in defining the parameters around this compromise.

One consequence of these facts is that the sensitivity of a trial to detect a statistically significant efficacy effect for a new drug depends in part on sample size. All other things being equal, the larger the sample size, the less effective a drug must be to show a significant, and potentially approvable, result. Financial investment in the clinical trial process can be an important determinant of ultimate marketing approval. It is often not clearly understood that this statistical fact has important societal implications.

Recommendations

Although a major paradigm shift would be required in our thinking about statistical gold standards for approval of new drugs, it would be consistent with sound statistical principles to abandon the rigid and ubiquitous alpha = 0.05 hurdle for regulatory approval. In its place could be an a priori process for establishing the treatment effect size consistent with clinically meaningful benefit, coupled with an agreement as to both the acceptable width of a confidence interval around that benefit and the degree of assurance required for that confidence interval. The latter could be specified for several confidence intervals, designed to show how differences in required precision affect the width of the interval. These parameters would be established based on known or expected risks, as well as the severity of the disease and the availability of alternative, effective, and safe therapies.

For example, a novel oncology therapy with a relatively good (expected) safety profile relative to currently available therapies might be required to show a 20% improvement in median survival in subjects who have shown progression of disease after treatment with the best currently approved therapies. Because of the lack of effective alternatives for these subjects and assuming a clean safety profile is established, an 80% confidence interval may be deemed adequate providing the lower bound does not include 0% improvement.

On the other hand, consider a trial versus placebo on a new product with no claimed advantage over existing drugs in a therapeutic area already crowded with safe, effective products that use the same mechanism of action and have well-known safety profiles. Here the minimum therapeutic benefit could be based on known competitors, even if the clinical trial compared against placebo, due to public health concerns of exposing subjects to unknown risks when a variety of safe and effective therapies already exist. The required confidence interval width may be quite narrow, and the assurance as to the width may need to be very high. Implications for sample size would clearly be very different as well. The challenge, of course, would be establishing a more flexible set of boundaries while maintaining objective decision parameters and repeatable decision processes. While these challenges are daunting in the face of the need to provide a regulatory atmosphere that encourages new drug development and predictable standards over the large number of years between compound discovery and marketing, the need for a more rich and thoughtful approach to the evaluation of efficacy and safety is clear, and the simplistic reliance on a single industry-wide standard p-value must be challenged.

Random Sampling

Underlying all of inferential statistics and the ability to forecast population benefits from clinical trials are two requirements with regard to random processes. First, it is necessary that the subjects in clinical trials represent a randomly chosen and representative sample of the population of future subjects in the total population eligible for the use of the drug, should it be approved. Second, it is essential for comparative trials that treatments be randomly assigned to clinical trial subjects. While most major trials carefully adhere to the second requirement, few if any follow the first.

In practice, medical professionals are selected to participate as investigators in clinical trials based on a number of factors, none of which reflect any element of random selection. Many self-select once they learn of a trial in their area of specialization. Others are selected because of the sponsor's past experiences with them in similar trials. Others are recruited for reasons ranging from their willingness to assure the recruitment of large numbers of subjects to their prominence as opinion leaders in a therapeutic area. Investigators and/or their institutions often receive financial grants for their participation. Subjects may be informed of the trial by a physician who is participating as an investigator, or they may be recruited through targeted advertisement or other means. Again, there is no random component to this process. Unlike statistical survey research where careful, stratified random sampling is used to assure the sample both represents the population of interest and is drawn within each stratum using a random process, the subjects in a typical clinical trial cannot be said to be representative of the target population for the drug in any statistical sense.

While this may seem to be an esoteric concern, it has an important consequence. As discussed earlier, the purpose of a clinical trial is to forecast outcomes for the population, not to focus on the results of the sample itself. Inferential statistics is the discipline used to make this forecast. Virtually all the commonly used statistical inferential analysis techniques for clinical trials require that the sample is drawn from the population using a random process. The p-value itself only has meaning in this framework, where it reflects the probability that two samples (subjects treated with the new drug vs. those treated with control) could have achieved the results seen in the trial if the two treatments in fact had the same effectiveness. This is often rephrased as the probability that the apparent benefit of the new drug over the comparator, as seen in the sample results of the trial, could have happened by chance alone. If this probability is very low (i.e., $p < = 0.05$), we are willing to conclude that chance alone cannot account for the difference, and the drug must therefore have greater efficacy than the comparator. This is what is meant by "statistical significance."

When subjects are not drawn from the population using a random process and therefore cannot be said to represent a population, inferential statistics lose their meaning. Although it may be impractical to select either investigators or subjects for clinical trials at random, it is not generally understood that the p-value of 0.05, mandated by regulatory authorities as the standard alpha level and hurdle for approval, does not measure the relationship between the subjects in a clinical trial and the target population for the new drug.

There is a critical need for statisticians to develop inferential analysis models that are valid in the face of the realities of nonrandom subject recruitment. In addition, there is a need to consider whether the current trend toward highly selective inclusion and exclusion criteria for clinical trial subjects should be reversed to allow a more representative sampling frame.

Sponsors of new drugs are tending toward increasing restrictions to reduce variability in subject's baseline characteristics, to minimize and standardize their use of concurrent medications, and to therefore ensure their likelihood to demonstrate consistently the benefits of the new therapy. However, a less restrictive trial design would not only lead to more rapid recruitment, but would also result in a sample more closely matching the intended population.

The pattern of nonrandom subject selection will likely to become even more prominent for a number of reasons. Trials in many therapeutic areas are designed with inclusion criteria that require subjects who have never received an increasing number of standard therapies. Because of health care practices in the industrialized countries, this often means a search for subjects in less-developed countries, and a resulting sample that does not resemble the majority of the population for whom the drug is targeted. This trend seems to be increasing, limiting the generalizability of trial results to target populations.

Another factor that will soon create more pressure toward highly selected samples of subjects for clinical trials is the future development of therapeutics that are narrowly targeted to benefit subjects with certain genetic characteristics. Advances in genomics and proteomics promise a new world of pharmaceutical products, but products requiring even tighter selection of subjects to show benefits. This will likely provide breakthrough therapies in certain areas. However, the implications for clinical trials are yet to be understood. Many new therapies will be particularly effective when used in combination with other therapies, yet our current practice is generally to trial them in isolation even when future use will likely be in combination. Experimental designs and statistical analysis models will both need to be reconsidered in light of these new developments. Certainly, the requirements of random sampling of subjects will not be easily met.

Recommendations

In a prospective randomized comparative clinical trial, the biostatistician should be primarily concerned with the ability to generalize from the results of the trial to the future population of subjects who may receive the new therapeutic product. To do so, the sampling frame must be constructed to represent the characteristics of that future population, and some element of random selection must be present when investigators and subjects are identified for the trial. If this is not possible in a strict sense due to limitations on available subjects, then techniques such as advanced approaches to stratified sampling may be used. Note that if relative sizes of strata do not match those of the population to which inferences will be made, adjustments will be required at the time of the analysis to achieve the correct balance. This type of analysis is not commonly accepted, however, for pivotal trials; hence, a good deal of work must be done by the statistical community to improve the relevance of trials to the population of subjects for whom drugs are intended. Trials targeting subjects who are not representative of the target population, such as some types of "treatment-naïve" subjects or subjects with an unusual set of inclusion criteria, should be avoided during phase III, as they are more applicable to establishing proof of concept in earlier phases.

DATA REFINEMENT

Pivotal trial designs in general, and the design of the data collection instruments in particular (usually called case report forms or CRFs), have been developed to maximize the likelihood that the final clinical database will meet the needs of the statistician for analysis and reporting, and of the sponsor to establish sufficient evidence for approval. While a clinician treating a subject thinks in terms of that individual's detailed and unique medical history and prognosis, the statistician must look at groups of subjects in the aggregate. Paradoxically, the very uniqueness of each individual that the clinician is trained to observe and analyze gets in the way of aggregate analysis. Individual variation to a statistician is often called "error variance"; using the metaphor above, it is the "noise" that may mask a "signal." To the clinician, it is the signal.

It is therefore understandable that statisticians and the data managers who prepare databases for statistical analysis prefer to collect data in a way that minimizes individual variation. The question, "What percentage of subjects dropped out of the trial due to an experience?" can only be answered if there is an explicit question on the CRF that requires a "yes" or "no" answer. Even though a paragraph written by a clinician describing the circumstances leading to a subject's withdrawal from the trial would be far more revealing from a medical perspective, the statistician cannot tabulate a paragraph of text and must instead have a clear binary answer to tabulate.

This simple logic leads to a forced categorization and structuring of efficacy and safety data in many of the more medically interesting and complex areas of information about how a subject fares under an experimental therapeutic regimen during a clinical trial. Questions on the CRF that lead to statistical analysis range from objective (blood pressure) to subjective (physician's global assessment), from immediate (pulse) to delayed (severity of pain last week), and from office-based (erythema score) to home-based (urinary incontinence diary) to laboratory-based (hematocrit count).

The nature of the data is related to the degree to which "data refinement" or "data cleaning" activities may in fact change the intended message. If on the vital signs CRF page, the subject's weight is recorded as 1.90 pounds, a query may be raised suggesting this is an error, and that based on the subject's previous visit CRF pages, the value should perhaps be 190 pounds. The clinician agrees and signs the correction. This seems unlikely to create a biased result in the database. However, here is a more worrisome hypothetical example. The physician is asked to categorize the subject's response on a five-point scale, from "much worse" to "much better," but the physician responds "much better in terms of overall symptoms but prognosis is actually worse." This response does not fit into the analysis scheme, and through a process of structured interrogation called "data cleaning," the physician does eventually agree (after some protest) to select a single category on the prescribed five-point scale. That category will however obscure the message that was intended. What if many subjects actually show improvement in symptoms, but something else about their condition raises concerns by their physicians regarding prognosis? Will the "filters" through which statisticians "refine" the data block this critical finding from our view?

Categorization of free-text data fields provides another important source of bias, particularly critical in the area of experiences. In some areas where verbatim text is accepted in the CRF, there is a post hoc process called "coding" that maps a very wide variety of verbatim text strings into a much smaller number of categorized responses. So-called coding dictionaries such as MedDRA, ICD-10, and WHO-ART provide the basis for mapping experiences, diseases and conditions, and medications to a standard set of codes. These codes are then further mapped to broader categories, such as body systems for experiences. Codes and categories can be tabulated, summarized, and analyzed by statisticians, whereas thousands of unique verbatim text strings are only used when reading an individual subject's case history. However, the act of coding and categorizing inevitably discards a great deal of information. Depending on the way they are created and used, coding schemes can create order out of chaos and reveal important patterns in the data, or obscure critical findings. The relevance of data tabulations and analyses is limited by the nature of the coding schemes and activities.

Entire syndromes can be broken into multiple codes, and after such disassembly, they may disappear entirely. Here is a hypothetical example that shows what can happen if an important verbatim term is either missing from a coding system or judged to be too vague for accurate coding.

A subject in a clinical trial visits the clinic and describes a complex experience that occurred two months ago to a physician who records it simply as "flu-like symptoms" and added a sentence of further details. These include the subject's report of general weakness, light-headedness, headache, nausea, vomiting, and possible fever. During the subject visit, the physician asked the types of questions consistent with years of training and experience. The physician took all this into account, along with the timing and relationship to other events such as trial drug dosing and the use of concurrent medications. Three months later, after the data have been submitted and entered into a database, this visit is reviewed handed over to coding experts who capture the primary term "flu-like symptoms." The physician is then asked in a written communication to please be more specific and concise. After a few iterations, and more than six months past the occurrence of the event itself, it is agreed to be resubmitted as two experiences—"nausea" and "vomiting"—each with its own indication of start date, stop date, severity, and outcome categorization. Yet the description the subject gave the physician at the visit plus the physician's own questions to the subject for clarification revealed much more information. Much of this has now been lost entirely from the perspective of the statistician, who will now focus only on the coded values for purposes of analysis and summarization.

What if this very syndrome, though not available in the coding system, is an important clue as to how the drug under trial affects a small but important subgroup of subjects?

The following recommendations arise from examples such as these and are intended as directions toward possible solutions to a broad set of problems that can lead to bias through data refinement and categorization activities:

1. Categorize data captured during a clinical trial in terms of its objectivity/subjectivity, immediacy or delay of collection, and source (clinician, subject, or machine). Categorize it further as to whether it is hypothesis testing, or hypothesis generating, or neither. For example, a predefined efficacy criterion such as reduction in serum cholesterol is hypothesis testing and has a predefined success criterion and known variance. In the same trial, body weight may be hypothesis generating if, whether suspected previously or not, the test drug is responsible for slight losses in body weight. Vegetarian diet (diet preference in general) may also be hypothesis generating. The question "Which meal would you choose on an airplane given the following five choices?" may help understand variability in response to the drug. Safety data will usually be hypothesis generating, and will be hypothesis testing for those areas targeted a priori based on reasonably foreseeable risk as discussed elsewhere in this chapter.
2. For objective data, especially when collected in an automated fashion, apply objective data cleaning criteria such as range checks and consistency comparisons. If apparent errors are found that are not simply transcription errors, delve deeply into the reasons and look for systematic errors such as incorrect units, miscalibrated devices, carelessness, or data fraud.
3. For subjective data, especially when a good deal of time has elapsed since its collection, exercise extreme caution when questioning values. (For diary data provided directly by subjects, do not make any changes no matter how unlikely the values may appear—the integrity of this type of data hinges on a reliance on the unaltered values provided directly by subjects.) When such data are either critical hypothesis testing or hypothesis generating, use the required audit trail to perform two types of analyses. The first is based on the final values after data cleaning. The second is a sensitivity analysis, based on the initial values before data cleaning. If there are differences in direction or trend or significance between the two analyses, look harder at the biases that may have been introduced. Report both sets of results.
4. Formalized coding schemes such as MedDRA should be augmented by a second classification based on syndromes, groupings, concurrent drug categories, types of medical conditions, and so on, that are identified a priori as being particularly relevant to the drug or class of drug under trial. Creation of this trial-specific classification scheme should be led by a medical expert intimately familiar with

the drug under trial, the preclinical and early human data available on it, and the disease or condition in question. In addition to experiences, concurrent medications, and concurrent conditions, laboratory data should also be considered in the identification of relevant syndromes, and so on. In some cases, other types of safety data such as ECGs and specialized laboratory data are relevant. The use of this information for safety surveillance and signal detection throughout the trial will be discussed below. At the end of the trial, analyses based on formalized coding systems should be compared with analyses based on the trial-specific system above. Differences must be explored and thoroughly understood before conclusions are drawn regarding the outcomes of the trial. This is far from a simple exercise and will require a great deal of thought by members of several disciplines. Yet without an adjunct to conventional coding, some of the most important information from the trial can be lost from the final analysis.

5.   Data cleaning efforts for variables that are not identified as critical hypothesis generating, testing, safety, or subject identification and classification variables should be minimized. Further, the detailed audit trails mentioned earlier should be used to create a new type of quality assurance benchmark—perhaps it should be called the Data Refinement Index (DRI). The proportion of data fields that were changed from their original values at least once should be tabulated for each category of data above. Categories of fields with an unusually high degree of data "refinement" would have a high DRI, would be highlighted, and could then be investigated in detail for the possibility of bias. Just as a high error rate between CRF and database is cause for concern regarding the integrity of the data, an unusually high amount of refinement should cause an even greater concern. The overall average DRI for each category of data, and for the data as a whole, would become an important indicator of the reliability of the database. The goal would be to minimize DRI, while still delivering analyzable data. Bear in mind that every data "correction" carries with it some probability that new value will introduce bias into the results of the trial. We should therefore rely more on the randomization process, the sampling frame, and the control group, than on individual data point "refinement" to lead to aggregate results that reflect the truth about the drug under trial. Note that this philosophy will also require analytic approaches that are more tolerant of the types of data irregularities that characterize medical information but are not particularly compatible with current analysis techniques.

SAFETY SIGNAL DETECTION AND EDA

Ongoing individual subject safety monitoring is routinely managed in a clinical trial by the investigator, the medical monitor, drug safety specialists, the CRAs, Institutional Review Boards (IRBs) or other human safety committees, and often by trial-specific Data Safety Monitoring Boards (DSMBs) that meet according to a predefined schedule (typically anywhere from quarterly to annually). However, with the exception of DSMBs, the daily ongoing review of safety data is normally done on a subject-by-subject basis. This practice is consistent with the needs of each subject in conjunction with the management of the disease, but it does not provide a sensitive method for detecting subtle trends or emerging safety warning signals that are only seen when the data are viewed across subjects.

DSMBs are well suited to see both the forest and the trees with regard to safety; however, they meet infrequently and they are far from a standard feature of the average clinical trial. In addition, they are often focused on predefined decision rules and hypotheses of interest, whereas the critical under-recognized need is for a more standard approach to looking for that which is not standard—the unexpected safety problem.

Fortunately, today's clinical trial technology can make available a wealth of detailed and timely safety data. These near-real-time globally available data feeds include highly precise central laboratory evaluations of blood and urine samples that can be available electronically from 24 to 48 hours after each subject visit, digitized ECGs that are remotely captured but centrally analyzed and available within 24 hours of the visit, serious experience reports prepared within a few days of the event, electronic subject diary information that is often transmitted daily to a central repository, and e-CRF data available from a few days to a few minutes after a subject visit. With this wide array of near-real-time safety data, there is no longer any reason why the health of a trial cannot be monitored just as closely and frequently as the health of a subject who is in intensive care. Indeed, the health of hundreds or thousands of subjects is affected by the quality and intensity of this ongoing aggregate safety data monitoring.

There are several good reasons normally given to explain why aggregate subject safety data review is not done with the frequency or approach suggested above. During the typical trial, the assignment of treatments to subjects is blinded and must remain so to protect the integrity of the trial. Conventional final unblinded analysis of safety data requires comparison between the groups, which is not possible during the trial unless a DSMB has been formed and has in its charter the ability to become unblinded without impacting the trial's scientific validity. Yet a DSMB adds cost and meets infrequently. Second, in the event a possible safety concern is raised during the trial, it could impact the conduct of the rest of the trial in such a way as to bias the results. Investigators may change their behavior and their evaluation of subjects' responses based on the suggestion of a safety issue. This change in behavior could lead to a self-fulfilling prophecy effect on the data. Third, the appearance of subtle trends or signals may be illusory or transient, and may not reflect a real problem. An early termination may preclude the collection of enough solid data to draw any clear conclusions from the trial.

Recommendations

Solutions do exist that avoid the problems above, yet they provide more sensitivity to detect safety signals throughout the trial. There are three categories that will be covered here: (*i*) ongoing review of all pooled data irrespective of treatment group assignment, but with an understanding of what would be expected from similar subjects not participating in the clinical trial as a comparison; (*ii*) the use of data displays borrowed from the discipline of EDA; and (*iii*) reasonably foreseeable risk projections to highlight in advance the hypotheses of interest.

1. *Pooled data review*: When we do not know which subjects are in which group, we can still look at the subjects in a trial as a single group without breaking the blind. There are always sources to reference to establish reasonable expectations for typical ranges of laboratory parameters, ECGs. experiences, and so on, for subjects like those in the trial. Further, the tracking of changes from baseline or changes visit-by-visit is a powerful indicator of effects over time that are often caused by the trial drug or the comparator. Ongoing review of the data

based on preestablished thresholds of concern that take into account the dilution effect of looking at pooled data from all combined treatment groups can lead to the identification of potential safety signals. These can then be followed up in more detail, and even taken to an ad hoc safety monitoring committee with the authority to perform unblinded analyses when required. This multi-tier process can be both efficient and sensitive, yet avoid false alarms that would impact the trial needlessly.

If, for example, the trial has two equal-sized groups and we expect subjects with the disease under trial to show liver enzyme values 20% higher than normal individuals, we would expect the overall pooled average laboratory data to have this characteristic, if the trial drug itself did not further increase liver enzyme abnormalities. An average value of +20% would not be seen as a safety signal. However, if we learned that the trial drug further increased liver enzyme abnormalities by an additional 10 percentage points, that would presumably show up in the final analysis as a difference between groups of 10% (20% in placebo subjects vs. 30% in the trial drug group). Under this circumstance, the pooled result while we are still blinded would be expected to be 25% (average of 20% and 30% given equal subject numbers per group). Therefore, we would know that a deviation from the expected "normal" results from subjects with this disease might show up in the aggregate pooled review as a deviation only half as large as experienced by the trial drug-treated subjects. This knowledge can be used to set a threshold for concern, even though we have not broken the blind. The same process can be used for quantitative and categorical data, whether from a laboratory, an ECG, an incidence of end points, a survival analysis of median time to a specified event, or an incidence of experiences.

2. *EDA*: While much of the work of the biostatistician in late-stage clinical development revolves around inference, testing of established hypotheses, and interpretation of p-values, some of the most interesting exploratory statistical methodology is designed to help understand experimental results, detect unexpected patterns, and develop new hypotheses to be tested and confirmed in future studies. One of the first lessons to be learned in this area is that the shape of the distribution of individual data points is more important to observe than the mean, or average, of the distribution. The latter is called a measure of central tendency and is a convenient one-number summary of a large amount of data. However, it hides much of the critical information about the pattern of results. The mean is also influenced heavily by even a few outliers in the distribution, and distributions with widely disparate shapes can share exactly the same mean.

Graphical displays have become a standard, simple yet powerful way to show the shape of the actual distribution of the results, as well as several important summary values that round out the information carried in the mean value. The use of graphical displays of scatterplots of the actual individual subject visit values versus baseline values is a quick way to spot overall trends as well as groups of subjects or areas on the scatterplot that differ from other groups or areas. Looking at the distribution will show at a glance whether it looks quite "normal," following the well-known symmetrical bell-shaped curve, or whether the distribution is skewed with a long tail containing extreme outliers, or even bimodal with evidence of two distinct groups of subjects, each with its own distribution. Each type of distribution can be an important clue to a clinical scientist or a statistician as to the effect of the trial drug on various types of subjects at different time points in the trial. As the data accumulate, the ability to see trends and patterns increases in a way that is visually obvious even to the nonstatistician.

Variables plotted may be continuous or discrete; however, plots of continuous variables generally contain more information. Sometimes it makes sense to plot one variable against time—for example, change in cholesterol versus trial day. Or the plot of one variable against another may be more important, such as WBC versus dose. Scatterplots are the first graphical display to consider. A useful addition to the scatterplot is often the regression line, showing the statistical relationship between one variable and another. The addition of confidence bounds on either side of the regression line can help distinguish between random fluctuation and true outliers. Dividing a scatterplot into quadrants may also add to the ability to see at a glance the concentration of subjects who are high on one parameter and low on the other, vice versa, high on both, or low on both. Next, there are various summary displays that do not show any individual data points, but still show evidence of the shape of the distribution of results. These include so-called box-and-whisker plots that reflect mean, median, upper and lower quartile points, confidence limits, and outliers, all at a glance.

The list of available graphical displays goes beyond the scope of this chapter. The clear recommendation is to establish at the beginning of a trial the safety parameters of possible interest (see next point below), set the thresholds of expectation based on subjects not receiving the trial drug, create thresholds of concern by adjusting those thresholds of expectation to take into account the pooled sample, select graphical displays that will be sensitive to the clinical safety issues of interest and display the threshold data, and make updated displays available on a continuous basis to clinical, medical, and/or statistical experts. These individuals should be given the explicit ongoing responsibility not only to look for the expected issues but also to scan for the unexpected. Finally, some mechanism must be established to review any suspected signals in a blinded fashion at first, then if the information warrants, there must be an unblinded team available to further pursue what appear to be stable patterns of concern. Technology is no longer a limitation, and the issues normally raised during a discussion of ongoing data-driven safety surveillance can be managed as outlined above.

3. *Reasonably foreseeable risk*: Finally, it is important to point out that safety surveillance for the unexpected should always be an adjunct to a diligent and disciplined attempt to forecast areas of risk based on what we already know prior to the beginning of a trial. Phase II/III clinical trials are usually preceded by earlier human clinical trials, the results of which should be studied closely for indications of possible safety issues. Even phase I first-in-man clinical research is done after thorough laboratory research that forms the basis for the determination that the drug is safe enough for initial testing in normal adults. The point is that there is always a great deal of data available before the start of a clinical trial that points to safety concerns, organ systems at risk, the potential for drug–drug interactions, and so on. This information should be used to identify key variables for safety surveillance and circumstances that lead to heightened risk to subjects in a trial.

The a priori identification of specific risk hypotheses leads to the ability to take some of the methodology normally applied to hypothesis testing of efficacy results, and apply it to safety assessment. The most important difference between these two analysis domains is that in the case of efficacy, outcomes of interest are identified a priori with great specificity, and clear statistical hypotheses are laid out in advance with complete analysis and decision rules documented in the clinical protocol. In practice, only a few efficacy variables are identified as "primary," and only a few others as "secondary." Sensitivity, statistical power, and sample size are all carefully analyzed in advance to assure the trial will have a high probability of detecting differences of interest in these few, critical variables.

Safety analyses live at the other end of the spectrum, with very little if any prespecified hypotheses to test, no a priori specification of sensitivity or statistical power, and few if any clear decision rules. At a recent industry conference, the Head of Biostatistics at FDA suggested that this disparity may be one of the major reasons why a number of drugs were recently withdrawn from the market due to safety issues not detected during phase III clinical trials. It is time to apply the focused spotlight of efficacy analysis to the broad but critical area of safety assessment, both at the end of the trial and in safety surveillance throughout the trial. Statisticians must address this challenge, using both old and new tools and concepts to protect subjects in the trials as well as those who would receive the new therapy upon approval.

SUMMARY

The primary focus of late-stage clinical trials is to forecast accurately the benefits and risks of new therapies for the broad population of subjects seeking better therapies, while protecting the safety of those subjects who volunteer to participate in the process. Our present approach has steadily evolved and, for the most part, improved over time. However, a number of challenges must be addressed and changes implemented for clinical trials to continue to deliver on their promise.

The current approach to clinical trials does not properly address the basic need to forecast the outcomes of the use of a new therapy for the intended population. Rigid and simplistic standards with regard to p-values and the assessment of inferential analyses do not allow the needed flexibility to address the enormous variety of therapeutic products and the circumstances of their intended use. Data cleaning, and the more general practice of categorizing raw trial information, can lead to systematic bias and a loss of critical outcome information. Safety assessments do not yet take advantage of the flood of near-real-time data coupled with exploratory aggregate data analysis tools. Pretargeted safety hypotheses based on reasonably foreseeable risk assessments of existing information are not normally established to assure that aggregate safety issues and trends are detected as early as possible in a trial and addressed appropriately.

Biostatistics as a discipline is at the heart of the issues discussed in this chapter. The development of the tools, techniques, and practices to address these issues is well within the scope and capabilities of the discipline. Some of these issues are already visible and important topics for pharmaceutical sponsors and regulators. Others will become more visible as new types of therapeutics approach the stage of development requiring human clinical trials. Applicability for many of the new therapeutics will be much narrower than in the past, stretching our current practices well beyond their limits. The challenge for biostatistics is to take the lead in forging the future of clinical trial design and analysis so that society's need for better, safer therapies will continue to be met while protecting the safety of those subjects who volunteer to make this process possible.

21 CFR/ICH/EU GCP Obligations of Investigators, Sponsors, and Monitors

Richard A. Guarino

Oxford Pharmaceutical Resources, Inc., Totowa, New Jersey, U.S.A.

INTRODUCTION

The Good Clinical Practices (GCPs) regulations section (21 CFR 312 Subpart D) in the Code of Federal Regulations, International Conference on Harmonization (ICH E6) Guideline for GCP and the European Clinical Trial Directive (2001/20/IEC on GCP), outlines the responsibilities and obligations of the clinical investigator, the drug sponsor, and the clinical trial monitor in the conduct of investigational new product development. In addition to the regulated conduct of clinical investigations, each participant has a moral and ethical responsibility for the safety of subjects who voluntarily participate in clinical trials. GCP has long been the norm in the United States for the investigator, as included in the Form FDA 1572. However, the first proposed regulations pertaining to investigators, sponsors, and monitors were circulated in U.S. Federal Register in 1977 and 1978. In 1987, 10 years later, GCP were published as final regulations in the Code of Federal Regulations. In ICH guidelines, these were proposed in 2001 and in the European Directives finalized in 2004 as regulations in the EU. Today, investigators, sponsors, and monitors are obligated by law to follow GCP.

In order to conduct clinical research that meets global regulations for new product approval, it is essential to understand the importance of these regulations and their subsequent impact on the clinical development process of drugs, devices, and biologics. Not only do investigators have a key responsibility in assessing subjects' efficacy and safety response to new drugs, devices, or biologics, but also sponsors and monitors have equal responsibility for the subjects' safety and welfare.

This chapter will be devoted to the regulatory obligations of investigators, sponsors, and monitors. Each one are defined as follows:

1. *Investigator*: The individual who conducts a clinical investigation (i.e., under whose immediate direction the drug is administered or dispensed to the subject). If an investigation is conducted by a team of individuals, the principal investigator (PI) is the responsible leader of the team. The subinvestigator is any other individual member of that team. These individuals are usually licensed physicians or individuals working under the direction of a licensed physician.
2. *Sponsor/investigator*: An individual who both initiates and conducts an investigation and under whose immediate direction the investigational drug is administered or dispensed. This category refers mostly to physician investigators who are conducting clinical research under an investigator IND (see chap. 8).
3. *Sponsor*: An individual or organization that takes responsibility for and initiates a clinical investigation. This may be an individual, pharmaceutical company, governmental agency, academic institution, a private or other organization.

4. *Monitor*: The person selected by the sponsor who is qualified by training and experience to facilitate and oversee the progress of an investigation in order to assure that the sponsor's and investigator's regulatory obligations are executed.

INVESTIGATOR OBLIGATIONS

In 21 CFR 312.53, the regulations contain the descriptive information provided on Form FDA 1572, the Statement of Investigator form, see ICH and EU directives on GCP. Also included in 21 CFR 312.53 are the selection requirements for clinical investigators. Historically, in the U.S. to conduct trials designated as phases 1 and 2, investigators were required to complete a Statement of Investigator (Form FDA 1572); investigators conducting phase 3 or phase 4 trials completed a different Statement of Investigator (Form FDA 1573). As a result of the IND rewrite regulations, Form FDA 1573 is no longer used for any clinical trials. As of this date, only Form FDA 1572 is required to be signed by all investigators conducting all phases of clinical research. This form commits the investigator under federal law to comply with GCP. Other information required on Form FDA 1572 includes the name and address of any clinical laboratory facility and address of the Institutional Review Board (IRB) or Independent Ethics Committee (IEC) that is responsible for the review and approval of the individual investigators participating and listed on Form 1572. It also states that the sponsor is charged with the responsibility of selecting qualified investigators who are defined as those capable of conducting the clinical trial by virtue of their training and experience. By using the phrase "training and experience," FDA implied that clinical investigators who are conducting a clinical trial evaluating a particular disease should have enough experience in the clinical specialty to observe correctly the signs, symptoms, and progress of that disease while experimenting and evaluating a new investigational drug, biologic, or device. For example, if a new pharmaceutical product is designed for an OB-GYN practice, a pediatrician would not be expected to have the expertise to assess this product nor would a cardiologist have expertise in evaluating a gastrointestinal drug.

Investigators are defined as those who have signed and completed Form FDA 1572, or sub- or coinvestigators listed on that form, and who are considered to have the academic and experiential qualifications for participating in the clinical program.

The "fine print" on the reverse side of Form FDA 1572 is a written agreement whereby the investigators assure the FDA and the sponsor that they will conduct the trial in accordance with the appropriate trial plan (i.e., the protocol) and will observe the GCP tenets. Implicit in this agreement is the fact that the investigator will have obtained signed informed consent (IC) forms from patients or subjects participating in the clinical research trial and they will be under the investigators jurisdiction. In other words, the investigator is taking full responsibility for the subjects' safety and welfare. Form 1572 also charges the investigator with the reporting of adverse experiences that occur during the investigation and provides assurance that the investigator has read and understood the Investigator's Brochure. In addition, the investigator assures that all individuals participating in the supervision or administration of any test during the course of the clinical trial are doing this under the direction of the investigator, and are aware of their GCP responsibilities. Once Form 1572 has been signed by investigators, they further assure compliance with the requirements of providing trial materials, protocols, and other pertinent information to an authorized IRB/IEC for review. A CV of the investigators and subinvestigators along with assurance that the investigational plan set forth in the trial protocol will be followed should accompany these documents.

Once the legal documents are completed, the investigators must understand that their primary responsibility in participating in clinical trials is the ethical and moral obligations to all the participating patients and subjects that commit to being administrated the investigational product. The investigators must provide measures of safety for each participant in the trial so that the subject is protected ethically and morally from any endangerment that might occur during the evaluation of an investigational product. After the investigator's responsibilities and obligations are clearly understood and they have signed Form FDA 1572, any additional information that investigators might need or concerns that they have about any procedure or evaluation of the clinical trial should be clarified from the sponsor.

Investigators obligations and responsibilities include the following:

(a) Ensuring that an investigation is conducted according to the signed investigator statement (1572).

(b) The investigational plan (the protocol) is agreed to be followed.

(c) Assuring the protection of the rights, safety, and welfare of the subjects/patients participating in the clinical trial.

(d) The experimental product will not be administered to participating subjects in a clinical trial with obtaining the IC of each participant.

(e) Maintaining complete control and accountability on all experimental products and that the experimental product will only be administered to the subjects who have signed an IC and have met the requirements of the protocol.

(f) Adequate records be maintained of the disposition of the experimental product, including dates of administration, quantity, and use by participating subjects.

(g) Upon completion or termination, suspension, or discontinuation of the trial, the accountability of used and unused trial supplies will be submitted to the sponsor.

(h) That the investigational plan protects the rights, safety, and welfare of subjects participating in a clinical investigation. An investigator shall obtain the IC of each human subject to whom the drug is administered and shall administer the drug only to subjects under the investigator's supervision or under the supervision of a subinvestigator responsible to the investigator. The investigator shall not supply the investigational drug to any person not participating in the clinical program.

(i) An investigator is required to maintain accurate case histories designed to record all observations and other pertinent data on each individual treated with an investigational product. (Usually, this is accomplished by completing case report forms and maintaining medical records.)

(j) Investigators shall retain records of all subjects enlisted in an investigational trial for two years after a marketing application for the drug is approved for the indication being investigated. If no application is to be filed, or if the application is not approved for such indication, records must be maintained for two years after the investigation is discontinued and the FDA has notified the sponsor of the status of the application.

(k) Investigators shall furnish all reports on the investigational product to the sponsor. The sponsor is responsible for collecting and evaluating the results obtained. The sponsor is also required to submit annual reports to FDA on the progress of the clinical investigations.

(l) Investigators shall promptly report to the sponsor any adverse effect that may reasonably be regarded as caused by, or probably caused by, the investigational product. If the adverse effect is serious, the investigator shall report the adverse effect immediately according to the regulations stated in the CFR, ICH, and EUD (see ADR Reporting, chap. 19).

(m) Investigators shall notify the IRB/IEC and provide the sponsor with an adequate report of the trial outcome shortly after completion of the investigator's participation in the trial.

OTHER INVESTIGATOR RESPONSIBILITIES

Prior to signing a 1572, the investigator must have a good understanding of the content in the Investigator's Brochure (see chap. 8). Based on this document, an investigator is usually assured that sufficient pharmacology and toxicology data allow trial subjects to be prescribed and administered an investigational product. However, it does not guarantee that subjects can tolerate the pharmaceutical product. Animal models often do not respond to products the same way as humans.

The investigator must assure that an IRB/IEC who reviews the clinical investigational protocol and the IC comply with the regulations established in CFR/ICH and EU Directives (see chap. 24). In addition, the IRB/IEC is responsible for the continuing review and approval of the proposed clinical trial and any amendments that take place after the original documents have received approval. The investigator must also ensure that he or she will promptly report all changes in the research activity, amendments, and all unanticipated problems involving risk to human subjects (AEs and SAEs) and any other reported problems to the IRB/IEC. The investigator will not deviate from the protocol without IRB/IEC approval, except where necessary to eliminate apparent immediate hazards to human subjects.

An investigator shall, upon request from any properly authorized officer or employee of FDA, at reasonable times, permit such an officer or employee to have access to, copy, and verify any records or reports made by the investigator. The investigator is not required to divulge subject names unless the records of particular individuals require a more detailed trial of the cases, or unless there is reason to believe that the records do not represent actual case trials, or do not represent actual results obtained.

Investigator Penalties

What are the results if an investigator has repeatedly or deliberately either failed to comply with GCP regulations, or has submitted false information on any report to the sponsor? In the United States, the Center for Drug Evaluation and Research (CDER), the Center for Biologics Evaluation and Research (CBER), or the Center for Devices and Radiological Health (CDRH) will furnish the investigator with written notice of the matter complained of and offer the investigator an opportunity to explain the matter in writing. On the other hand, at the option of the investigator, an informal conference could be requested. If the explanation offered by the investigator is not accepted by these FDA divisions, the investigator will be given an opportunity for a regulatory hearing. At this hearing, the issue of whether the investigator is entitled to receive investigational drugs will be addressed. After evaluating all available information, including any explanation presented by the investigator, the FDA commissioner determines whether the investigator has repeatedly or deliberately failed to comply with GCP requirements or has deliberately or repeatedly submitted false information to the sponsor in any communication or required report. The commissioner will then notify the investigator and the sponsor of any investigation in which the investigator has been named, as a participant is not entitled to receive investigational products. If there is reasonable cause for this action, the investigator becomes subject to further investigation for each IND and each approved application submitted to the FDA containing data reported by this investigator. Therefore, every investigational trial conducted by this investigator will be examined to determine whether the investigator has submitted unreliable data. Other investigations that are conducted under the same protocol may be temporarily put on hold.

Conversely the commissioner may determine, after eliminating the unreliable data by the investigator under examination, the remaining data coming from other sites conducting similar trials may continue with their trials. However, if a danger to the public health exists, the commissioner will terminate the IND immediately. The sponsor will be notified and will have an opportunity for a regulatory hearing before the FDA on the question of whether the IND should be reinstated. If the commissioner determines that the data submitted are unreliable and data submitted by the investigator cannot be justified, the commissioner will proceed to withdraw approval of the investigational product in accordance with the provisions of the FD&C Act. As a result, an investigator who has been deemed to be ineligible to receive investigational drugs will be blacklisted and unable to participate in any experimental trials. This investigator may be reinstated when the commissioner determines that he or she has presented adequate assurances that the investigator will use investigational products in compliance with FDA regulations. Presently, no penalties for investigators are stated in the ICH guidelines or the EU Directives.

In conclusion, before an investigator accepts the responsibilities to conduct a clinical investigation for a drug, biologic, or device, he or she must be aware of the legal obligations and responsibilities as directed by GCP. When Form FDA 1572 is signed by an investigator in any country, especially when the data are to be used for a U.S. submission, it is expected that the investigator will abide by and pursue the clinical investigation following GCP. ICH guidelines and the European Directives are the guide used to follow GCP in other countries. The investigators must realize that they are subject to a federal offense in the United States and may be criminally charged in other countries when GCPs are not followed. The results of violation of GCP can jeopardize their reputation and ultimately their ability to conduct further clinical research. Investigators must know that precise collection of data is mandatory in the conduct of clinical research. Experimental clinical research under GCP demands that before the efficacy of a product is evaluated, the protocol design must ensure that the safety of the subjects who consent to participate in a clinical trial remains the primary concern.

SPONSOR OBLIGATIONS

The sponsor's primary responsibility is clearly delineated in 21 CFR 312.50 of the CFR, the ICH, and the European Directives. The sponsor is responsible for selecting qualified investigators and for providing them with the information they need to conduct an investigation in accordance with the published regulations. Usually, the sponsor accomplishes this task by supplying the potential investigator with an Investigator's Brochure (IB) and a protocol of the clinical investigation on the product to be investigated (see chaps. 8 and 16). An IB contains all the information from nonclinical trials and reports (pharmacology and toxicology), and any previous human efficacy and safety trial reports that reflect previous experiences of subjects on the investigational agent. In addition, it gives enough chemistry, manufacturing, and control (CMC) on the product being investigated giving the investigator the assurance that the product manufactured is safe to be introduced into humans.

Of primary interest in the obligations is the option of a sponsor to transfer total or partial responsibility for the conduct of a clinical trial to a contract research organization (CRO). CROs play a significant role in new drug development (see chap. 8). However, CROs who are contracted by sponsor companies are obligated under the same GCP regulations as defined in this chapter. A CRO may be the sponsor or the monitor with equal obligations as defined in 21 CFR 312, ICH, and EU Directives. The current regulations are specific and require that any transfer, whether in total or in part, be described in writing and agreed to by both parties. The FDA states that any obligations not specifically described by the sponsor in the written transfer of responsibilities will be considered as not transferred to the CRO; the liability for these undefined responsibilities therefore remains with the sponsor. The regulations further require the CRO (once any transfer of responsibilities has been made by the sponsor) to comply with all applicable regulations and that the CRO is subject to the same regulatory actions as a sponsor. A CRO must assure complete GCP compliance with the responsibilities assigned in writing to them. However, the sponsor continues to have the overall responsibility to ensure the quality and integrity of data generated under the supervision of a CRO. In this situation, the sponsor would be expected to act as a quality assurance auditor of the data, even though assignment for the conduct of a trial has been delegated to the CRO. The regulations also charge the sponsor with responsibility for the inventory and control of the drug. Only investigators participating in a clinical trial may receive and have access to investigational drug and materials. It must be emphasized that the sponsor, no matter what is assigned to a CRO, is always ultimately responsible for the safety of the subjects participating in the clinical trial, the conduct of the investigator and their staff, and the overall reporting of data for every clinical investigation under their auspices.

SPONSOR AND MONITOR OBLIGATIONS

One of the most important responsibilities of a sponsor is to monitor the progress of every clinical investigation conducted under their auspices. Primary is to ensure the safety of the subjects recruited for the clinical trial. A monitor's obligation, under the direction of the sponsor, is to ensure that any deficiencies created during the conduct of clinical investigations are corrected or justified by the investigator and that the investigator adheres to the investigational plan (the protocol; see chap. 16). The obligations of the appointed monitors for all clinical investigations are to assure that an investigator is complying with their obligations and the general investigational plan, for example, the clinical protocol is being adhered to, that there are not deviations from the protocol, that all safety assessments are followed, that every AE or SAE was reported in the required timelines, and that the investigators are not violating their GCP obligations. Investigators and their staff at times record data that must be changed or corrected, either due to miss-entries, mistakes in transposing data from medical charts to case report forms, and so on. These corrections or changes, if justified, must be noted and corrected by the investigator, checked by the monitor, and should not be repeated in future data recordings. If investigators cannot justify their miss-entries or errors of their data recordings and they continue to commit these errors during the progress of the trial, the monitor shall promptly secure compliance or discontinue shipment of the investigational product to the investigator and end the investigator's participation in the clinical program. During the monitoring visits, monitors should evaluate the data relating to the drug's safety and effectiveness, for example, look for inconsistencies in the data, and laboratory and mechanical evaluations that seem suspicious (ECGs that all look alike, BPs that are all the same at each evaluation, etc.). The obligations of a clinical research monitor go far beyond the compliance of the investigators obligations for GCP. Monitors should be looking for trends in the data, especially safety evaluations that appear to be detrimental to the subjects' safety and welfare.

Monitors have a special duty in ensuring that any adverse experience (see chap. 19) is reported to the sponsor's medical person in charge of the investigational trial. It is the sponsor's obligation to determine whether there is an unreasonable and significant risk to the subject or patient. At that time, the sponsor medical representative must determine if the investigational trial is to be discontinued. Important among the procedures of reporting adverse experiences is the sponsor's obligation to the FDA, and to all investigators who, at any time, participate in clinical trials and who are prescribing the experimental drug. It is the investigators obligation, as noted above, to report any AEs or SAEs to the IRB/IEC. However, the monitor should assure that this has been done.

The sponsor should report to FDA or the competent authority (CA) of each country any AEs or SAEs that are unexpected, fatal, or life threatening within seven calendar days of receipt of information. ADRs that are both serious and unexpected and related to drug administration should be reported within 15 calendar days of receipt of information. Subsequent to this, the sponsor should furnish FDA/CA with a complete report no later than seven days from the time of the report. The decision to discontinue the investigation will be contingent on the severity of the product-related reports and the number of similar reports as compared to the overall subject population being evaluated (see AE and SAE Reporting, chap. 19).

It is important to understand that the obligations of monitors include the responsibility for assuring that all records and data recorded on case report forms reflect valid data gathered by the investigator, and that they coincide with corresponding medical and hospital records of the subject participating in the investigational trial. Detailed auditing and documentation of the audit assure the sponsor that the monitor is overseeing the clinical data collected by the investigator and that GCP are being followed. It is extremely important to reemphasize the misconception that monitors who audit clinical investigations are box checkers and that their only task is to assure correct recording of data. However, one of the monitor's primary obligations is to note any adverse effects or deviations in laboratory values that could signify a safety problem in investigational trial subjects. This is especially true in large multiclinic trials, when many centers are conducting investigational trials following the same protocol, and many monitors are auditing data. If any abnormal reactions or laboratory deviations are noted from center to center, the monitors should compare observations and assess an accumulative percentage of occurrence of these deviations. At times, a sporadic, apparently minor deviation can turn out to be significant when calculated across all centers. If monitors are astute, they can often prevent recurrence of adverse experiences that might jeopardize the safety of the subjects participating in investigational drug trials or discuss a protocol amendment that might decrease or eliminate the adverse effect.

Another responsibility of the monitor is to assure maintenance of accurate records showing the receipt, shipment, or other disposition of the investigational drug. These records are required to include, as appropriate, the name of the investigator to whom the drug is shipped, the date, the quantity, and the batch number of each shipment. Regulations state that a sponsor shall retain these records and reports for two years after a marketing application is approved for the drug, or, if an application is not approved, until two years after shipment and delivery of the drug for investigational use is discontinued and the regulatory agencies have been notified (sponsor usually keep these records indefinitely). The sponsor shall also assure the return and accountability of all unused supplies of the investigational product from each investigator whose participation in the investigation is discontinued or terminated. The sponsor may authorize alternative disposition of unused supplies of the investigational product providing this alternative disposition does not expose humans to risks. Although the overall responsibility of drug inventory is assigned to sponsors, it is the monitors' underlying responsibility for drug accountability as they represent the sponsor.

In turn, the investigators, during experimental research, are also responsible for record retention similar to that of the sponsor. They are required to maintain adequate records of the disposition of the drug, including dates, quantity, and use by the subjects or patients. The investigator is also obligated if he is terminated, suspended, or discontinued, or if he has completed a trial, to return all unused supplies of the drug to the sponsor or otherwise provide documentation of how the unused supplies of the drug were disposed. (It is recommended to always return the unused trial medication to the sponsor to assure drug accountability.) An investigator is required to prepare and maintain accurate case histories (designed to record all observations and other data pertinent to the investigation) on each individual treated with the investigational drug. An investigator shall retain records from the trial for a period of two years after a marketing application is approved for the product for the indication for which it was being investigated; again, if no application is to be filed or if the application is not approved for the indication, an investigator must retain records for two years after an investigation is discontinued and FDA has been notified. Although these investigator obligations have been previously discussed, the monitor should assure that these procedures are adhered to and reported in a timely fashion.

Another responsibility of a monitor is to assure that the investigator fulfills their GCP obligations. An often neglected investigator responsibility is their requirement to submit periodic reports to the sponsor. Many investigators assume that the case report forms are sufficient in providing periodic reports. However, an investigator should be prepared to provide the sponsor with progress reports. As this task is rarely accomplished by investigators, it usually falls under the monitor's responsibility to assure that progress reports are on file. These should include an update of the ongoing investigational trial. Reports on the progress of the clinical investigations are required to be submitted by the sponsor and are usually included in the annual reports to the regulatory authorities. These reports contain information based on the investigators' progress reports. The monitor should make sure that the safety reports are promptly reported to the sponsor including any adverse experiences that may reasonably be regarded as caused by or likely caused by the investigational drug. Alarming adverse experiences (i.e., severe adverse reactions that jeopardize a subject's safety in any way) must be reported immediately by the investigator to the sponsor. Lastly, when an investigator has completed or terminated an investigational trial, a final report should be submitted to the sponsor. This comprehensive report should be completed shortly after an investigator's participation in the investigation is over. The report summarizes the final observations of the trial and any adverse experiences that occurred during the course of the clinical investigation. Monitors should be responsible for encouraging investigators to complete and submit these reports. In this case, constant follow-up may be necessary. In most cases, the clinical monitor will provide the investigator with these reports. They are usually based on the summary of findings in the closeout visit (see page 400).

Legal repercussions can occur from any neglect of GCP obligations by investigators, sponsors, or monitors. The Code of Federal Regulations stipulates in 21 CFR 312.58 that FDA can inspect the sponsor's records or reports upon request from any properly authorized officer or employee of the FDA. These inspections normally occur at reasonable times and permit FDA to have access to copy and verify any records or reports relating to a clinical investigation conducted under an IND or NDA/CTD. Upon written request by FDA, the sponsor may be asked to submit the records, reports, or copies of them to the FDA. Under these regulations, the sponsor is also obligated to discontinue shipments of the drug to any investigator who has failed to maintain or make available records or reports of the investigation. Subsequently, an investigator shall, upon request from any properly authorized officer or employee of the FDA, at reasonable times, permit such an officer or employee to have access to or copy and verify any records or reports made by the investigator. The investigator is not required to divulge subject or patient names unless the records of particular individuals require a more detailed trial of the cases. The monitor must assure that all these investigator responsibilities are fulfilled. In foreign countries practicing and implementing the EU Directives, Member States abiding by these directives are also obligated to allow inspections of investigators and clinical sites conducting clinical research. In these EU countries, the CA appoints inspectors who will visit investigators and the sites where the clinical research was conducted to ensure that the clinical trials were executed under GCP.

Investigators', sponsors', and monitors' obligations must be followed by complying with GCP rules and regulations. Sponsors' and monitors' consistent and persistent managing roles are vital in assuring that each person involved in conducting investigational clinical trials meet their legal obligations. The success of any clinical program will depend on the cooperation, understanding, and compliance of this triad of professionals working together. With this agreement and a well-organized clinical plan, the combination can only result in valid data to successfully support a new product application.

22 Quality Assurance

Helena M. Van den Dungen
Novartis Pharma AG, Basel, Switzerland

Earl W. Hulihan
Medidata Solutions Worldwide, New York, New York, U.S.A.

Richard A. Guarino
Oxford Pharmaceutical Resources, Inc., Totowa, New Jersey, U.S.A.

INTRODUCTION

To enable appropriate decision making on the safety, and efficacy and value of new and marketed medicinal products, it is clearly of the utmost importance that the available information and data on these products should be of high quality. Throughout the life cycle of a product, it is essential to ensure that the clinical trials that form the basis for product approval by the Regulatory Authorities are conducted with the highest degree of safety for the subjects participating in the clinical trials. In addition, the results reported must reflect the highest quality of data. Likewise, the same level of quality and safety should be applied post marketing through pharmacovigilance activities. An important instrument to ensure the quality, safety, and completeness of the essential information is the implementation of quality control (QC) and quality assurance (QA) processes throughout the drug's life cycle.

The term "assurance" is mostly used to indicate a hierarchy of quality assessment. The term QA reflects audit activities, implicating self checks, and includes QC. The QA activities are conducted outside the clinical trial process itself. But QA also includes activities directed at training, applications of standard operating procedures (SOPs), source document verification (SDV), and templates; these are all aimed at ensuring evidence of data integrity (validation).

It is therefore obvious that QC and QA systems and activities should be highly visible in drug development organizations. The intricacies, organizations, and procedures of QA functions and responsibilities in the clinical environment will be the focus of this chapter.

CHALLENGES OF QA

Traditionally, in the pharmaceutical industry, QA oversight was implemented through the activities of a QA department, functioning strictly independent from the clinical trial operations. The QA department was mostly involved in the performance of audits, SOP review, and training on quality matters. Until recently, separate pharmacovigilance QA groups were seldom established and pharmacovigilance QA was conducted mostly from the clinical QA or the GMP QA departments. In addition, QC processes were considered to be strictly and visibly separated from QA activities and to be implemented *within* the clinical trial and pharmacovigilance operational organizations. The QA department as recognized today is often organized as a staff function to management and is *independent* from the operational development and postmarketing activities. This gives rise to the challenge of the QA groups' responsibilities and at the same time ensures an operational, effective, and independent QA department. It is important that the QA department keeps a close relationship with the preclinical and clinical trial departments, thus allowing the benefit of insight and knowledge in their research operational procedures.

QA AND LEGISLATION

One of the principles of GCP (ICH E6: Section 2.13) requires "the implementation of systems that assure the quality of every aspect of a clinical trial" (1). Despite the fact that full compliance with the ICH GCP guideline has not been made a mandatory legal requirement in all global regions, the FDA, EU, and some of the Far East countries acknowledge the QA department and its importance with respect to the implementation of quality systems (2). The European Union has formally implemented the requirement to comply with the *principles* of ICH GCP (and hence the requirement for QA) for all clinical trials conducted in the EU region, through the issuing of the EU Directive 2005/28 (3). This same requirement also applies to clinical trials conducted in "third countries" (i.e., all non-EU countries) that are submitted as part of a marketing application in the EU. Also, effective through Volume 9A (4) of the European Union compilation of pharmaceutical legislation [Eudralex (5)]. The EU has required quality systems to be in place that cover the pharmacovigilance activities. These enhanced QA requirements for assuring the quality of clinical research data and the protection of the subjects participating in clinical trials will result in expediting valid data that can be relied on in the new drug approval process.

DEFINITION OF QA

The definition of QA within the context of the ICH GCP guidance document (1) refers to "all planned and systematic actions that are established to ensure that clinical trials are conducted and data are generated, documented (recorded), and reported in compliance with the protocol, GCP, and the applicable regulatory requirements." In this text, the term QA is extended to mean a quality assurance system, and is used closely associated with the term QC, which refers to the "operational techniques and activities undertaken within the QA system to verify that the requirements for quality of the trial-related activities have been fulfilled." In fact, ICH GCP promotes the idea to apply a *quality systems* approach to QA and QC, rather than ad hoc measures to ensure the quality of clinical trials and safety evaluation/pharmacovigilance activities. QA activities are an ongoing operation and must be implemented before, during, and after product development.

QA FUNCTION

In line with the quality systems approach, the QA function should play a role in the evaluation of compliance with the regulations, internal documentation such as policies, quality manuals and SOPs, current good practices, and other requirements that govern the clinical trial and pharmacovigilance activities and systems in place within the organization it serves.

The QA function in the pharmaceutical industry faces many challenges. True to its nature, the QA function will have to evaluate and report on the quality and safety compliance. Therefore, robust processes and procedures should be put in place. The attributes of the auditing role are ethical conduct, impartial reporting, and due professional care need to be coupled with independence and evidence-based conclusions. The challenges particular to the auditing facets of QA have been comprehensively described in the Engage Auditing Guideline (5).

To deal with these challenges, a solid and clear reporting line into management of the organization at a suitably high level should be established, in order to ensure independence and effectiveness. It is often a challenge to find the right level of reporting structure in major pharmaceutical companies because of the enormous staffs and generally complex reporting structures. In addition, management must be fully aware of the importance in supporting the QA function, and an appropriate process for follow-up should be implemented.

The "independence" of the QA function must be clearly established within the organization. Independence, for QA purposes, is defined as not being involved in the operational activities that are subject to the QA audits and to have a reporting line outside of the management of the operations subject to the QA audits. This independence will guard against any potential conflicts of interest and ensure that QA functions can be performed without bias. In addition, they should be able to report their findings to the appropriate management level in order to be effectuate actions to correct any deficiencies or errors that could potentially invalidate data and safety.

Some organizations have a corporate oversight compliance group, overseeing the audit and general QA activities at a corporate level. Others may have separate QA functions for GCP, GMP, GLP, and PV QA. Some companies prefer a central QA organization covering the GCP. Small companies are faced with the opposite problem in securing suitable independence for the QA functionary when there are a limited number of personnel for QA positions. In such cases, it might prove to be advantageous to hire a QA CRO so as to guard against the potential conflict of interest situation of being both the QA and research personnel.

QA DEPARTMENT

Traditionally, a QA department would consist of a group of specialists, each having a high degree of knowledge and many years of experience in drug development. There main focus would be to audit all aspects of drug development and train research personnel on GCP, GLP, and GMP. Their backgrounds would allow them to provide practical advice to the drug development departments with whom they interact. Auditors within a QA group need very good interactive and cognitive skills developed over many years from experiences with successes and failures within various aspects of the drug development process. Their knowledge and experience is to provide assistance and practical applications and suggestions to their colleagues, contributing to expedite and efficient development of new products.

The QA departments presently get involved in many more ways to improve or implement quality systems, more in the ways of GXP consulting. The QA function is coming away from merely assessing and evaluating the compliance level with respect to safety and quality, becoming an intrinsic linking factor for the improvement cycle. This expectation requires even more qualities of the QA professional. Training, quality system maintenance, early detection through supply of self-evaluation systems, quality system building, and so on, may all be part of daily activities in the QA group as a whole. Root cause analysis and corrective and preventive actions (CAPA), including follow-up, need to be a major responsibility of the QA department. This requires highly organized analytical skills as well as the ability to be a tutor.

Coping with these highly varied capabilities and attributes for QA professionals within one department is often solved by having distinguished divisions within the QA department, each covering a complementary function, while avoiding conflicting interests.

QA ACTIVITIES

QA personnel, due to the complexity of their function, will use many different techniques to fulfill their roles. Activities range from ensuring basic GXP knowledge in their customers, conducting interviews, quality review of documentation and performing audits, and generally ensuring that QA practices, that is, regulations, guidelines, procedures, and QC activities, are implemented by the various audiences with which they interact. They have to ensure that the organization is and remains compliant with the good practices (cGCP, cGLP, and cGMP as well as state-of-the-art pharmacovigilance). In addition, they must confirm that internal SOPs are complete and valid and give clear directions to guarantee that these practices will be adhered to.

In order to not only have a successful and smooth but also demonstrably operational QA department, it is extremely important that the QA functions are based on internal written policies and procedures defining the scope of QA activities within the organization (QA SOPs). These policies and procedures should specifically guide the activities of the QA department.

A selective application of directed and evidence-based as well as routine- and systems-oriented audits of each aspect in the process of drug development forms the basis of the QA program. The development of the QA program not only should be based on the information to be reviewed by the QA team but also should be done with the knowledge and understanding of the material to be audited. The limitation of resources and the independent approach to QA requires that an assessment of risk is the basis of each QA program.

The approach of continuing quality improvement will provide the most assurance that the safety and integrity are implemented in the entire drug development process independent of the QA audits. In fact, internal QA procedures generally should be sufficient in scope to utilize a thorough sampling process to determine internal operations' effectiveness in completing corporate objectives, policies, and procedures at all levels.

The principles and practices of QA procedures do not really differ from early development to the postmarketing environment of products. However, development of the various tools and techniques that are used in the QA procedures may vary. For example, the more strictly organized phase I environment is coupled with a large uncertainty with regard to the safety profile of a drug, whereas in post-marketing surveillance studies, with a more comprehensive knowledge of safety protocols and records are often less structured as in structured clinical trials. In the development of the QA programs, these differences should be accounted for, and, clearly, how audits are accomplished should be approached differently, but the processes used in QA activities during the various audits and quality sampling are basically similar.

An extensive description of the audit and higher level QA activities can be founding the Engage Audit Guideline (5).

QA TOOLS AND TECHNIQUES

With the change in technologies that are being implemented in conduct of clinical trials and safety reporting, the potential tools and techniques available for the assessments of compliance have been vastly enriched. Electronic data capture, for instance, allows early access to safety, efficacy, and compliance data, through audit trails and data locks. Conversely, the validation of data through these electronic technologies can take "nightmarish proportions" when trying to determine the validity and integrity of a set of clinical trial or data capture system. QA professionals should stay on top of these developments in order to be quality leaders in their organization. QA personnel must be constantly apprised of how these systems are operated and proactively seek information on any changes during the course of clinical research programs. Recent surveys have shown that the larger QA groups have employed their own e-compliance specialists. These experts are involved not only in the evaluation of the quality and safety compliance status, but are also an intrinsic part of the development organization as a whole. This ensures that the necessary requirements for QA and safety are built in from the start of a program. These computerized systems used to support the product development life cycle will be a major part of validating clinical data.

The availability of audit trails in properly validated computerized systems used in clinical trials offers great potential in closer monitoring of compliance by QA personnel. Remote monitoring of clinical trial data at the time these data are being developed has become an integral part of the daily activities of the QA departments. This allows QA personnel the opportunities for implementing remedial activities at a time when this still affects the quality and integrity of the clinical trial. These developments, clearly, have implications for the structure and day-to-day activities of the QA department.

In-house audits of clinical operations by QA personnel can also enhance and complement the remote data monitoring. Early scrutiny of data collected gives the opportunity to identify noncompliance situations and prevention of miss-entries of data. QA personnel can play a major part in preventing delays in correcting or reentering data that does not meet GCP.

QA DURING THE PRODUCT LIFE CYCLE

As was briefly mentioned, typical aspects of QA activities in early product development are focused on the evaluation of safety and establishing a safety profile of a compound. In many relatively small clinical trials designed for the early phases of clinical trials, small-scale manufacturing is employed. Often, the manufacturing of the product never reaches large-scale production if the product does not demonstrate safety as well as efficacy. As the product life cycle grows, the completion of safety and efficacy profiles requires further investigation with larger scale trials. This increases the need for more robust safety data capture, and if the product is approved for market, a pharmacovigilance database will be established.

With each developmental phase, emphasis on QA must change. Many aspects and categories of activities in the QA group should mirror the developmental stages of the products' life cycle; hence, the change in approach is more with respect to focus and priority of the QA orientation than the actual activities themselves. The value of QA activities should also reflect the organizations concern in not only meeting global regulatory requirements but also to constantly be aware of the safety aspects of all products as they relate to the safety of the consumers. QA programs must focus on these issues and revolve around the confirmation that appropriate regulatory requirements and corporate procedures are carried through as confirmed by the SOPs established for the QA department.

REGULATORY INSPECTIONS

A specific aspect of activities of the QA group in a pharmaceutical company is the assistance with regulatory inspection. Whereas in most pharmaceutical companies, the regulatory departments are ultimately responsible for the contacts with regulators and, hence, for the regulatory inspections that are requested by agencies throughout the world. It is often the QA department that is the point of contact for the conduct of the inspections and is instrumental in ensuring a smooth running of such inspections. When an inspection is announced, the QA associates are usually involved in the preparation of the inspection site, ensuring that all documents are in readiness and are available for inspection. This inspection preparation also includes training of the inspectees. During an inspection, the QA associates can facilitate the organization and retrieval of documents requested by the agencies inspectors ensuring that the right documents are provided and the information requested is correct.

After the inspection, the QA department is often instrumental in ensuring a smooth resolution of inspection findings. This may include leading the compilation of an appropriate reply to the inspection findings and inspection report, including corrective and preventive action plans, as well as general follow-up on inspection activities or on queries that need clarification.

FUTURE VALUE OF QA

The product development process is rapidly becoming more difficult. Regulations are more restrictive and the costs of new product development are soaring. Global product development will be the focus of companies to bring new products to market. Regional disciplines will require more intense justification of the validity of data. QA is one way that companies can ensure that the development of products can occur more efficiently, economically, and expeditiously. The regulatory environment is ever tightening, and the public demands on the quality and safety and availability of medicinal products are ever increasing.

QA resolutions in the process of product development can resolve questionable situations and save time and costs. QA cannot guarantee success in every difficult regulatory situation. The appropriate placing of QA resources requires a clear oversight of the needs of the organization to enable a risk-based approach. In addition, the use of the electronic tools that come with the use of remote data entry, e-CRFs, and electronic subject reported data can be optimized to focus the resources needed to on-site as well as remote QA activities. However, if the personnel comprising the QA staff have the experience and the knowledge to identify and resolve (potential) problems already at the time of the clinical trial process, this would significantly reduce delays in new product development. Evidently, it is to their benefit if companies are there to invest in a substantial QA department.

REFERENCES

1. ICH GCP Note for guidance on Good Clinical Practice, CHMP/ICH/135/95, ICH Topic E6.
2. FDA Regulation 21 CFR Part 820-Quality system regulations.

3. Directive of the European Community 2005/28/EC.
4. Volume 9A of the Rules Governing Medicinal Products in the European Union— Guidelines on Pharmacovigilance for Medicinal Products for Human Use.
5. Revised Engage Auditing Guideline (2005). V12 050222.doc.

Appendix   Main aspects to be considered in QA reviews, evaluations, or audit activities provided during the life cycle of a product

1. Institutional review committee
    (a) Document review prior to study initiation
    (b) Investigator qualifications by a CV
    (c) Continuing review of investigation
    (d) Financial, coercion/undue influence
    (e) Membership
    (f) Written procedures
2. Investigator
    (a) Investigation products
    (b) Randomization procedures
    (c) Informed consent of trial subjects
    (d) Records and reports
    (e) Safety reporting
    (f) Trial termination or suspension
    (g) Qualifications
    (h) Agreements
    (i) Resources
    (j) Medical care of trial subjects
    (k) Communication with IRC compliance with protocol
3. Sponsor
    (a) QCs
    (b) Medical expertise
    (c) Trial design
    (d) Trial management, data handling, and records
    (e) Investigator selection
    (f) Allocation of responsibilities, compensation to subjects
    (g) Notification to regulatory authorities, confirmation of review by IRC
    (h) Information on investigation products, manufacturing, packaging, labeling
    (i) Supply and handling of products
    (j) Record access
    (k) Safety information
    (l) Adverse drug reaction reporting, monitoring
    (m) Noncompliance reporting
    (n) Clinical trial reports
    (o) Training and development
4. Data management
    (a) Procedures
    (b) Document design (e.g., CRF), document tracking
    (c) CRF correction
    (d) Data entry

    (e) Data coding
    (f) QC system, computer system, software, data reporting
    (g) Record keeping
    (h) Record retention
    (i) Training initiatives
5. Regulatory submissions
    (a) Protocol review
    (b) Clinical study report review
    (c) Text consistency, grammar, spelling headers, footers, pagination, and spacing
    (d) Compare CRF data points with report
    (e) Protocol statements with report statements
    (f) Data validity and verification
    (g) Appropriate signatures
6. Compliance with validation requirements
    (a) System overview
    (b) Validation test environment including hardware and software and HLRA of the systems
    (c) System security including passwords, network rights, functional security, physical security, modem access, and virus protection
    (d) Validation test environment including related documents, along with SOPs, user manuals, and system development/maintenance and documentation
    (e) Validation assumptions, exclusions, and limitations
    (f) Responsibilities matrix
    (g) Validation data sets
    (h) Acceptance criteria
    (i) Expected results
    (j) Execution of the validation plan
    (k) Resolution of errors
    (l) Documentation
    (m) Training records
    (n) Archives, storage, backup, and recovery procedures
    (o) Methodology and change control
    (p) Disaster, recovery, and contingency planning
7. Contract vendors
    (a) Previous experience
    (b) Facilities
    (c) Affiliations
    (d) Qualifications of personnel, services available
    (e) Offered procedures
    (f) Capability to complete project, QCs program, QA program, review and approve contracts, future compliance audits, database management, validation/verification needs, contract laboratories, procedures, facilities/equipment, personnel qualification, training
    (g) Methodology
8. Contract laboratories
    (a) QC program
    (b) QA program

    (c) Computer validation procedures, results acceptance procedures, documentation
    (d) Maintenance calibration
    (e) Record keeping/retention
    (f) Computer system/software
    (g) Specimen handling/storage
    (h) Specimen analysis/reporting
    (i) Result reporting
    (j) Accreditation licenses
    (k) Software system vendors/suppliers
    (l) Appropriate understanding of procedures
9. Contract research organizations
    (a) Organization staffing/resources
    (b) Experience
    (c) Controls/assurance
    (d) SOPs
    (e) Other items as identified above

23 Managing and Monitoring Clinical Trials

Andrea Proccacino

Johnson & Johnson Pharmaceutical Research & Development, L.L.C., Titusville, New Jersey, U.S.A.

OVERVIEW

What is a clinical trial? In its purest form, it is an activity designed to test a hypothesis to ultimately reach a conclusion as to whether or not a drug, biologic, medical device, or combination product has any effect on the human body and the disease condition in which it is being tested. The ultimate goal is to demonstrate that the product will improve the subject's health or quality of life, have an advantage over the current treatment available for that disease or condition, and can be administered safely to the subject.

Clinical trials can be the most timely and costly part of new product development. They require thoughtful planning in trial design and careful consideration of the types of subjects to be enrolled.

Above all, every evaluation must ensure the subjects' safety and well-being while participating in the trial. Therefore, it is critical that all personnel involved in the conduct of clinical trials understand the regulations and guidelines that govern the protection of human subjects while evaluating the efficacy of experimental products.

Timelines for product development are continually being shortened by sponsor companies in an effort to get a product to the market as quickly as possible for a sales competitive advantage. Current and future trends and industry paradigm shifts are changing the face of clinical trials so that the pharmaceutical industry can look forward to global approvals of new and old pharmaceutical products. Global approvals hopefully will reduce the drug lag that appears in some regions of the world.

At times, insufficient preparation and management of the clinical trials and inadequate on-site monitoring and correction of subject data fall by the wayside. This creates delays in timelines for market launches. This chapter will focus on the components of clinical trial management and the monitoring of clinical trials from execution to closure.

REGULATIONS AND GUIDELINES

The conduct of clinical trials is regulated by regulatory authorities around the world such as the U.S. Food and Drug Administration (FDA), the European Medicines Agency (EMEA), the State Food and Drug Administration in China, and so on. In the United States, the U.S. government has codified into law the rules that govern clinical research conducted in the United States or data submitted to the U.S. government for approval to market approval in the United States. They can be found in the U.S. Code of Federal Regulations (CFR). The FDA has the authority to ensure that the CFR containing good clinical practices (GCPs) are adhered to by every-one involved in the conduct of clinical trials in the United States. Europe previously had the International Conference on Harmonization (ICH) that set guidelines on the conduct of clinical research using GCPs as the "gold standards." However, in May 2004, the European Clinical Trial Directives went into effect, requiring the European Union (EU) Member States to codify the ICH guidelines into their national laws. Of late, there has been a lot of regulatory activity by the State Food and Drug Administration (SFDA) of China to establish their drug and medical device regulations. They have tried to pattern them after the U.S. FDA, where appropriate. Also, in September 2007, the Japanese Health authority, Pharmaceutical and Medical Device Agency (PMDA), issued its guidelines for conducting global studies in order to address Japan becoming more involved in global studies. Considerations of intrinsic and extrinsic ethnic factors in global studies will also be addressed in these guidelines. Depending on where drug trials are conducted around the world and to what countries marketing applications will be submitted will dictate what regulations need to be followed. Many countries have their own local laws and regulations that also govern clinical trials. Countries such as Jordan and the United Arab Emirates are also starting to seek participation in global trials and have begun to create appropriate governmental controls for clinical trials. No matter where the research is done, a thorough understanding of the applicable regulations and how to apply them is vital in the process of the conduct of clinical trials. These regulations and guidelines detail government requirements that must be followed by the investigators, their staff, sponsor companies, and research monitors. Noncompliance of these regulations can result in the termination of a clinical study or program, penalties, and, in some countries, criminal prosecution. In the United States, the FDA imposes these regulations to protect consumers' safety from drugs, biologics, devices, foods, and cosmetics that are marketed in the United States. The U.S. GCP regulations can be found in 21 CFR Parts 11 (electronic records/signatures), 50 (protection of human subjects), 54 (financial disclosure), 56 (Institutional Review Boards), 312 (investigational new drug processes), 314 (application for FDA approval to market a new drug), and 812 (medical devices) in the United States. There are also additional regulations in the United States that address federally funded studies and they can be found in 45 Part 46. Internationally, there are the ICH guidelines on GCP that are found in Section E6. For the EU Clinical Trial Directive, the requirements can be found in Directive 2005/28/EC of the European Parliament and of the Council of April 8, 2005.

CLINICAL TRIAL MANAGEMENT

There are key elements in managing clinical programs that must be considered. Among them are investigator selection, preinvestigational site visits (PISVs), study initiation visits (SIVs), trial conduct and execution, legal aspects, privacy laws, periodic monitoring visits, product accountability, adverse experience or adverse drug reaction reporting, financial disclosure, study closeout visits (SCVs), and final recommendations to the investigator on record retention and inspections. These important components of managing clinical investigations and how a practical application of these regulations and guidelines can lead to a successful completion of clinical research trials are detailed in this chapter.

INVESTIGATOR SELECTION

U.S. and EU GCP regulations and ICH/GCP guidelines mandate that a sponsor select only investigators qualified by training and experience as appropriate experts to evaluate an investigational product (21 CFR 312, ICH GCP 4.1). As investigator selection is a critical step in conducting clinical trials, the following recommendations to identify potential investigators are the most frequently used:

- Experience with investigators who conducted other studies for the sponsor.
- Literature searches in the therapeutic area or disease state under study. These searches can be done in key medical publications/journals such as the Journal of the American Medical Association (JAMA), the New England Journal of Medicine, and so on, or via general searches on the Internet.
- Medical or scientific meetings such as the American Psychiatric Association, American Dermatology Association, and so on.
- Clinical research professional organizations directories such as the Association of Clinical Research Professionals (ACRP), the Association of Pharmaceutical Physicians and Investigators (APPI), Drug Information Association (DIA), and Regulatory Affairs Professional Society (RAPS).
- Referrals from other investigators with whom a sponsor company is already working on a particular project.
- Disease foundations (e.g., American Cancer Society, Lymphoma Research Foundation).
- *Site management organizations (SMOs)*: These are organizations that act as a brokerage for investigators for certain therapeutic areas and often have a large geographic selection of investigators available.

It is important to remember, in the investigator selection process, that the sponsor company is entrusting this individual to research their investigational product that will result in quality, reproducible trial data. Most importantly, this individual will be managing the study subject's safety and medical care during the trial and must have the proper credentials and specialty experience to do so. Other items to carefully consider during the investigator selection process are as follows:

- Experience in clinical research and human clinical trials of the disease under study (e.g., a gynecologist would not be appropriate for a study of a product for brain cancer).
- *Location of the site*: Is it in an area that is easily accessible to subjects? Is it in a center of excellence for the therapeutic indication under study?
- Does this investigator have the appropriate subject population available to him or her to be able to adequately recruit study subjects for the trial in a timely fashion? (A heterogeneous subject population is always more desirable.)
- Is the budget proposal from this investigator appropriate or is it cost prohibitive? Does the institution require an overhead cost that is beyond budgetary restrictions?
- Has the investigator been previously inspected by the U.S. FDA or another global health authority, and if so, what was the outcome of the inspection?

NB: The U.S. FDA may disqualify an investigator from receiving investigational drugs, biologics, or devices if the FDA determines that the investigator has repeatedly or deliberately failed to comply with regulatory requirements for conducting clinical studies or has submitted false information to the study sponsor. Investigators may agree to certain restrictions on their conduct of future studies. The FDA publishes the list of those investigators that have at one time been disqualified, restricted, have made assurances in their use of investigational products, or have been prosecuted or had a criminal conviction. This list can be found on the FDA Web site (1). When an investigator has been reinstated or restrictions have expired, this too is also noted on the list. The list can be found on the FDA Web site (2). The sponsor should check this list to make sure that the investigator is not on it before they are selected to participate in a clinical program. Many sponsor companies have Standard Operating Procedures (SOPs) that require that they do not use any investigator who has ever appeared on this list. It is also prudent not to use investigators who have been reinstated from this list by the FDA. Industry often refers to this list as the FDA "black list."

- Can they complete the trial in the given time frame?
- What methods will they have to employ to recruit subjects? Will they require extra assistance to recruit subjects?
- Does the investigator have the appropriate staff available to assist with the conduct of the trial? Does the staff have the appropriate education and experience to conduct the trial?
- Is there a dedicated and experienced study coordinator in place to assist the investigator with the conduct of the study?
- Has the investigator ever worked with the sponsor company in the past, and if so, how was their conduct during the course of the trial?
- Do the investigators have any other current research commitments that would compete with the trial you are trying to place at their site in terms of the study staff's time and subject population?

These questions are posed to potential investigators to examine the feasibility of their participation in the clinical program.

CLINICAL MONITORS

Once a potential investigator has been identified, the sponsor company will continue to be in contact with the investigator and the site to make additional assessments of their continued interest and capabilities to participate in the clinical program. This responsibility is assigned to personnel within sponsor companies that carry many different titles. Site Managers (SMs), Medical Research Associates (MRAs), Clinical Research Associates (CRAs), or Clinical Research Monitors (CRMs) are among the names used. For the purpose of this chapter, personnel with these responsibilities will be called "monitor."

The monitor is the individual appointed by the sponsor who is familiar with the investigational product and the protocol developed for the clinical program and is responsible for coordinating, initiating, and overseeing the conduct of the clinical trial. They ensure adherence to the protocol, regulatory requirements, and act as a liaison between the investigator and their staff and the sponsor company. It is important that monitors have the scientific and medical knowledge needed to oversee the clinical research program. They must understand the condition under evaluation and assure that all data recorded are entered correctly and reflected in the medical/hospital records. In addition, they should also have exceptional interpersonal skills.

The sponsor may contract the monitoring or the entire execution of the trial out to a contract research organization (CRO). A CRO is defined as a person or an organization (commercial, academic, or other) contracted by the sponsor to perform one or more of the sponsor's trial-related duties and functions (ICH 1.20). Although the CRO assumes the sponsor's obligations, the sponsor is still ultimately responsible for the clinical trial [21 CFR 312.52(b); ICH 5.2].

After the investigator and site have been selected to participate in the clinical program, preliminary documentation is sent to the investigator. This includes

- a confidentiality statement (which must be signed prior to receiving any study-related documents);
- an Investigator's Brochure;
- a copy of the protocol and case report form;
- a sample informed consent form;
- a contract with budget information.

Once the site has had the opportunity to review these materials, the monitor will again contact the site by phone to answer any questions and schedule a PISV.

PISV

After prescreening of potential investigators is completed, it is vitally important that the monitor or an authorized individual appointed by the company conducts a PISV at the investigational site with the investigator and their staff to continue to assess their ability to conduct the trial. The sponsor representative(s) will have a "face-to-face" meeting with the principal investigator (PI) and their staff to ensure that they clearly and fully understand and accept their obligations in conducting clinical trials. Each person's qualifications will be reviewed and their curricula vitae (CV) and medical licenses will be confirmed.

Among the staff members, it is essential that an investigator appoints a study coordinator [sometimes referred to as a Research Nurse, Clinical Research Coordinator (CRC), or Study Nurse] who is dedicated to the study and plays a key role in the execution of the clinical trial as a direct support to the PI. Therefore, careful consideration should be given to their qualifications and research experience.

If an investigator does not have a study coordinator, it is recommended that they should not be selected to participate in the clinical research program or the monitor should suggest that they hire or train one immediately.

The study coordinator will have continuous interaction with the investigator and monitor during the trial. After the PISV, the monitor will also assess the qualifications of any subinvestigators or other physicians who will be evaluating the subjects. It should be stressed that subinvestigators will have the same regulatory responsibilities as the PI; however, the PIs must assure that they will oversee the entire clinical investigation including the involvement of the subinvestigators.

During the PISV, the facility should be toured to ensure that all of the necessary equipment is available to fulfill the required study procedures and that the same examination rooms are available throughout the study to evaluate the study subjects. The equipment being used for the trial should be state of the art and fully calibrated. The facilities should be clean and orderly, and storage of the investigational product must be established. The storage area should be in a secure and locked area or cabinet with access granted only to those personnel assigned to dispense the product by the investigator. (The investigational products have not been approved by a regulatory authority for general market use. Therefore, tight control over their availability and distribution must be adequately maintained.) Over-the-counter (OTC) medications that may also be required for use in a clinical trial should be stored under the same conditions. If the investigator does not have a storage facility to house investigational products appropriately, one can be purchased by the sponsor company for them. If the investigational product is considered a "controlled substance," there are additional regulatory safeguards required in its storage above and beyond what is required for other investigational products. The sponsor company will review these additional requirements with the investigator.

It is critical that the investigator understands their regulatory obligations and agrees to conduct the study accordingly. The FDA requires that each investigator signs a "Statement of Investigator" or FDA 1572 document. This lists the investigator's legal/regulatory obligations during the trial. An investigator conducting an investigational drug trial under a U.S. Investigational New Drug (IND) application must complete Form 1572. This form is not required by countries outside of the United States; however, if the sponsor plans to submit the data from a foreign clinical trial in support of a product for U.S. marketing, this document should be signed by the PI from that country. Presently, this form is not required for trials conducted outside of the United States that will not be filed in a U.S. IND application. This federal regulatory document is a binding contract between the investigator and the U.S. FDA. Failure to comply with any of the obligations listed on this document could result in a citation on an FDA inspection report, a warning letter, or regulatory action by the FDA. Monitors should emphasize the seriousness of violating the requirements on the Form 1572 to all who participate in a clinical program and whose names are listed on the document. By signing this document, the investigator agrees and commits to the following obligations required by the U.S. CFR in 21 CFR Part 312:

- Will personally conduct or supervise the investigation.
- Obtain informed consent.
- Report adverse experiences to the sponsor within the specified time.
- Read and understand the Investigator's Brochure.
- Ensure that the study staff is informed of their obligations in meeting these requirements.
- Maintain adequate and accurate study records.
- Ensure that the Institutional Review Board (IRB) complies with requirements.
- Agrees to comply with all other requirements regarding the obligations of clinical investigators.

NB: IND applications are a U.S.-only submission. In the EU, its equivalent is an Investigational Medicinal Product Dossier or IMPD. An IMPD has information on the quality and manufacturing of the investigational product, any available pharmacological and toxicological study data, and results from previous clinical studies. It was adopted by the CHMP and published in Volume 10, "Clinical Trials—Notice to Applicants," the rules governing medicinal products in the EU, in July 2006.

The document also contains general information: title of the clinical trial, names of the investigator and subinvestigators, the laboratory to be used for the trial, the IRB responsible for ethical oversight, and the name of the CRO if one is appointed.

Since many trials are being conducted in all regions of the world and submitted to a U.S. IND application, the FDA is working on a separate type of Form 1572 to be used for these sites. The reason for this is because an ethical committee (EC), the international version of the U.S. IRBs, reviewing the research protocols and informed consents are composed slightly differently from IRBs in the United States. Independent Ethics Committees (IECs) follow ICH/GCP guidelines and EU Clinical Trial Directives (if located in the EU) that differ slightly from U.S. CFR regulations.

The Investigator's Brochure (IB) and the clinical protocol are reviewed at the PISV. The IB is a compilation of all of the nonclinical, preclinical, and clinical data collected to date on the investigational product. The investigator must review and understand this document in detail because it provides information on the pharmacology, toxicology, and other pertinent data confirming that the starting dosage to be administered to the subjects is reasonably safe. The protocol is reviewed and discussed in detail with the investigators and their staff during this visit. The protocol's objective, inclusion/exclusion criteria, study visit procedures, product accountability requirements, adverse experience reporting procedures, and all logistical procedures are presented. Any questions that arise should be clarified.

At the completion of the PISV, the monitor will complete a written PISV report. This report will document any observations or findings from this visit as well as any agreements reached with the investigator and/or staff. All information gathered from this visit will be reviewed by the sponsor, and based on the PISV assessment, a decision is made to include or exclude this investigator. A follow-up letter will be sent to the investigator informing him or her of the sponsor's decision. When the investigator has been selected, they will be required to submit the following documents to the sponsor:

- *Signed protocol page*: This must be signed and dated by the PI to document their agreement to conduct the trial as per the protocol.
- Signed and completed Form FDA 1572 Statement of Investigator (if the trial is to be filed in support of a U.S. IND).
- CVs of the PI and any subinvestigators listed on the FDA Form 1572. Some sponsors even request that a CV be submitted for the study coordinator, although this is not required by regulation. It is also worthy to note that the CVs should be current within two years and list the investigator/subinvestigator's current position at the institution or medical facility. Some sponsor companies will also request a copy of the PI and subinvestigators' medical licenses.
- A signed and dated Clinical Trial Agreement or study contract between the investigator and the sponsor detailing any financial remuneration to be paid to the investigator for his or her participation in the trial; the study contract should include an indemnification clause that indemnifies the investigator and the institution against claims arising from the trial (not including claims that may arise from malpractice and/or negligence by the investigator or institution).
- *IRB/IEC approval letter*: This letter must clearly state that the protocol, informed consent, and any advertisement materials to be used for recruitment were reviewed and approved by the IRB/IEC. (This may take time, as these committees do not meet on a regular basis.)
- List of the IRB/IEC members and their qualifications or, in the United States, an IRB Assurance number to ensure that the IRB was properly constituted as per the requirements.

- Laboratory license or certification, laboratory normal values, and a CV for the Laboratory Director for each laboratory to be used in the trial. If a central laboratory is used, the sponsor will obtain this document directly from the central laboratory and copies will be sent to the investigator site for their files.
- *Prestudy financial disclosure information*: This will be explained further in this chapter.

Investigator Meetings

When the sponsor company has selected all of the investigators and the investigative sites (a multicenter program) to participate in a clinical trial, they usually will hold an investigators meeting. Representatives from each site (usually the PI and study coordinator) will attend the meeting along with representatives from the sponsor's clinical team, regulatory affairs, data management, and quality assurance departments. If a central laboratory or central imaging group is being used for the trial, representatives from the laboratory will also participate in the investigators meeting. Investigator meetings can be conducted in three ways. One type of investigator meeting is a preparatory or peer group meeting where the protocol is being reviewed for comments by the investigators prior to being finalized. The second type is more common/standard where the protocol has already been finalized and this face-to-face meeting is a training session for the participants. A complete understanding of the protocol and how to conduct the clinical trial are usually the main objectives of this meeting. This is an excellent opportunity for the investigators and their staffs to ask questions about the trial and trial conduct. The following topics are typically addressed during the investigator meeting:

- Review of preclinical/clinical findings on the product
- Protocol review
- Case report form review and completion
- Laboratory procedures for collecting specimens and how to properly ship them
- Review of GCPs, and investigator and staff obligations
- AE and ADR reporting
- Recruitment techniques
- Record retention

Attendance should be carefully monitored throughout the duration of the meeting to ensure that the investigator and staff personnel are present. The CFR regulations, ICH/GCP guidelines, and EU Clinical Trial Directives as well as many other national regulations require that the sponsor company train the investigator and his or her staff on the protocol and protocol requirements. A new trend is for sponsor companies to hold "virtual" investigator meetings. Web 2.0 collaborative technologies and interactive portals are used to allow the investigators and their staffs to obtain vital information with which to run the studies remotely without having to travel to a face-to-face meeting. This is also more cost effective for the sponsor companies in today's challenging financial environment because they do not have to incur the expense of flying investigative staff to one location.

NB: Investigators should pursue in-depth training on GCPs. Many clinical research professional organizations offer such training programs on GCPs for clinical investigators, CRAs, and CRCs [e.g., the DIA, the ACRP, the Academy of Pharmaceutical Physicians and Investigators (APPI), Barnett International, etc., to name a few]. Some even offer certification programs for investigators, CRAs, and CRCs (ACRP and APPI). This is one of the new paradigm shifts in the clinical research arena. Sponsor companies are now being held responsible by regulatory authorities for investigator training in GCP obligations and the ethical conduct of clinical trials. Countries in the emerging market areas of the world such as China, Taiwan, and so on, are also pursuing GCP training and certification for their government officials as well as their investigators in order to show their commitment to participating in global trials and to ensuring they have the appropriate knowledge and training to do so.

The third option for an investigator meeting is starting to become more fashionable as sponsor companies become more comfortable and savvy in using technology for learning. In this option, a blended approach of e-learning modules delivered prior to the meeting on a secure-access Web site must be taken by the investigator and coordinator on key topics such as adverse event reporting, record retention, and so on, and completed prior to attending the meeting. The actual meeting itself can be either face-to-face but in a shortened time frame than usual because of the training prerequisites they have taken online prior to the meeting, or the meeting can be "virtual." Virtual learning technologies can be used to hold the meeting simultaneously in many locations around the world via the computer with "live meeting" capabilities in order to reduce the high costs for the sponsor company associated with these meetings and in order to minimize the investigator and his or her staff's time away from their practice and patients. As we see Web 2.0 technologies continue to evolve, this option will become more of the norm rather than the exception.

SIV

Once the PISV has been completed, an SIV is the next step. Some sponsor companies will combine the PISV and the SIV into one visit to compress the timelines and to be more cost-effective. This occurs especially when the investigator has worked previously with the sponsor on other trials. The monitor will schedule the SIV with the investigator and study coordinator via telephone or e-mail and will send a follow-up letter in writing to confirm the date and time of the visit and the staff's availability for the visit. All study staff personnel participating in the study should be in attendance at this important meeting. The investigator and their staff must be present for the entire meeting. Prior to this meeting, the monitor will also arrange for the initial shipment of investigational product to be sent to the site along with any additional ancillary supplies that are required (e.g., syringes, alcohol swabs, sharps, containers for syringe disposal, etc.). The site should await the monitor's review of the shipment at the SIV prior to logging the product and storing it. The monitor will review the product and its storage at the initiation visit. The monitor will also send the Investigator Trial Binder with copies of all required study documentation received to date in it. This binder will act as the central storage and filing of all required documentation for the duration of the trial.

The SIV is also a training meeting. This is the last training on the protocol that the investigators and their staff will have before beginning to recruit and enroll subjects into the trial. During this meeting, the monitor will review the following in detail:

* *Protocol*: Rationale, study design, inclusion/exclusion criteria, visit schedule and study procedures required at each visit, diagnostic tests and procedures, concomitant medications, and publication requirements.

- *Adverse experience and serious adverse experience (SAE) reporting*: Documentation, reports, whom to notify of SAEs and within what time frame and reporting requirements to the IRB/IEC. The obligation of the investigator and sponsor to report AEs and ADRs to the FDA or other application regulatory authorities in a required time frame is mandatory. (See chap. 19 on safety reporting topics.)
- *Product dispensation and accountability*: The PI is responsible for product accountability. He or she may delegate this responsibility to another qualified individual, for example, pharmacist, subinvestigator, and study coordinator; however, the investigator is ultimately accountable for prescribing the investigational product to the study subjects, and maintaining and assuring that dispensation and storage records account for all investigational products. The monitor is responsible for reviewing the documentation for product accountability prior, during, and at study closure.
- *Case report form (CRF) completion*: The CRF is the data collection tool for the trial. The monitor will review in detail how to complete each evaluation on the CRF. Monitors should demonstrate proper correction procedures to ensure that data are not obliterated or that whiteout is not used and what medical abbreviations are acceptable to be used. For example, if paper CRFs are used, when an error occurs, the person completing the CRF will put a line through the incorrect information, record the correct information next to it, and initial and date the new entry. It must be emphasized that the same person who entered the original data be the one to enter, sign, and date any corrections if at all possible. The sponsor company may also have created CRF completion guidelines to give to the site, which detail page by page how each data field should be completed. For a multicenter trial, this helps to ensure consistency in data collection and reporting. However, the current trend many monitors are using now is electronic data capture or eDC. Each sponsor company chooses a system or technology platform to use at the sites to capture the data electronically at the site with immediate transmission into the sponsor company's database where they can begin to immediately review or clean the data. If eDC is used, the monitor, and potentially a data specialist present with the monitor during the SIV, will show the appropriate site staff how to collect the data electronically using a laptop provided by the sponsor as well as the system itself, security/password measures, audit trail features, how to make corrections electronically, and so on.
- *Review of regulatory documents*: The monitor will review what type of documentation should be collected during the trial and how and where to store it. These documents can be stored in a centrally located binder supplied by the sponsor or in a designated file drawer. Company-specific documents are also filed with the trial documents. Examples of company-specific documents are a monitoring or screening log. The monitoring log is used by the monitor to sign in at each monitoring visit, including the initiation and closeout visits. This tracks how and when the sponsor company monitored the trial. Upon an inspection by a regulatory authority, there is evidence that the sponsor met their obligations and that the sponsor monitored the progress of the clinical trial [21 CFR Part 312.56(a); ICH 5.18.2]. The screening log keeps track of all of the subjects that are screened for the trial, identifying them only by a screening number and their initials. Any other correspondence received by the investigator from the sponsor company and all correspondence to or from the investigator and IRB/IEC should be maintained in this binder.

- *Source documentation*: Source data, as defined by ICH guidelines 1.51, are all the information in original office or hospital records, and certified copies of original records of clinical findings, observations, and other activities in a clinical trial necessary for the reconstruction and evaluation of the trial. Original data are contained in source documents. Source documents are composed of hospital records, office charts, laboratory data sheets, subject diaries, pharmacy dispensing records, recorded data from automated instruments, X rays, and so on. Source documents should be legible and should document that the subjects are participating in a clinical trial. Some of the key areas to cross-reference source documents to CRFs and regulatory criteria are the informed consent process, inclusion/exclusion criteria, adverse experiences, investigational product administration, concomitant medications administered to the subject during the trial, withdrawal from the study for any reason, and subjects lost to follow-up.

The investigator is responsible for the accuracy and completeness of their trial records and any discrepancies found in these records during an audit (ICH 4.9.1). The monitor will review the source documents for accuracy and completeness against the CRFs at each monitoring visit and will provide feedback on their acceptability to the investigators and their staff. Once the initiation visit has occurred, the study site is considered officially started and subject recruitment can begin.

Periodic Monitoring of a Clinical Trial

The CFR, ICH/GCP guidelines, and EU Clinical Trial Directives as well as many other national regulations require that the sponsor monitor the progress of the clinical trial at the site where the trial is being conducted. How frequently these monitoring visits should occur is not specified in the regulations and guidelines. It is up to the sponsor to make the determination of what the frequency should be. Most companies will have SOPs for monitoring that require periodic visits to occur at a set frequency that is appropriate for the difficulty of the trial and will verify 100% of all data fields against the source documentation. This is not required under regulations or guidelines. The overall purpose of these periodic monitoring visits by the sponsor's monitor or authorized representative (e.g., CRO) is to assure that the investigators and their staffs follow GCP regulations/guidelines, local regulations, adhere to the protocol to assure that the rights of the subjects participating in the clinical trial are being protected, and that the data reported are complete, accurate, verifiable, and reproducible. Therefore, it is extremely important to schedule monitoring visits based on the objective of the trial, the rate of enrollment, and the quality of the data emanating from the investigational site. The first monitoring visit should occur soon after the enrollment of the first few study subjects into the trial and subsequent monitoring visits are then scheduled on a regular basis according to the SOPs of the sponsor. During these visits, the monitor must meet with the investigator to review any issues that need clarification or explanation and to entertain any questions that may arise on the general progress of the trial. The study coordinator must also readily be available during these visits to assist the monitors by retrieving source documents as needed, making any necessary corrections to the CRFs that come under their jurisdiction, and provide any needed regulatory documents. The site must ensure that it has a suitable area available to monitor as a workspace during their visit and that the CRFs and their supporting source documents are readily available for review. After each monitoring visit, the monitor will complete a detailed monitoring visit report for internal use within the sponsor company. This report should contain information as to whom the monitor met during the visit, any issues noted and the resolutions that were discussed, and any corrections made by the investigator, research coordinator, or any other staff person.

The monitor is the main line of communication between the sponsor and the investigator. The following checklist can be used as a guide to underline the main responsibilities of the monitor at each site visit:

- Ensure the investigator is using their qualification and resources to conduct the trial.
- Ensure the investigational product is stored, dispensed, returned, and disposed of properly.
- Ensure that the investigator is adhering to the protocol and amendments.
- Ensure the appropriate CFR/ICH laws, national regulations, and guidelines are being followed.
- Confirm all the subjects screened have signed and informed consent prior to undergoing any study-related procedures.
- Verify only eligible subjects were enrolled in the clinical trial.
- Ensure the data on the CRFs are reflected in the source documents, and are accurate and complete.
- Review all adverse experiences and serious adverse reactions for each subject and ensure that the investigator reported them to the sponsor and IRB/IEC appropriately and in a timely fashion.
- Review the regulatory documents and check that they are being maintained at the site.
- Perform product accountability, ensure that the storage of the product is maintained and the amount of drug/device shipped to the sites, dispensed to the subjects, returned to the site and disposed of are all accountable.

Trial Conduct/Execution

There are several other key components to trial execution that will require special attention: subject recruitment, the informed consent, IRBs/IECs, product accountability, adverse experience and adverse reaction reporting, financial disclosure, and record retention. Each is critical in the overall success of a clinical trial. If one of these is not handled or processed appropriately, the clinical trial will not be used in support of a new product application or many resources (time, people, and money) will be needed to correct the deficiencies so that the trial can be used in support of the application. Many of these components have been discussed previously in the context of monitoring. Adverse experience and adverse reaction reporting, also collectively referred to as "safety reporting," informed consent, and IRB/IEC issues are detailed in this book in chapters 17 and 19. The remaining key components relative to managing clinical trials will now be addressed.

Subject Recruitment

One of the surest ways to decrease the overall time to complete a clinical trial is to recruit the right subjects into the trial in the shortest amount of time. However, the demand for these subjects meeting protocol criteria can be very challenging, especially when there are competing trials at a given site. Regulatory agencies are also taking a closer look at how a site recruits and enrolls subjects. Questions arise such as: is the site coercing the subjects into entering a trial? Is the site influencing them inappropriately with money or gifts? The secret to effective subject recruitment is planning on how and where to recruit a subject population in the most efficient and cost-effective manner. The earlier in the trial process that a site or sponsor company does this, the more successful the outcome. Sponsor companies and sites sometimes wait until a clinical study is ready to begin before they address recruitment planning. In doing so, they find themselves in "rescue mode." ("Rescue mode" is a term used when one waits until the last minute to address a lagging recruitment rate with hopes to resolve it by allocating large budgets to it in an effort to "rescue" the recruitment.) In planning for recruitment, you must know and understand the subject population that will meet the protocol criteria. What motivates these subjects to participate in the clinical trial? What kind of medical treatment are they presently receiving and whom are they seeing to get this treatment? What is the present state of their medical condition? Do they make their own medical decisions or does a caregiver handle these decisions?

The type of disease that a subject is being treated for and the severity of that condition effect recruitment rates. For example, cancer subjects are highly motivated to receive promising therapies because of the seriousness of their condition and their enthusiasm for new therapies. They educate themselves very quickly about their disease via the Internet and various disease foundations for information. On the other hand, migraine subjects act very differently and are more apt to have discussions with their physicians about other experimental treatments. These factors should be considered in the overall plan for subject recruitment. Other considerations are the resources needed to complete the recruitment, that is, money, time, and people. Also, a subject's confidence in the physician and his/her staff as well as in the clinical research process also can affect recruitment rates. Today's environment is such that the general public is very wary of clinical research and therefore is not quick to enroll in a clinical study without a lot of information being provided to them to allay their fears.

Once a strategy is created for subject recruitment and the trial has begun, the site must periodically review its success in recruiting subjects. If it is not working as planned, the reasons should be examined as to why the plan is not working and alternative methods should be discussed and implemented. The old paradigm in clinical research was to plan lavish advertising campaigns that included newspaper, radio, and television advertisements. These methods are no longer very effective or efficient. The new paradigm is psychographics . . . the study of how a subject behaves, where they shop, what they do, how they deal with their condition emotionally, and so on. Sponsors now are testing the feasibility of subject recruitment before a clinical trial begins. By asking this question, in the protocol development stage, it can save both the company and the site from expending precious time and resources in seeking subjects that will never meet protocol criteria. Future studies will experience even another paradigm shift, as genomics will play an important role in how subjects are recruited. Also as Web 2.0 technologies continue to develop and become more widespread in their use, they will also play a role in helping sites recruit subjects (Internet sites, patient portals, etc.).

Product Accountability

Clinical trials evaluate new investigational drugs, biologics, and devices that have not yet received marketing authorization from the appropriate health care authority. Therefore, it is mandatory that strict control be maintained on any investigational product. The investigator is responsible for the accountability of the test product. Investigational products should only be prescribed by the investigator or authorized subinvestigators. The sponsor is responsible for retrieving/verifying the disposition of all used and unused product. Detailed records of product accountability must be maintained throughout a trial with information of date dispensed, quantity dispensed, subject identifier (subject number), and batch number of product prescribed.

When a health care authority inspects the site's product accountability records, every detail will be examined, that is, dispensing, unused, and final disposition of product. Auditors will examine the product accountability procedure and evaluate its acceptability. What they are really looking for is that the site has control of the investigational product because of the simple fact that it is investigational and cannot be available to the general public. At the end of the trial, the monitor will ensure the accountability of all investigational products that were shipped to the site throughout the trial. Any discrepancies will be investigated and documented accordingly in the source document data, the product accountability records, and/or in the monitoring visit reports.

Financial Disclosure—U.S. Requirement Only

One of the newer components of a clinical trial that is submitted to the U.S. FDA for inclusion in a new drug application (NDA) is financial disclosure. This regulation initiated in the United States on February 2, 1999 is required on all current or ongoing clinical trials filed in an IND. It is not retroactive to studies completed prior to this date. Financial disclosure is defined by the FDA as compensation related to the outcome of the study, proprietary interest in the product (e.g., patent), significant equity interest in the sponsor of the study, and significant payments of other sorts to the investigator or institution (e.g., equipment, honorariums). The reason for this regulation is to assure that the appropriate steps are taken to minimize bias in the design, conduct, reporting, and analysis of the studies even when the investigator has a financial gain or interest in a new product. The investigator's responsibilities with respect to financial disclosure are to provide the sponsor company with sufficient and accurate information to allow for disclosure or certification to the FDA of no or any financial interests with the investigational product or with the sponsor. Therefore, the sponsor company will collect the required financial disclosure information from the investigator. This information is required at the start of the study and one-year post completion of the trials. Some sponsor companies may even request it at study completion. Any time that this information changes for an investigator, they should send updated information to the sponsor company. The FDA will evaluate the financial disclosure information for each trial to determine its impact on the reliability of the trial data. Disclosure of any financial information in and of itself does not prohibit an investigator from participating in a clinical program. The FDA will consider both the size and nature of the financial information disclosed as well as what steps were taken during the conduct of the trial minimize potential bias. The FDA will also look at the design of the trial as well as the number of centers that participated in the trial and at what percentage of the overall subject population was enrolled at that site where financial disclosure information was revealed. If the FDA feels that there is a question about the integrity of the data or with the information disclosed, they can initiate agency audits for the investigator whose data are in question, request that the sponsor company submit further analyses of the data, and request that the sponsor company conduct additional studies to confirm the study results or refuse to treat that study as providing data that can be supportive of the agency approving the compound's application and hence "throw out" those data. If the sponsor company refuses to reveal this information, the FDA can refuse to file their NDA.

Closely related to financial disclosure is *conflict of interest*. Individuals involved in clinical research have the responsibility to maintain objectivity in research. Investigators and their staff must take precautions to prevent employees, consultants, or members of governing bodies from using their positions for purposes that are or give the appearance of being motivated by the prospect of financial gain. This is an area of growing concern and one the industry will most definitely be hearing more about in the future. Examples of conflict of interest would be a situation where a chairman of a department at a university acts as PI on many studies and then appoints every faculty member of his staff to the IRB/IEC to review his studies. Another example would be if an FDA advisory panel had a consumer representative reviewing a product application and that same person happens to serve in an advisory capacity to the sponsor company submitting the NDA to the FDA. As a result of heightened concern with conflict of interest, there have been very controversial proposals discussed in editorials in industry publications such as blocking investigators from participating in clinical trials when they have a financial link to the sponsor company, having independent experts who have no financial investment in a product do the design of the protocols, execute the trials, and analyze the data. These debates are among many that have arisen in the past few years about conflict of interest and are a growing concern in the new product development industry, especially as public scrutiny around clinical research continues to rise.

Record Retention

Record retention is critical in the ongoing viability of the study data. The FDA or other health care authorities may possibly conduct an on-site inspection to verify the data from a given site at some time after submission of the NDA. This information must be readily available at the site. Both the CFR regulations and ICH guidelines require that the records be retained for two years after the date a marketing application is approved. If the application is not approved or the file is rejected, the records must be retained for two years after the investigation is discontinued or withdrawn and the FDA or regulatory authority is notified. Records can be maintained as paper files, microfilm or microfiche, or as scanned documents in an electronic or Web-based document management system. If the investigator should move or retire during the retention period, records can be transferred and can be the responsibility of another person as long as the sponsor company is notified in writing of who is now responsible for the records and that new person is aware of his or her responsibilities in retaining these records.

Study Closure Visit (SCV)

Once a trial is completed at an investigational site, the study must be appropriately "closed." This cannot occur until all of the subjects have either completed the course of the trial, were dropped or withdrawn, and all data queries and issues have been addressed and resolved in the final evaluations. Only when this is done can the monitor proceed to a "close out visit." The following list will guide the monitor in completing the SCV:

- All subjects entered in the trial have been accounted.
- All CRF pages have been completed and retrieved.
- All data queries have been resolved.
- All AEs and ADRs have been reported and followed up.
- All investigational products have been accounted for and disposed of or returned to the sponsor.
- All remaining supplies (CRFs, ancillary supplies, etc.) are returned or disposed of properly.
- Regulatory records are complete and organized in the Trial Binder.
- All outstanding issues are addressed. The monitor will meet with the investigator to conclude any outstanding issues and to review any lasting requirements such as the IRB/IEC notification in writing of study closure (with a copy sent to the sponsor as well as filed in the site's Trial Binder).
- Review record retention requirements for investigator and staff for all study-related records.
- Review of the sponsor's publication policy.
- What to do in the event the site is notified of a health authority audit.

SUMMARY

Managing clinical trials requires a great deal of patience, integrity, and hours of attention to critical details. However, knowing that one has contributed in some way to the improvement of a life or the treatment of a disease or condition can be very gratifying. With this comes an overwhelming responsibility to abide by and instill the rules and regulations and guidelines to ensure the protection of subjects' safety. Everyone involved in clinical trials plays a key role in the product development process. They must take that role seriously and be educated on the regulations and guidelines designed to evaluate products safely and effectively for all global submissions. New product development contributes not only to science and medicine but also to the improvement of the overall health care of the world population.

REFERENCES

1. http://www.fda.gov/ora/compliance_ref/bimo/dis_res_assur.htm.
2. http://www.fda.gov/ora/compliance_ref/debar/default.htm.

European CT Directive: Implementation and Update

Kent Hill

Biopharma Consulting Ltd., Colwyn Bay, U.K.

Richard A. Guarino

Oxford Pharmaceutical Resources, Inc., Totowa, New Jersey, U.S.A.

GLOSSARY

AE	Adverse experience
CA	Competent authority
CPMP	Committee for Proprietary Medicinal Products
CT	Clinical trial
EEA	European Economic Area
EMEA	European Agency for the Evaluation of Medicinal Products
EU	European Union
Eudra	European Drug Regulatory
EUDRACT	European Drug Regulatory Affairs Clinical Trial
FDA	Food and Drug Administration
GCP	Good Clinical Practice
GMP	Good Manufacturing Practice
HVT	Healthy Volunteer Trials
IC	Informed consent
ICH	International Conference on Harmonisation of Technical Requirements for Registration of Pharmaceuticals for Human Use
IEC	Independent Ethics Committee
IMP	Investigational medicinal product
IND	Investigational New Drug (United States)
MAA	Marketing Authorization Application (EU)
MS	Member States
QP	Qualified person
SAR	Serious adverse reaction
SUSAR	Suspected unexpected serious adverse reaction (Eudravigilance CT module)

BACKGROUND

Since finalization in 1996, the International Committee on Harmonisation Tripartite Guideline for Good Clinical Practice (ICH GCP) underpinned by the ethical principles of the Declaration of Helsinki have been the cornerstones upon which most clinical research has been conducted outside the United States (1,2). However, in such a widely disparate and expanding territory as the European Union (EU) and the Far East, the differences in complying with local national requirements have presented an increasing administrative workload for sponsors and regulators.

In the EU, countries known as "Member States" (MS) currently present a formidable challenge to sponsors wishing to conduct a research trial with the same protocol in many centers. The submission process in each MS is mostly governed by regulatory agencies known as "competent authorities" (CA) and Independent Ethics Committees (IEC). The approval process may be conducted in parallel or in sequence, in some cases with IEC first and CA second, or in other countries in reverse order. In some MS, a single national IEC may grant an approval for all sites without a local IEC approval. In other MS, local IEC approval may be required even if the protocol is representing a multicenter study. Clearly, this creates varying time-lines to approvals in each MS.

Another obstacle is the need for drug import permits. These require additional IEC requirements and may vary with each MS as do export licenses if trials are not conducted under a U.S. Investigational New Drug (IND) Application. This variance of each MS translates into different delays from initiation to receiving approvals to the start-up of clinical trials and the time has varied between 2 and 26 weeks (3).

The initiation and management of multinational clinical trials in the EU and other parts of the world therefore require considerable coordination and effort. The centralized coordination of the international procedures is essential to make sense of the complexity, ensure consistency, and to avoid duplication of effort, saving time and money. Therefore, to transform the cumbersome disparate situation through the EU CT Directive and the interpretation of the ICH guideline into a single set of legally enforceable set of procedures is commendable in its purpose and desirable economically.

May 1, 2004 heralded the beginning of implementation as law for all the MS of the EU Directive 2001/20/EC on GCP in clinical trials (4). Thus, for the first time, we could expect to witness a common legally binding and comprehensive set of laws supported by detailed guidance documents covering all aspects of clinical research on medicinal products covering the largest single pharmaceutical market of the world of over 450 million citizens (5).

The full title of the Directive is "Directive of the European Parliament and of the Council on the approximation of the laws, regulations and administrative provisions of the MS relating to implementation of good clinical practice in the conduct of clinical trials on medicinal products for human use." Other Directives previously implemented and in force in MS concerning medicinal products cover matters such as licensing requirements, manufacturing, distribution, classification for supply, labeling, and advertising.

Agreement on this Directive was reached in February 2001 and the final version was published in the Official Journal of the European Communities on May 1, 2001 by the European Commission. After that point, MS have had to transpose the requirements of the Directive into national legislation by May 1, 2003 and had to implement them into domestic law by May 1, 2004.

Although other international countries that are not part of the EU are not required to follow the EU Directives, they are conscientiously following the ICH guidelines for GCP that are well incorporated into the EU Directives.

PURPOSE

The overall purpose of the EU Directive was to unify the standards and procedures of ICH GCP as a common legally enforceable process for the protection of subjects participating in clinical trials within the EU. In addition, it was envisaged that the

Directive would allow the harmonisation of regulatory requirements and country-specific nuances to be addressed, thus permitting a standardized approach to clinical trials to be adopted throughout the EU. The European Agency for the Evaluation of Medicinal Products (EMEA) referred to in the Directive as the "Agency" is a London-based decentralized regulatory agency assisted by the Committee for Proprietary Medicinal Products (CPMP) set up in 1995 to coordinate all clinical research applications leading to marketing authorizations, subsequently granted by the Commission.

SCOPE

The Directive covered all current EU MS and European Economic Area (EEA) members (Norway, Iceland, and Liechtenstein). The scope of the Directive was very wide as the conduct of all CT in the EU on human subjects involving medicinal products as defined in Article I of Directive 65/65/EEC were covered. The term "investigational medicinal product (IMP)" applied whether it is either medicinal by function, or presented as treating or preventing disease in human beings. In effect, every CT involving medicinal products was covered, irrespective of who sponsored it, that is, industry, government, research council, charity, or university.

In medical terms, the Directive encompassed clinical research in all citizens of the EU. It covered trials from phase I in normal healthy subjects, via small phase II dose ranging efficacy trials in subjects expected to derive medicinal benefit, through large efficacy and safety phase III trials leading to Marketing Authorization Application (MAA), the European equivalent to a U.S. New Drug Application (NDA).

The Directive set standards for protecting clinical trial subjects, including incapacitated adults and minors. Importantly, it also established Ethics Committees [equivalent to an U.S. Institutional Review Board (IRB)] on a legal basis and provide legal status for certain procedures, such as times within which an opinion must be given. In addition, it covered certain CA procedures for commencing a clinical trial, laid down standards for the manufacture, import, and labeling of IMPs and provided for quality assurance of clinical trials and IMPs. However, not all unlicensed chemical entities would be considered as IMPs as the regulations (United Kingdom) would apply only to those that were medicinal products and to be tested or used as a reference in a clinical trial. To ensure compliance with these standards, it required MS to set up inspection systems for GCP and good manufacturing practice (GMP). The Directive provided for safety monitoring of subjects in trials, and set out procedures for reporting and recording adverse drug experiences and adverse drug reactions. To help with the exchange of information between MS, secure networks have been established linked to European databases for information about approved CT and for pharmacovigilance.

The provisions of the Directive do not distinguish between commercial and noncommercial clinical trials, that is, those conducted by academic researchers without the participation of the health care industry. Furthermore, "noninterventional" trials where the medicinal product is prescribed in the usual manner in accordance with the terms of the marketing authorization are not within the scope of the Directive. In these cases, the assignment of a subject to a particular therapeutic strategy is not decided in advance by a trial protocol, but falls within current practice, and the prescription of the medicine is clearly separated from the decision to include the subject in the trial. Also, no additional diagnostic or monitoring procedure is applied to the subjects, and epidemiological methods are to be used for the analysis of the collected data.

Notable changes in the United Kingdom as a result of the Directive included abolition of the "Doctors and Dentists Exemption (DDX)" scheme whereby hitherto practitioners had been allowed to prescribe novel agents which they believed on balance to have efficacious advantages that outweighed the risks to their subjects, not on behalf of a commercial organization or other non-EU party (6). Furthermore, phase I trials in the EU are now subject to exactly the same regulatory agency scrutiny as other types of trials.

The Directive laid down significant new legislation affecting clinical research and development of medicinal products in each MS and their national health services.

Theoretically, the currently notable heterogeneous central or regional IEC and regulatory agency hurdles are reduced to more readily manageable levels under the Directive with the order and format of applications reduced to levels more acceptable to and welcomed by applicants.

DEFINITIONS

The Directive provides detailed definitions for terms in common use within clinical research; the reader is urged to refer to the original document for details (4) with the multilingual glossary in European languages (7). These include "noninterventional trial" as trials outside the scope of the Directive and "IMP" as a pharmaceutical form of an active substance or placebo being tested or used as a reference in a CT, including products already having a marketing authorization but used or assembled (formulated or packaged) in a way different from the authorized form, or for an unauthorized indication, or to gain further information about the authorized form.

PRINCIPAL ELEMENTS OF DIRECTIVE ARTICLES, DETAILED GUIDELINES, AND GUIDANCE DOCUMENTS

In brief, the Directive sets standards for protecting CT subjects, establishes IECs on a legal basis, and provides the legal status for certain procedures. It is largely structured as for ICH GCP but with some notable additions. The Directive compels all IEC to operate within a detailed legal framework to provide a consolidated central approach to the ethical review of clinical trials. It also lays down standards for the manufacture, import, and labeling of an IMP, and provides for quality assurance of both CT and IMP. Notably, the provisions of the Directive do not distinguish between commercial and noncommercial clinical trials, and the 1996 rather than the then latest 2000 version of the Declaration of Helsinki is specifically referenced.

While the Directive as reasonably expected covers all aspects of the clinical research process, it is underpinned by the principles of ICH GCP, and as such, only main definitions, modifications, and additions of note are described in the following sections.

Protection of Clinical Trial Subjects, Minors, and Incapacitated Adults

MS must legislate to protect from abuse individuals who are incapable of giving informed consent. Thus, a CT may be only undertaken if in particular the foreseeable risks and inconveniences have been weighed against anticipated benefit for individual trial subjects. The CT may only proceed if the IEC and/or the CA conclude that anticipated therapeutic and public health benefits justify the risks and continued only if compliance with this requirement is permanently monitored.

A clinical trial may only be undertaken if the informed consent of the minor's parents or incapacitated subject's legal representative has been obtained, representing the subject's presumed will and may be revoked at any time without detriment to the subject. The subject must receive information on the trial with risks and benefits in an understandable form from appropriately experienced staff. Investigators must heed the wishes of minors capable of forming an opinion or their legal representatives to refuse or discontinue participation at any time. No incentives or financial inducements except compensation are allowed. Some direct benefit to this class of subject and relating to the clinical condition suffered by or uniquely in the subjects must be demonstrable. Particular attention is made to minimize pain, discomfort, fear, and to ensure potential benefits of the IMP outweigh any foreseeable risks or produce no risk in relation to the disease and developmental stage; the risk threshold and degree of distress must be specifically defined and constantly monitored. The IEC having specialized expertise or after taking specialist advice on clinical, ethical, and psychosocial problems associated with these subjects must endorse the protocol in which the interests of the subject always prevail over those of science and society.

Ethics Committee, Single Opinion, and Detailed Guidance
A Member State must take all necessary measures for establishing and operating IECs that must give its opinion on any issue before a trial commences. In preparing its opinion, the IEC must particularly consider the relevance of the trial and its design, whether anticipated benefits and risks are satisfactory and justified in terms of the protocol, suitability of investigator and staff, quality of facilities, adequacy and completeness of the information to subjects and the informed consent form and procedures to be followed for obtaining informed consent, justification of research on persons incapable of giving consent.

Provision for indemnity or compensation in the event of injury or death of subjects attributable to the clinical trial, and for insurance or indemnity to cover liability of the investigator and sponsor, must be described. The financial arrangements for rewarding or compensating investigators and trial subjects and relevant aspects between the sponsor and site and arrangements for recruiting subjects are documented.

Importantly, a MS may decide that the IEC is responsible for giving an opinion on the indemnity, insurance, and remuneration aspects; when this provision is applied, the MS must notify the Commission, other MS, and the EMEA.

The IEC will be limited to 60 days from date of receipt of a valid application to give its reasoned opinion to the applicant and to the CA. Within this period of examination, the IEC may send a single request for supplemental information to the applicant; the timeline is suspended until receipt of the information.

Extension to the 60-day period is only permissible for trials of gene therapy or somatic cell therapy or medicinal products containing genetically modified organisms. In such a case, an extension of 30 days is permitted with a further extension of 90 days in the event of local MS consultation with a group or committee also allowed for, bringing the total to 180 days. There is no time limit for xenogenic cell therapy applications.

MS have established procedures for managing multicenter trials limited to the territory of a single MS, irrespective of the number of IEC, in order to adopt a single opinion. Where the CT is to be conducted simultaneously in more than one MS, a single opinion is given by each MS.

The Commission in consultation with MS has published detailed guidance documents on the application format, documentation to be submitted in an application for an IEC's opinion paying particular attention to the information given to subjects, and on appropriate safeguards for the protection of personal data. Some MS already have data protection legislation in place and the reader is encouraged to check this within each MS under consideration.

Commencement of a Clinical Trial

MS employ the following measures to ensure that the IEC and the CA have issued favorable opinions on the application before a clinical trial is allowed to start; the opinions can be sought in parallel. If the CA notifies the sponsor of grounds for nonacceptance, the sponsor may on one occasion only amend the content of the request to take due account of the grounds given. If the sponsor fails to amend the request accordingly, the request is rejected and the CT not permitted to start.

Consideration of the request by the CA is expected as rapidly as possible and is limited to 60 days but the MS may lay down periods shorter than 60 days if in compliance with current practice; the CA may notify the sponsor of the approval at any time before the end of this specified period.

Written authorization is required before starting clinical trials on an IMP not having a marketing authorization and other IMPs with special characteristics such as those having as their active ingredient(s) or components or the manufacturing that is a biological product(s) of human or animal origin.

Specific reference is made to the application of 1990 Council Directives on the contained use of genetically modified microorganisms (8) and on the deliberate release into the environment of genetically modified organisms (9). Gene therapy trials, which could result in modifications to the germ line genetic identity of the subject, are not allowed.

Conduct of a Clinical Trial

These relate to amendments to conduct of a CT that is underway. Thus, the sponsor may make amendments to the protocol, which if substantial and likely to impact on safety of the trial subjects or change the interpretation of the scientific documents in support of the conduct of the trial, or if are otherwise significant, the sponsor must advise the CA of all MS and all IEC.

In response, the IEC must give an opinion within a maximum of 35 days of receipt. If this opinion is unfavorable, the sponsor is disallowed from implementing the amendment to the protocol; under these circumstances, the sponsor should either take account of the grounds for nonacceptance and adapt the proposed amendment accordingly or should withdraw the proposed amendment. But, if the IEC and CA approve the amendment, the sponsor is clear to proceed with its clinical application.

Should a new event likely to affect the safety of the subjects, the sponsor must take appropriate urgent safety measures to protect subjects from any immediate hazard and inform all CA and IEC accordingly of the new events and the measures taken.

Within 90 days of the end of a CT, the sponsor must notify all CA and IEC; if the CT is terminated early, this period is reduced to 15 days and the reasons for termination clearly explained.

Exchange of Information, Suspension or Infringements, European Clinical Trials EUDRACT Database

The CA in whose territory the CT takes place enters the details into the European Drug Regulatory Affairs Clinical Trial (EUDRACT) database. It allocates a unique EUDRACT number that cannot be reallocated to another trial if the original one does not proceed; if an International Standard Randomized Controlled Trial Number (ISRCTN) is available, this detail is also entered. These EUDRACT entry data are accessible only to the CA, the EMEA, and the Commission and details the request for authorization, the protocol, any proposed protocol amendments, approvals by the CA and IEC, any suspension, the declaration at the end, and reference to any GCP inspections.

Upon request by any MS, the EMEA, or the Commission, the CA to which the request for authorization was submitted must supply all further information concerning the CT in question other than the data already in the European database.

In consultation with the MS, the Commission has published detailed guidance documents on the relevant data to be included in the database, which is operated with the assistance of the EMEA as well as methods for its secure and confidential electronic communication.

A MS having objective grounds for considering the conditions in the request for authorization at the outset are no longer met or has information raising doubts about the safety or scientific validity of the trial may suspend or prohibit the trial and notify the sponsor. Except where there is imminent risk, the MS would ask the sponsor and/or the investigator for their opinion to be delivered within one week. In this case, the CA advises other involved CA, the IEC concerned, the Agency, and the Commission of its decision with reasons to suspend or prohibit the trial.

Manufacture, Import, and Labeling of Investigational Medical Products

All appropriate measures to ensure manufacture or importation of the IMP by MS are subject to applicants and subsequent "holder of the authorization" satisfying requirements in accordance with procedures referred to in a 2003 Council Decision (10).

The holder of the authorization must have at its disposal at least one "qualified person" (QP) who is authorized in the particular MS to continue working permanently and continuously and providing expert services as laid down in the GMP Directive and detailed guidelines (Table 1). The QP is directly and independently responsible for satisfying himself or herself of the purity and quality of production batches of the IMP manufactured locally or in a non-EU country. Where an IMP is a comparator product from a non-EU country having a marketing authorization, the QP is responsible for ensuring that the certification of each production batch has been manufactured under conditions at least equivalent to GMP standards. IMP(s) imported from another MS will not have to undergo further analytical checks if received together with batch release certification signed by the responsible QP.

TABLE 1 EU Clinical Trials Directive: Principal Elements of Articles and Primary Applicable Documents

Principal element	Article title	Guidance document* title date and document no.
1. Protection of clinical trial subjects	1. Scope 2. Definitions 3. Protection of clinical trial subjects 4. Clinical trials on minors 5. Clinical trials on incapacitated adults not able to give informed legal consent	Request for authorization of clinical trial to competent authorities, notification of substantial amendments, and declaration of the end of the trial.
2. Independent Ethics Committee	6. Independent Ethics Committee 7. Single opinion 8. Detailed guidance	Application format and documentation to be submitted in an application for an IEC opinion on the clinical trial on medicinal products for human use.
3. Commencement	9. Commencement of a clinical trial	As for Articles 3 and 6.
4. Conduct	10. Conduct of a clinical trial	Principles of GCP in the conduct in the EU of clinical trials on medicinal products for human use. Detailed guidelines on the trial master file and archiving for the Directive on Clinical Trials on Medicinal Products for Human Use.
5. Exchange of information	11. Exchange of information	Details on the European clinical trials database (EUDRACT Database). April 2003. ENTR 6101/02. Details on inspection procedures for the verification of GCP compliance to implement the Directive on Clinical Trials on medicinal products for human use.
	12. Suspension of the clinical trial or infringements	
6. Manufacture and import	13. Manufacture and import of investigational medical products 14. Labeling	Principles and guidelines of GMP for medicinal products for human use, as required by Directive details on the community basic format and the contents of the application for a manufacturing and/or import authorization of an investigational medicinal product for human use in clinical trials on medicinal products for human use. Good Manufacturing Practices Annex 13 for Clinical Trials on medicinal products for human use.

7. Inspections		
15. Verification of compliance of investigational medical products with good clinical and manufacturing practice	Details on the qualifications of inspectors who should verify compliance in clinical trials with the provisions of good clinical practice for an investigational medicinal product.
	Details on inspection procedures for the verification of GCP compliance for clinical trials on medicinal products for human use.
	Details on the qualifications of inspectors who should verify compliance in clinical trials with the provisions of good manufacturing practice for an investigational medicinal product.
8. Adverse experiences	
16. Notification of adverse experiences	
17. Notification of serious adverse reactions	Details on the collection, verification, and presentation of adverse reaction reports arising from clinical trials on medicinal products for human use.
18. Guidance concerning reports	Detailed guidance on the European database of suspected unexpected serious adverse reactions (Eudravigilance—Clinical Trial Module).
9. General provisions	
19. General provisions	
20. Adaptation to scientific and technical progress	
21. Committee procedure	
22. Application	
23. Entry into force	
24. Addressees	

The QP must certify in an up-to-date register available to CA or their agents for the period specified in the provisions of the MS concerned and not less than five years that each production batch satisfies the provisions of the Article.

Readers are also urged to refer to the "Commission Directive on the requirements to obtain an authorization to manufacture or import an IMP and the requirements to be met by the holder of this authorization to implement the directive on Clinical Trials on medicinal products for human use" (10).

Labels must be in the official language(s) of the MS on the outer or immediate packaging of the IMP and published in accordance with existing regulations to ensure protection of the subjects, traceability, and proper use.

Inspections, Verification of Compliance of Investigational Medical Products with Good Clinical Practice and Good Manufacturing Practice

Duly qualified community inspectors appointed by the MS inspect the CT sites, manufacturing facilities for the IMP, laboratories used for analysis, and/or the sponsor's premises in accordance with the Directive on behalf of the community. Inspection findings are recognized by all other MS, coordinated by the Agency within the existing regulatory framework (Table 1) and reports given to the sponsor/inspectee and at their reasoned request to other MS, the IEC, and the Agency. Should verification of compliance reveal differences between MS, the Commission may request further inspections. Inspections are not limited to MS but may be conducted upon request at sponsor's premises, trial sites, and/or the manufacturer in non-EU countries.

Detailed guidelines are available for CT documentation constituting the trial master file (TMF) and archiving (11), qualifications of inspectors (12), and inspection procedures (13) to verify compliance is in accordance with published procedures laid down in Article 21.

Adverse Experiences (AEs) and Serious Adverse Reactions (SARs) Notification, Collection, Verification, Presentation and Reporting, SUSAR Database, Eudravigilance Clinical Trial Module Database

SARs must be reported immediately either verbally or in writing except where the protocol or IB identify as not required. Subsequent follow-up reports must be detailed and in writing; any further information on deaths of subjects must be provided by the investigator to the sponsor and IEC. Subject's anonymity will be preserved by a unique code numbering system.

AEs and/or laboratory abnormalities identified in the protocol as critical to safety evaluations must be reported in accordance with requirements and timelines specified in the protocol. Sponsors must maintain detailed records of all AEs, which are to be submitted upon request by the MS in whose territory the trial was conducted.

All relevant information on suspected unexpected SARs considered life threatening or fatal must be reported to CA in all MS and to the IEC as soon as possible or within seven days of the sponsor learning of them and all follow-up information within a further eight days. All other reactions are to be advised within 15 days of knowledge by the sponsor. MS are responsible for recording all AEs and SARs and it is the sponsor's responsibility to advise all investigators.

The sponsor must make an annual safety update to MS and the IEC of all AEs and SARs, outcomes, and safety aspects for all subjects. All MS must update the

Eudravigilance database (see Article 11) and the Agency disseminates this information to all CA.

The Commission in consultation with other parties drew up two detailed guidance documents on the collection, verification, and presentation of AEs/SARs with decoding procedures for SARs (Table 1).

General Provisions, Adaptation to Scientific and Technical Progress, Committee Procedure, Application, Entry into Force, and Addressees

The Directive came in to force on its 2001 publication date reaffirming that sponsors and investigators have "without prejudice" civil and criminal liabilities; the sponsor must be established in the community and provide the IMP and any administration devices free of charge.

As intended, the Directive was adapted by MS and CA in line with scientific and technical progress, the removal of technical barriers to trade. Should any amendments become necessary, this is through the existing "Standing Committee on Medicinal Products for Human Use," which the Commission must consult; if the Commission disagrees with this Committee, the matters are referred to the Council.

IMPLEMENTATION

The principles of the Directive have removed the complexity of clinical trial application, authorization, and regulation in existing, new, and future MS. Thus, substantial amendments to protocol that impact on safety of the subjects or where there is a change in the interpretation of data on the IMP must be notified under the legislation underpinning the Directive. This common process obviates any disparate national procedures that range from a simple notification scheme to a complex authorization procedure. Implementation of the Directive could be expected to alter national requirements for provision to examiners of information to subjects and informed consent forms in local languages.

A common clinical trial application form is used and accompanied by data on the quality, safety, and efficacy of the IMP to the CA. The application process is an implicit approval within a maximum 60-day review period with one exception, for clinical trials with biotechnology IMPs, for example, gene therapy, somatic cell therapy, and genetically modified organisms. In this case, written approval is mandatory and a 90-day review period applies.

IMPLICATIONS FOR FUTURE RESEARCH

Although the Directive is aimed at providing an environment for conducting clinical research that transparently protects participants without hampering the discovery of new medicines, several parties expressed concern that this may not be the case and publication of their viewpoints were wide and unrelenting. The entire sector was anxious as to how well the MS are abiding the rules and the local effect by some parties believing there were grounds for believing they will not make it easier to conduct international trials but could have made them still harder.

The effect of the May 1, 2004 EU Directives and to assess the actual effects on clinical research within the EU and whether these anxieties for its global competitiveness in the marketplace were in the event largely groundless. Strategically, this was an attempt by the EU to boost local medicines research, keep the industry buoyant and actively able to supply the new products that patients need to be safely developed.

Implementation of the Directive has lead to the better acceptability of EU clinical data not only by the FDA but also globally.

REFERENCES

1. ICH E6 Guideline for Good Clinical Practice (July 1996), CPMP/ICH/135/95/Step 5.
2. World Medical Association, Declaration of Helsinki, Ethical Principles for Medical research Involving Human Subjects, 5th revision. 48th WMA General Assembly, Somerset West, Republic of South Africa, October 1996 and the 52nd WMA General Assembly, Edinburgh, Scotland, October 2000.
3. Mermet-Bouvier P, de Crémiers F (2002). Clinical trial initiation in Europe: current status. Regul Aff J 13(7):571–578.
4. Directive 2001/20/EC of the European Parliament and of the Council of April 4, 2001 on the approximation of the laws, regulations and administrative provisions of the Member States relating to the implementation of good clinical practice in the conduct of clinical trials on medicinal products for human use. OJ 2001, L121, 34–44.
5. EU Member States. Integration Office DFA/DEA. Available from http://www.europa.admin.ch/eu/expl/staaten/e/index.htm
6. The Medicines (Exemption from Licences) (Special Cases and Miscellaneous Provisions) Order 1972. Available from www.mca.gov.uk.
7. Vander Stichele R (2000). Multilingual glossary of technical and popular medical terms in nine European Languages. Available from http://allserv.rug.ac.be/~rvdstich/eugloss/welcome.html.
8. Council Directive OJ L 117 (May 8, 1990), p. 1 Directive as last amended by Directive 98/81/EC (OJ L 330, December 5, 1998, p. 13).
9. Council Directive OJ L 117 (May 8, 1990), p. 15. Directive as last amended by Commission Directive 97/35/EC (OJ L 169, June 27, 1997, p. 72).
10. Commission Directive on the requirements to obtain an authorisation to manufacture or import an investigational medicinal product and the requirements to be met by the holder of this authorisation to implement the directive on clinical trials on medicinal products for human use. OJ L 262 (October 14, 2003), p. 22.
11. Detailed guidelines on the trial master file and archiving. Available from http://pharmacos.eudra.org./F2/pharmacos/docs/Doc2002/june/tmf_06_2002.pdf.
12. Detailed guidelines on the qualifications of inspectors who should verify compliance in clinical trials with the provisions of good clinical practice for an investigational medicinal product to implement the directive on clinical trials on medicinal products for human use (June 2002). Available from http://pharmacos.eudra.org./F2/pharmacos/docs/Doc2002/june/ins_gcp_06_2002.pdf.
13. Detailed guidelines on inspection procedures for the verification of GCP compliance to implement the directive on clinical trials on medicinal products for human use (June 2002). Available from http://pharmacos.eudra.org./F2/pharmacos/docs/Doc2002/june/dtld_06_2002.pdf.

25 | Combination Products

Evan B. Siegel

Ground Zero Pharmaceuticals, Inc., Irvine, California, U.S.A.

Advances in drug, biologic, and medical device development deal with both single entities and combinations of each type of medical product. A desire for new modes of administration of therapeutics, enhancement of long-term delivery of drugs and biologics, new routes of administration, and commercial/competitive reasons have led to a veritable explosion of requests for review of experimental combination products. These developments continue to be enhanced by advances in technology and materials science, as well as biotechnological sophistication of manufacturing processes. All of these factors have generated requests for the FDA to review combination investigational drug and device applications for human clinical testing. Eventually, these programs will lead to NDAs for marketing approval, where a drug is involved.

The formal definition of "combination product" for FDA purposes involves a product comprising two or more regulated components (e.g., drug/device, biologic/device, or biologic/drug) provided as a single entity, single package, intended for use with an approved product, or intended for use with an investigational product. We will also use the term to connote drug/drug, biologic/biologics, and so on, active principles either incorporated into a single entity or copackaged. This situation might be called "combined therapy."

Examples of combination products where the components are physically, chemically, or otherwise combined include the following:

- A monoclonal antibody combined with a therapeutic drug.
- A device coated or impregnated with a drug or biologic, for example,
  - drug-eluting stent, pacing lead with steroid-coated tip, catheter with antimicrobial coating, and condom with spermicide;
  - skin substitutes with cellular components, orthopedic implant with growth factors.
- Prefilled syringes, insulin injector pens, metered-dose inhalers, and transdermal patches.

Examples of combination products where the components are packaged together include

- a drug or biological product packaged with a delivery device;
- a surgical tray with surgical instruments, drapes, and lidocaine or alcohol swabs.

Examples of combination products where the components are separately provided but labeled for use together include

- a photosensitizing drug and activating laser or other light source;
- an iontophoretic drug delivery patch and controller.

Regulatory review of these combination products is complicated by the fact that while drugs are regulated primarily under Section 505 of the Food, Drug, and Cosmetic Act (1) and reviewed by the Center for Drug Evaluation and Research (CDER), biologics are regulated under the Public Health Service Act (Section 351) (2) and reviewed by CDER [therapeutic biologics, synthetic peptides and proteins (e.g., monoclonal antibodies), except for vaccines] (3) or the Center for Biologics Evaluation and Research (CBER: vaccines, blood and blood products and medical devices used for collection, processing, administration of biological products and blood products or components, cell sorters and in vitro tests and other medical devices involving retroviruses). The Center for Devices and Radiological Health (CDRH) regulates certain biological products and many combination products, including wound dressings with antibiotics or antiseptics, antimicrobial coated catheters and implants, bone cements with antibiotics, drug-eluting stents, photodynamic therapy, orthopedic implants with therapeutic drugs or biologicals, dermal replacement devices with living cells, and drug delivery devices (pumps, inhalers, and pen injectors). Please see Table 1 for a delineation of jurisdictions of products across centers. Combination product review at the FDA involves differing histories and philosophies at the various centers. For example, for evaluation of effectiveness, devices

TABLE 1   FDA Centers with Jurisdiction over Drugs, Biological Products, and Medical Devices

Center for Drug Evaluation and Research (CDER)
Nonbiological (e.g., chemically synthesized) drugs
Therapeutic biological products except those specifically assigned to CBER (e.g., blood and
 vaccines) including
  monoclonal antibodies for in vivo use
  proteins intended for therapeutic use
  immunomodulators
  growth factors, cytokines, and monoclonal antibodies intended to mobilize, stimulate, decrease,
   or otherwise alter the production of hematopoietic cells in vivo

Center for Biologics Evaluation and Research (CBER)
Biological and related products not regulated by CDER including
  cellular products
  gene therapy products
  vaccines
  allergenic extracts
  antitoxins, antivenins, and venoms
  blood, blood components, plasma-derived products including recombinant and transgenic
   versions of plasma derivatives, blood substitutes, plasma volume expanders, human or animal
   polyclonal antibody preparations including radiolabeled or conjugated forms, certain
   fibrinolytics such as plasma-derived plasmin, and red cell reagents
Medical devices related to licensed blood and cellular products including all HIV tests and test kits

Center for Devices and Radiological Health (CDRH)
Medical devices including in vitro diagnostic products that are not regulated by CBER
Radiation-emitting products

require "valid scientific evidence," drugs require "substantial evidence," and biologics must be "safe, pure, and potent." Thus, when a sponsor submits an NDA for a combination product for review, the cross-jurisdictional coverage may enter into the submission, review, and approval process.

CLINICAL INVESTIGATION AND PREMARKET REVIEW REQUIREMENTS FOR DRUGS AND MEDICAL DEVICES

FDA has not established clinical investigation and premarket review requirements specifically applicable to combination products, so combination products are regulated using the requirements that have been established for the components. These are described in regulation. They are similar with regard to their overall intent to assure that clinical investigations are designed to be scientifically sound and adequately protect human subjects, and that products approved or cleared for marketing are safe and effective for their intended use. There are differences with regard to their specific requirements, however, and this can have an impact on the marketing application(s) that are submitted for review. Please seec Table 2 for a description of these issues.

The level of premarket review required for devices is risk based. Devices are classified by regulation into one of three regulatory classes: I, II, or III. Most Class I and certain Class II devices are exempt from premarket approval or clearance requirements. Most Class II devices require a 510(k) premarket notification to the CDRH. The 510(k) submission must contain information and data establishing that the device is substantially equivalent to one or more identified "predicate devices" that may be legally marketed in the United States for the same intended use. In most instances, clinical data are not required to support the 510(k) premarket notification submission. The device may not be marketed until FDA responds to the 510(k) submission that the device is cleared for marketing.

TABLE 2 Clinical Investigation and Premarket Submission Requirements for Drugs, Biological Products, and Medical Devices

Product	Clinical investigation requirements[a]	Premarket review requirements
Drug	IND (21 CFR Part 312)	NDA
Generic drug	IND[b]	ANDA
Biological product	IND	BLA[c]
Medical device		
Class I	IDE[d]	510(k)[e]
Class II	IDE[d]	510(k)[e]
Class III	IDE[d]	510(k)[f] or PMA

[a] The clinical investigation of drugs, therapeutic biological products, and medical devices must be conducted in compliance with the requirements for institutional review set forth in 21 CFR Part 56 and with the requirements for informed consent set forth in 21 CFR Part 50.
[b] Clinical data are normally not required to support an ANDA; however, an IND is required to conduct clinical investigations of any unapproved new drug.
[c] A BLA is required for any biological drug product regardless of the FDA center with jurisdiction over the product.
[d] Clinical data are not required to support most 510(k) premarket notification submissions. When clinical studies are conducted, an IDE approved by an institutional review board (IRB) is required unless exempted. If the study involves a significant risk device, the IDE must also be approved by the FDA.
[e] For device classifications not exempted by regulation from premarket notification requirements.
[f] Class III "preamendment" device classifications for which FDA has not established an effective date for the submission of PMA applications may be cleared for marketing via the 510(k) substantial equivalence process.

If FDA responds to the 510(k) submission that the device is not substantially equivalent to a predicate device, the device is automatically considered a Class III device requiring an approved premarket approval (PMA) application before it can be marketed (4).

To market most Class III devices, a PMA application must be approved by FDA. The PMA application is similar to an NDA or a BLA in that it must contain sufficient valid scientific evidence from nonclinical and clinical studies to show that the product is safe and effective for its intended use(s). Devices that were on the market prior to the date of enactment of the medical device amendments to the FD&C Act (May 28, 1976) are called preamendment devices. Sponsors of Class III preamendment devices require a PMA application only after FDA publishes a final regulation calling for a PMA for the types of devices covered by that regulation, and establishes an effective date for submission of the PMA application. Devices that are of the same type as a Class III preamendment device for which FDA has not yet established an effective date for a PMA submission require 510(k) clearance prior to marketing. The majority of devices that are subject to premarket requirements (Class I reserved, Class II, and Class III) are cleared for marketing via the 510(k) substantial equivalence process.

The implications of a jurisdictional assignment for a combination product with respect to its primary mode of action can be significant (5,6). For example, user fees for medical device marketing applications are substantially lower than those for products regulated as drugs. Expected time for FDA to review marketing applications is also a factor. The target review time for a device 510(k) premarket notification, for example, can be as little as 30 days while target review times for an NDA can be 6 to 10 months. Also, companies that are used to dealing with a certain product type (e.g., devices) may not be familiar with the regulatory requirements and options applicable to other types of products (e.g., device companies may not be familiar with IND requirements for drug products or Fast Track designation for qualifying drug products) that may be applicable to the combination product based on its jurisdictional assignment. Table 3 presents examples of jurisdictional determinations for combination products.

The electronic (eCTD) marketing application requirements for NDAs are also detailed, complex, and expensive, and developers of combination products must take this into account. The sponsor's strategic regulatory and product development approach may be to seek marketing approval or clearance of a component of their combination product as well as for the combination product as a whole by submitting separate marketing applications. The sponsor of a drug–device combination regulated by CDER may, for instance, in addition to seeking approval of an NDA for the drug–device combination, intend to submit a separate PMA or 510(k) application to CDRH for approval or clearance, respectively, of the device component as a separate or stand-alone product. In this case, the sponsor would likely wish to assure that all communications with FDA regarding both development programs are appropriately coordinated between reviewing centers to assure that the safety and effectiveness issues associated with the device component of the combination and the stand-alone device can be addressed as efficiently as possible, and that the required timing of each marketing application is understood (7). In such instances, communication with FDA should be initiated as early as possible in the development program so that FDA can provide guidance on how best to proceed.

TABLE 3 Examples of Jurisdictional Determination in Accordance with 21 CFR Part 3

Example 1

Product: *Spinal fusion device coated with a therapeutic protein* intended to treat degenerative disc disease. A spinal fusion cage soaked in a solution of a therapeutic protein to coat the inside surfaces of the device. In this hypothetical example, the fusion cage, a permanent implant, maintains the spacing and stabilizes the diseased region of the spine, while the protein is used to encourage the formation of bone within the fusion cage to further stabilize this portion of the spine as well as the cage itself.

Modes of action (MOA)/primary mode of action (PMOA): The PMOA is attributable to the device component's MOA to mechanically maintain the intervertebral spacing and stabilize the diseased region of the spine, while the therapeutic protein's MOA to encourage bone formation within and around the cage plays a secondary role. In this hypothetical example, the therapeutic protein does not have the mechanical properties necessary to maintain the spacing and stabilize the spine if used alone. Furthermore, clinically successful spinal fusion (pain reduction and stability of the spine) can be achieved even in the absence of bone growth within the cage. The device component provides the most important therapeutic action of the combination. It is unnecessary to proceed to the assignment algorithm because it is possible to determine which MOA provides the most important therapeutic action of this combination product.

Assignment algorithm criteria: Not applicable.

Jurisdictional assignment: CDRH.

Example 2

Product: Chemotherapeutic drug and monoclonal antibody for targeted cancer treatment. The monoclonal antibody is intended to improve the drug's effectiveness by directly targeting the drug to receptors on cancer tumor cells.

MOA/PMOA: The PMOA is attributable to the drug component's MOA (cytotoxic action on cancer cells), while the biological product component's MOA to target the drug to the receptors on the cancer cells enhances the efficacy of the drug. The drug component provides the most important therapeutic action of the combination. It is unnecessary to proceed to the assignment algorithm because it is possible to determine which MOA provides the most important therapeutic action of this combination product. Note that in June 2003, FDA transferred to CDER the regulation of certain therapeutic biological products that had been regulated by CBER, including monoclonal antibodies. Although CDER now has regulatory responsibility over both the chemotherapeutic drug and monoclonal antibody described in this hypothetical example, this example is provided for illustrative purposes.

Assignment algorithm criteria: Not applicable.

Jurisdictional assignment: CDER.

Example 3

Product: Scaffold seeded with autologous cells for organ replacement. The hypothetical product has the shape of the target organ, and the autologous cells are intended to allow the product to ultimately function like the target organ in the patient.

MOA/PMOA: The PMOA is attributable to the biological product component's MOA to help form new organ tissue that will ultimately function like the native organ. The device component's MOA to provide a scaffold upon which the new tissue will form is secondary. Although the scaffold is necessary to create the new tissue and provide the necessary shape, the creation of a functioning organ is primarily dependent upon the role of the cells to provide the tissue organization and muscular layer needed to function like the native organ. The biological product component provides the most important therapeutic action of the combination. It is unnecessary to proceed to the assignment algorithm because it is possible to determine which MOA provides the most important therapeutic action of this combination product.

Assignment algorithm criteria: Not applicable.

Jurisdictional assignment: CBER.

(Continued)

TABLE 3   Examples of Jurisdictional Determination in Accordance with 21 CFR Part 3 (*Continued*)

Example 4

Product: Menstrual tampon impregnated with genetically modified bacteria. The hypothetical product is intended for use throughout menstruation both in the collection of menstrual fluid and to treat and/or prevent recurrence of bacterial vaginosis.

MOA/PMOA: The product has two MOAs: the action of the biological product component to act upon the vaginal mucus membrane to produce antimicrobial factors that will control opportunistic pathogens and the device component's action to collect menstrual fluid. Both actions are independent and neither appears to be subordinate to the other; so it is necessary to apply the assignment algorithm.

Assignment algorithm criteria: (*i*) Is there a center that regulates other combination products that present similar questions of safety and effectiveness with regard to the combination product as a whole? CDRH regulates tampons and CBER regulates bacterial products and genetically modified cells. In this example, no combination product intended to collect menstrual fluid and to treat and/or prevent recurrence of bacterial vaginosis through the actions of a genetically modified organism has previously been reviewed by the agency. Although both CDRH and CBER regulate products that raise similar safety and effectiveness questions with regard to the product components, neither center regulates combination products that present similar safety and effectiveness questions with regard to the product as a whole; so it is necessary to apply the second criterion.

(*ii*) Which center has the most expertise related to the most significant safety and effectiveness questions presented by the combination product? Because there is no center that regulates combination products that present similar safety and effectiveness issues with regard to the product as a whole, FDA would consider which center has the most expertise related to the most significant safety and effectiveness questions presented by the product. In this case, the menstrual tampon component presents generally routine safety and effectiveness questions, similar to those of other menstrual tampons. In contrast, the biological product component raises more significant safety and effectiveness questions, such as those related to bacterial strain selection and dose; bacterial purity, potency, and metabolic activity, including the impact of genetic modifications; bacterial adherence potential, microbial strain interactions, and constitutive production of ancillary antimicrobial substances.

Jurisdictional assignment: CBER.

Example 5

Product: Interferon and ribavirin combination therapy. The product is intended for use in the treatment of chronic hepatitis C. Interferon is approved under the licensing provisions of the Public Health Service Act as a single-entity product for treatment of chronic hepatitis C. Clinical studies show that ribavirin when used alone to treat chronic hepatitis C can improve liver function, but most patients relapse with treatment of ribavirin alone. Data show that when used in conjunction with interferon, ribavirin produces a more efficacious response than when interferon is used alone to treat chronic hepatitis C. The drug and biological product components may be copackaged or are provided separately but cross-labeled for use together.

MOA/PMOA: The PMOA is attributable to the biological product component's MOA to treat chronic hepatitis C, which produces a dose-dependent decline in hepatitis C virus ribonucleic acid (RNA) titers, while the drug component's MOA is to enhance the efficacy of the biological product. Note that interferons are now reviewed in CDER following the transfer of therapeutic biological products to CDER in 2003.

Assignment algorithm criteria: Not applicable.

Jurisdictional assignment: CDER.

(*Continued*)

TABLE 3 Examples of Jurisdictional Determination in Accordance with 21 CFR Part 3 (*Continued*)

Example 6

Product: Implantable device with local chemotherapeutic drug. Embolization device coated with a chemotherapeutic agent intended to treat hypervascularized tumors.

MOA/PMOA: In this hypothetical example, the embolization device is a permanent implant, while the drug component is a short-term acting chemotherapeutic. The PMOA is attributable to the device component's MOA to physically occlude the blood supply to the tumor site through embolization, while the drug component's MOA plays a subordinate role in causing apoptosis in any remaining proliferating tumor cells. Data indicate that the effectiveness of the embolization device alone for the stated indication is much greater than the effectiveness of the drug component when delivered directly to the tumor site without use of the embolization agent. It is unnecessary to proceed to the assignment algorithm because it is possible to determine which MOA provides the most important therapeutic action of this combination product. In this hypothetical example, the PMOA was attributable to the device component; however, such a product used for another indication, or with another drug, could have a drug PMOA depending on the relative effectiveness of the drug and device components in providing the most important therapeutic action for the new use.

Assignment algorithm criteria: Not applicable.

Jurisdictional assignment: CDRH.

Example 7

Product: Vertebroplasty implant with extended-release analgesic. This hypothetical product is intended to provide spinal stabilization in patients with spinal bone metastases who also require palliative relief of pain.

MOA/PMOA: The product has two MOAs: the device action to stabilize the fractured spinal vertebral body bone and the drug action to provide for extended analgesic delivery as an alternative to oral medication in patients expected to continue to require long-term pain management despite the stabilization implant. Both actions of the product are independent, and neither is clearly subordinate to the other; so it is necessary to apply the assignment algorithm.

Assignment algorithm criteria: (*i*) Is there a center that regulates other combination products that present similar questions of safety and effectiveness with regard to the combination product as a whole? CDRH regulates vertebroplasty implants and CDER regulates analgesic drug products. No product combining a vertebroplasty implant and an extended-release analgesic has yet been submitted to FDA for review; therefore neither center regulates combination products that present similar safety and effectiveness questions with regard to the product as a whole and it is necessary to apply the second criterion of the algorithm.

(*ii*) Which center has the most expertise related to the most significant safety and effectiveness questions presented by the combination product? Although important safety and effectiveness questions are presented by this new route of administration of an analgesic and its extended release from the device that would need to be addressed, in this hypothetical example, the most significant safety and effectiveness questions associated with the combination product as a whole are related to the mechanical strength, wear, and clinical performance of the vertebroplasty implant.

Jurisdictional assignment: CDRH.

The number of marketing applications that FDA may require or that the sponsor would like to submit should be included among the topics covered in early discussions with FDA early in the development process. Sponsors should keep in mind that the regulation of combination products is evolving as FDA deals with new issues presented by innovative combination products. Sponsors should review current regulations and guidance documents, recent jurisdictional determinations, proposed rules, and other information FDA makes available on its Web site before contacting FDA with questions or to discuss specific issues that may be applicable to the sponsor's combination product development program.

User Fees

One significant result of the assignment of regulatory jurisdiction for combination products is the user fee schedule that will be applied to the combination product for FDA review of marketing applications and for other FDA regulatory activities associated with the product. In general, combination products for which a single marketing application is submitted will be subject to the fee associated with that type of application (8). Thus, combination products reviewed by CDRH will normally be subject to device user fees (under MDUFMA) and perhaps other fees (e.g., establishment registration fees) that may be assessed pursuant to legislative changes. Similarly, combination products assigned to CDER or CBER for review will be subject to Prescription Drug User Fee Act (PDUFA) fee requirements. PDUFA establishes NDA application fees as well as annual fees on establishments, and renewal fees on products. Sponsors may be eligible for fee waivers or reductions (e.g., for small businesses and orphan drug products) under PDUFA. Table 4 provides an overview of applicable fees and waivers for combination products.

As noted above, a sponsor may elect to submit two applications when only one would be required by FDA if it believes there is a benefit from doing so (e.g., new drug product exclusivity, orphan status, proprietary data protection when two firms are involved, and additional market for a component combination product as a stand-alone product). The review of the additional application places an extra burden on FDA resources so the sponsor will generally be required to pay a fee for each application. Similarly, when the FDA requires two applications for a combination product, two application fees will be assessed to help defer FDA's review costs.

A PDUFA "barrier to innovation" waiver may be appropriate to reduce the additional fee burden associated with the FDA's requirement for two marketing applications. PDUFA provides for a fee waiver or reduction when the assessment of the fee would present a significant barrier to innovation because of limited resources available to the sponsor or other circumstances. The FDA has stated that such "other circumstances" may exist in the relatively few instances where two marketing applications are required, and will consider the following as appropriate in determining eligibility for this fee reduction (8):

- The combination product [as defined in 21 CFR 3.2(e)] as a whole is innovative.
- FDA is requiring two fee-eligible marketing applications for the combination product.
- The applications only request approval of the two components of the combination product for use together. Applications that include independent uses of one or both components outside the combination product generally would not be eligible for this waiver. However, applications for combinations of already approved, independent products generally would be eligible if two applications are required for approval of the new combined use.
- The applicant does not qualify for a PDUFA small business waiver or have limited resources. Applicants who qualify for a PDUFA small business waiver receive a full waiver of their first PDUFA application fee. In addition, applicants with an innovative combination product who do not qualify for a PDUFA small business waiver but who have limited resources may be eligible for a standard PDUFA barrier to innovation waiver, which may provide a full waiver of the PDUFA application fee because of the applicant's financial need. More

TABLE 4 Combination Product Application Fees and Available Waivers or Reductions

Single application/fees[a]	Available waiver/reduction	Amount of reduction
NDA/PDUFA fees BLA/PDUFA fees	Waivers applicable to single PDUFA applications: Small business[b] Barrier to innovation Necessary to protect the public health Fees will exceed the anticipated present and future review costs incurred by FDA	PDUFA provides for a waiver of the fee for the first human drug application from a small business upon request. FDA will either deny or grant a fee waiver or reduction request based on the PDUFA public health or barrier to innovation provisions after assessing the financial burden placed on the applicant by fees. If FDA determines that the fees paid have exceeded the actual costs to review the application (using standard cost figures), the excess may be refunded upon request.
PMA, BLA, or 510(k)/MDUFMA fees	Waivers applicable to single MDUFMA applications: Small business Humanitarian device exemption (HDE)[c] BLA for a product licensed for further manufacturing use only Third-party 510(k) Any application for a device intended solely for pediatric use Any application form a state or federal government entity	A small business may receive a one-time waiver of the MDUFMA fee that would otherwise apply to a PMA, BLA, PDP, or premarket report (premarket approval application for a reprocessed single use device—see Ref. 22). There is no fee for an HDE application, a BLA for a product licensed for further manufacturing use only, an application for a device intended solely for pediatric use, or any application from a state or federal government entity.
Additional NDA or BLA[d]/PDUFA fees	PDUFA barrier to innovation	In applying the waiver to combination products requiring two PDUFA applications, FDA would expect to reduce each PDUFA fee by half. In the case where two full PDUFA fees would otherwise be required, the total amount paid under this waiver would be equivalent to one PDUFA fee.

(Continued)

TABLE 4 Combination Product Application Fees and Available Waivers or Reductions (*Continued*)

Single application/fees[a]	Available waiver/reduction	Amount of reduction
Additional PMA or 510(k)[d]/MDUFMA fees	PDUFA barrier to innovation	In applying the waiver to products requiring a MDUFMA application and a PDUFA application, FDA would expect to reduce the PDUFA fee by the amount of the MDUFMA fee. Thus, a sponsor would pay the full MDUFMA fee associated with the type of MDUFMA application, and a PDUFA fee reduced by the paid MDUFMA fee. The total amount paid would be equivalent to one PDUFA fee.

[a] PDUFA applications (NDA or BLA) not requiring clinical data for approval are assessed half the fee that is assessed for applications that do require clinical data for approval. NDA or BLA supplements that require clinical data for approval are assessed half the full application fee; however; NDA or BLA supplements that do not require clinical data for approval are not assessed a fee.

[b] The criteria for qualifying as a small business under PDUFA are different than those under MDUFMA. Under PDUFA, it is an entity that has fewer than 500 employees for the small business and its affiliates. Under MDUFMA, it is a firm with gross receipts or sales less than $30 million. In FY 2007, firms with annual gross sales and revenues of $100 million or less, including gross sales and revenues of all affiliates, partners, and parent firms, may qualify for lower rates for PMAs, premarket reports, and supplements. A similar reduction may be available for subsequent fiscal years.

[c] A HDE is an application to market a humanitarian use device (HUD). The HED application is similar to a PMA, but exempt from the effectiveness requirements of the FD&C Act. An HUD is a "medical device intended to benefit patients in the treatment or diagnosis of a disease or condition that affects or is manifested in fewer than 4000 individuals in the United States per year."

[d] May be required by FDA or submitted at the discretion of the sponsor. FDA has indicated that when multiple applications are submitted at the discretion of the sponsor, FDA will take the sponsor's financial status into consideration in determining if a waiver or reduction will be granted.

information about the standard barrier to innovation waiver is available on the FDA Web site. Applicants who believe they qualify are encouraged to explore their eligibility for the PDUFA small business or barrier to innovation waivers first.

FDA has indicated that it expects to consider several factors in determining whether a combination product is innovative for the purposes of this waiver, and notes that these are similar to those used in determining the eligibility of a product for expedited or priority review, where such factors are relevant to a determination of a combination product's innovativeness. A product need not be "life saving" or for use in critical conditions to satisfy these factors, although the benefits of such innovation are sometimes more evident in these circumstances. The factors include the following:

- The product addresses an unmet medical need in the treatment, diagnosis, or prevention of disease, as demonstrated by one of the following:
  - No approved alternative treatment or means of diagnosis exists.
  - The combination product offers significant, meaningful advantages over existing approved alternative treatments.
- Factors such as whether one of the two applications includes a new molecular entity, has been designated as a priority drug or eligible for expedited device review, or has been granted Fast Track status (9), may also be considered in determining whether a product is considered innovative for the purposes of this waiver.
- The existence of treatment alternatives would weigh against deciding that a product is innovative.

The sponsor of a combination product is urged to avail himself of the FDA consultation process in dealing with these and other issues (10,11).

NONCLINICAL RECOMMENDATIONS FOR SUCCESSFUL CHARACTERIZATION AND DEVELOPMENT OF COMBINATION DRUG PRODUCTS

Many pharmaceutical and biotechnology companies have successfully developed drug candidates [both small organic molecules or novel chemical entities (NCEs) and macromolecules or biologicals, both of which will be designated in this chapter as novel molecular entities (NME)] that have been approved for marketing by the U.S. Food and Drug Administration (FDA) or other regulatory authorities. Most of these NMEs have been studied as single therapeutic agents for the treatment of a human disease or disorder. The regulatory recommendations for the characterization and development of these NMEs are described in various FDA regulations, FDA guidance documents, and International Conference on Harmonization (ICH) guidelines and have been documented elsewhere (12–14). Table 5 summarizes these requirements.

For the successful treatment of many human diseases and disorders, however, a single therapeutic agent is not the "optimal" choice and combination therapy is necessary to provide the desired biological or therapeutic response with an acceptable human safety or toxicity profile. The development requirements for a combination therapy or combination drug product (CDP) differ from those for a single agent since the pharmacologic activities and toxicologic profiles of the marketed drugs

TABLE 5 Recommended Pharmacology and Safety Pharmacology Activities for CDPs Containing Marketed Drugs and/or NMEs

Nonclinical area	Recommended activity
Pharmacology	
Marketed drug	Evaluate available pharmacology database and prepare appropriate summaries of results for inclusion in regulatory submissions
NME	Conduct necessary pharmacology studies to define dose level and regimen for desired activity in animal models
CDP with only marketed drugs	If considered desirable, conduct animal studies to evaluate pharmacology profile when components in a CPD are dosed using established clinical routes and frequency of administration for each drug
CPD with marketed drugs and one NME	Conduct animal studies to evaluate pharmacology profile of CPD and to determine optimal dose levels and frequency of dosing for NME when administered concurrently with marketed drugs
CPD with more than one NME	Conduct animal studies to evaluate pharmacology profile of CPD and to determine optimal dosage regimen for each NME when administered concurrently with another NME
Safety pharmacology (SP)	
Marketed drug	Evaluate available SP database, and if necessary, conduct SP studies to meet current regulatory standards
NME	Conduct recommended ICH SP studies (standard battery and where appropriate, supplemental battery)
CDP with only marketed drugs	If one or more marketed drugs has incomplete SP assessments or if the marketed drugs produce adverse SP effects for the same organ system, design and conduct appropriate SP studies on CDP to determine if SP results are adversely affected when marketed drugs are administered in combination
CPD with marketed drugs and one NME	If SP studies on the individual components indicate possible adverse SP effects for the same organ system, design and conduct appropriate SP studies on CDP to further evaluate and extend the findings for that organ system
CPD with more than one NME	If SP studies on the individual NMEs show adverse effects on the same organ system, design and conduct appropriate SP studies on the CDP to further evaluate and extend the findings for that organ system

and/or NMEs in a CDP may be substantially different from those observed for each of the single agents alone. The changes in biological potency for a CDP may include, but are not limited to, synergism (desirable) or enhanced or prolonged pharmacologic activity in combination compared to the activity (extent and/or duration) of the single agents alone; additive effects (desirable) when the therapeutic effects of the single agents combined provide more effective treatment; or antagonism (usually undesirable) when the therapeutic effects of one or more of the single agents in a CDP are reduced when administered concurrently with other marketed drugs and/or NMEs. The changes in the toxicologic profile for a CDP may include, but are not limited to, reduction (desirable) of adverse effects because lower doses of one or more of the single agents in a CDP can be administered with a similar or improved pharmacologic profile; mediation (desirable) of adverse effects caused by one or more of the single agents in a CDP by another marketed drug and/or NME; similar (acceptable) adverse effect profile for each marketed drug and/or NME in the CDP; or increased (undesirable) adverse effects because the safety or toxicity profile of one or more of the single agents in a CDP is changed when administered in combination with other agents.

In addition to defining and characterizing the pharmacologic and toxicologic profiles of the marketed drugs and/or NMEs in a CDP, another important area that needs to be evaluated is potential changes in the pharmacokinetic (PK) and drug metabolism (DM) profiles of each of the single agents to be included in a proposed CDP. Possible desirable or undesirable (depending on why the CDP is being developed) changes in PK profiles include, but are not limited to, increases or decreases for one or more of the single agents in a CDP in the rate and/or extent of absorption, in plasma protein binding characteristics, in the tissue distribution profiles, and in the rate and/or route of elimination. Changes in the extent and type of metabolism for any of the single agents in a CDP may also be desirable or undesirable. Increased metabolism may not only reduce the adverse effect profile of one marketed drug or NME but could also cause more rapid clearance and thus decrease the pharmacologic effectiveness of a second agent. Decreased metabolism may not only provide longer exposure to a pharmacologically active compound and thus produce enhanced effectiveness but could also cause accumulation of one or more of the single agents in a CDP in one or more tissues and/or organs and thus potentially cause increased adverse effects. Table 6 summarizes recommended PK, toxicokinetic, and DM suggestions for combination products containing marketed drugs and/or NMEs. Table 7 provides an overview of recommended nonclinical safety or toxicology support for such products.

NDAs for combination products must take into account these issues, and strategies for developing these products should include the content of the eventual marketing application stemming from the development program.

CLINICAL PHARMACOLOGY AND CLINICAL DEVELOPMENT OF COMBINATION PRODUCTS

Safety testing of the components of combination products should be integrated with planning for the clinical pharmacology studies and the clinical studies that will generate data supporting substantial evidence of safety and efficacy. The interaction of combination products with the human body is often more complicated than that of a single-entity drug, biologic, or medical device. Sponsors should strategically approach pharmacology and clinical testing as a continuum with a staged,

TABLE 6 Recommended Pharmacokinetic/Toxicokinetic and Drug Metabolism Activities for CDPs Containing Marketed Drugs and/or NMEs

Nonclinical area	Recommended activity
Pharmacokinetics	
Marketed drug	Evaluate available PK and TK database, and if necessary, conduct additional studies to further characterize the PK profile of the marketed drug
NME	Conduct the necessary PK and TK studies to characterize the absorption, distribution, metabolism, and elimination profiles of the individual NME
CDP with only marketed drugs	Provide TK support for the recommended toxicology studies (bridging and developmental toxicology) on the CDP and if potential PK interactions between the components in a CDP are expected, design and conduct animal PK studies to evaluate and characterize these possible drug–drug interactions
CPD with marketed drugs and one NME	Conduct recommended PK and TK studies on the NME alone, provide TK support for the recommended toxicology studies on the CDP, and if potential PK interactions between the components in a CDP are expected, design and conduct animal PK studies to evaluate and characterize these possible drug–drug interactions
CPD with more than one NME	Conduct recommended PK and TK studies on each NME alone, provide TK support for the recommended toxicology studies on the CDP, and if potential PK interactions between the components in a CDP are expected, design and conduct animal PK studies to evaluate and characterize these possible drug–drug interactions
Drug metabolism	
Marketed drug	Evaluate available DM database [e.g., tissue distribution, protein binding, metabolism (including enzyme systems involved and potential for enzyme inhibition or induction), and routes and rates of elimination] on each marketed drug, and if necessary, conduct additional DM studies to further characterize the DM profile of a marketed drug to meet current regulatory standards
NME	Conduct recommended DM studies on the NME alone to characterize how the NME is handled by the body
CDP with only marketed drugs	Compare the available and sponsor-generated DM information on each marketed drug in the CDP, and if necessary, design and conduct DM studies on the CDP to determine if the DM profiles of the individual components are changed when administered in combination
CPD with marketed drugs and one NME	Compare the DM information on the marketed drugs with the DM information generated by the sponsor on the NME, and if necessary, design and conduct DM studies on the CDP to determine if the DM profiles of the individual components are changed when administered in combination
CPD with more than one NME	Compare the DM information generated by the sponsor on the NMEs alone (and on any marketed drugs), and if necessary, design and conduct DM studies on the CDP to determine if the DM profiles of the individual NMEs (and any marketed drugs) are changed when administered in combination

TABLE 7 Recommended Nonclinical Safety or Toxicology Activities for CDPs Containing Marketed Drugs and/or NMEs

Nonclinical area	Recommended activity
General toxicology	
Marketed drug	Evaluate available toxicology database to ensure sufficient data are available to meet current regulatory recommendations for acute and repeated dose toxicology, genotoxicity, carcinogenicity, reproductive and developmental toxicology, and local tolerance, and if necessary, conduct additional studies to further characterize the toxicology profiles of the marketed drug in rodent and nonrodent species
NME	Conduct the recommended toxicology studies, which may be different for a NCE and a biological, to characterize the animal safety profiles of the individual NME in rodent and nonrodent species
CDP with only marketed drugs	After the toxicology database for each marketed drug in a CDP is complete, compare the toxicology profiles of each component in the CDP to determine if additional toxicology studies, other than the toxicology bridging study and a developmental toxicology study (discussed below), are necessary to evaluate and characterize a potential toxicological interaction between two or more of the components in a CDP
CPD with marketed drugs and one NME	After the toxicology database for each marketed drug is complete and the recommended toxicology studies on the NME have been conducted, compare the toxicology profiles of each component in a CDP to determine if additional toxicology studies, other than the toxicology bridging study and a developmental toxicology study (discussed below), are necessary to characterize a potential toxicological interaction between the components in a CDP
CPD with more than one NME	After the recommended toxicology studies on each NME in a CDP have been conducted and the toxicology database for any marketed drugs in the CDP is considered complete, compare the toxicology profiles of each component in a CDP to determine if additional toxicology assessments are needed to further characterize the toxicology profiles of components administered concurrently
Recommended bridging toxicology study	
CDP with only marketed drugs	Design and conduct the recommended toxicology bridging study in the most relevant animal species using multiple dose levels of the CDP, the projected clinical route and frequency of dosing for each marketed drug, and dose groups for each of the marketed drugs alone
CPD with marketed drugs and one NME	Design and conduct the recommended toxicology bridging study in the most relevant animal species using multiple dose levels of the CDP, the projected clinical route and frequency of dosing for the NME and for each marketed drug, and dose groups for the NME alone and for each of the marketed drugs alone

(Continued)

TABLE 7 Recommended Nonclinical Safety or Toxicology Activities for CDPs Containing Marketed Drugs and/or NMEs (*Continued*)

Nonclinical area	Recommended activity
CPD with more than one NME	Design and conduct the recommended toxicology bridging study in the most relevant animal species using multiple dose levels of the CDP, the projected clinical route and frequency of dosing for each NME in the CDP, and if included, for each marketed drug in the CDP, and dose groups for each of the NMEs alone, and if included, in the CDP, for each of the marketed drugs alone
Recommended developmental toxicology study	
CPD with only marketed drugs	Unless one or more of the marketed drugs in a CDP is known to have significant risk for developmental toxicity, design and conduct (at the appropriate time in the CDP development program) the recommended embryo—fetal developmental toxicology study on a CDP
CPD with marketed drugs and one NME	Unless one or more of the marketed drugs in a CDP is known to have significant risk for developmental toxicity or if the NME alone is shown to cause reproductive and developmental toxic effects in rodents or nonrodents, design and conduct the recommended embryo—fetal developmental toxicology studies on a CDP
CPD with more than one NME	If any of the NMEs alone in a CDP is shown to cause reproductive and developmental toxic effects in rodents or nonrodents and unless any marketed drugs, if included, in the CDP is known to have significant risk for developmental toxicity, design and conduct the recommended embryo—fetal developmental toxicology studies on a CDP

integrated, and logical plan that will minimize expenditure of scarce funding, time, and resources, and yet satisfy the needs of the regulatory authorities to protect the public from the unknown effects of such products. Bioavailability, bioequivalence, and efficacy combined with acceptable safety in the human population of interest should be covered, with the NDA content foremost in mind.

An increased understanding of the regulatory review process may decrease sponsor hesitancy to develop innovative combination products. Previously, there has been concern that the advantages of being first-to-market with a new therapeutic class are more than offset by the complications and delays associated with being the test case as FDA determines the best approach to review the given product type. Even when efforts between reviewing divisions are coordinated, the need to involve multiple divisions increases FDA review time. Reviewing divisions have been less responsive to the mandated response time periods when they are not the primary reviewing division than when they are a consulting division, resulting in delays for a complete review of combination product data and plans.

One challenge for clinical development of a combination product is the lack of specific guidance. The Office of Combination Products (OCP) has issued guidance documents on preclinical and chemistry, manufacturing, and controls (CMC) considerations. For clinical programs, however, the amount of data and approach to development depend heavily on the reviewers' previous experience with the components as well as any unique issues raised by the combination. A recent series of guidances covering drug-eluting stents represent FDA's first attempt to provide global and detailed guidance on an important class of combination products that are widely used in the general population (15,16). These guidances cover suggested development pathways for these specific products, safety support for drug substance and combination product, finished product handling (e.g., sterilization, package integrity, and shelf life) and clinical assessment, and CMC information required.

One common factor among the more successful (and rapid) combination product approvals is early and frequent communication among developers, FDA reviewers, and, as appropriate, the OCP. Organized teleconferences with the decision makers in all reviewing divisions (and with all sponsors, when there are more than one) have been especially beneficial in establishing consensus, avoiding weeks and even months of e-mail and letter "loops." Complete reviewer buy-in on the development program (e.g., appropriateness of surrogate end points, number of studies, and indications) and individual trial issues (e.g., study design, sample size, and end points) can avoid extended review periods and unnecessary duplication of research efforts. New combination product developers can especially benefit from obtaining FDA guidance on how to approach unique issues such as techniques to measure drug levels in tissues not typically accessible (for targeted therapies), or techniques to evaluate drug–device interactions (17). Tables 8 and 9 provide examples of common drug/delivery system and drug/active device combination products, respectively, with the advantages and challenges of each type.

While the safety and effectiveness of drug and biologic products are mainly intrinsic to the products themselves, the safety and effectiveness of devices often have a human-use component that should be examined in clinical development. For example, improper patient use of a metered-dose inhaler can drastically reduce the efficacy of the inhaled drug. Studies of how patients operate the device in "realistic, stressful conditions" should be conducted early in development, as

TABLE 8   Drug–Delivery System Combinations

Examples	Advantages	Challenges
Metered-dose inhalers	Streamlined regulatory process possible	Altered pharmacodynamic effects
Transdermal patches	Improved efficacy over previously approved delivery routes	Route-dependent metabolic profile
	Noninjection bioavailability for peptides and proteins	Inherent delivery site sensitivity
		Safety of excipients in novel delivery routes
		Possible immune system reactions
		Bridging effects specific to human physiology
		Formulation changes

they will provide insight into possible device improvements prior to substantial evidence studies (17).

CDER has a long history of reviewing products that combine two active drugs at fixed doses. As both active drugs carry the risk of side effects, CDER requires developers to demonstrate in clinical studies that each component contributes to the overall efficacy. CDER will often want to see data to justify each component in a drug/device combination, which can increase the size, cost, and complexity of a clinical program. Instead, it is often advantageous to have the product regulated as a device and assigned to CDRH, which reviews often complex device systems, and reviews the safety and efficacy of the product as a whole (18).

Table 10 provides a summary of advantages and challenges for drug/in vitro diagnostic combination products with two examples of such products.

While all FDA centers require that products be demonstrated to be both safe and effective to be approved, the amount of clinical support each requires is different. CDRH requires a single high-quality substantial evidence study for approval while, in most cases, CDER requires two independent substantial evidence trials. In situations where a disease is serious or life threatening and there is an unmet medical need (i.e., no product approved in the United States for the specific indication), or the prevalence of the disease state is very low, CDER may approve a product with one well-controlled substantial evidence trial plus strong supporting information from earlier, smaller, trials. A typical NDA approved by CDER contains approximately 60 clinical studies (including dose-finding, PK, drug-interaction, and special population studies), while a PMA approved by CDRH may only contain 2 or 3 studies. Streamlined approvals are critical for devices, which can become obsolete within 6 to 12 months.

TABLE 9   Drug–Active Device Combination

Examples	Advantages	Challenges
Coronary drug-eluting stents	Increased efficacy over device alone	Often requires request for designation process
Antibiotic bone cement	Localized drug can reduce systemic adverse effects	Localization of drug can alter safety profile

TABLE 10 Drug–In Vitro Diagnostic Combination

Examples	Advantages	Challenges
Helicobacter pylori	May permit approval for products without limited general efficacy	Biomarker development and validation
Detection test	May expand use of pharmaceuticals with significant safety concerns	Possible limiting of target population
	Smaller clinical studies possible	Increased complexity of development program

Of course, the amount of clinical trial data required to support approval of a multiactive combination product (under either a PMA or an NDA) depends on whether device or drug components of the product have been previously approved. If the drug to be used is unapproved, or is an analog of an approved drug, it is considered a new molecular entity by both CDER and CDRH, and manufacturers will need to provide information in the investigational device exemption (IDE) equivalent to the content of a phase 1 investigational new drug (IND) exemption for CDER. The eventual NDA for a CDER-regulated combination product must similarly include results of a robust clinical program that establishes substantial evidence of safety and effectiveness for the new product.

The number of combination products developed in the future will depend heavily on the success of products approved for marketing. Of concern for developers are the delays involved in being an innovator product, where the regulatory approval path is not well established. The approval process may remain challenging as regulators require the developers of follow-on products to consider safety issues of the innovator products in their development programs.

Even with the FDA's efforts to make the approval process consistent and transparent, the developers of combination products will have to consider the expectations and review culture of the different divisions in their positioning of the primary mode of action for the product. Developers should maximize opportunities for meetings (and/or teleconferences) that include both the main reviewing division and the consulting division(s). These meetings are critical in developing a streamlined clinical program that will address the needs of all reviewers, and in addressing unique issues that arise from the interaction of the combination product components.

REGULATORY STRATEGY CONSIDERATIONS FOR CMC

Compliant combination product development, leading to a successful NDA, is designed to meet the requirements of a product's development throughout its life cycle by incorporating into the planning and execution of work all requisite elements of traceability to assure the validity and retrievability of information. The building blocks of this approach are planning, performing, recording, reporting, monitoring, and change control. Since both cGMP and quality system issues are involved in the typical combination product manufacturing controls arena, a careful approach to this area will lead to a more successful regulatory outcome for an otherwise safer and effective combination product during the marketing application review cycle (19,20).

Regulatory compliant product development is built upon the basic tenet of pharmaceutical development that product quality is by design. Utilizing good

TABLE 11   Key Current Good Manufacturing Practice Provisions to Consider During and After Joining Together Copackaged and Single-Entity Combination Products

---

If the operating manufacturing control system is Part 820 (QS Regulation)[a]:
    Section 211.84: Testing and approval or rejection of components, drug product containers, and
       closures
    Section 211.103: Calculation of yield
    Section 211.137: Expiration dating
    Section 211.165: Testing and release for distribution
    Section 211.166: Stability testing
    Section 211.167: Special testing requirements
    Section 211.170: Reserve samples
If the operating manufacturing control system is Part 210/211 (CGMP Regulation)[a]:
    Section 820.30: Design controls
    Section 820.50: Purchasing controls
    Section 820.100: Corrective and preventative actions

---

[a] Including all subsections, as appropriate.

documentation practices, a sponsor can demonstrate an understanding that product and process knowledge will be gained throughout the life cycle of a product. Regulatory compliant product development activities are designed to gain insight and understanding of the effects that sources of variability will introduce to product quality. These insights and understandings form the basis of quality risk management programs. The information and process knowledge garnered through development activities and manufacturing experiences form the basis of specifications and manufacturing controls that assure that product is consistently manufactured to established standards of quality. If properly designed and implemented, a strategic CMC plan with the appropriate tactical execution will assist the CDP sponsor in meeting the requirements of parallel drug and device manufacturing systems.

The FDA has acknowledged that drug and device manufacturing regulations overlap, are generally similar, and have the same objectives, that is, to allow the manufacture of safe and effective products. To date, FDA has not promulgated CGMPs for combination products; until it does, each component of a CDP is subject to its governing CGMP regulations. For CDPs produced as single entities or packaged together, all applicable CGMP regulations are relevant (19). Table 11 provides a delineation of key cGMP provisions to consider for copackaged and single-entity combination products involving small molecule or biological drugs and medical devices.

Components of a CDP are identifiable and assignable to specific FDA centers, CFR sections, and applicable guidelines. In developing an approach to regulatory compliance, sponsors are well served by understanding that the different centers have varying regulatory approaches. CDRH is most concerned with design controls, documentation supporting the administration of quality systems during development and manufacturing, and the application of ongoing risk assessments. Conversely, CDER is more focused on the characterization and control of changes to CDP development that may potentially affect the quality, strength, purity, or potency of the product. A primary challenge for a CDP sponsor is to understand both the divergent and convergent perspectives of the centers on the regulatory processes.

For CDP developers and manufacturers, attention must be appropriately focused to provide FDA with the necessary CMC information. The organization of this information may be broadly categorized into the two primary areas of drug and device, keeping in mind that the effects of the drug on the device performance and the device's potential impact on the impurity profile, safety, and efficacy of the drug will be of primary importance to the regulatory review process.

Effective regulatory submissions for CDPs require that the sponsors present information that details the evolution of process and product knowledge from the perspective of CMC development. The approaches taken should be integrated at the foundational level of planning, performing, recording, reporting, and monitoring of the CDP development activities to communicate to CMC reviewers that the application of well-documented change control has resulted in the identification, understanding, and control of sources of variability. The sponsor should demonstrate that the resultant continual improvements in the design and manufacturing of the CDP are associated with reductions in manufacturing and performance variability, which in turn underlie the sponsor's risk management program.

The framework for the CMC section of regulatory submissions remains constant throughout the life cycle of a CDP. The information required to be detailed in the framework is influenced by the stage of the product's development and risk-based considerations pertaining to the safety and effectiveness of its use (21). The sponsor, if submitting an NDA as the end result of a CDP development program, must take into account the incorporation of all of these elements in planning for the marketing submission.

REFERENCES

1. Federal Food, Drug and Cosmetic Act, 21 USC Section 321 (2007). Available from http://www.fda.gov/opacom/laws/fdcact/fdcact1.htm.
2. Public Health Service Act, 42 USC Section 201 (1999). Available from http://www.fda.gov/opacom/laws/phsvcact/sec201.htm.
3. Drug and biological product consolidation (2003). Federal Register 68(123), 38067–38068. Available from http://www.fda.gov/OHRMS/DOCKETS/98fr/03-16242.pdf.
4. US Department of Health and Human Services, FDA, CDRH, Office of Device Evaluation. New Section 513(f)(2)—Evaluation of Automatic Class III Designation: Guidance for Industry and CDRH Staff (February 19, 1998). Available from http://www.fda.gov/cdrh/modact/clasiii.pdf.
5. Definition of primary mode of action of a combination product (2005). Federal Register 70(164):49848–49862. Available from http://www.fda.gov/ohrms/dockets/98fr/05-16527.htm.
6. US Department of Health and Human Services, FDA, OCP. Guidance for Industry and FDA Staff: How to Write a Request for Designation (RFD) (August 2005). Available from http://www.fda.gov/oc/combination/Guidance-How%20to%20Write%20an%20RFD.pdf.
7. US Food and Drug Administration (June 18, 2004). Manual of standard operating procedures and policies, general information—review, intercenter consultative/collaborative review process. Version 4.
8. US Department of Health and Human Services, FDA, OCP (April 2005). Guidance for Industry and FDA Staff: Application User Fees for Combination Products. Available from http://www.fda.gov/oc/combination/userfees.html.
9. US Department of Health and Human Services, FDA, CDER, CBER (July 2004). Guidance for Industry: Fast Track Drug Development Programs—Designation, Development, and Application Review. Available from http://www.fda.gov/cder/guidance/5645fnl.htm.

10. US Department of Health and Human Services, FDA, CDER, CBER (February 2000). Guidance for Industry: Formal Meetings with Sponsors and Applicants for PDUFA Products. Available from http://www.fda.gov/cder/guidance/2125fnl.htm.
11. US Department of Health and Human Services, FDA, CDRH (February 28, 2001). Early Collaboration Meetings under the FDA Modernization Act (FDAMA): Final Guidance for Industry and for CDRH Staff. Available from http://www.fda.gov/cdrh/ode/guidance/310.html.
12. Lakings DB (2004). Nonclinical drug development: pharmacology, drug metabolism, and toxicology. In: Guarino RA, ed. New Drug Approval Process, Accelerating Global Registration, 4th ed. New York: Marcel Dekker, 19–61.
13. Siegel EB, Lakings DB (2008). Preclinical Drug Development Handbook: Regulatory Considerations. In: Gad SC, ed. Pharmaceutical Development Handbook: Toxicology, New Jersey: Wiley-Interscience, 945–964.
14. US Department of Health and Human Services, FDA, CDER (March 2006). Nonclinical Safety Evaluations for Drug or Biologic Combinations. Available from http://www.fda.gov/cder/guidance/6714fnl.htm.
15. US Department of Health and Human Services, FDA, CDRH, CDER (March 2008). Guidance for Industry: Coronary Drug-Eluting Stents-Nonclinical and Clinical Studies. Available from http://www.fda.gov/cder/guidance/6255dft.htm.
16. US Department of Health and Human Services, FDA, CDRH, CDER (March 2008). Guidance for Industry: Coronary Drug-Eluting Stents-Nonclinical and Clinical Studies Companion Document. Available from http://www.fda.gov/cder/guidance/6255companion.doc.htm.
17. US Department of Health and Human Services, FDA (September 2006). Guidance for Industry and FDA Staff: Early Development Considerations for Innovative Combination Products. Available from http://www.fda.gov/oc/combination/innovative.html.
18. US FDA (October 2002). Regulation of Combination Products: FDA Employee Perspectives. Available from www.fda.gov/oc/combination/perspectives.html.
19. US Department of Health and Human Services, FDA, Office of the Commissioner, OCP (September 2004). Guidance for Industry and FDA: Current Good Manufacturing Practice for Combination Products.
20. US Department of Health and Human Services, FDA, CDER, CBER, CVM, ORA (September 2006). Guidance for Industry: Quality Systems Approach to Pharmaceutical CGMP Regulations. Available from http://www.fda.gov/cder/guidance/7260fnl.htm.
21. US Department of Health and Human Services, FDA, CDER, CBER (May 2006). Guidance for Industry: Q8—Pharmaceutical Development. Available from http://www.fda.gov/cder/guidance/6746fnl.htm.
22. http://www.fda.gov/cdrh/reprocessing/.

The Current State of GXP in China

Earl W. Hulihan
Medidata Solutions Worldwide, New York, New York, U.S.A.

Daniel Liu
Medidata Solutions Worldwide, Beijing, P.R. China

Cai Cao
Center for Certification of Drugs, State Food and Drug Administration of China, Beijing, P.R. China

Qingshan Zheng
Shanghai University of Traditional Chinese Medicines, Shanghai, P.R. China

Good Clinical Certificate Practice in Clinical Trials in China

INTRODUCTION

For thousands of years, China was known for its system of traditional Chinese medicine (TCM). Until 100 years ago, Western drugs began to be used in China. Since then, some local companies began to produce Western drugs, but most of these drugs are generics, and no substantive clinical trials were conducted prior to approval.

Pharmaceutical administration, including clinical pharmacology research, started in China around 1960 because of the mushrooming development of the modern pharmaceutical industry. Some regulations were introduced at that time, but most of them were not carried out because of the Cultural Revolution. As a result, the discipline of clinical pharmacology, especially in human clinical trials, did not take shape until the 1980s, when the previous China Drug Administration Law was issued in 1984.

Since the 1990s, good clinical practice (GCP) has found access to China through international academic communications and exchanges as well as the investments of many multinational pharmaceutical companies in China, resulting in the increase of clinical trials. With the growing globalization of the economy in the 1990s, more and more pharmaceutical joint ventures, wholly owned enterprises, and global contract research organizations (CROs) were established in China, and most of them requested China to conduct clinical trials according to the international standard, which established a favorable atmosphere for the appearance of GCP in China.

SFDA STRUCTURE AND REGULATORY RESPONSIBILITIES

Historically, the Chinese drug regulatory system has developed as followed below:

☐ 1949—Bureau of Drug Affairs administered by Department of Medical Affairs of the Ministry of Health (MOH)

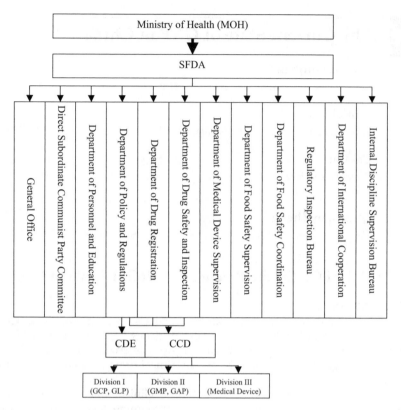

FIGURE 1   SFDA organization structure.

☐ 1953—Department of Drug Affairs, MOH
☐ 1998—State Drug Administration
☐ 2003—State Food and Drug Administration (SFDA)
☐ 2008—Effective in March 2008, SFDA was placed under the State MOH. The SFDA had been incorporated within the MOH again. This should be understood when reference is made to SFDA.

Structurally, SFDA contains one executive office, one Communist Party office and ten functional departments (Fig. 1). As the drug regulatory body, according to the Drug Administrative Law of People's Republic of China, SFDA as a comprehensive and affiliated institution is responsible for the following:

• To organize relevant authorities to draft laws and regulations on the safety management of food, health food, and cosmetics; organize relevant authorities to formulate comprehensive supervision policy, work plan, and supervise its implementation.
• To exercise comprehensive supervision on the safety management of food, health food, and cosmetics in accordance with laws; organize and coordinate supervision work on safety of food, health food, and cosmetics carried out by relevant authorities.

- To organize and carry out investigation and impose punishment on serious safety accidents of food, health food, and cosmetics; delegated by the State Council, organize, coordinate, and conduct specific law-enforcement campaigns over safety of food, health food, and cosmetics nationwide; organize, coordinate, and collaborate with relevant authorities in carrying out emergency rescue work on serious safety accidents of food, health food, and cosmetics.
- To comprehensively coordinate the testing and evaluation for the safety of food, health food, and cosmetics; formulate provisions on releasing of supervision information for safety of food, health food, and cosmetics in conjunction with relevant authorities and monitor their implementation; sum up safety information of food, health food, and cosmetics from relevant authorities and release it to the public regularly.
- To draft law and administrative regulations on drug administration and supervise their enforcement; carry out protection system for certain traditional Chinese medicinal preparations and administrative protection system for pharmaceuticals in accordance with law or regulations.
- To draft law and regulations on administration of medical devices and supervise their enforcement; take charge of registration and regulation of medical devices; draft relevant national standards; draw up and revise professional standards of medical devices, manufacturing practice and supervise their implementation.
- To be in charge of drug registration, draw up, revise, and promulgate national standard of drugs; draw up criteria for marketing authorization of health food; review and approve health food; set up classification system for prescription drugs and OTC drugs; establish and improve ADR monitoring system; be responsible for drug reevaluation, review drugs to be withdrawn and formulate national essential medicines list.
- To draft and revise good practices for drug research, manufacturing, distribution and use, and supervise their implementation.
- To control the quality of drugs and medical devices in manufacturers, distributors, and medical institutions; release national quality bulletin on drugs and medical devices on a regular basis; investigate and punish illegal activities of producing and selling counterfeit and inferior drugs and medical devices in accordance with law.
- To regulate radioactive pharmaceuticals, narcotics, toxics, psychotropics, and other controlled drugs and devices in accordance with law.
- To draw up and improve qualification system for licensed pharmacist; supervise and direct the registration of licensed pharmacist.
- To direct national drug regulation and comprehensive supervision on the safety management of food, health food, and cosmetics.
- To carry out exchanges and cooperation in drug regulation, relevant safety management of food, health food, and cosmetics with foreign governments and international organizations.
- To undertake other work assigned by the State Council.

Under the functional departments, SFDA has a variety of affiliated organizations and centers that play technical and administrative roles in support of SFDA regulatory activities. For example, the Center for Drug Evaluation (CDE) under the Department of Drug Registration (DDR) is in charge of all technical and scientific reviews of NDA applications and provides technical recommendations of clinical trials and new drug marketing applications to SFDA. The Center for Certification of Drugs (CCD) is responsible to develop and modify the National Act and Guidance of GLP, GCP, GMP, GAP, and GSP; review and validate the qualification of pharmaceutical companies and investigator sites with GLP, GMP, GAP, GCP, and quality of medical device; and conduct on-site inspections on certified pharmaceutical companies and investigator sites.

ESTABLISHMENT OF A GCCP SYSTEM IN CHINA
The implementation of Good Clinical Certification Practice (GCCP) is one of intrinsic GCP efforts in China for SFDA to cooperate and motivate Chinese regulatory rules more consistent with international guidelines. In China, under this GCCP system, any institutions that wish to qualify as a "clinical institution" must be accredited by SFDA. Any clinical trial must be conducted in a qualified clinical institution with the corresponding accreditation. Prior to March 1998, the MOH of the People's Republic of China was authorized to assign the regulatory accreditation to a "Base for Clinical Pharmacology." Historically, clinical institutions had different names due to the changes of their executive administration. Between March 1998 and March 2003, the authorization of such regulatory accreditation to a "National Base for Drug Clinical Study" was granted by the SFDA, which was established in 1998. Currently, the clinical institutions are named as drug clinical study institution (abbreviated as clinical institution).

Administration Office at Clinical Institution
SFDA does not have a detailed requirement for the administration pattern of the clinical institutions, which means that SFDA does not intervene in the management model of the institutions. What SFDA requires is that the institution should set up a special administrative office with full-time staff to oversight behaviors and outcomes of clinical trials. It is required that the office should strictly implement relevant laws and regulations and establish a quality assurance (QA) system for the clinical trials according to GCP.

A QA person at the office is responsible to audit the authenticity and standardization of the clinical research, guarantee the SOPs and the scientific compliance in the clinical trials, the protection of safety and rights of the subjects and the reality, accuracy, and completeness of the clinical data obtained.

Independent Ethics Committee
As part of GCCP criteria, SFDA requires that clinical institutions set up the Independent Ethics Committee (IEC or EC) system. The IEC is responsible to review and approve the protocol. Prior to the SFDA's approval, any clinical trials may be initiated only after the approval by IEC is received at the clinical institution. The requirements by SFDA for the IEC of the drug clinical trial institutions are as follows:

• The institutions should establish an IEC, which is independent to the investigators and the sponsor.
• IEC is directed by the Declaration of Helsinki and bound by the laws and regulations of China.
• IEC should review the clinical trial protocol and informed consent form for clinical trials to be conducted in the institution and audit the clinical trial process during the trials to ensure the compliance of investigators with the ethical requirements, and to appropriately resolve and record any issues and/or findings.

- IEC must make certain that all elements of informed consent, including the procedure of clinical projects, the benefit/risk of the clinical trial, the compliance of subjects on protocol, and the rights and privacy of subjects, are provided to research subjects.
- Members of IEC should learn and master the principles of the Declaration of Helsinki and other relevant requirements, and understand that "the most priority is the health care of patients by physicians," "any medical measures that may impact psychological or physical conditions by a physician should not be acted unless they meet the medical needs of patients," and "medical progresses are based on researches that ultimately must rest in part on experimentation involving human subjects."

The composition of IEC is consistent with international criteria, that is, IEC must be composed of

- at least one member whose primary area of interest is not in a medical or pharmaceutical area;
- at least one member who is working in legal field;
- at least one member who is independent to the institution/trial site;
- a diversity of gender among its members;
- at least five members with varying backgrounds.

When necessary, experts outside IEC could be invited to participate in the meeting, but they will not have a voting right. In China, there are usually five to seven members with one veto system in the IEC.

Certified Clinical Institution
In order to be qualified, clinical institutions must follow regulatory procedures to submit their application to SFDA and get the certificate when they pass the on-site regulatory inspection. Major regulatory steps for clinical institutions to obtain the certificate are as follows:

1. A medical institution that meets certain preconditions must submit an application to the local provincial health administrative departments. After the local health administrative departments' review and approval, the application will be transferred to the local provincial drug administration departments.
2. After reviewing and approving the application, the local drug administrative departments will pass the application package to the Administrative Acceptance Center of SFDA (AAC).
3. The AAC will conduct a format review of the application file. Applications that passed the format review will receive an acceptance notice with an acceptance number. The application will then be transferred to the CCD of SFDA.
4. CCD will conduct a technical evaluation to the application file. For those institutions that meet the necessary requirements, CCD will organize an on-site inspection. If the on-site inspection confirms that the site meets necessary requirements, CCD will then transfer the on-site inspection report and relevant documents to the DDSI of SFDA.
5. DDSI will review the application with MOH and report the final approval to the SFDA commissioner.
6. After the SFDA commissioner signs the approval document, the AAC will develop a certificate. At the same time, the SFDA will publish the result of the site evaluation on its Web site (1).

Currently, for the conduct of "Western pharmaceutical clinical research," 134 clinical institutions and 1030 subspecialty areas are certified by the SFDA through the first quarter of 2008. In addition to these certified sites, 33 institutions and 128 subspecialties have also been certified for TCM clinical research.

Institution Qualifications
In order for an institution to be qualified as the investigative site to initiate clinical studies in China, it should meet the following nine prerequisites:

1. The applicant's clinical institution should have a medical license to practice medicine.
2. The medical subspecialty being examined must be a part of the institution's medical license to practice medicine and be certified to undertake the clinical studies by SFDA.
3. The institution at which the investigator works should have relevant equipment and facilities necessary to support clinical trials.
4. The investigator should have the capacity and experience for the diagnosis and treatment of the condition(s) to be studied under the relevant clinical trial.
5. The institution should have the appropriate number of hospital beds and access to subjects necessary to meet clinical trial requirements.
6. The institution at which the investigator works should have the relevant administrative office and staff for clinical trials.
7. The investigator's research staff should be trained in the technical and regulatory aspects of clinical trials.
8. The institution at which the investigator works should have an administrative system and SOPs for clinical trials.
9. The institution's administrative system should have a process/system for preventing and managing emergency situations that may arise during clinical trials.

Auditing Clinical Institution
The qualification of a GCP-certified clinical institution is divided into hardware and software together with qualification of staffs. Hardware refers to the level and area of the hospitals/medical institutions, construction area, number and quality of hospital beds and wards, facilities and equipments, equipments for emergency, other research conditions, and quality of staff. Software has five requirements, that is,

• integrity and workability of the management system;
• management team, which is responsible for the daily management for the ongoing trial;
• documents management, which should be managed in the whole processing;
• overall quality of clinical personnel, including education background, experiences, management ability, familiarity of the laws and regulations, members of Ethics Committee, and management staff and standards;
• subject resource, such as diverse disease type, patient population.

During the on-site inspection, a special focus is on if the site has a Clinical Research Office besides the hardware required, how much the power resides in the office, and whether it can control the whole clinical trial and ensure the quality of the trial as well as the roles and procedure of IEC in the management and supervision of clinical trials. Furthermore, daily supervision and follow-up inspections are paying special attentions to the following three parts:

- Corrective action and outcomes of the identified issues during qualification validation
- Any changes or updates since certification awarded
- GCP compliance of investigators in clinical trials

Some inspections (also called as flying inspection) are targeting on irregular cases and special reporting of issues. The flying inspection normally includes reality of whole data and source documents, behavior and compliance evidence of all investigators who undertake the clinical trials; the existence and protocol compliance evidence of subjects who participate in the clinical trials; and the audit traceability of all source data, submitted data, lab data, and PRO reports collected in the clinical trials, ensuring that all data are authentic, accurate, and integrated.

Certification Requirements for Trial Drugs
The investigational drugs shall be produced in a GMP-certified institution and the production process shall be strictly in accordance with the requirements of GMP. If the study drugs are locally manufactured, the drug manufacturer should receive the drug manufacturing license issued by corresponding provincial SFDA after they pass the on-site GMP inspection. If the study drugs are manufactured overseas and imported into China for the purpose of the clinical trial, a drug importing license should be applied for and approved by the SFDA after the foreign sponsors are recognized to be compliant with the Chinese regulatory standards.

Certification Requirements for Preclinical Data
Any preclinical data associated with the NDA application should be collected from an SFDA-certified GLP lab.

IMPLEMENTATION OF GCCP IN CHINA
Both China GCP and ICH/GCP have the same principles. However, China GCP has its own features as follows:

- Clinical trial should be approved by SFDA.
- Clinical trial could be only conducted at certificated clinical institutions by SFDA.
- Principle investigator must have the medical license.
- Clinical trial documents must be maintained five years after the completion of the study.

The reasons for China to insist on these principles are that China is a country with a large and diverse population with many medical institutions. For example, there are more than 8000 large-scale hospitals, and more than 4000 pharmaceutical enterprises with GMP certification in China. Provided there were no strict limitations on certification, it might result in unqualified hospitals participating in the trials without compliance of regulations. As a result, subject right could not be protected, and verifiable, reliable, integrated, and accurate data of clinical trials could not be guaranteed.

When the institution's clinical investigator is certified, the China GCP standard stipulates the following responsibilities for investigators who undertake clinical trials:

- An investigator must be qualified by training and experience and have a certificate of GCP training from one of the SFDA-recognized training programs.

- An investigator shall be familiar with the characteristics, therapeutic activities, and efficacy and safety information of the investigational drug.
- An investigator shall read and understand the details of the protocol, and conduct the trial strictly according to the protocol.
- An investigator should conduct a clinical trial in a clinical institution with a certificate of qualification to conduct a clinical trial and that has a history of GCP compliance and appropriate facilities, laboratory equipment, and clinical staff.
- An investigator should take full responsibility for educating the clinical site staff regarding the protocol and the regulations that must be followed during the trial.
- An investigator must show that he or she has sufficient time to undertake and complete the clinical trial within the period the clinical study is to be conducted, and that he or she has sufficient access to patients to meet the demands of the clinical trial.
- An investigator should explain the detailed clinical procedures, the benefits and risks of the clinical trial, and indemnification and insurance information to participating subjects. He or she should also personally sign and date the informed consent after a subject signs and dates the form.
- An investigator's priority should be to care for the subjects' safety and rights, and to ensure that any medical measures that impact psychological or physical conditions should not be acted upon unless they meet the medical needs of patients.
- An investigator is responsible for making medical treatment decisions about the clinical trial, and for ensuring that the human subjects receive proper treatment when adverse events occur during the trial.
- An investigator is responsible for the use of the investigational drug, for ensuring that the investigational drug is used only by study subjects and for ensuring that the drug's dosage and the drug's use are in accordance with the clinical study protocol. The investigators shall not provide the drug to any person not participating in the clinical study, and shall not sell the drug to any party.
- An investigator has an obligation to adopt and make a record of necessary measures, and to take all necessary measures to ensure the safety of the subjects.
- An investigator shall carefully monitor subjects for adverse events, adopt appropriate measures, and keep a record during the clinical trial. If a serious adverse event occurs during a clinical trial, the investigator shall immediately provide appropriate medical treatment to the human subject and report the event to PDA and SFDA within 24 hours of the SAE's occurrence, and immediately report the SAE to the Ethics Committee.
- An investigator shall ensure that the data are appropriately recorded on the case report form in an accurate, complete, and legal manner with signing and dating the CRF.
- An investigator has an obligation to reply to the concerns and questions of the IEC, and to permit necessary access to a sponsor's monitors/auditors as well as the auditors/inspectors from the drug administration authorities in order to ensure the quality of the clinical trial.
- An investigator shall submit the clinical study information to the IEC and obtain an approval before he or she initiates the clinical study.
- An investigator must submit a progress report or annual report to the IEC during the clinical study and prepare and sign/date the final report and then forward it to the sponsor after the clinical trial is completed.

- An investigator notifies SFDA, IEC, human subjects, and/or the sponsor when a clinical trial is terminated.

A number of measures have been taken to ensure that GCCP is used in the management of clinical trials. These include the following:

- The verification of qualification of clinical institutions. For all applicants intending to conduct a clinical trial, their institutions and the corresponding medical facilities must pass an on-site inspection (as laid out by the legislation) jointly performed by MOH and SFDA. Such inspection emphasizes that the institutions should meet the admittance criteria of hardware and software as well as qualification of staffs.
- On a yearly basis, routine regulatory inspections on the certified clinical institutions are performed by local and provincial representative of SFDA. This inspection is to examine if the staff in the institution have follow the GCP, clinical trial protocols, and clinical trial SOPs. Most common approach is randomly selecting a fixed percentage of investigator institutes (typically 15–30% samples). In general, the first task of the inspection is a thorough review of the in-house documentation, and then reviews the overall compliance of GCP, SOPs, and regulatory guidelines in the conduct of clinical studies by investigator. Once new issues are found, investigator institutes are requested to make a corrective action plan. At the next inspection, inspector will examine if the corrective actions are implemented and how improvement or corrections have been made. The routine inspections are conducted due to
  - randomized to choose a clinical trial;
  - too high or too low randomization rate;
  - simultaneously more projects at one site;
  - abnormal safety and efficacy outcome;
  - monitors address special concerns or questions;
  - indication of clinical trial is out of medical expertise at the site;
  - geographic reason;
  - black list;
  - suspect to have protocol violation.
- Under certain circumstances, a flying inspection (unannounced inspection) is performed. Such inspection is to target abnormal situations, impeached issues, or a suspicion of study misconduct existed at the certified clinical institutions. The flying inspection is usually triaged due to
  - suspicious data in the submission for drug registration;
  - public reporting to SFDA on fraudulent clinical study or involvement of questionable research practice;
  - simultaneous submissions of the same product from different applicants for drug registration;
  - the number of the clinical trials projects an institution undertook exceeding the capacities the institution has.
- Two-dimensional (country-level and local-level) drug GMP quality inspection system ensures the quality and safety of trial drugs used in the clinical trial. In addition, all quality inspectors should receive extensive trainings and certified by SFDA.

As mentioned above, the NDA technical review and approval are conducted by the CDE SFDA in China. Before any NDA approval is granted, CCD should conduct an on-site inspection to verify the NDA data. The eight aspects of such on-site regulatory inspections for NDA submission are as follows:

1. Verification of data reality and integrity
2. Science of protocol and protection of subjects in clinical trials
3. Responsibilities of IEC, including review and approval of protocol and monitoring of clinical trials performances
4. Compliance of investigators on relevant acts, rules, protocols, and operational standard
5. Compliance of subjects on protocols
6. Compliance of sponsors on relevant acts and rules and GCP
7. Audit Trail and source document integrity of all trial data
8. Maintenance records of equipments and facilities used

Regarding site inspections, any laboratory working with the clinical institution, the manufacturing line of drug entity, the company or offices of the study sponsors as well as CRO involved may receive relevant inspections.

CONCLUSION

The SFDA has made great efforts to regulate the process of clinical trials on the basis of GCP standards, strengthen international communications, and learn from advanced experience of international experts brought in to advise the SFDA, ensuring consistence with compulsory regulations and industry expectations for the global pharmaceutical community. Overall, the SFDA has started to realize it can no longer be nontransparent in its regulated activities.

As well-known, both the breadth and level of clinical research activity are on the rise in China. It is viewed that the improved regulatory environment in China would encourage more sponsoring companies can now be confident that they can derive value from data obtained in studies in China. As the Olympic spirit "One World One Dream" embodies, the SFDA would further improve the measures for drug administration of inspection and supervision in the clinical kingdom, making their progresses together with the world.

The NDA Registration Process and Critical Tips in the Conduct of Clinical Trials in China

BACKGROUND

Global drug development, as part of globalization phenomena, is coming to Asia, the emerging markets in particular. The regulatory bodies in emerging markets need to study it and understand it in order to better carrying out public health mission to their citizens.

The pharmaceutical industry is probably the most regulated industry in the world. The Chinese government has taken some actions to follow up the ICH/GCP guidelines in the administration of drug research and development processes, including the NDA application process in China. A series of broad regulatory requirements, standards, and recommendations that apply to the full fields of drug research and development have been published by SFDA of China. Given connections between the detailed nature of clinical processes and tasks and the general NDA application requirements, it is not surprising that the understanding and implementation of the NDA registration requirements in China continue to represent challenges for the pharmaceutical, biotechnology, and medical device industries, especially for the foreign pharmaceutical industry that plans to step into China pharmaceutical markets.

As well-known, the Chinese population is spread over a vast area, and its population varies greatly socioeconomically and educationally. In addition, China has a diverse history in medicine (with its unique mix of TCM and modern medical science), which presents its own intrinsic situations that makes SFDA taking a leadership to encompass not only the process modifications and other endeavors that are necessary to leverage the global regulatory standards, but also the implementation of its own NDA regulatory system that fits China's unique features.

Recognizing these factors, this text is to provide international peers with more background information on the NDA registration process in China, which has not been widely introduced outside of China.

BASICS OF AN NDA APPLICATION IN CHINA

Law and Regulation
When apply for new drug application in China, following laws and regulations should be followed:

(a) *Drug Administrative Law, People's Republic of China (DAL)*: The basic law to govern all the drug registration, distribution, and surveillance activities in China.
(b) *Regulations for implementation of the Drug Administration Law of the People's Republic of China*: More detail explanation for how to follow the DAL.
(c) *Drug Registration Regulation (DRR)*: Detail process and requirement for drug registration in China (Table 1).

Other regulations related to drug registration in China include China GCP, China GMP, and so on.

Health Authority
SFDA is the state drug regulatory body under the MOH in charge of comprehensive supervision on the safety management of food, health food, and cosmetics, and is the competent authority of drug regulation. In drug registration process, SFDA is responsible for final administrative approval for all the new drug applications, including clinical trials permission and all drug marketing applications in China. For domestic drug products, 31 provincial Food and Drug Administration, which is subsidiary body under SFDA, is responsible to accept the drug application in its administrative region. For import drug products, SFDA is responsible for acceptance of the applications. DDR is the responsible department within SFDA for the final approval and registration of an NDA application (1). Moreover, in the phase of the NDA registration, CDE, the technique review body under SFDA for all the technique dossier review, is involved (2).

National Institute for Control of Pharmaceutical and Biological Products (NICPBP) is the central official institute who takes the responsibility to assess and verify the drug quality and specifications during drug registration process. For import products, the drug assays and specification verification should be directly handled by NICPBP. For domestic products, the drug assays and specification verification may be performed by a provincial NICPBP. It is recommended to check

TABLE 1   SFDA Procedures for the Administration of an NDA Registration

Chapter 1	General Principles
Chapter 2	Basic Requirements
Chapter 3	Clinical Study of Drugs
Chapter 4	Application and Approval of New Drugs
Chapter 5	Application and Approval of Generic Drugs
Chapter 6	Application and Approval for Import Drugs
Chapter 7	Application and Approval for OTC Drugs
Chapter 8	Supplemental Application for Drug Registration
Chapter 9	Reregistration of Drugs
Chapter 10	Inspection During Drug Registration
Chapter 11	Drug Registration Standards and Insert Sheet
Chapter 12	Prescribed Timeline
Chapter 13	Reconsideration
Chapter 14	Legal Liability
Chapter 15	Miscellaneous
Annex 1	Registration Categories and Application Information Requirements of TCM and Natural Drugs
Annex 2	Registration Categories and Application Information Requirements of Chemical Drugs
Annex 3	Registration Categories and Application Information Items Requirements of Biological Products
Annex 4	Registration Items and Application Information Requirements of Supplemental Application of Drug Registration
Annex 5	Application Information Items of Drug Reregistration
Annex 6	Time Frame for Monitoring Period of New Drugs

the appropriate policy on whether the products are assayed by the local or central NICPBP at its Web site (3).

Qualification of the Foreign Applicant

According to the DRR, the applicant (foreign pharmaceutical company) should be a legally established pharmaceutical company outside of China. At the same time, to apply a drug registration application for an imported drug, the foreign applicant should use its office in China, or authorize an agent in China to handle the application. SFDA do not accept the application directly from outside of China. For a foreign drug to be accepted for submission of an application to receive approval, the drug company must conduct at least one phase II and/or phase III clinical trial in China. The clinical trial requirement may be an international multicenter trial with at least one trial center being within China and certain Chinese subject populations, which is determined by the SFDA. The SFDA also retains the right to further require a China-based phase I clinical trial before the NDA is approved for foreign drug.

TYPES AND MATERIALS OF AN NDA APPLICATION TO SFDA

Type of the Application and New Application Category

An application of drug entities that is seeking to gain SFDA approval includes applications for new drug, generic drug and imported drugs, supplemental application as well as renewal applications.

Due to the different complexity of technique requirements, there are six categories for drug applications as follows:

- *Category 1*: New chemical entity never marketed in any country, which includes the following:
  - Drug substance and its preparations made by synthesis or semisynthesis.
  - Chemical monomer (including drug substance and preparation) extracted from natural sources or by fermentation.
  - Optical isomer (including drug substance and preparation) obtained by chiral separation or synthesis.
  - Drug with fewer components derived from marketed multicomponent drug.
  - New combination products.
  - A preparation already marketed in China but with a newly added indication not yet approved in any country.
- *Category 2*: Drug preparation with changed administration route and not marketed in any country.
- *Category 3*: Drug already approved in other country, but not yet approved in China, which includes the following:
  - Drug substance and its preparation, and/or with changed dose form, but no change of administration route.
  - Combination preparations and/or with changed dose form, but no change of administration route.
  - Preparations with changed administration route and marketed ex-China.
  - A preparation already marketed in China but with a newly added indication approved ex-China.
- *Category 4*: Drug substance and its preparation with changed acid or alkaline radicals (or metallic elements), but without any pharmacological change, and the original drug entity already approved in China.
- *Category 5*: Drug preparation with changed dose form, but no change of administration route, and the original preparation already approved in China.
- *Category 6*: Drug substance or preparation following national standard. This category refers to generic drug application.

Any applications of import drugs should follow either category 1 or category 3.

Dossier Requirements

According to the features of an NDA application to be submitted by a sponsor, SFDA requires the sponsor to submit the application, supportive documentation, and material package for review and approval of the drug application. All the submitted dossiers should be written or translated into Chinese. The application dossier should follow the required format of the dossier list. A CTD dossier can be accepted by SFDA, but is mandatory to be translated into Chinese. The major dossiers must be submitted to SFDA and categorized as major four modules, which include

1. *Module 1*: Summary documents.
   (a) Name of the drugs.
   (b) *Certified documents*: These documents include the following:

     (i) Certificate document to demonstrate the drug product registration status in the manufacturer country with notarization and embassy legalization.

     (ii) GMP of the manufacturer with notarization and embassy legalization.

     (iii) Letter of Authorization to local application agency (notarized).

     (iv) Patent declaration.

  (c) Objectives and basis for research and development.

  (d) Summary of main study work.

  (e) Draft of packaging insert, note to the draft, and latest literature.

  (f) Design of packaging and labeling.

2. *Module 2*: Pharmaceutical data.

  (a) Summary of pharmaceutical study.

  (b) Research information and relevant literature of the production process of the drug substance, research information, and relevant literature of formula and process of the preparations.

  (c) Study information and relevant literature for the chemical structure and components determination.

  (d) Study information and literature for quality specification.

  (e) Draft of quality specification and notes, and providing reference standard.

  (f) Test report of drug sample.

  (g) The source, test report, and quality specification of drug substance and excipient.

  (h) Stability study and relevant literatures.

  (i) Selection basis and quality specification of immediate packing material and container.

3. *Module 3*: Pharmacology and toxicology study information.

  (a) Summary of pharmacology and toxicology study.

  (b) Primary pharmacodynamics study and literatures.

  (c) General pharmacology study and literatures.

  (d) Acute-/single-dose toxicity study and literature.

  (e) Repeated-dose toxicity study and literatures.

  (f) Special safety study and literatures of hypersensitive (topical, systemic, and phototoxicity), hemolytic, and topical irritative (blood vessel, skin, mucous membrane, and muscle) reaction related to topical and systemic use of the drugs.

  (g) Study and relevant literatures on pharmacodynamics, toxicity, and pharmacokinetics change caused by the interactions among multiple components in the combination products.

  (h) Study and literature of mutagenicity test.

  (i) Study and literature of reproductive toxicity.

  (j) Study and literature of carcinogenicity test.

  (k) Study and literature of drug dependence.

  (l) Study and literature of preclinical pharmacokinetics.

4. *Module 4*: Clinical study information.

  (a) Summary of global clinical study information.

  (b) Clinical study protocol.

  (c) Investigator's Brochure.

  (d) Draft of informed consent form, approval of the Ethics Committee.

  (e) Clinical study report.

NDA APPLICATION PROCESS IN CHINA

Current registration process for new entities in China is a two-submission and two-approval process. In the DRR, chapter 3 provides a framework for the conduct of clinical trials within China, and authorizes clinical trials to be conducted in China in accordance with GCP. Generally speaking, the applicant should firstly register a new drug with SFDA, and receive approval to conduct phase I, phase II, and phase III clinical trials, and conduct those trials within China prior to submitting a final NDA application. Until the clinical trial required is finished, the NDA applicant may submit the clinical trial report to SFDA for Import Drug License/Local Manufacturer License.

The detailed process is as follows:

1. Before application of the new entity in China, the applicant should review the DRR and its annexes to find out the correct drug category of the product and prepare the package of registration dossiers according to the requirements. Specific electronic application form can be downloaded from SFDA Web site and then filled, signed, and sealed by the company or authorized agency.
2. The agency then submits the package of application dossiers to the acceptance office of SFDA for format checking. If the format checking is passed, an acceptance notice and a notice for drug registration assay are issued.
3. The package of the application dossiers is then handled by CDE for technique review.
4. Meanwhile, the applicant should submit the three batches of the drug samples used in the clinical trials to NICPBP for assays and specification verification. The acceptance and failure report of the quality evaluation by NICPBP will be used as part of the technique reviews.
5. After technique review, CDE will submit the review conclusion report to the DDR for final administrative approval. Following then, SFDA issues the clinical trial permission or Import Drug License.
6. Regarding the NDA application for locally manufacturing license of the new entities, an on-site regulatory GMP inspection on the drug manufacturing facilities should be passed before the CDE makes its positive recommendation to the executive department of SFDA. The acquirement of local manufacturing license means the approval of the new entity for marketing in China.

The Import Drug License is usually suggested in two ways. The foreign sponsor is permitted to import the trial drugs into China for the purpose of clinical study only. For those drugs that are approved to market both outside and inside of China, the foreign sponsors may import the drugs into China for marketing. It should be aware that raw materials for the new drug manufacturing should be approved respectively by SFDA when the NDA is approved. This is involved with the GMP individual validation for each raw material. Moreover, the Import Drug License is effective for five years. At least six months before the expiration date, the license should be renewed by SFDA.

LOGISTICAL REQUIREMENTS OF THE NDA REGISTRATION IN CHINA

Clinical Trial Requirement

It is important to know that the clinical trials should be only conducted at the local certified clinical institutions in China. Any clinical data collected from the uncertified clinical institutions will be rejected by SFDA. For the new drugs under the category 1 and 2, numbers of subjects who participate in the clinical trials should be reached to meet the statistical criteria and the minimal cases required. The minimal subject cases involved in the drug treatment arm of the clinical trials are accounted for 20 to 30 in phase I, 100 in phase II, 300 in phase III, and 2000 in phase IV.

For the new drugs under the category 3 and 4, a human pharmacokinetic study and a randomized controlled clinical trial involved with at least 100 pairs of subjects should be conducted. Once the new drug is applying to claim more than one indication, it is mandatory respectively to enroll no less than 60 pairs of subjects in clinical trials with each indication.

For the category 5 and 6, clinical bioequivalence studies may be replaced to clinical trials depending on the drug characteristics.

Specific Review and Approval Process

SFDA may use specific approval process (fast track) for the following new drugs:

- New active ingredients and its preparation extracted from TCM, natural drugs, or preparation made of material from plant, animal, and minerals, which have not been marketed in China.
- Drug raw material and its preparations, and biological products that have not been marketed domestically or outside of China.
- New antiviral drug for AIDS and drug used for diagnosis and prevention of AIDS, cancer, and orphan drug.
- New drugs that treat diseases for which there is no effective therapy.
- According to an application by sponsor, SFDA shall decide whether to use specific approval for the drug application.

NDA Application Fee

Currently, the application fee for the import drug application is at 45,300 RMB, which is about $5850. For the clinical trial permission, the application fee is at 3500 RMB (around $452), and local manufacturing license at 25,000 RMB for category 1 and 2 new entity (around $3227), 20,000 RMB for category 3 and 4 new entity (around $2580), 10,000 RMB for category 5 new entity (around $1290), and 1500 RMB for me-too entity (around $195).

NDA Reviewing Timeline

According to China's DRR, the technical review should be in accordance with the following prescribed timelines:

- Ninety days for a new clinical study, and 80 days if a drug meets the requirements of special approval from SFDA to expedite. This can be granted if the drug in question addresses unmet medical needs within China.
- One hundred and fifty days for production of new drug, and 120 days if a drug meets the requirements of special approval.
- One hundred and sixty days for registration of generic drugs or a change in dosage form of a marketed drug.
- Forty days for a supplemental application if a technical review is needed.
- SFDA administrative review timeline is 20 to 30 days.

All these days are referred to actual working days, which exclude public holidays and nonworking off days.

Currently, the review duration for the NDA application may take longer as expected. This factor should be considered from two sides of the story. In some cases of technique reviews, the package of the NDA application contains incomplete materials, which triggers the inquiry process to the applicants by CDE. The inquiry process usually takes additional working days depending on the length of feedback cycles. On the other hand, it is recognized that the quantities of the NDA application cases SFDA and CDE are reviewing exceed much their resources. However, it is expected that the late unusual situation would be improved soon. It is suggested that an appropriate plan would be better made when the NDA registration timeline is scheduled accordingly.

CRITICAL TIPS IN THE CONDUCTION OF CLINICAL TRIALS IN CHINA

Legal and Regulatory Basis for Drug Researches
Major laws, regulations, and guidelines related to drug researches in China should be followed, which include the following:

- Drug Administration Law of People's Republic of China
- Regulations for Implementation of the Drug Administration Law of the People's Republic of China
- DRR
- Regulation for Drug GCP
- Provisions for Handling Malpractices in Drug Research and Registration (interim)
- Rules for Drug Clinical Study
- Provisional Rules for Drug Research Record
- Measures for Clinical Research Supervision
- Guideline of Drug Clinical Trial
- Rules for Statistics in Clinical Study

Characteristics of Clinical Trials Conductions in China
Although China's GCP standards are essentially the same as those in the ICH E6 guideline, there are some differences. Some examples of such differences between China GCP standards and the ICF E6 guideline include the following:

- ICH E6 GCP calls for investigators to report only unexpected and serious AEs to IRB/ECs, but the GCP standards in China (chap. 3, Article 10) state that, "any serious events that occur during the trials shall be reported to the Ethics Committee."
- The Chinese GCP standard states that the investigator must sign the informed consent form, while the ICH E6 GCP states that the subject and "the person who conducted the informed consent discussion" need to sign the informed consent.
- SFDA requires the clinical institution to set up a special administrative office with full-time staff to provide oversight on clinical trial activities and outcomes. The office must strictly implement relevant laws and regulations and establish a QA system for the clinical trials according to GCP. QA is responsible for auditing the authenticity and standardization of the clinical research, for ensuring that SOPs are adhered to, for ensuring the science and compliance in the

clinical trials are adhered to, for ensuring that the safety and rights of the subjects are protected, and for ensuring the accuracy and completeness of the clinical data obtained. Some elements of these responsibilities are directly assigned to the investigators in ICH E6.

- All clinical trials in China should be conducted within clinical institutions (hospitals) that obtained, from SFDA, a certificate of qualification to serve as an authorized clinical trial site in relevant medical specialties.
- Without a certificate of qualification to conduct a clinical trial (issued by SFDA), a clinical institution cannot undertake a clinical trial in China. Such a certificate is granted after an application and then the pass after an on-site regulatory inspection.
- The drug products used in the clinical trials must be submitted to NICPBP for an assay. Without the certificate of analysis issued by NICPBP, the Institutional Ethics Committee (IEC) will not approve the clinical study.
- Clinical studies cannot be initiated at clinical institutions until the sponsor and investigator receive the approval letter issued by SFDA.
- Clinical studies must be initiated only after the IEC issues an approval letter. The IEC should be registered to SFDA. The submission package provided by the investigators and sponsors to the IEC generally includes the following:
  - The SFDA approval letter
  - Certificate of Analysis for the drug issued by NICPBP or corresponding institutes
  - Investigator's Brochure
  - Clinical Protocol (attached with the list of principal investigator and clinical staff members and their resumes)
  - Sample of informed consent form
  - Case report form

It is noted that imported drugs, biological products, and blood products should be tested by NICPBP; other chemical products or TCM products may be tested by corresponding provincial drug control institutions or by sponsors themselves.

Major Provisions to Run a Clinical Trial in China
Before Clinical Trials
While the clinical trial permission is applied to SFDA, the sponsor may prepare the initiation of clinical studies. First of all, the sponsor should look up for the certified clinical institutions that meet the medical specialty and other logistic requirements of the clinical trial. A prestudy site visit is necessary for sponsor to verify the qualification of the clinical institutions that will undertake the clinical trial. The sponsor shall sign a clinical trial agreement with the leading and the participating institutes selected for the clinical study, and then provide the SFDA approval document, the draft informed consent form, Investigator's Brochure, and jointly improve the clinical trial protocol with reference to the technical guidelines. When a clinical trial agreement is negotiated with a clinical institution, a number of documents must be collected from the clinical institutions. Most of these are required by the SFDA regulations and the IEC submission, although some sponsors may require their own additional documents. Both the sponsor and the investigator must have copies of

each of these documents. The conclusion after IEC reviews the clinical studies could be

- agreed;
- agreed after necessary revision;
- disagreed;
- terminated or suspended previous approved clinical trial.

Once the agreed conclusion is obtained, the sponsor may initiate the trials at the selected clinical institutions.

Trainings on the investigator and relevant staffs who participate in clinical trials are mandatory and should be completed before the trial is initiated. These trainings include, but are not limited to, the following:

- GCP
- Clinical protocol
- Trial flow procedure
- Relevant SOPs
- ICF requirements and procedure
- Establishment and maintenance of source documents and study files
- CRF completion
- Trial milestone expectation

During Clinical Trials

If a sponsor discovers that an institution conducting clinical study is in violation of relevant regulations, or is not following the clinical study protocol, the sponsor shall try to correct the situation. For serious violation, the sponsor may request to suspend or stop the clinical study and shall submit a written report to SFDA and the relevant IEC.

SFDA may request the sponsor to amend the clinical study protocol, suspend or stop the clinical study in any of the following circumstances:

- The Ethics Committee has failed to perform its duty.
- The safety of the subjects cannot be effectively ensured.
- Serious adverse event was not timely reported.
- The clinical study progress report was not timely submitted.
- The completion of the clinical study is more than three years behind the original completion date and there are still no results that can be evaluated.
- Evidence that the investigational drug is not any effective.
- Quality problems in the drug used for clinical trials.
- Fraud in the clinical study.
- Other circumstances violating GCP.

Study monitoring the conduction of clinical trials is one of regulatory requirements sponsor should take. The focus of the study monitoring should be placed on

- protection of rights, safety, and well-being of human subjects;
- subjects status, including enrolment rate, eligible rate, and compliant rate to the approved protocol/amendments;
- principal investigator behaviors, including compliance with the approved protocol/amendments, SOPs, GCP, and other regulatory requirements;

• reporting data integrity, including accuracy, completeness and reliability, adequate informed consent process, and consistency of medical records and lab results relative to CRF.

The frequency of the study monitoring should be dependent on the actual length and needs of clinical trials.

During the clinical study, in case a large range or unexpected adverse reaction or serious adverse event occurs, or there is evidence to prove that the investigational drug has significant quality problems, SFDA or PDA may adopt emergency mandatory administrative measures to suspend or stop the clinical study, and the sponsor and institutions must immediately stop the study. Any SAE should be reported promptly to SFDA. A national safety Web report system has been set up.

At the End of Clinical Trials

It is important that the reported data completely and accurately reflect the findings and events of the clinical trials. It is well recognized that the good data management practice is the foundation of GCP. The key areas of the good data management practice have been regulated by SFDA as follows:

• Procedures for the entry, verification, and validation management of reported data
• Management for data queries of any errors, omissions or items requiring clarification or changes to collected data detected during the trial, by computer edits or during the data analysis
• Expected requirements for database lock
• Measures for statistical analysis of the reported data
• Generation of a clinical study report

Outcomes of any clinical trials should mandatorily be reported to SFDA in the clinical study report setting. When the CDE is technologically reviewing the NDA application, the sponsor or relevant investigators may be invited to have defenses on the questions and give information about the project and/or the outcomes.

Preparation of Investigational Drugs

• The sponsor shall provide the institutions with the investigational drugs and comparator drugs (expect for phase IV clinical trials) together with drug samples, at no charge. The sponsor shall bear the costs related to conducting the clinical study.
• The investigational drugs shall be produced in a workshop that meets GMP requirements and the production process shall be strictly in accordance with the requirements of GMP.
• The sponsor may inspect the investigational drug itself in accordance with the drug's standards approved by SFDA. But vaccine, blood products, and other bioproducts designated by SFDA as well as investigational drugs produced overseas must be inspected by a drug control institute designated by SFDA. The drug may not be used before it has passed the inspection. The sponsor assumes all responsibility for the quality of the investigational drug.

Time Demand of Starting Trial

A clinical study shall start within three years of approval. The approval date of IEC is a starting day. Otherwise, the approval certificate shall automatically become null and void. A reapplication shall be submitted to resume the study.

International Multicenter Clinical Study

A foreign sponsor who wants to conduct an international multicenter clinical study shall apply at SFDA in accordance with the following provisions:

- The drug used for an international multicenter clinical study shall be one already registered in a foreign country or in phase II or phase III clinical trials. An application for an international multicenter clinical study of new preventive vaccine from a foreign sponsor still not registered outside of China shall not be accepted.
- In approving an international multicenter clinical study in China, SFDA may first request the sponsor to firstly conduct the phase I clinical trials in China, if needed.
- During a study conducted in China, the sponsor shall, in accordance with the relevant regulations, report to SFDA any serious adverse events or unexpected adverse events that occur in any country.
- Upon the completion of the study, the sponsor shall submit the complete clinical study report to SFDA.
- Data generated from an international multicenter clinical trial used for drug registration in China shall be in accordance with the relevant provision of this regulation, and the sponsor shall submit the complete research information of the study.

CONCLUSION

The SFDA has made efforts to regulate Chinese pharmaceutical industry based on global GCP standards. Thus, the process and results of clinical trials are ensured to be more scientific, reliable, and integrated. The improved regulatory environment would encourage international pharmaceutical regulators can now be confident to conduct global mutual recognition of the drug researching data. The Chinese authorities clearly realize that there is a long way to go before they may achieve the objective. They are thus continuing to intensify international exchange, learn advanced techniques, and experiences, making their regulations more synergetic with global standard practice.

Medical Devices and Clinical Research in China

Earl W. Hulihan

Medidata Solutions Worldwide, New York, New York, U.S.A.

Daniel Liu

Medidata Solutions Worldwide, Beijing, P.R. China

BACKGROUND

The introduction and implementation of GCP in the field of medical devices in China has not been widely published outside of China. China has a vast population and area, which has given attractive marketing baits in the field of medical devices.

Although its population and area vary greatly socioeconomically and educationally, the improved health and quality of life of population and updated public health and therapeutic interventions support the idea that the stronger overall economic status of China is substantial.

The regulatory administration of medical devices in China has a shorter history compared with the drug regulations. Much not to our surprise, the existence in the issues and imperfect regulatory system in the field of medical devices in China has brought the SFDA of China more sharpened attentions and increase in the regulatory administration and guidelines developments covering this field. Most recent evidences of regulatory processes for medical devices in China have demonstrated the popular perceptions and promising value of medical devices developments and applications. This paper is intended to be a brief introduction of the regulatory registration and requirements of clinical trials in the field of medical devices in China. Of course, it should be realized that no article can be a substitute for regular interaction and passive consultations with regulators during the planning stages of medical devices regulatory registration. The regular consultation to SFDA may facilitate accurate and timely keeping of the most recent regulations.

LEGAL BASIS FOR MEDICAL DEVICES SUPERVISION

Regulations Basis

Since 1996, a series of regulatory guidelines, acts, and instructions have been respectively come into force during the establishment and development of Chinese medical devices administration system. These regulatory documents are constructing the historical trail of the medical device administration system by SFDA in China. When a new medical devices registration was or is submitted to SFDA in China, laws and regulations promulgated by SFDA and followed by sponsors include the following:

- The first guideline "Interim rule for clinical tests of medical devices" in March 1996.
- "Guideline of medical advice regulatory administration" in April 2000.
- "Regulations for medical device registration" (interim) in April 2000. This 2000 version was retired while the 2004 version below was implemented.
- "Rule for the classifications of medical devices" in April 2000.
- "Administrational provisions for medical devices standardization" in May 2002.
- "Measures for ADR reporting and monitoring of medical advices" in January 2004.
- "Provisions for clinical trials of medical devices" in April 2004.
- "Administration guideline of medical device GMP" in July 2004.
- "Provision for the administration of instruction, labeling, and package mark of medical devices" in July 2004.
- "Provision for administration of medical device registration" in August 2004.
- "Guideline on the format and requirements of submission documents" in March 2005.

Other regulations related to medical devices registration and applications in China include GLP, GCP, GMP, and so on. Currently, SFDA is planning to

- expedite the revision of medical devices standards;
- revise the existing regulations to harmonize more the Chinese regulatory practices with global standards;

- intensify instruction, coordination, and supervision to standard revision;
- improve registration approval program;
- enforce regulatory programs by instructing and supervising the national registration process;
- encourage to learn and adapt advanced administration and techniques of medical devices registration;
- strengthen the training and education programs on monitors and inspectors of medical devices;
- enforce the priority concept and consciousness of device safety.

In China, medical device classification is the basis to determine regulatory requirements. There are three categories of medical devices set by SFDA, which are as follows:

- *Class I*: Any devices whose safety and effectiveness can be ensured through routine administration.
- *Class I*: Any devices that further control is required to ensure their safety and effectiveness.
- *Class III*: Any devices that are implanted into the human body, or used for life support or sustenance, or pose potential risk to the human body and thus must be strictly controlled in respect to safety and effectiveness.

In the Chinese regulatory environment, it should be essential that more technique files required by SFDA, mandatory submission of Chinese product specifications for review and approval by SFDA, and conduction of sample testing at certified testing centers are expected. Moreover, all of foreign-manufactured medical device, including Class I medical devices, are required to have registration and approval by SFDA before they are marketed.

Regulatory Body System
Within SFDA body, Department of Medical Device (DMD) (Fig. 2) is composed of five divisions, direct and indirect affiliated centers. The Division of Research Evaluation has responsibilities for

- organizing to draft and revise the official standard for medical devices (including medical dressing, chemical and biochemical diagnostic reagents in vitro), and undertaking the assignments related with International Organization for Standardization;
- formulating the list of classified medical devices in consultation with health department under the State Council, and organizing the management of classification of medical devices;
- assessing the qualification of testing institutions;
- formulating the list of medical measuring products.
- supervising and inspecting medical device manufacturers and investigator sites;
- assessing the qualification of institutions and good manufacturing practice for medical devices;
- implement medical device adverse event monitoring and re-evaluation

The Division of Product Registration I is responsible for active medical instruments and II for passive medical instruments. Both divisions take leaderships in

- approval and registration of medical devices (including import medical dressings, chemical and biochemical diagnostic reagents in vitro);
- assessment of the qualification of medical device clinical trial bases;

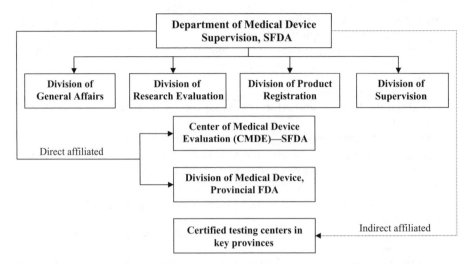

FIGURE 2 Structure of DMD SFDA.

- approval of clinical trials of medical devices;
- management of the database of medical device review experts;
- issuing of the medical device export certificates;
- application acceptance and certificate issue for medical devices.

The Division of Manufacture and Marketing Supervision plays a key role in

- drafting and revising the provisions for implementation of medical device manufacturing and marketing practice and supervising their implementation;
- implement and supervise the certificate process for medical device manufacturing and marketing affairs
- implement and supervise the exportation of designated medical devices
- execute the examination and evaluation process for manufacturing quality control of medical devices

Those affiliated centers play technique and administrative roles in supports of DMD regulatory activities. The strategy of medical devices registration in developed countries is to centralize the review and approval of devices submission and dispersed supervision of device management. However the Chinese medical devices regulatory registration feature a model of three-line parallel way, that is, medical devices registration (Fig. 3), manufacturing line certificate and marketing permit are managed by SFDA and provincial FDA, respectively, as predefined regulatory responsibilities. The China model benefits the direct and real regulatory managements but leads to discrepancy of approval standard and unbalanced supervision on medical devices by provinces.

Authorization Requirements on Device Registration for Foreign Companies in China

According to the Provision for administration of medical device registration, the applicant (foreign devices company) should be a legally established devices company outside of China. At the same time, to apply a device registration application as an imported device, the foreign applicant should use its office in China, or

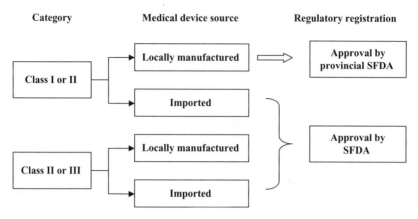

FIGURE 3 Medical devices regulatory approval in China.

authorize an agent in China to handle the device registration. When a Chinese registration agent is contracted, this foreign device company should issue an authorization letter to the agent on the assistance of the device registration in China. Also, this
agent must be a legal company located in China, and have a valid business license.
The copy of business license of this Chinese agent with its official company's seal
must be attached with the device submission, together with an acceptance letter
with its company's seal from the Chinese agent. SFDA does not accept the application directly from outside of China. For a foreign device that is required to conduct
a clinical trial before it is approved for marketing, the foreign device company must
plan to conduct at least one phase II and/or phase III clinical trial in China. If a Chinese agent is contracted for the clinical trial, the authorization letter to this Chinese
agent must be attached, including the transfer of responsibility to report the adverse
events to the SFDA and act as the contact person on the AE with the SFDA. When a
Chinese agent is appointed as the Chinese distribution agent for the foreign device
company, the original authorization letter issued from the foreign device company
and the acceptance letter from the Chinese agent must be attached with the official
company's seal together with the copy of the business license of the Chinese agent
to SFDA for the review and approval of the device registration. The registration
filing requirements for a Chinese agent to be appointed to provide the after-sale services in China by the foreign device company to SFDA are the same as the one for
the Chinese distributor agent.

TYPES AND MATERIALS OF A MEDICAL DEVICE REGISTRATION
APPLICATION TO SFDA

Process of the New and Renewal Application for Medical Devices
Registration
Generally speaking, a device that meets the following criteria should be registered
as a new device product:

* The first time entering the Chinese market or the new device product
* Change to a new manufacturing location
* Adding new models or new accessories

- Technical improvements that impact device specifications
- Adding a new indication or intended use

Changes in manufacture's name, device trade name, and after-sale services agent in China should be registered as the amendment device registration to SFDA.

The Class I device registration from the foreign companies should be following the process as given below:

- Sponsor drafts Chinese specifications based on international and Chinese national standards and format.
- Sponsor submits a set of application dossiers to the acceptance office of SFDA for format checking. If the format checking is passed, an acceptance notice is issued.
- The set of application dossiers is transferred to CMDE for technical review.
- The set of the application dossiers is then handled by CMDE for technique review.
- CMDE issues supplement notice, if necessary.
- The sponsor prepares and submit supplement dossier as required.
- After technique review, CMDE will submit the approval or nonapproval conclusion to the SFDA for final administrative approval.
- SFDA issues the import device license if no supplement dossier is required.

Total timelines for Class I device registration is usually taken for five months or so. The Class II and III device registration that does not require clinical trials should follow the similar process as the Class I above. However, before submission of the set of application dossiers to SFDA, the sample testing at the SFDA-certified testing centers should be completed and the testing reports should be attached with the Class II or III filing. The timeline for Class II or III device registration that does not require the clinical trials would take about seven to eight months. Any new Class II or III devices, which have not been approved anywhere in the world and are implant products, or the first medical device product of the foreign country applying for Chinese registration (even it was already approved in the foreign countries), must complete the sample testing at the SFDA-certified testing center and then clinical trials before they are submitted to SFDA for the review and approval. In addition, CMDE would organize clinical experts review meeting to go through the clinical trials report when CMDE is doing technical reviews (Fig. 4). Total timeline for the Class II or III that require clinical trials may normally need around 15 to 18 months (closely depending on clinical trials period).

In China, every device registration is valid for four years and renewal application must be submitted six months before the license expires. The whole renewal process is similar to the new application. When the renewal application is submitted to SFDA, the sample testing should be repeated again and the postmarket quality and safety surveillance report should be attached with the application.

Dossiers Requirements for the Medical Device Registration in China

According to the features of a device registration to be submitted by a sponsor, SFDA requires the sponsor to submit the application, legal and technical documents, and testing report issued by SFDA-certified testing center (if applicable) for review and approval of the device application. All the submitted dossiers should be written or translated into Chinese. The application dossier should follow the required format of the dossier list. The English specification and documents is

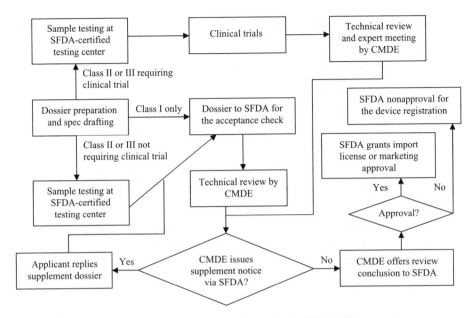

FIGURE 4 General process for medical device registration by SFDA in China.

accepted by SFDA, but are mandatory to be translated into Chinese simultaneously. The major dossiers to be submitted to SFDA may be categorized as three parts of 12 items, which includes

- Legal documents
  - *SFDA registration application*: Information in the application form must contain correct sponsor's name, address, contact numbers of the manufacturer, product name, models accessories name, catalog numbers, registration agent, and after-sale agent in China, and also be consistent with the one in the marketing approval certification from foreign countries.
  - *Legal production qualification*: All files of legal production qualification should be valid and notarized by notary public, which include
    - For U.S. device product, the Form FDA 2891 (annual registration of device establishment) should be attached.
    - For other countries, the business license of the foreign company should be enclosed as well as relevant device product certificate.
  - *Authorization on registration in China*: If a foreign company is not using its own office to submit the device application, the original authorization letter from the foreign company to a Chinese registration representative on product registration in China should be attached. This Chinese registration representative must be a legal company with a valid business license located in China. The copy of business letter of the Chinese representative with its official seal and acceptance letter from this Chinese registration representative with its official seal should be enclosed with the application.
  - *Marketing approval from foreign government*: The marketing approval evidences include U.S. approved device file, such as FDA 510(k) letter, original CFG

(Certificate to foreign government), EU-approved devices files, such as CE approval certificate and original declaration of conformity letter, and other countries files or equivalent, such as free sales certificate, and so on. All files submitted should be notarized by a notary public. Also, a list containing all device product information, such as models, components, accessories, and so on, should be attached.

- *Quality guarantee letter*: The original copy of the quality guarantee letter issued by the foreign device company, which certifies that the device product being registered and sold in China is identical to the one already approved and sold in the foreign countries.
- *Authorization letter to a Chinese agent*: If a distributor and/or representative is appointed to conduct the clinical trial and/or sales of the device product in China, the original transfer letter or authorization letter of responsibility to a Chinese agent, including the reporting of adverse event to the SFDA and acting as the contact person with the SFDA, should be attached. The acceptance letter from the Chinese agent with its official seal and a copy of business license of this Chinese agent should be enclosed, too.
- *Authorization letter for after-sale services in China (if applicable)*: When a Chinese agent is appointed as the after-sale service for the foreign company in China, an original authorization letter to the Chinese agent from the foreign company, an acceptance letter from the Chinese agent with its official seal, and the copy of business license of the Chinese agent must be submitted with the device application to SFDA.
- *Self-guarantee declaration letter*: This original letter from the foreign company certifies to guarantee the accuracy and reliability of submitted documents with a legal responsibility for the statement enclosed in the submission. This letter should indicate the full list of all documents to be guaranteed.
- Technical documents
  - *Chinese specification*: Any original specification should be translated into Chinese. The Chinese specification must comply with the National and International Standards (ISO, IEC, or GB). An authorization letter with a list of all model specification and information of components, catalog numbers/codes, and accessories should be enclosed. When a Chinese registration agent is appointed, the original authorization letter issued by the foreign company to the Chinese agent should be attached, claiming that the Chinese agent may draft the Chinese specification, but the foreign company will take full responsibility for the device quality guarantee.
  - *Package inset*: One real sample of the package insert in the original language should be enclosed together with Chinese label or insert information. The sample includes, but is not limited to, instruction book or inset, user's guide, label or product brochure, and so on. The real sample should be signed on the front page to verify the validity of all documents with the notary public. The Chinese label or insert must comply with the provisions for the administration of instructions, labeling, and package mark of medical devices issued by SFDA.
  - *Clinical trial report (if applicable)*: Any devices that require conduction of clinical trials in China should provide clinical contract, protocol, IEC approval, and clinical report to SFDA. For those devices that do not require clinical trials, the clinical report or published literatures that were submitted to

the foreign government for the purpose of the device registration must be enclosed.
- *Testing report issued by SFDA-certified testing center (if applicable)*: The certified testing center may be freely selected from SFDA list for applicants to complete the testing process. Only testing report issued by the SFDA-certified testing center within one year will be valid and acceptable to SFDA. When a series of similar models is to be tested, applicant may select one of models to conduct the testing, but this mode must be typical and the applicant should provide the rationales for such selection.

LOGISTICAL REQUIREMENTS OF MEDICAL DEVICE CLINICAL TRIALS IN CHINA

In China, there are two types of device' clinical uses, that is, clinical investigational use and clinical validated use of medical devices. Any medical devices that are newly created, developed, or invented should conduct the investigational use to confirm their safety and effectiveness as well as the mechanism principles, basic structure, and functions of medical devices. Applicants who wish to conduct these investigations may be granted exemptions from clinical trials as per the SFDA regulations, and undertake clinical trials by filing an applications to SFDA. Any medical devices that imitate or copy the existing device product should complete clinical validation use to verify that their safety and effectiveness as well as relevant functions and structures parameters are clinically equivalent to the existing device products approved. The validation use may be performed by either filing a clinical trial application or granting exemptions from clinical trials as per SFDA regulations. Any clinical trials should be approved by SFDA and IEC before the trials are initiated. It is important to know that the clinical trials should be only conducted at the SFDA-certified clinical institutions in China. Any clinical data collected from the uncertified clinical institutions will be rejected by SFDA. The clinical trial process should comply with the global GCP and SFDA regulatory requirements. Table 2 summarizes the clinical dossier requirements of clinical and nonclinical trials-required device registration.

Before a clinical trial application of medical devices is planned to submit to SFDA, the sponsor should ensure that the following requirements have been met for the device product to be registered:

- Complying with the existing standards, or state and professional criteria of the same type of other device products approved.
- Having self-testing reports.
- Completing the qualification assay report with "pass" conclusion issued by an SFDA-certified testing center.
- Having an animal trial report for the innovated implanted device product to be used in human first time, or any type of other device products that need to confirm the safety via the animal studies.
- For the Class III implanted device or any device that is innovated based on the theory of Chinese traditional medicine, the protocol should be set up in a file in the CMDE.

TABLE 2 Clinical Trial Dossier Requirements for Medical Device Regulatory Registration in China

Category	Status of device companies	Basic conditions	Clinical dossiers required
Class III	No matter what type of device products.	Neither SFDA nor foreign government approves the device product to be registered for marketing.	Must submit the clinical trial data conducted in China.
Class III implanted devices	Company has no device products marketed in China.	Devices never approved by SFDA but approved by foreign regulatory agency for marketing.	Must submit the clinical data conducted in China.
	Company has device products marketed in China.	A. Meeting all criteria as given below: Devices never approved by SFDA but approved by foreign regulatory agency for marketing. The QA system of the company has passed the regulatory inspection, but the device products are not covered.	Submissions for device products locally manufactured must contain the relevant clinical data required. Submissions for device products foreign company manufactures must contain the clinical data that were submitted to foreign governments for the purpose of the device registration for marketing. Such clinical data should be reviewed and approved by the authorized experts SFDA appoints.
		B. Meeting all criteria as given below: Devices never approved by SFDA but approved by foreign regulatory agency for marketing. The QA systems for both the company and the device product category have passed the regulatory inspection and are still valid. The company has not received any complaints of its products marketed in the passing four years in China (if there is a complaint, the criteria A above should be followed).	Submissions for device products locally manufactured must contain the relevant clinical data required. Submissions for device products foreign company manufactures must contain the clinical data that were submitted to foreign governments for the purpose of the device registration for marketing.

Company has device products marketed in China, and the device product to be registered is the similar type approved but not the same model of device product.	A. Meeting all criteria as given below: Devices never approved by SFDA but approved by foreign regulatory agency for marketing. The QA system of the company has passed the regulatory inspection but the model to be registered is not covered. B. Meeting all criteria as given below: Devices never approved by SFDA but approved by foreign regulatory agency for marketing. The QA systems for both the company and the device product model have passed the regulatory inspection and are still valid. The company has not received any complaints of its products marketed in the passing four years in China (if there is a complaint, the criteria A above should be followed)	Submissions for device products locally manufactured must contain the relevant clinical data required. Submissions for device products foreign company manufactures must contain the clinical data that were submitted to foreign governments for the purpose of the device registration for marketing. Such clinical data should be reviewed and approved by the authorized experts SFDA appoints. Submissions for device products locally manufactured must contain the relevant clinical data required. Submissions for device products foreign company manufactures must contain the clinical data that were submitted to foreign governments for the purpose of the device registration for marketing.

(Continued)

TABLE 2 Clinical Trial Dossier Requirements for Medical Device Regulatory Registration in China (*Continued*)

Category	Status of device companies	Basic conditions	Clinical dossiers required
	Company has device products marketed in China, and the device product to be registered is the same model but there are different specifications of the device product.	A. Meeting all criteria as given below: Devices never approved by SFDA but approved by foreign regulatory agency for marketing. The QA system of the company has passed the regulatory inspection but the specification to be registered is not covered. B. Meeting all criteria as given below: Devices never approved by SFDA but approved by foreign regulatory agency for marketing. The QA systems for both the company and the device product model/specification have passed the regulatory inspection and are still valid. The company has not received any complaints of its products marketed in the passing four years in China (if there is a complaint, the criteria A above should be followed).	Submissions for device products locally manufactured must contain the relevant clinical data required. Submissions for device products foreign company manufactures must contain the clinical data that were submitted to foreign governments for the purpose of the device registration for marketing. Such clinical data should be reviewed and approved by the authorized experts SFDA appoints. Submissions for device products locally manufactured must contain the relevant clinical data that were submitted for the regulatory registration of the same type of the existing device product by the company. Submissions for device products foreign company manufactures must contain the clinical data that were submitted to foreign governments for the purpose of the device registration for marketing.

Other Class III device product			
Company has no device products marketed in China.	Devices never approved by SFDA but approved by foreign regulatory agency for marketing.		Submissions for device products locally manufactured must contain the relevant clinical data required. Submissions for device products foreign company manufactures must contain the clinical data that were submitted to foreign governments for the purpose of the device registration for marketing. Such clinical data should be reviewed and approved by the authorized experts SFDA appoints.
Company has device products marketed in China, but the device product to be registered is the new product in China.	A. Meeting all criteria as given below: Devices never approved by SFDA but approved by foreign regulatory agency for marketing. The ultrasound, microwave, laser, X ray, gamma ray, or other radio particles are used as the treatment source of the device product to be registered.		Submissions for device products locally manufactured must contain the relevant clinical data required. Submissions for device products foreign company manufactures must contain the clinical data that were submitted to foreign governments for the purpose of the device registration for marketing. Such clinical data should be reviewed and approved by the authorized experts SFDA appoints.
	B. Meeting all criteria as given below: Devices never approved by SFDA but approved by foreign regulatory agency for marketing. The ultrasound, microwave, laser, X ray, gamma ray, or other radio particles are not used as the treatment source of the device product to be registered. The company has not received any complaints of its other products marketed in the passing four years in China (if there is a complaint, the criteria A above should be followed).		Submissions for device products locally manufactured must contain the relevant clinical data required. Submissions for device products foreign company manufactures must contain the clinical data that were submitted to foreign governments for the purpose of the device registration for marketing.

(Continued)

TABLE 2 Clinical Trial Dossier Requirements for Medical Device Regulatory Registration in China (*Continued*)

Category	Status of device companies	Basic conditions	Clinical dossiers required
	Company has device products marketed in China, and the device product to be registered is the same type of device product to be approved.	A. Meeting all criteria as given below: Devices never approved by SFDA but approved by foreign regulatory agency for marketing. The ultrasound, microwave, laser, X ray, gamma ray, or other radio particles are used as the treatment source of the device product to be registered.	Submissions for device products locally manufactured must contain the relevant clinical data required. Submissions for device products foreign company manufactures must contain the clinical data that were submitted to foreign governments for the purpose of the device registration for marketing. Such clinical data should be reviewed and approved by the authorized experts SFDA appoints.
		B. Meeting all criteria as given below: Devices never approved by SFDA but approved by foreign regulatory agency for marketing. The company has not received any complaints of the same type of other device products marketed in the passing four years in China (if there is a complaint, the criteria A above should be followed).	Submissions must contain the relevant clinical data the company used in the regulatory registration for the same type of other device products.
Class II	No matter what type of device products. First time to be registered in China for marketing.	Neither SFDA nor foreign government approves the device product to be registered for marketing. Devices approved by foreign regulatory agency for marketing.	Must conduct the clinical trials in China. Submissions for device products foreign company manufactures must contain the clinical data that were submitted to foreign governments for the purpose of the device registration for marketing.
		SFDA approved the same type of device product marketed in China.	Submissions must contain the relevant clinical data of the same type of device product as well as the validation trial information.
		Other device product complying with national and professional standards of quality assays.	No clinical data are required.

PREREQUISITES OF CLINICAL TRIAL WAIVER

Based on the administration guideline of medical device registration, the following is a summary for the prerequisites of the clinical trials waive of medical devices in China.

For the Device Product Manufactured Overseas

1. *Class III*
   (a) Implanted device
       (i) The conduction of clinical trials in China may be waived but the clinical data that were submitted to the foreign regulatory agency for the purpose of marketing approval should be attached.
           (I) The device has already been approved by the foreign regulatory agency for marketing.
           (II) The company has device products marketed in China.
           (III) Certificates for the QA system of the company and the device products to be registered granted by the regulatory inspection are still valid.
           (IV) The company has not received any complaints of other device products marketed in China for four years or more.
       (ii) The conduction of clinical trials in China may be waived but the clinical data that were submitted to the foreign regulatory agency for the purpose of the marketing approval should be enclosed and also be reviewed and approved by the authorized experts SFDA appoints.
           (I) The device has already been approved by the foreign regulatory agency for marketing.
           (II) The company has device products marketed in China.
           (III) Certificate for the QA system of the company has been granted by the regulatory inspection but not covered for the device product to be registered.
           (IV) Certificate for the QA system of device product to be registered is still valid and the company has not received any complaints of other device products marketed in China for four years or more.
   (b) *Other device products*: The conduction of clinical trials in China may be waived but the clinical data that were submitted to the foreign regulatory agency for the marketing approval should be attached:
       (i) The device has already been approved by the foreign regulatory agency for marketing.
       (ii) The company has device products marketed in China.
       (iii) Diagnostic devices or the device products not used ultrasound, microwave, laser, X ray, gamma ray, or other radio particles as the treatment source.
       (iv) The company has not received any complaints of other device products marketed in China for four years or more.

Conduct of clinical trials for other Class III device products, which have been approved for marketing by foreign regulatory agency but not meeting the prerequisites above, may be waived when the clinical reports submitted at the point of marketing registration to foreign regulatory agency are enclosed and also reviewed and approved by the authorized experts SFDA appoints.

2. *Class II*: Those devices that have been approved for marketing by foreign regulatory agency may be given with exemption of the conduction of clinical trials in China. However, the clinical reports that were used to support the marketing registration by the foreign regulatory agency should be attached.

For Device Products Locally Manufactured
1. *Class III*
   (a) *Implanted device products*: The conductions of clinical trials in China may be an exemption but the relevant clinical reports that were previously used in the regulatory registration by SFDA for the same type of device products approved in China should be submitted for the device product to be registered.
      (i) The company had obtained the approval for the same type but not the same model of device products for marketing in China.
      (ii) The company had obtained the approval for the same model but not same specification of the device products for the marketing in China.
      (iii) Certificate for the QA system of the company and the device products to be registered are still valid.
      (iv) The company has not received any complaints of other device products marketed in China for four years or more.
   (b) *Other device products*: Only clinical reports submitted to support the regulatory approval for the same type of device products marketed in China should be required for the device product to be registered by SFDA.
      (i) The company has the same type of device products marketed in China.
      (ii) Diagnostic devices or the device products not used ultrasound, microwave, laser, X ray, gamma ray, or other radio particles as the treatment source.
      (iii) The company has not received any complaints of other device products marketed in China for four years or more.
2. *Class II*: Generally, the regulatory registration for the Class II device products locally manufactured is executed by provincial FDA. Thus, the standards and list of the Class II device products not necessary to conduct clinical trials should be stipulated by the relevant provincial FDA. The consultation with provincial FDA on the clinical trial exemption for the Class II device products locally manufactured in China is highly recommended.
   The general rules to waive clinical trials for the Class II device products are as follows:
   (a) Those device products with the exemption of the clinical trial clearly defined by SFDA.
   (b) Those device products with less risk.
   (c) Those device products that have clear mechanism, well-developed manufacturing techniques, and extensive clinical application as well as common recognition for their functions in the corresponding medical area.
   (d) Those device products that show equivalent features with the same type of existing device products, including materials made, basic mechanism, major functions, components, prospective application, manufacturing techniques, sterile procedure and operation way, and so on, and no postmarketing ADR records of the existing device products.

(e) Those device products that demonstrate better prospective application, and well-recognizable effectiveness although their therapy index is hard to be clinically verified. Their safety and effectiveness may be easily validated via a testing process.

(f) Those diagnostic devices that execute the lab tests of state and professional standards.

SPECIAL ATTENTIONS TO BE PAID IN THE MEDICAL DEVICE REGISTRATION IN CHINA

When the device application is processed and submitted, the company and device information should be consistent in CFG/CE certificate, authorization letters and SFDA application forms, such as company's address, manufacturer plan address, OEM plant address, device brand name, device product model, product code, accessories, and so on. Any change in the application form, such as manufacturing plan address or model or accessories, and so on, will be considered a new registration. Any inconsistency will be rejected by the SFDA.

The cost and time to complete the sample testing are different at testing centers. It should be sure that testing report by the testing centers complies with the SFDA standards. Otherwise, retesting is unavoidable. All clinical trials should be conducted in accordance with the GCP standards. The protocol and clinical report for medical device clinical trials are regulated in China, which requires special format. The previous experiences of similar device products are helpful to develop the protocol and clinical trial report.

Careful selection of the Chinese distributor is critical. The original import license usually is held by the Chinese distributor, since its name was listed on the import license. The Chinese distributor may require the original license to process the device import affairs, such as clearance from customs, the hospital listing, and so on. Once the foreign device company plans to change the Chinese distributor or after-sales service agent, it is mandatory to return the original license and apply a new one to SFDA through license amendment procedure. If the previous distributor or agent is unlikely to return or hold up the original license, it is impossible for foreign company to complete the license amendment process. Therefore, a professional and independent registration agent and/or distributor agent with a good reputation and capability to complete an accurate and professional dossier, having experiences on medical device clinical trials and selection of high quality of testing center, may play active roles in the device registration and distribution in China.

Chinese specification is the most important document in the device registration in China. CMDE will review the draft Chinese specification after the sample testing report is submitted. It might be requested to revise the Chinese specification or redo the sample testing if the testing outcomes are deemed inconsistent. The detailed information of device products including technical parameters and technical information on raw materials (imported device product) is suggested in the Chinese specification. Any standards or requirements mentioned in the Chinese specification, such as sterility test report, stability testing report, biocompatibility, general requirements for electronic safety, and so on, should be attached with a relevant full report as the supportive evidence to SFDA. Moreover, the determination of other difference models' registration under one import device license by SFDA will be based on the Chinese specification approved.

Finally, it is worthy noted that the CCC mark review is executed by the China Quality Certification Center of General Administration of Quality Supervision, Inspection, and Quarantine (AQSIQ). Under this 3C mark reviews, seven categories of medical devices (medical diagnostic X-ray equipment, hemodialysis equipment, hollow fiber dialysis, extracorporeal blood circuit for blood purification equipment, electrocardiographs, implantable cardiac pacemakers, and artificial heart–lung machine) should be certified except the SFDA's review and approval. Without the 3C mark, the device products may be held at the Chinese custom and be a subject to heavy penalties.

CONCLUSION

The Chinese regulation of medical device has its own features. SFDA has been making efforts to regulate the development and registration of medical devices in China based on global regulatory standards. Clear understanding of Chinese regulations may be beneficial for foreign device company to make the best strategy and creative way in the registration and market of medical devices in China. Although China's regulatory system on monitoring medical device needs more improvements, it is expected that the new efforts on improving legislation of medical device industry SFDA is putting may make China more compliant with global GXPs standards, and ensure the clinical data and supervision of medical devices are more accredited.

Registration Information Requirements of Natural Drugs in China

Qingshan Zheng
Shanghai University of Traditional Chinese Medicines, Shanghai, P.R. China

Daniel Liu
Medidata Solutions Worldwide, Beijing, P.R. China

Earl W. Hulihan
Medidata Solutions Worldwide, New York, New York, U.S.A.

INTRODUCTION

For thousands of years, China was known for its system of TCM. Until 100 years ago, Western drugs began to be used in China. Since then, some local companies began to produce Western drugs, but most of them are generics, and no clinical trial conducted. However, the introduction and implementation of GCP on the TCM in China has not been widely published outside of China. Chinese diverse history in medicine with its unique mix of TCM and modern medical science gives more challenges when the GCP is to be implemented successfully. Chinese government has been making efforts to streamline the GCP requirements and managements of TCM development with the international regulatory standards on the Western medicines. In China, natural drugs refer to the natural substances and its pharmaceutical preparations derived from plants, animal, and minerals, and medically used in the treatment of patients based on the combination of modern medical theory with the TCM rationales, which includes some of TCM themselves. The following registration information requirements of natural drugs are presented based on DRR approved on June 18, 2007 by SFDA.

REGISTRATION CATEGORIES AND NOTES

Registration Categories
An application of natural drug entities that is seeking to gain SFDA approval includes applications for active ingredients, active botanical part, and preparations. Based on the features of natural drugs, there are nine types of natural drug categorizes as follows:

1. Active ingredients and its preparation extracted from plant, animal, and minerals, which have not been marketed in China.
2. Newly found drug materials and preparations.
3. New TCM substitutes.
4. New part of drug materials to be used as drugs.
5. New active part of materials to be used as drugs and its preparations, which are extracted from plant, animal, and minerals, and have not been marketed in China.
6. TCM, natural drugs, and its combined preparations not yet marketed in China.
7. Preparations with change in route of administration of the TCM or natural drugs already marketed in China.
8. Preparations with change in dosage form of the TCM or natural drugs already marketed in China.
9. Generic drugs.

Notes
Drug under category 1 to 6 refers to as new drugs, while procedure for new drugs is applicable for the new drug under category 7 and 8.

1. "Active ingredients and its preparations extracted from plant, animal, and minerals, which have not been marketed in China," refer to the single component or its preparation, which are extracted from plant, animal, and minerals, and not yet collected into National Drug Standards, where the content of this single component should be more than 90% of the extraction.
2. "Newly found drug materials and preparations" refer to the drug materials and preparations not yet collected into National Drug Standard or provincial drug formulary (statutory standards).
3. "New TCM substitutes" refer to drug materials used to substitute the toxic drug materials of the formula in the National Drug Standard or the endangered drug materials, which are not yet collected by statutory standards.
4. "New part of drug materials to be used as drugs" refers to the new part of existing drugs of animals or plants, which is to be used as drug, while the existing drugs are already in the statutory standards.
5. "New active part of drug materials to be used as drugs and its preparation, which are extracted from plant, animal, and minerals, and have not been marketed in China," refers to active parts of similar or multiple component and its preparations, which are extracted from plant, animal, and minerals, and not yet collected in National Drug Standards, where the active part should be more than 50% of the extraction.

6. "TCM, natural drugs, and its combined preparations not yet marketed in China" include the following:
   (a) *Combined preparations of TCM*: The combined preparations of TCM should be formulated under traditional Chinese medical theory, including combined preparations of TCM from ancient classic formula, combined preparations with indication of ancient term, or combined preparations with combined term.
   (b) *Combined preparations of natural drugs*: The combined preparations of natural drugs should be formulated under modern medical theory, where indication should be in modern medical term.
   (c) *Combined preparations of TCM, natural drugs, and chemical drugs*: The combined preparations of TCM, natural drugs, and chemical drugs include combined preparations of TCM and chemical drugs, combined preparations of natural drugs and chemical drugs, and combined preparations of TCM, natural drugs, and chemical drugs.
7. "Preparations with change in route of administration of the TCM or natural drugs already marketed in China," refer to the preparations with transfer between route of administration or absorption location.
8. "Preparations with change in dosage form of the TCM or natural drugs already marketed in China" refer to the preparation of change in dosage form but with no change in route of administration.
9. "Generic drug" refers to the registration application of TCM or natural drug already approved being marketed in China with expired branding drug entity.

APPLICATION CONTENT ITEMS AND NOTES
See Table 3.

Application Content Items
The following are the summary items that should be included in the application dossier of natural drugs to SFDA:

1. Name of the drugs.
2. Certified documents.
3. Objectives and basis for the application.
4. Summary and evaluation of main research results.
5. Sample draft of insert sheet, notes to the draft, and literatures.
6. Sample design for packing, label.
7. Pharmaceutical study results:
   (a) Summary of pharmaceutical study information.
   (b) Source and identification of the original botany.
   (c) Ecological environment, identity, description, cultivation, growing method, local processing, and preparing.
   (d) Draft of standard of drug material, and note of drafting, with provision of drug standard material and related information.
   (e) Vouches of plants, including flower, fruit or seeds, or mineral.
   (f) Research information of production process, verification information, literature, source of excipients, and standards.
   (g) Experiment data and literature of chemical content study.
   (h) Experiment data and literature of quality study.

TABLE 3 Summary of Application Information Items for TCM and Natural Drugs

Information category	Information items	Registration category and information item required										
		1	2	3	4	5	6.1	6.2	6.3	7	8	9
Summary information	1	+	+	+	+	+	+	+	+	+	+	−
	2	+	+	+	+	+	+	+	+	+	+	+
	3	+	+	+	+	+	+	+	+	+	+	+
	4	+	+	+	+	+	+	+	+	+	+	+
	5	+	+	+	+	+	+	+	+	+	+	+
	6	+	+	+	+	+	+	+	+	+	+	+
Pharmaceutical information	7	+	+	+	+	+	+	+	+	+	+	+
	8	+	+	+	+	+	+	+	+	+	+	+
	9	−	+	+	−	▲	▲	▲	▲	−	−	−
	10	−	+	+	+	▲	▲	▲	▲	−	−	−
	11	−	+	+	−	▲	▲	▲	▲	−	−	−
	12	+	+	+	+	+	+	+	+	+	+	+
	13	+	+	±	+	+	+	+	+	+	+	−
	14	+	+	±	+	+	+	±	±	±	±	−
	15	+	+	+	+	+	+	+	+	+	+	+
	16	+	+	+	+	+	+	+	+	+	+	+
	17	+	+	+	+	+	+	+	+	+	+	+
	18	+	+	+	+	+	+	+	+	+	+	+
Pharmacology and toxicology	19	+	+	*	+	+	+	+	+	+	±	−
	20	+	+	*	+	+	±	+	+	+	±	−
	21	+	+	*	+	+	±	+	+	−	−	−
	22	+	+	*	+	+	+	+	+	+	±	+
	23	+	+	±	+	+	+	+	+	+	±	+
	24	*	*	*	*	*	*	*	*	*	*	*
	25	+	+	▲	+	+	+	+	+	+	−	−
	26	+	+	*	*	*	*	*	*	*	−	−
	27	*	*	*	*	*	*	*	*	*	−	−
	28	+	−	*	−	−	−	−	−	−	−	−
Clinical trial information	29	+	+	+	+	+	+	+	+	+	+	−
	30	+	+	+	+	+	+	+	+	+	*	−
	31	+	+	+	+	+	+	+	+	+	*	−
	32	+	+	+	+	+	+	+	+	+	*	−
	33	+	+	+	+	+	+	+	+	+	*	−

1. The symbol + denotes the information must be submitted.
2. The symbol ± denotes literatures can be used instead of test information, or may be exempted by regulation.
3. The symbol − denotes the information may be exempted.
4. The symbol ▲ denotes the information may not be provided for those TCM of natural drug listed in statutory standards, and if not listed, data must be submitted.
5. The symbol * denotes the information shall be submitted according to the requirement.

    (i)   Draft of the drug standards, with notes to the draft and verification with provision of drug standard material and related information.
    (j)   Test report of sample.
    (k)   Experiment data and literature of stability study.

(l) Basis for selection and quality standards of immediate packing materials and container.
8. Pharmacology and toxicology study results:
   (a) Summary about the pharmacology and toxicology study information.
   (b) Experimental outcomes and literature of pharmacodynamic.
   (c) Experimental outcomes and literatures of regular pharmacology study.
   (d) Experimental outcomes and literatures of acute toxicity.
   (e) Experimental outcomes and literatures of long-term toxicity.
   (f) Special safety studies and literatures of hypersensitive (topical, systemic, and phototoxicity), hemolytic and topical irritative (blood vessel, skin, mucous membrane, and muscle) reactions related to topical and systemic uses of the drugs.
   (g) Research information and literatures of genotoxicity.
   (h) Studies and literatures of reproductive toxicity.
   (i) Studies and literatures of carcinogenicity test.
   (j) Studies and literatures of animal pharmacokinetics.
9. Clinical study results:
   (a) Summary of clinical study(ies).
   (b) Clinical study plan(s) and protocol(s).
   (c) Relevant Investigator's Brochure.
   (d) Sample draft(s) of informed consent form, approval of the Ethics Committee.
   (e) Summary report(s) of the clinical study.

Notes to Application Content Items

Relevant to the application content items above, the following are the points to be further explained in details:

1. Name of drugs includes
   (a) Chinese name,
   (b) phonetic name,
   (c) nomenclature of the drug.
2. Certified documents includes the following:
   (a) Lawful registration of the applicant, copies of *Drug Manufacturing License*, GMP Certificate. For the application of production of new drugs, copies of *GMP* Certificate for the workshop where the sample product of the drugs was manufactured should be provided.
   (b) The documents stating patent status and ownership of this drug entity and formula, production process of the drug, and letter of guarantee stating no infringement upon the patent rights of others.
   (c) Copies of official approvals of the research proposal of narcotics, psychotropic, medical-use toxic drugs, and radioactive drugs.
   (d) For the application of production of new drugs, copy of *Approval of Clinical Study of New Drug.*
   (e) Copies of the *Drug Packing Material and Container Certificate* or *Import Drug Packing Material and Container Certificate* for the immediate packing material and container.
   (f) Other certified documents.
As regulations, the import drug entities are also required:

(a) Certified documents, notarized document for the free sale certificate (FSC) issued from the competent authorities of the local country or region where the manufacturer is located, and the GMP Certificate of the manufacturer, and the Chinese translation.

(b) Applications of the drugs under registration category 1 of the NDA registration, the above certified documents can be submitted together with the clinical study report upon the completion of the clinical study in China. However, at the point of the application of clinical trails, certified documents of *GMP Certificate* of the manufacturer issued by local competent drug administration where the drugs are manufactured must be provided.

(c) When the registration by a foreign drug manufacturer is conducted through its own office in China, copies of Registration Certificate of Resident Office of Foreign Enterprise should be provided.

(d) When a foreign drug manufacturer authorizes a domestic agent to conduct the registration, copies of the authorization document, notarized document, the Chinese translation, and the Business License of the domestic agent shall be provided.

(e) For preclinical safety data, a related GLP certificate that undertook the preclinical safety studies should be provided.

(f) A GMP Certificate should be provided for investigative drugs produced for clinical trails.

3. In the objectives and basis of the application, ancient and modern literatures should be provided related to TCM and natural drug; source of formula and basis for the application, current development of R & D (research and development) in China and overseas, current clinical use and production summary, necessary analysis as for the innovation, feasibility, and rationale of dosage form, including the comparison with similar drug already with National Standard, should be provided for preparation of TCM and natural drug. For TCM, traditional medical theory and ancient drug books should also be referred.

4. Summary and evaluation of main research results mean the summary of main research results by the applicant, including a comprehensive analysis of safety, efficacy, and quality controllability of the drugs to be registered.

5. Sample of insert sheet, notes to the draft, and latest literatures includes the draft template of packaging insert sheet in accordance with the relevant regulations, notes on how each items of the insert sheet were drafted, and latest relevant literatures cited.

6. In the summary of pharmaceutical studies, it is required that a self-study report of the drug entity (at least one batch) should be included when the clinical trial permission is applied; upon completion of clinical trial, self-test reports of clinical study projects with three batches of drug entity should be provided when the application dossier is submitted.

7. Regarding the summary of pharmacology and toxicology studies, it is referred that varieties of toxic studies (if applicable), including hypersensitive (topical, systemic, and phototoxicity), hemolytic, and topical irritative (blood vessel, skin, mucous membrane, and muscle) reactions as well as literature related to studies, should be covered. Experiments information related to the preparation safety should also be provided compatible with the details of the appropriate route of the drug administration. When there is a tendency of drug dependence, the relevant outcome data should be described.

8. Special efforts should be made for experiments information and literatures related to genotoxicity, when the formulas contain the drug materials not yet collected in statutory drug standards, or the active part of drug materials not yet collected in statutory drug standards, or new drug is to be used for the child bearing patient population, where it acts on reproductive system (e.g., contraceptives, sexual hormones, drugs for sexual function disorder, drugs for maturation promoting of sperm, and the new drugs with positive result in mutations test or drugs with cytotoxicity).

9. It is mandatory for new drug to be used for the child bearing patient group where it may act on reproductive system (e.g., contraceptives, sexual hormones, drugs for sexual function disorder, drugs for maturation promoting of sperm, the new drugs with positive result in mutations test or drugs with cytotoxicity) to provide experiments data and literatures related to reproductive toxicity in consistency with the specific situation.

10. During long-term toxicity test of a new drug, investigations and literatures related to carcinogenicity must be performed if cytotoxic effects were shown or extraordinary activation on the growth of cells in certain visceral organs and tissues was caused, or there is a positive test result during mutagenicity test.

Special Attentions on Application Dossiers of the Natural Drug Registration

1. Application of clinical trial permission should usually be summated with items 1 to 4, 7 to 8, and 9 (a–c).

2. When an NDA is submitted upon completion of clinical trial, the full items above plus any changes and supplemental information should be submitted with detailed explanation of reason and basis.

3. The application of generic drugs should be covering with the items 2 to 6 and 7a, b, f, i, and l (except for TCM or natural drug injection where clinical trail is needed).

4. When all technical information and certified documents from local authority used for importation application are submitted, they should be in Chinese attached with original documents, where Chinese version of quality standard should be complied and submitted according to the format specified by Chinese National Drug Standards.

5. As for the complexity and diversity of TCM and natural drugs, when making the application, necessary researches should be completed based on the relevant drug specifications. If there is need for reduction or exemption of tests, there should be sufficient justified reasons.

6. Technical requirements of TCM and natural drug injection should be separately promulgated.

7. For the natural drugs meeting the category 1 of the new drug entity, the investigational data and literatures related to carcinogenicity must be provided; if active ingredients and its preparations extracted from plant, animal, and minerals have not been marketed in China, the active ingredients are related to the known carcinogen; the metabolite of the new drugs is similar to the known carcinogen; the expected treatment period is longer than six months, or used for treatment of chronic and recurrent diseases, or intermittent use for a regular period of time, then. For those that have not been marketed in China, there should be comparison between the drugs and the existing part to evidence the advantage of the new drug, if there is similar drug or preparation made from

active part extracted from single plant, animal, and mineral, which have been marketed in China.

8. For the substitutes of TCM materials meeting the category 3 of the new drug entity, in addition to the preclinical data requirements of the category 2 of the drug registration, the comparisons of pharmacodynamic parameters between this drug and the substitutes should also be included, while experimental outcomes of human tolerance tests and clinical bioequivalence evidences of the related preparations should be provided as well. If the substitute is a single component, experiments and literatures of pharmacokinetic features may be provided. After the approval of the substitute of the TCM materials, application of corresponding preparations for this substitute should be followed with the procedure of supplemental application, and must be strictly within the approved scope of substitution.

9. For those new active part of materials to be used as drugs and its preparations, which are extracted from plant, animal, and mineral, have not been marketed in China, and belong to the category 5 of the new drug entity, in addition to the required data to be submitted, the following information is necessary in the application dossier:

   (a) Research information or literatures related to the screening of the active parts by the item 7f and to major chemical contents of the active parts by the item 7g.

   (b) If the active parts are composed of multiple components, each of the components should be assayed, where there should be lower limit of representative value for each component (upper limit should be added for the toxic component as well).

   (c) When applying for new active part of materials to be used as drugs and its preparations that have not been marketed in China, appropriate comparison investigations including pharmacodynamic parameters should be conducted with this active ingredient to evidence the advantage and merit, if this active part is comprised of the similar sources extracted from plant, animal, and mineral that were already marketed in China.

10. The essential information for those under the category 6 of the new drug entity, in which TCM, natural drugs, and its combined preparations are not yet marketed in China, is dependent on individual situation, respectively:

    (a) Combined preparations of TCM, the exemption of some experiment data are adjusted based on the source of formula, indication, and preparation process.

    (b) Investigational data and literatures of efficacy and interaction studies of multiple components should be provided for combined preparations of natural drugs.

    (c) If the combined formula contains a drug not listed in the statutory drug standards, additional investigational information may be necessary to be submitted according to the requirements of the corresponding registration category.

    (d) There must be statutory standards for any material medically used in the combinations of TCM, natural drug, and chemical entity, where comparison of experimental data and literatures set as of efficacy and interaction (improvement in efficacy, reduction in toxicities, or complimenting of bioavailability) between TCM, natural drugs, and chemical entity should

be included in the submission dossier of clinical trials. When the application is involved with the production of the natural drugs, evidences from
clinical trial should be offered to prove the necessity of the formula, where
the experimental data of interaction in bioavailability between TCM, natural drug, and chemical entity should be attached. The chemical entity
used in formula (single or combined setting) must have been referred in
the National Drug Standards.

11. For those under the category 6 of the new drug entity, which involves with
preparations with change in dosage form of the TCM or natural drugs already
marketed in China, the advantage and merits of the new preparations should
be described. The indication of the new preparations should in principle be
the same with that the existing preparation, unless there is a new evidence to
verify the new efficacy by clinical trials, whose related information should be
attested.

12. For those under the category 9 of the new drug entity, generic drugs should be
consistent with the drugs they imitate in the standpoints of PK/PD views, and
if necessary, the quality standards should be improved.

13. Certain criteria and requirements of clinical study are as follows:

    (a) Sample size of patients in clinical trials should meet the statistical expec-
    tations and the minimal cases required.

    (b) The minimal cases required (trial group) of clinical trials are as follows: 20
    to 30 for phase I, 100 for phase II, 300 for phase III, and 2000 for phase IV.

    (c) Phase IV clinical trial should be conducted for any new drug, and the
    drugs where there is a significant change in processing line or solvent.

    (d) Normally, 18 to 24 cases should be required in bioequivalence trials.

    (e) Phase I clinical trials of the contraceptives should be conducted as per rel-
    evant regulations. In phase II trials, a randomized controlled clinical study
    should be completed with at least 100 pairs of subjects for at least six men-
    struation cycles. In phase III trials, an open trial with at least 1000 cases for
    12 menstruation cycles should be accomplished. In phase IV trials, vari-
    able factors of such kind of drugs should be carefully assessed to meet the
    trial objectives with adequate numbers of cases.

    (f) For a new indication of the TCM substitute, preparations of the substitute,
    in which the preparations' application are sufficiently consistent with indi-
    cation of the substitute, should be chosen from the drug standards. In the
    comparison study, it should be used as the comparative drug; for each
    indication, more than two TCM preparations should be used to verify the
    new claim and subjects' cases for each preparation should not be less than
    100 pairs.

    (g) For those with a change in dosage form, clinical trails may be exempted or
    be conducted with no less than 100 pairs of cases according to the change
    in process and specific drugs.

    (h) For generic drugs, the clinical trails should be performed with no less than
    100 pairs of cases according to specific situation.

    (i) For imported TCM or natural drugs, application dossier should be pro-
    vided according to the corresponding requirement of the registration cat-
    egory, where the historical preclinical data and clinical trials data of the
    human pharmacokinetic study conducted in China may be required with

no less than 100 pairs of clinical cases. For multiple indications, clinical cases for each major indication should not be less than 60 pairs.

CONCLUSION

SFDA wishes to establish and implement GCP standards in the development of TCM area, ensuring the processes of the clinical trials and reviews and approval of the TCM NDA in compliance with the international regulatory standards. Having been achieved with this goal, the results of the clinical data for new TCM entities are more scientific and reliable. However, we also realize that due to the differences from the Western medicines, unique and complicated features of TCM bring us more intrinsic challenges to regulate and implement the GCP better in the TCM field. With the formulation practice of relevant guidelines in the passing years, it is more optimistic that the creation of China-featured TCM GCP regulations makes quality and credibility of these ancient Chinese medicines best fitting and progresses together with the world.

REFERENCES

1. www.sfda.gov.cn.
2. www.cde.org.cn.
3. www.nicpbp.org.cn.

Acronyms and Initialisms

AAAS	American Association for the Advancement of Science
AABB	American Association of Blood Banks
AACR	American Association for Cancer Research
AADA	Abbreviated Antibiotic Drug Application (FDA) (used primarily for generics)
AAFP	American Academy of Family Physicians
AAI	American Academy of Immunologists
AAP	American Association of Pathologists
AAPP	American Academy of Pharmaceutical Physicians
AAPS	American Association of Pharmaceutical Scientists
ABPI	Association of the British Pharmaceutical Industry
ABS	Absolute
ACCP	American College of Clinical Pharmacology
ACE	Adverse Clinical Event
ACIL	American Council of Independent Laboratories
ACP	Associates of Clinical Pharmacology (USA), a group that certifies Clinical Research Associates (CRAs) and Clinical Research Coordinators (CRCs)
ACPU	Association of Clinical Pharmacology Units
ACRA	Associate Commissioner for Regulatory Affairs (FDA)
ACRPI	Association for Clinical Research in the Pharmaceutical Industry (UK)
ACS	American Chemical Society
ACT	*Applied Clinical Trials* magazine
ACTG	AIDS Clinical Trials Group (NIAID)
ACTU	AIDS Clinical Trials Unit (NIH)
AD	Alzheimer's disease; antidepressant
ADAMHA	Alcohol, Drug Abuse, and Mental Health Administration (no longer exists)
ADAS	Alzheimer's Disease Assessment Scale
ADAS COG	Alzheimer's Disease Assessment Scale, Cognitive Subscale
ADE	Adverse Drug Experience/Effect/Event
ADI	Acceptable Daily Intake
ADME	Absorption, Distribution, Metabolism, Elimination
ADP	Automated Data Processing
ADR	Adverse Drug Reaction
ADRS	Adverse Drug Reporting System
AE	Approvable
AE	Adverse Experience

AE	Adverse Event
AED	Antiepileptic Drug
AEGIS	ADROIT Electronically Generated Information Service
AERS	Adverse Event Reporting System (FDA)
AESGP	Association Européenne des Specialités Grand Public (European Proprietary Medicines Manufacturers Association)
AFCR	*See AFMR.*
AFDO	Association of Food and Drug Officials
AFMR	American Federation for Medical Research, formerly known as the American Federation for Clinical Research (AFCR)
AHA	Area Health Authority (UK)
AHCPR	Agency for Health Care Policy Research (NIH)
AICRC	Association of Independent Clinical Research Contractors (UK)
AIDS	Acquired Immune Deficiency Syndrome. *See also HIV and SIDA.*
AIM	Active Ingredient Manufacturer
AIP	Abbreviated Inspection Program
AMA	American Medical Association
AMA-DE	AMA Drug Evaluations
AMC	Academic Medical Centers
AMF	Administrative Management of the Files
AmFAR	American Foundation for AIDS Research
AMG	Arzneimittelgesetz (German Drug Law)
AMI	Acute Myocardial Infarction
ANADA	Abbreviated New Animal Drug Application
ANDA	Abbreviated New Drug Application (for a generic drug)
ANOVA	Analysis of Variance
AOAC	Association of Official Analytical Chemists
AOAC	Association Pharmaceutique Belge (Belgium)
AP	Approved (COMIS term)
APhA	American Pharmaceutical Association
APHIS	Animal and Plant Health Inspection Service
AQL	Acceptable Quality Level
ARC	AIDS-Related Complex
ARDS	Adult Respiratory Distress Syndrome
ARENA	Applied Research Ethics National Association
ASA	American Statistical Association
ASAP	Administrative Systems Automation Project (FDA)
ASCII	American Standards Code for Information Interchange (computer files)
ASCO	American Society for Clinical Oncology
ASCPT	American Society for Clinical Pharmacology and Therapeutics
ASM	American Society for Microbiology
ASQC	American Society for Quality Control
AT	Active (COMIS term)
ATF	Bureau of Alcohol, Tobacco, and Firearms
AUC	Area Under the Curve (an expression of exposure)
AZT	Zidovudine (HIV treatment)
BARQA	British Association of Research Quality Assurance
BB	Bureau of Biologics (now CBER)

BCE	Beneficial Clinical Event
BDS	Bulk Drug Substance
BEUC	European Bureau of Consumer Unions
BfArM	Bundesinstitut für Arzneimittel und Medizinprodukte (Federal Institute for Drugs and Medical Devices, Germany)
BGA	Bundesinstitut für gesundheitlichen Verbraucherschutz und Veterinärmedizinn (Federal Institute for Health Protection of Consumers and Veterinary Medicine, Germany)
BGVV	Bundesgesundheitsamt (former German public health agency)
BID	Two Times Per Day
BIND	Biological Investigational New Drug
BIO	Biotechnology Industry Organization
BIRA	British Institute of Regulatory Affairs
BLA	Biologic License Application
BMB	Bioresearch Monitoring Branch
BMI	Body Mass Index
BPAD	Bipolar Affective Disorder
BPI	Bundesverband der Pharmazeutischen Industrie EV (Germany)
BPM	Beats Per Minute
BrAPP	British Association of Pharmaceutical Physicians
BRB	Biomedical Research Branch
BSA	Body Surface Area
BUN	Blood Urea Nitrogen
BVC	British Veterinary Codex
C & S	Culture and Sensitivity
CA	Chemical Abstracts
CA	Competent Authority (regulatory body charged with monitoring compliance with European member state national statutes and regulations)
CAC	Carcinogenicity Assessment Committee
CACE	Committee for Advancement of Chemistry Education
CAD	Coronary Artery Disease
CANDA	Computer-Assisted New Drug Application. *See NDA.*
CAPLA	Computer-Assisted Product License Application. *See PLA.*
CAPLAR	Computer-Assisted Product License Agreement Review (FDA)
CAPRA	Canadian Association of Pharmaceutical Regulatory Affairs
CAS	Chemical Abstracts Service
CBC	Complete Blood Count
CBCTN	Community-Based Clinical Trials Network
CBER	Center for Biologics Evaluation and Research (FDA)
CBF	Cerebral Blood Flow
CCASE	Coordinating Committee for Advancement of Scientific Education
CCC	Compliance Coordinating Committee (CDER)
CCD	Canadian Drugs Directorate
CCDS	Company Core Data Sheets
CCI	Committee on Clinical Investigations. *See also IRB.*
CCRA	Certified Clinical Research Associate. *See also ACP.*
CCRC	Certified Clinical Research Coordinator. *See also ACP.*

CDC	Centers for Disease Control (Atlanta, GA)
CDER	Center for Drug Evaluation and Research (FDA)
CDRH	Center for Devices and Radiological Health (FDA)
CE	Continuing Education
CE	Mark signifying compliance with EU harmonized standards and directives
CEN	Comité Européen de Normalisation (European Committee for Standardization)
CESS	CDER Executive Secretariat Staff
CFR	*Code of Federal Regulations* (usually cited by part and chapter, as 21 CFR 211)
CFSAN	Center of Food Safety and Applied Nutrition
CGMP	Current Good Manufacturing Practices
CH	Clinical Hold
CHD	Coronary Heart Disease
CIB	Clinical Investigator's Brochure
CID	CTFA Cosmetic Ingredient Dictionary
CIOMS	Council for International Organisations of Medical Sciences (postapproval international ADR reporting, UK)
CIR	Cosmetic Ingredient Review
CIS	Commonwealth of Independent States
CLIA	Clinical Laboratory Improvements Amendments
C_{max}	Maximum Plasma Concentration
CMC	Chemistry, Manufacturing, and Controls
CMCCC	Chemistry and Manufacturing Controls Coordinating Committee (CDER)
CME	Continuing Medical Education
CNS	Central Nervous System
COA	Commissioned Officers Association
COA	Certificates of Analysis
COE	Code of Ethics
COIMS	Centerwide Oracle Management Information System (FDA)
COMIS	Center Office Management Information System
COSTART	Coding Symbols for a Thesaurus of Adverse Reaction Terms
CP	Compliance Program
CPMP	Committee for Proprietary Medicinal Products (EU)
CPSC	Consumer Product Safety Commission (USA)
CR	Cross Reference (COMIS term)
CRA	Clinical Research Associate
CRADA	Cooperative Research and Development Agreement (with NIH)
CRC	Clinical Research Coordinator. *See also CCRC.*
CRF	Case Report Form
CRO	Contract Research Organization. *See also IPRO.*
CS	Civil Service
CS	Clinically Significant
CSDD	Center for the Study of Drug Development
CSI	Consumer Safety Inspector

CSM	Commission for Safety of Medicines (UK Regulatory Agency)
	Committee on Safety of Medicines (UK)
CSO	Consumer Safety Officer (FDA) – Project Manager
CSR	Clinical Study Report
CSSI	Company Core Safety Information
CT	Computerized Tomography
CT	Clinical Trial
CTC	Clinical Trial Certificate
CTEP	Clinical Therapeutics Evaluation Program (NCI)
CTX	Clinical Trial Exemption Certification (MCA)
CV	Curriculum Vitae
CVM	Center for Veterinary Medicine (FDA)
CXR	Chest X-ray
DAS	Drug Abuse Staff
DAWN	Drug Abuse Warning Network
DB	Double-Blind
DCF	Data Clarification Form
DD	Department of Drugs (Swedish regulatory agency)
ddC	dideoxycytidine, a cytidine nucleoside analogue
ddC	didanosine, a purine nucleoside analogue
DDIR	Division of Drug Information Resources
DDMAC	Division of Drug Marketing, Advertising, and Communications
DEA	Drug Enforcement Administration (USA)
DEN	Drug Experience Network
DES	Division of Epidemiology and Surveillance
DESI	Drug Efficacy Study Implementation Notice (FDA, to evaluate drugs in use before 1962)
DGD	Now OGD (formerly CBER's Division of Genetic Drugs)
DHEW	Department of Health, Education, and Welfare (USA, now split into HHS and Department of Education)
DHHS	Department of Health and Human Services (USA)
DIA	Drug Information Association
DISD	Division of Information Systems Design
DLT	Dose-Limiting Toxicity
DMF	Drug Master File
DoD	Department of Defense (USA)
DPC-PTR Act	Drug Price Competition and Patent Term Restoration Act of 1984 (also known as Waxman-Hatch bill)
DRG	Diagnosis Related Groups
DRG	Division of Research Grants (NIH)
DSI	Division of Scientific Investigations (FDA)
DSM	Diagnostic and Statistical Manual (of the American Psychiatric Association)
DSMB	Data and Safety Monitoring Board
DSNP	Development of Standardized Nomenclature Project (FDA)
DUR	Drug Utilization Review
EA	Environmental Assessment
EAB	Ethical Advisory Board (term used in some nations for groups similar to IRBs and IECs)

EBSA	European Biosafety Association
EC	European Commission (in documents older than the mid-1980s, EC may mean European Community)
EC	Ethics Committee
ECG	Electrocardiogram
ECJ	European Court of Justice
ECPHIN	European Community Pharmaceutical Products Information Network
ECU	European Currency Unit
ED	Effective Dose
EEC	European Economic Community (old term for EC, now EU)
EEG	Electroencephalogram
EEO	Equal Employment Opportunity
EER	Establishment Evaluation Request
EFGCP	European Forum on Good Clinical Practice (Evere, Belgium)
EFPIA	European Federation of Pharmaceutical Industries' Associations
EFTA	European Free Trade Association
EIA	Establishment Inspection Reports
EIR	Establishment Inspection Report (FDA)
ELA	Establishment License Application (biologics)
EMEA	European Medicines Evaluations Agency (UK)
EMS	Electronic Mail Service
EO	Executive Order
EOP1	End-of-phase 1
EOP2	End-of-phase 2
EORTC	European Organization for Research and Treatment of Cancer
EOS	End of Study
EP	European Parliament
EPA	Environmental Protection Agency
EPAR	European Public Assessment Report
EPL	Effective Patent Life
EPMS	Employee Performance Management System
EPO	European Patent Office
EPRG	European Pharmacovigilance Research Group
ER	Essential Requirements (EU)
ESRA	European Society of Regulatory Affairs
ESS	Executive Secretary and Staff
ETT	Exercise Tolerance Test
EU	European Union
EUDRACT	European Drug Regulatory Affairs Clinical Trial
EUP	Experimental Use Permit
FACA	Federal Advisory Committee Act 1972
FÄPI	Fachgesellschaft der Ärzte in der Pharmazeutischen Industrie e.V. (German Association of Physicians in the Pharmaceutical Industry)
Farmindustria	The Association of the Italian Pharmaceutical Manufacturers
FAX	Facsimile
FCC	Federal Communications Commission

FCCSET	Federal Coordinating Council for Science, Engineering and Technology
FD&C Act	Federal Food, Drug and Cosmetic Act
FDA 1571	Form Used to Submit IND
FDA 1572	Statement of Investigator Form (accompanies IND)
FDA 1639	Form Used to Submit Drug Experience Report
FDA 2252	Form Used to Submit NDA Annual Report
FDA 2253	Form Used to Promotional Advertising or Labeling
FDA 3500A	Form Used to Submit Drug Experience Report
FDA 356H	Form Used to Submit NDA
FDA 483	Form Issued by FDA upon Adverse Findings of Inspection
FDA	Food and Drug Administration (USA)
FDA-SRS	Spontaneous Reporting System of the Food and Drug Administration
FDLI	Food and Drug Law Institute
FDP	Finished Drug Product
FFDCA	Federal Food Drug & Cosmetic Act
FFPM	Fellow of the Faculty of Pharmaceutical Medicine (UK)
FMD	Field Management Directives
FOI	Freedom of Information
FOIA	Freedom of Information Act
FONSI	Finding of No Significant Impact
FPIF	The Finnish Pharmaceutical Industry Association
FPL	Final Printed Labeling
FR	Federal Register
FRC	Federal Records Center (Suitland)
FRCP	Fellow of the Royal College of Physicians, sometimes followed by a place name—for example, FRCP (Edin.)—that indicates a university medical school
FSIS	Food Safety and Inspection Service
FTC	Federal Trade Commission (USA)
FUR	Follow up Request
GAO	General Accounting Office (US government)
GATT	General Agreement of Tariffs and Trade
GC	General Counsel (FDA)
GC	Gas Chromatography
GCP	Good Clinical Practice
GI	Gastrointestinal
GLP	Good Laboratory Practice
GMP	Good Manufacturing Practice
GP	General Practitioner
GPRA	Government Performance and Results Act
GRAS	Generally Recognized as Safe
GRASE	Generally Recognized as Safe and Effective
GRP	Good Review Practice
HAACP	Hazard Analysis and Critical Control Point (inspection technique)
HAI	Health Action International
HC	Health Canada (Canada's equivalent to the FDA)

HCFA	Health Care Financing Administration (HHS)
HF	Routing code for mail to the Office of the Commissioner of the FDA
HFD	Routing code for mail to CDER
HFM	Routing code for mail to CBER
HFS	Routing code for mail to CFSAN
HFT	Routing code for mail to NCTR
HFV	Routing code for mail to CVM
HFZ	Routing code for mail to CDRH
HHS	Department of Health and Human Services (USA, also called DHHS)
HIMA	Health Industry Manufacturer's Association (devices)
HIPAA	Health Insurance Portability and Accountability Act
HIS	Indian Health Service
HIV	Human Immunodeficiency Virus
HIV+	HIV-positive; HIV-infected
HIV−1	Human Immunodeficiency Virus Type 1
HMO	Health Maintenance Organization
HPLC	High-Pressure Liquid Chromatography
HRG	Health Research Group
HRRC	Human Research Review Committee
HRSA	Health Resources and Services Administration
HX	History
IB	Investigator's Brochure
IBD	Inflammatory Bowel Disease
i.v.	Intravenous
IACUC	Institutional Animal Care and Use Committee
IARC	International Agency for Research on Cancer
IC	Informed Consent
IC	Chemistry Information Amendment (COMIS term)
ICD	Informed Consent Document
ICH	International Conference on Harmonisation of Technical Requirements for Registration of Pharmaceuticals for Human Use
ICPEMC	International Commission for Protection Against Mutagens and Carcinogens
ICTH	International Committee on Thrombosis and Hemostases
IDB	Investigational Drug Brochure
IDE	Investigational Device Exemption (FDA)
IDR	Idiosyncratic Drug Reaction
IDSMB	Independent Data Safety Monitoring Board
IEC	Independent Ethics Committee. *See also EAB, IRB, NRB.*
IFPMA	International Federation of Pharmaceutical Manufacturers' Associations
IG	Office of the Inspector General (HHS)
IKS	Interkantonale Kontrollstelle für Heilmittel (Switzerland)
IM	Clinical Information Amendment (COMIS term)
IM	Intramuscular

INAD	Investigational New Animal Drug
IND	Investigational New Drug application (FDA). *See also TIND.*
INDA	Investigational New Drug Application
INDC	Investigational New Drug Committee
INN	International Nonproprietary Name
IOM	Institute of Medicine (National Academy of Science, USA)
IPCS	International Program for Chemical Safety
IPRA	International Product Registration Document
IPRO	Independent Pharmaceutical Research Organization. *See also CRO.*
IRB	Institutional Review Board, sometimes Independent Review Board. *See also IEC, EAB, NRB.*
IRC	Institutes Review Committee
IRD	International Registration Document
IRG	Initial Review Groups
IRS	Identical, Related, or Similar
IS	Information Systems
ISCB	International Society for Clinical Biostatistics
ISO	International Organisation for Standardisation
ISPE	International Society for Pharmacoepidemiology
IT	Toxicology Information Amendment (COMIS term)
IT	Information Technology
ITCC	Information Technology Coordinating Committee (CDER)
IV	Interview
IVD	In Vitro Device; In Vitro Diagnostics
IVF	In Vitro Fertilization
IVF/ET	In Vitro Fertilization/Embryo Transfer
JCAH	Joint Commission for the Accreditation of Hospitals
JCAHO	Joint Commission of Accreditation of Health Care Organizations
JCPT	Journal of Clinical Pharmacology and Therapeutics
JCRDD	Journal of Clinical Research and Drug Development
JCRP	Journal of Clinical Research and Pharmacoepidemiology
JPMA	Japan Pharmaceutical Manufacturers' Association
KS	Kaposi's sarcoma
L&D	Labor and Delivery
LAN	Local Area Network
LD	Lethal Dose
LD50	Lethal Dose (50%)
LEAA	Law Enforcement Assistance Administration
LERN	Library Electronic Reference Network
LIF	Swedish Pharmaceutical Industry Association
LKP	Leiter der klinischen Prüfung, under the German Drug Law, the physician who is head of clinical testing
LNC	Labeling and Nomenclature Committee
LOA	Letter of Agreement
LOC	Level of Concern
LOCF	Last Observation Carried Forward
LOD	Loss on Drying
LRC	Lipid Research Clinic

LRI	Lower Respiratory Infection
LTE	Less Than Effective
LVP	Large Volume Parenterals
MA	Marketing Authorization
MAA	Marketing Authorization Application (EC)
MAH	Marketing Authorization Holders
MAPP	Manual of Policy and Procedures
MBC	Minimum Bactericidal Concentration
MCA	Medicines Control Agency (UK)
MDA	Medical Devices Agency (UK)
MDD	Medical Device Directives (EU)
MDI	Metered-Dose Inhaler; Manic-Depressive Illness
MDR	Medical Device Reporting
MDV	Medical Device Vigilance
MECU	Million ECU
MEDDRA	Medical Dictionary for Drug Regulatory Affairs
MEDLARS	Medical Literature Analysis and Retrieval System
MEDWATCH	MedWatch Adverse Event Reporting System
MEFA	Association of the Danish Pharmaceutical Industry
MEMO	Medicines Evaluation and Monitoring Organisation
MEP	Member of the European Parliament
MHW	Ministry of Health and Welfare (Koseisho, Japan's drug regulatory agency)
MI	Myocardial Infarction
MIC	Minimum Inhibitory Concentration
MOU	Memorandum of Understanding (between FDA and a regulatory agency in another country) that allows mutual recognition of inspections
MPCC	Medical Policy Coordinating Committee (CDER)
MRA	Medical Research Associate
MRI	Magnetic Resonance Imaging
MTD	Maximum Tolerated Dose
NA	Not Approvable
NABR	National Association for Biomedical Research
NADA	New Animal Drug Application
NAF	Notice of Adverse Findings (FDA postaudit letter)
NAFTA	North American Free Trade Agreement
NAHC	National Advisory Health Council
NAI	No Action Indicated (most favorable FDA postinspection classification)
NAS	National Academy of Sciences
NAS	New Active Substance
NAS-NRC	National Academy of Sciences—National Research Council
NATRIK	National Reporting and Investigation Centre (UK)
NCCLS	National Committee for Clinical Laboratory Standards
NCE	New Chemical Entity
NCHGR	National Center for Human Genome Research (NIH)
NCHS	National Center for Health Statistics (in CDC)
NCI	National Cancer Institute (NIH)

NCPIE	National Council on Patient Information and Education (Washington, DC)
NCRP	Northwest Clinical Research Professionals (Portland, OR)
NCRR	National Center for Research Resources (NIH)
NCS	Not Clinically Significant
NCTR	National Center for Toxicological Research
NCVIA	National Childhood Vaccine Injury Act (1986)
NDA	New Drug Application (FDA)
NDE	New Drug Evaluation
NDS	New Drug Study (Canada's new drug application)
NEFARMA	Dutch Association of the Innovative Pharmaceutical Industry
NEI	National Eye Institute (NIH)
NEJM	*New England Journal of Medicine*
NF	National Formulary
NHLBI	National Heart, Lung, and Blood Institute (NIH)
NHS	National Health Service (UK)
NHW	National Health and Welfare Department (Canada's equivalent of DHHS)
NIA	National Institute on Aging (NIH)
NIAAA	National Institute on Alcohol Abuse and Alcoholism (NIH)
NIAID	National Institute of Allergies and Infectious Diseases (NIH)
NIAMS	National Institute of Arthritis and Musculoskeletal and Skin Diseases (NIH)
NIAMSD	National Institute of Arthritis and Musculoskeletal and Skin Diseases
NICHD	National Institute of Child Health and Human Development (NIH)
NIDA	National Institute on Drug Abuse (NIH)
NIDCDD	National Institute on Deafness and Other Communication Disorders (NIH)
NIDDKD	National Institute of Diabetes and Digestive and Kidney Diseases
NIDR	National Institute of Dental Research (NIH)
NIEHS	National Institute of Environmental Health Sciences (NIH)
NIGMS	National Institute of General Medical Sciences (NIH)
NIH	National Institutes of Health (DHHS)
NIMH	National Institute of Mental Health (NIH)
NINDS	National Institute of Neurological Disorders & Stroke (NIH)
NINR	National Institute of Nursing Research (NIH)
NLEA	Nutrition Labeling and Education Act (1990)
NLM	National Library of Medicine (NIH)
NME	New Molecular Entity
NMR	Nuclear Magnetic Resonance
NOAEL	No Observed Adverse Effect Level
Non-Mem	Nonlinear Mixed Effect Model
NR	No Reply Necessary (COMIS term)
NRB	Noninstitutional Review Board, also known as an Independent Review Board. *See also EAB, IEC, IRB.*
NRC	National Research Council

NRC	Nuclear Regulatory Commission
NSAID	Nonsteroidal Anti-Inflammatory Drug
NSF	National Science Foundation
NSR	Nonsignificant Risk
NTP	National Toxicology Program
OAI	Official Action Indicated (serious FDA postinspection classification)
OAM	Office of Alternative Medicine (NIH)
OASH	Office of the Assistant Secretary for Health
OB-GYN	Obstetrics-Gynecology
OC	Office of the Commissioner
OC	Office of Compliance (CDER)
OCD	Office of the Center Director (CDER)
OCPB	Office of Clinical Pharmacology and Biopharmaceutics (CDER)
OCR	Office of Civil Rights
OCR	Optical Character Recognition
OD	Right Eye
ODB	Observational Database
ODE	Office of Drug Evaluation (CDER now has five such offices: ODE I, II, III, IV, and V)
OEA	Office of External Affairs
OEB	Office of Epidemiology and Biostatistics (CDER)
OECD	Organization for Economic Cooperation and Development
OGC	Office of the General Counsel
OGD	Office of Generic Drugs (CDER, formerly DGB)
OGE	Office of Government Ethics (formerly part of Office of Personnel Management, separate executive branch in 1989)
OHA	Office of Health Affairs
OHRM	Office of Human Resource Management
OJC	Office Journal of the EU-C Series (Information)
OJL	Office Journal of the EU-L Series (Legislation)
OLA	Office of Legislative affairs
OM	Office of Management (CDER)
OMB	Office of Management and Budget (USA)
ONDC	Office of New Drug Chemistry (CDER)
OP	Open (COMIS term)
OP	Office of Policy
OPA	Office of Public Affairs
OPD	Orphan Products Division Directorate
OPM	Office of Personnel Management
OPRR	Office of Protection from Research Risks (NIH)
OPS	Office of Pharmaceutical Science (CDER)
ORA	Office of Regulatory Affairs
ORM	Office of Review Management (CDER)
ORO	Office of Regional Operations
OS	Left Eye
OSHA	Occupational Safety Health Administration (USA)
OTA	Office of Technology Assessment (USA; abolished by Congress, Fall 1995)

OTC	Over-The-Counter (refers to nonprescription drugs)
OTCOM	Office of Training and Communications (CDER)
OTR	Office of Testing and Research (CDER)
OU	Both Eyes
P	Priority
PAHO	Pan American Health Organization
PAI	Preapproval Inspection
PAITS	Preapproval Inspection Tracking System
PAR	Postapproval Research
PB	Privacy Boards
PC	Personal Computer
PC	Protocol Amendment—Change (COMIS term)
PCC	Parklawn Computer Center
PCC	Poison Control Center
PCP	*Pneumocystis carinii* pneumonia
PD	Position Description
PD	Pharmacodynamics
PDA	Parenteral Drug Association
PDQ	Physicians' Data Query (NCI-sponsored cancer trial registry)
PDR	*Physicians' Desk Reference*
PDUFA	Prescription Drug User Fee Act (of 1992, USA)
PEM	Prescription Event Monitoring
PEP	Performance Evaluation Plan
PERI	Pharmaceutical Education & Research Institute, division of PhRMA
PET	Positron Emission Tomography
PFT	Pulmonary Function Tests
PHI	Protected Health Information
PhRMA	Pharmaceutical Research and Manufacturers of America (previously PMA)
PHS	Public Health Service (USA)
PI	Package Insert (approved product labeling)
PI	Principal Investigator
PI	Protocol Amendment—New Investigator (COMIS term)
PK	Pharmacokinetics
PLA	Product License Application (biologics) (UK)
PLA/ELA	Product License Application/Establishment License Application
PM	Project Manager
PMA	Premarket Approval Application (FDA); Pharmaceutical Manufacturers Association (now PhRMA) (equivalent to NDA for Class III Devices)
PMCC	Project Management Coordinating Committee (CDER)
PMDIT	Project Management
PMS	Postmarketing Surveillance
PN	Protocol Amendment—New Protocol (or Pending Review) (COMIS term)
PO	Per Os (by mouth)
PPA	Poison Prevention Act

PPI	Patient Package Insert
PPM	Physician Practice Management Organizations
PPO	Preferred Provider Organization; Policy and Procedure Order
PR	Pulse Rate
PR	Public Relations
PRIM&R	Public Responsibility in Medicine and Research (Boston, MA)
PRN	As Needed
PROG	Peer-Review Oversight Group (NIH)
PSUR	Periodic Safety Update Reports
PTCC	Pharmacology/Toxicology Coordinating Committee (CDER)
PUD	Peptic Ulcer Disease
QA	Quality Assurance
QAU	Quality Assurance Unit
QC	Quality Control
QD	Once Daily
QID	Four Times a Day
QL	Quality of Life
QNS	Quantity Not Sufficient
QOD	Every Other Day
QOL	Quality of Life
QSAR	Quantitative SAR
R&D	Research and Development
R&TD	Research and Technological Development
RAC	Reviewer Affairs Committee (CDER)
RADAR	Risk Assessment of Drugs—Analysis and Response
RAPS	Regulatory Affairs Professional's Society
RBC	Red Blood Cell
RCC	Research Coordinating Committee (CDER)
RCH	Remove Clinical Hold
RCT	Randomized Clinical Trials
RD	Response to Request for Information (COMIS term)
RDE	Remote Data Entry
RDRC	Radioactive Drug Research Committee
RDT	Rising-dose tolerance
RFA	Request for Approval
RIF	Reduction in Force
RKI	Robert-Koch-Institut, Bundesinstitut für Infektionskrankheiten und nich-über tragbare Krankheiten (Federal Institute for Infectious and Non-communicable Diseases, Germany)
RL	Regulatory Letter (FDA postaudit letter)
RMO	Regulatory Management Officer
RTF	The decision by the FDA to refuse to file an application
RTF	Refuse To File
RUG	Resource Utilization Group
Rx	Prescription
S	Standard
SAE	Serious Adverse Event
SAL	Sterility Assurance Level
SAR	Structure Activity Relationship

SAR	Serious Adverse Reaction
SBA	Summary Basis of Approval
SBIR	Small Business Innovative Research Program (USA)
SC	Subcutaneous
SC	Study coordinator. *See also CCRC, CRC.*
SCSO	Supervisory Consumer Safety Officer
SCT	Society for Clinical Trials
SD	Standard Deviation
SDAT	Senile Dementia of the Alzheimer's Type
SE	Standard Error
SEA	Single European Act of 1987
SEER	Surveillance, Epidemiology, and End Results (Registry of NCI)
SES	Senior Executive Service
SIDA	The Spanish (síndrome inmunodeficiencia adquirida), Italian, and French abbreviation for AIDS. *See AIDS.*
SMART	Submission Management and Review Tracking (FDA)
SMB	Safety Monitoring Board
SMDA	Safe Medical Devices Act (1990)
SME	Significant Medical Event
SMO	Site Management Organization
SmPC	Summary of Product Characteristics
SNDA	Supplemental New Drug Application
SNIP	Syndicat National de l'Industrie Pharmaceutique (France)
SoCRA	Society of Clinical Research Associates
SOMD	Safety of Medicines Department (UK)
SOP	Standard Operating Procedure
SPM	Society of Pharmaceutical Medicine
SQ	Subcutaneous
SRS	Spontaneous Reporting System
SSCT	Swedish Society for Clinical Trials
SSFA	Società di Scienze Farmacologiche Applicate (Italy)
SSM	Skin Surface Microscopy
STD	Sexually Transmitted Disease
STT	Short-Term Tests
SUD	Sudden Unexpected Death
SUPAC	Scale up and postapproval changes
SVP	Small Volume Parenterals
SX	Symptoms
$T_{1/2}$	Half-life
TB	Tuberculosis
TGA	Thermographic Analysis
TID	Three Times a Day
TIND	Treatment IND. *See also IND.*
TK	Toxicokinetics
TMO	Trial Management Organization
TOP	Topical
TSH	Thyroid Stimulating Hormone
UA	Urinalysis
UKCCR	UK Coordinating Committee on Cancer Research

UNESCO	United Nations Educational Science and Cultural Organization
USAN	US Adopted Names Council
USC	*United States Code* (book of laws)
USCA	U.S. Code Annotated
USDA	United States Department of Agriculture
USP	United States Pharmacopeia
USPC	U.S. Pharmacopeial Convention
USP-DI	United States Pharmacopeia-Drug Information
USP-NF	United States Pharmacopeia-National Formulary
USUHS	Uniformed Services University of the Health Sciences
VA	Veterans Administration (officially, United States Department of Veterans Affairs)
VAERS	Vaccine Adverse Event Reporting System
VAI	Voluntary Action Indicated (FDA postaudit inspection classification)
WBC	White Blood Cells
WD	Withdrawn (COMIS term)
WHO	World Health Organization (also used to refer to WHO glossary for coding AEs)
WHOART	World Health Organization Adverse Reaction Terminology
WI	Inactive (COMIS term)
WL	Warning letter (most serious FDA postaudit letter, demands immediate action within 15 days)
WNL	Within Normal Limits
WRAIR	Walter Reed Army Institute of Research (DoD)
WTO	World Trade Organization

Index